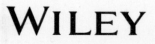

Fundamentals of

Anatomy and Physiology

For Nursing and Healthcare Students

This title is also available as an e-book. For more details, please see
www.wiley.com/buy/9781119055525
or scan this QR code:

Fundamentals of
Anatomy and Physiology
For Nursing and Healthcare Students

Second Edition

EDITED BY

IAN PEATE EN(G), RGN, DipN (Lond) RNT, BEd (Hons), MA (Lond) LLM
MURALITHARAN NAIR SRN, RMN, DipN (Lond) RNT, Cert Ed, BSc (Hons) MSc
(Surrey), Cert in Counselling, FHEA

WILEY Blackwell

Short contents

Contents

Chapter 2   **Cells, cellular compartments, transport systems, fluid movement between compartments**   **29**
Muralitharan Nair

Introduction	30
Cell membrane	32
Functions of the cell membrane	33
Cellular fluid compartments	34
Intracellular fluid	35
Extracellular fluid	36
Fluid movement between compartments	37
Composition of body fluid	38
Effects of water deficiency	38
Variation in body fluid content	39
Transport systems	40
Simple diffusion	40
Facilitated diffusion	41
Osmosis	42
Filtration	43
Active transport system	43
Electrolytes	46
Functions of electrolytes	47
Hormones that regulate fluid and electrolytes	50
Antidiuretic hormone	50
Aldosterone	51
Atrial natriuretic peptide	52
Parathyroid hormone	52
Conclusion	52
Glossary	53
References	54
Further reading	54
Activities	54

Chapter 3   **Genetics**   **61**
Peter S Vickers

Anatomical map	62
Introduction	62
The double helix	63
Nucleotides	63
Bases	64
Chromosomes	65
From DNA to proteins	67
Protein synthesis	67
Key steps in protein synthesis	69
Summary of protein synthesis	72
The transference of genes	74
Mitosis	74
Meiosis	76
First meiotic division	78

Chapter 6   The muscular system   **153**

Janet G Migliozzi

Chapter 10   **The renal system**   **299**
Muralitharan Nair

Chapter 14   The senses   439
Carl Clare

Chapter 15   The endocrine system   479
Carl Clare

Chapter 16 The immune system 513

Peter S Vickers

Contributors

About the Editors

Ian Peate EN(G), RGN, DipN (Lond) RNT, BEd (Hons), MA (Lond) LLM
Editor-in-Chief of the *British Journal of Nursing*
Head of School, School of Health Studies, Gibraltar
Ian began his nursing career in 1981 at Central Middlesex Hospital, becoming an enrolled nurse working in an intensive care unit. He later undertook 3 years' student nurse training at Central Middlesex and Northwick Park Hospitals, becoming a staff nurse and then a charge nurse. He has worked in nurse education since 1989. His key areas of interest are nursing practice and theory, men's health, sexual health and HIV. Ian has published widely. He is Visiting Professor, Kingston University London and St George's, University of London.

Muralitharan Nair SRN, RMN, DipN (Lond) RNT, Cert Ed, BSc (Hons) MSc (Surrey), Cert in Counselling, FHEA
Muralitharan commenced his nursing a career in 1971 at Edgware General Hospital, becoming a staff nurse. In 1975 he commenced his mental health nurse training at Springfield Hospital and worked as a staff nurse for approximately 1 year. He worked at St Mary's Hospital Paddington and Northwick Park Hospital, returning to Edgware General Hospital to take up the post of senior staff nurse and then charge nurse. He has worked in nurse education since 1989. His key interests include physiology, diabetes, surgical nursing and nurse education. Muralitharan has published widely in journals and co-edited a number of textbooks. He has now retired from being a full-time lecturer but is working as a nursing consultant.

About the Contributors

Carl Clare RN DipN, BSc (Hons), MSc (Lond), PGDE (Lond)
Carl began his nursing a career in 1990 as a nursing auxiliary. He later undertook 3 years' student nurse training at Selly Oak Hospital (Birmingham), moving to The Royal Devon and Exeter Hospitals, then Northwick Park Hospital, and finally The Royal Brompton and Harefield NHS Trust as a Resuscitation Officer and Honorary Teaching Fellow of Imperial College (London). He has worked in nurse education since 2001. His key areas of interest are physiology, sociology, cardiac care and resuscitation. Carl has previously published work in cardiac care, resuscitation and pathophysiology.

Louise McErlean RGN, BSc(Hons), MA (Herts)
Louise began her nursing career in 1986 at the Victoria Infirmary in Glasgow, becoming a registered general nurse. She later completed the intensive care course for registered general nurses while working in Belfast as a staff nurse. She then worked as a junior sister at the Royal Free Hospital and has worked in nurse education since 2005. Her key areas of interest are pre-registration nurse education and intensive care nursing.

Janet G Migliozzi RN, BSc (Hons), MSc (Lon), PGDE, FHEA

Janet is a senior lecturer in the School of Health & Social Work, University of Hertfordshire. Janet commenced her nursing career in London and worked at a variety of hospitals across London, predominantly in vascular, orthopaedic and high-dependency surgery before specialising in infection prevention and control. Janet has worked in higher education since 1999, and her key interests include medical microbiology and microbial resistance, healthcare-associated infection, patient safety, infection prevention strategies/education of healthcare professionals at both a UK and European level and the use of clinical simulation to minimise healthcare risk. Janet has previously published work in minimising healthcare-associated risk and pathophysiology. Janet is a member of the European Nurses Association and is also the research and development lead for the East of England branch of the Infection Prevention Society.

Peter S Vickers Cert Ed, DipCD, SRN, RSCN, BA, PhD, FHEA

Following a career in teaching, Peter commenced nursing in 1980, working at the York District Hospital and the Hospitals for Sick Children, Great Ormond Street, London, becoming the Clinical Nurse Specialist in Paediatric Immunology. Following a degree in Biosciences and Health Studies, in 1999, he was awarded his doctorate following research into the long-term development of children with severe combined immunodeficiency in the UK and Germany. He worked in nurse education for several years and has written books on children's responses to early hospitalisation and on research methodology; he has also written chapters for nursing bioscience and pathophysiology books, and presented papers at international conferences. His areas of interest are immunology and immunology nursing, infectious diseases, genetics and research. Now retired, he remains active in writing and was President of INGID (the international organisation for nurses working within the field of primary immunodeficiencies) from 2012 to 2014.

Anthony Wheeldon MSc (Lond), PGDE, BSc(Hons), DipHE, RN

Anthony began his nursing career at Barnet College of Nursing and Midwifery. After qualification in 1995 he worked as a staff nurse and senior staff nurse in the Respiratory Directorate at the Royal Brompton and Harefield NHS Trust in London. In 2000 he started teaching on post-registration cardio-respiratory courses before moving into full-time nurse education at Thames Valley University in 2002. Anthony has a wide range of nursing interests, including cardio-respiratory nursing, anatomy and physiology, respiratory assessment, nurse education, and the application of bioscience in nursing practice. In 2006 Anthony joined the University of Hertfordshire, where he has taught on both pre- and post-registration nursing courses. He is currently an associate subject lead for adult nursing.

Acknowledgements

Ian would like to thank his partner Jussi Lahtinen for his support, Mrs Frances Cohen for her ongoing assistance and the library staff at the Gibraltar Health Authority.

Muralitharan would like to thank his wife, Evangeline, and his daughters, Samantha and Jennifer, for their continued support and patience.

We would like to thank Magenta Styles at Wiley for her help and continued encouragement.

Preface

We were delighted when we were asked to write a second edition of the popular *Fundamentals of Anatomy and Physiology for Student Nurses*. The first edition has been a very popular choice not only with student nurses but also with students in other healthcare professions and this has been reflected in the title of this second edition. The second edition of *Fundamentals of Anatomy and Physiology for Nursing and Healthcare Students* retains all of the attributes in the popular first edition as well as a whole range of new features in this book and also through the companion websites.

Those contributing to the text are all dedicated to the provision of high-quality, safe and effective care. The authors are all experienced academics working in higher education, with many years of clinical experience, knowledge and skills, teaching a variety of multidisciplinary student groups at various academic levels. We are confident that after you have gained a sound understanding of anatomy and physiology you will be able to understand better the needs of the people you have the privilege to care for. High-quality, safe and effective care for all is something all of us should strive to provide; however, this will be a challenge if we do not fully appreciate the person in a holistic manner. Those who provide care have to take into consideration the anatomical and physiological elements, but they must also consider the psychosocial aspects of the person and their family, addressing the needs of the whole being, the whole person. This text has been devised in such a way as to encourage learning and understanding. We hope you enjoy reading it, and more importantly that you are hungry to learn more, that you will be tempted to delve deeper as you grow and develop into becoming a provider of healthcare that is world class, safe and effective.

The companion to this book, *Fundamentals of Applied Pathophysiology: An Essential Guide for Nursing and Healthcare Students* (Nair and Peate, 2013), also in its second edition, will help in your development and understanding. Within your programme of study which is related to the provision of care it is important that you are confident and competent with regards to pathophysiology and anatomy and physiology. It is not enough that you remember all of the facts (and there are many of these) that are linked with anatomy and physiology; you also have to relate these to those you care for. Some of those people may be vulnerable and at risk of harm, and it is your responsibility to ensure that you are knowledgeable and that you understand the complexities of care. This new edition of *Fundamentals of Anatomy and Physiology for Nursing and Healthcare Students* will help you.

It is a requirement of several programmes of study that lead to registration with a professional body that you demonstrate competence in a number of spheres, and this will include anatomy and physiology – for example, see The Standards for Pre-Registration Nursing Education (Nursing and Midwifery Council, 2010).

The human body is as beautiful on the inside as it is on the outside; when working in harmony the mind and body is an astonishing mechanism that has the capacity to perform a range of amazing things. Healthcare students practise and study in a number of healthcare settings, in the hospital and the primary-care setting and in the person's own home where they are destined to meet and care for patients with a range of altered anatomical and physiological problems. Employing a fundamental approach with a sound anatomical and physiological understanding will provide healthcare students with an essential basis on which to provide care.

Anatomy and physiology

Anatomy can be defined simply as the science related to the study of the structure of biological organisms; there are dictionaries that use such a definition. *Fundamentals of Anatomy and Physiology for Nursing and Healthcare Students* focuses on human anatomy, and the definition of anatomy for the purposes of this text is that it is a study of the structure and function of the human body. This allows for reference to function and also structure; in all biological organisms structure and function are closely interconnected. The human body can only operate through interrelated systems.

The term anatomy is Greek in origin and means 'to cut up' or 'to dissect'. The first scientifically based anatomical studies (credited to Vesalius, the 16th-century Flemish anatomist, doctor and artist) were based on observations of cadavers (dead bodies). Contemporary approaches to human anatomy differ, however, as they include other ways of observation; for example, with the aid of a microscope and other complex and technologically advanced imaging tools. Subdivisions are now associated within the broader field of anatomy, with the word anatomy often preceded with an adjective identifying the method of observation; for example, gross anatomy (the study of body parts that are visible to the naked eye, such as the heart or the bones) or microanatomy (where body parts such as cells or tissues are only visible with the use of a microscope).

Living systems can be defined from a number of perspectives:

- At the very smallest level, the chemical level, atoms, molecules and the chemical bonds connecting atoms provide the structure upon which living activity is based.
- The smallest unit of life is the cell. Specialised bodies – organelles – within the cell perform particular cellular functions. Cells may be specialised; for example, bone cells and muscle cells.
- Tissue is a group of cells that are similar and they perform a common function. Muscle tissue, for example, is made up of muscle cells.
- Organs are groups of different types of tissues working together to carry out a specific activity. The stomach, for example, is an organ made up of muscle, nerve and tissues.
- A system is two or more organs that work together to carry out a specific activity. The digestive system, for example, comprises the coordinated activities of a number of organs, including the stomach, intestines, pancreas and liver.
- Another system that possesses the characteristics of living things is an organism; this has the ability to obtain and process energy, the capacity to react to changes in the environment and the ability to reproduce.

As anatomy is associated with the function of a living organism it is almost always inseparable from physiology. Physiology can be described as the science dealing with the study of the function of cells, tissues, organs and organisms. Physiology is concerned with how an organism carries out its many activities, considering how it moves, how it is nourished, how it adapts to changing environments – human and animal, hostile and friendly. It is in essence the study of life.

Physiology is the foundation upon which we build our knowledge of what life is; it can help us to decide how to treat disease as well as help us to adapt and manage changes imposed on our bodies by new and changing surroundings – internal and external. Studying physiology will help you understand disease (pathophysiology) arising from this; physiologists working with others are able to develop new ways for treating diseases.

Just as there are a number of branches of anatomical study, so too are there a number of physiological branches that can be studied; for example, endocrinology, neurology and cardiology.

There are 17 chapters. The text is not intended to be read from cover to cover, but you may find reading chapters one to four first will help you come to terms with some of the more complex concepts; we would encourage you to dip in and out of the book. The chapters use simple and generously sized full-colour artwork in order to assist you in your understanding and appreciation of the complexities associated with the human body from an anatomical and physiological perspective. There are many features contained within each chapter that can help you to build upon and develop your knowledge base; we would encourage you to get the most out of this book.

The text takes the reader from the microscopic to macroscopic level in the study of anatomy and physiology. The contents demonstrate the movement from cells and tissues through to systems. This approach to teaching is a tried-and-tested approach, especially when helping learners understand a topic area that can sometimes be seen as complex.

This book has been written with these key principles in mind, to help inform your practice as well as your academic work. This second edition retains the features that have helped students bring to life the fascinating subject of human anatomy and physiology; there is also a range of new features provided to further enhance the student experience.

Each chapter begins with several questions that are posed to test your current knowledge; this allows you to pre-test. Learning outcomes are provided. These will cover the content within the chapter, but only you can do the learning; these outcomes are what are expected of you after reading and absorbing the information. This is a minimum of what you can learn; do not be constrained by the learning outcomes, they are only provided to guide you. Where appropriate an anatomical map is provided; this is related to the chapter you are reading, allowing you to 'situate or visualise' the anatomy being discussed.

Another feature in most of the chapters that is provided to help you consider people you care for, to help you make clinical links, is the 'Clinical considerations' box. These boxes demonstrate the application to your learning, citing specific care issues that you may come across when working with people in care settings.

A new addition is the feature called 'Medicines management'. In this feature the contributors discuss the administration of medicines, medicine management issues. This addition can help you appreciate the importance of understanding anatomy and physiology with the intention of administering medicines safely and effectively.

In most chapters there is a series of snapshots. This new addition relates the theory to practice, introducing you to the issues being discussed in a practical way.

At the end of the chapter you are provided with a bank of multiple choice questions. Some of the answers to the questions are not found in the text; in this case you are encouraged to seek out the answers and in so doing develop your learning further.

Other features provided will help you measure the learning that has taken place; for example, true or false, label the diagram, find out more, crosswords or word searches. These are meant to be fun, but they also aim to pull together the content of the chapter.

The feature 'Conditions' at the end of the chapter provides you with a list of conditions that are associated with the topics discussed in the chapter. You are encouraged to take some time to write notes about each of the conditions listed; this will help you relate theory to practice. You can make your notes taken from other textbooks or other resources – for example, the people you work with in a care area – or you may make the notes as a result of people you have cared for. It is important, however, that if you are making notes about people you have cared for you must ensure that you adhere to the rules of confidentiality.

At the end of every chapter a glossary of terms is provided. We present this to facilitate the learning of difficult words or phrases; understanding these words and phrases is important to your success as a healthcare student. When you have mastered the words your medical vocabulary will have grown and you will be in a better position to develop it further.

We have, in this new edition, included a list of prefixes and suffixes as well a table of normal values.

A myriad of features have been compiled to help your learning with two companion websites. The features include an interactive glossary and a series of case studies with the intention of bringing alive the subject matter. The electronic resources associated with this book are designed to help enhance your learning; they are varied and informative and are visually stimulating.

The advantages of these resources are that they can be used in your own place at your own pace. The aim is to encourage further learning and to build upon what you know already. There are also links to other resources via the further reading section at the end of the chapters.

Using the electronic resources alongside the book, as well as the human resources you will meet in practice, will enhance the quality of your learning. The electronic resources available cannot replace the more conventional face-to-face learning with other students, lecturers, registered practitioners and patients; they complement it.

We have enjoyed writing this second edition and we sincerely hope you enjoy reading it. We wish you much success with your studies, whether they are in the classroom or in the many care areas that you might find yourself working.

References

Nair, M. and Peate, I. (2013) *Fundamentals of Applied Pathophysiology: An Essential Guide for Nursing and Healthcare Students*, 2nd edn. Oxford: John Wiley & Sons, Ltd.

Nursing and Midwifery Council (2010) Standards for Pre-Registration Nursing Education. http://standards.nmc-uk.org/PublishedDocuments/Standards%20for%20pre-registration%20nursing%20education%2016082010.pdf (accessed 7 November 2015).

Prefixes, suffixes

Prefix: A prefix is positioned at the beginning of a word to modify or change its meaning. Pre means 'before'. Prefixes may also indicate a location, number, or time.

Suffix: The ending part of a word that changes the meaning of the word.

Prefix or suffix	Meaning	Example(s)
a-, an-	not, without	analgesic, apathy
ab-	from; away from	abduction
abdomin(o)-	of or relating to the abdomen	abdomen
acous(io)-	of or relating to hearing	acoumeter, acoustician
acr(o)-	extremity, topmost	acrocrany, acromegaly, acroosteolysis, acroposthia
ad-	at, increase, on, toward	adduction
aden(o)-, aden(i)-	of or relating to a gland	adenocarcinoma, adenology, adenotome, adenotyphus
adip(o)-	of or relating to fat or fatty tissue	adipocyte
adren(o)-	of or relating to adrenal glands	adrenal artery
-aemia	blood condition	anaemia
aer(o)-	air, gas	aerosinusitis
-aesthesi(o)-	sensation	anaesthesia
alb-	denoting a white or pale colour	albino
-alge(si)-	pain	analgesic
-algia, -alg(i)o-	pain	myalgia
all(o-)	denoting something as different, or as an addition	alloantigen, allopathy
ambi-	denoting something as positioned on both sides	ambidextrous
amni-	pertaining to the membranous foetal sac (amnion)	amniocentesis
ana-	back, again, up	anaplasia
andr(o)-	pertaining to a man	android, andrology
angi(o)-	blood vessel	angiogram

Prefix or suffix	Meaning	Example(s)
ankyl(o)-,ancyl(o)-	denoting something as crooked or bent	ankylosis
ante-	describing something as positioned in front of another thing	antepartum
anti-	describing something as 'against' or 'opposed to' another	antibody, antipsychotic
arteri(o)-	of or pertaining to an artery	arteriole, arterial
arthr(o)-	of or pertaining to the joints, limbs	arthritis
articul(o)-	joint	articulation
-ase	enzyme	lactase
-asthenia	weakness	myasthenia gravis
ather(o)-	fatty deposit, soft gruel-like deposit	atherosclerosis
atri(o)-	an atrium (especially heart atrium)	atrioventricular
aur(i)-	of or pertaining to the ear	aural
aut(o)-	self	autoimmune
axill-	of or pertaining to the armpit (uncommon as a prefix)	axilla
bi-	twice, double	binary
bio-	life	biology
blephar(o)-	of or pertaining to the eyelid	blepharoplast
brachi(o)-	of or relating to the arm	brachium of inferior colliculus
brady-	'slow'	bradycardia
bronch(i)-	bronchus	bronchiolitis obliterans
bucc(o)-	of or pertaining to the cheek	buccolabial
burs(o)-	bursa (fluid sac between the bones)	bursitis
carcin(o)-	cancer	carcinoma
cardi(o)-	of or pertaining to the heart	cardiology
carp(o)-	of or pertaining to the wrist	carpopedal
-cele	pouching, hernia	hydrocele, varicocele
-centesis	surgical puncture for aspiration	amniocentesis
cephal(o)-	of or pertaining to the head (as a whole)	cephalalgy
cerebell(o)-	of or pertaining to the cerebellum	cerebellum
cerebr(o)-	of or pertaining to the brain	cerebrology
chem(o)-	chemistry, drug	chemotherapy

Prefix or suffix	Meaning	Example(s)
chol(e)-	of or pertaining to bile	cholecystitis
cholecyst(o)-	of or pertaining to the gallbladder	cholecystectomy
chondr(i)o-	cartilage, gristle, granule, granular	chondrocalcinosis
chrom(ato)-	colour	haemochromatosis
-cidal, -cide	killing, destroying	bacteriocidal
cili-	of or pertaining to the cilia, the eyelashes	ciliary
circum-	denoting something as 'around' another	circumcision
col(o)-, colono-	colon	colonoscopy
colp(o)-	of or pertaining to the vagina	colposcopy
contra-	against	contraindicate
coron(o)-	crown	coronary
cost(o)-	of or pertaining to the ribs	costochondral
crani(o)-	belonging or relating to the cranium	craniology
-crine, -crin(o)-	to secrete	endocrine
cry(o)-	cold	cryoablation
cutane-	skin	subcutaneous
cyan(o)-	denotes a blue colour	cyanosis
cyst(o)-, cyst(i)-	of or pertaining to the urinary bladder	cystotomy
cyt(o)-	cell	cytokine
-cyte	cell	leukocyte
-dactyl(o)-	of or pertaining to a finger, toe	dactylology, polydactyly
dent-	of or pertaining to teeth	dentist
dermat(o)-, derm(o)-	of or pertaining to the skin	dermatology
-desis	binding	arthrodesis
dextr(o)-	right, on the right side	dextrocardia
di-	two	diplopia
dia-	through, during, across	dialysis
dif-	apart, separation	different
digit-	of or pertaining to the finger (rare as a root)	digit
-dipsia	suffix meaning '(condition of) thirst'	polydipsia, hydroadipsia, oligodipsia
dors(o)-, dors(i)-	of or pertaining to the back	dorsal, dorsocephalad

Prefix or suffix	Meaning	Example(s)
duodeno-	duodenum	duodenal atresia
dynam(o)-	force, energy, power	hand strength dynamometer
-dynia	pain	vulvodynia
dys-	bad, difficult, defective, abnormal	dysphagia, dysphasia
ec-	out, away	ectopia, ectopic pregnancy
-ectasia, -ectasis	expansion, dilation	bronchiectasis, telangiectasia
ect(o)-	outer, outside	ectoblast, ectoderm
-ectomy	denotes a surgical operation or removal of a body part; resection, excision	mastectomy
-emesis	vomiting condition	haematemesis
encephal(o)-	of or pertaining to the brain; also see **cerebr(o)-**	encephalogram
endo-	denotes something as 'inside' or 'within'	endocrinology, endospore
enter(o)-	of or pertaining to the intestine	gastroenterology
eosin(o)-	red	eosinophil granulocyte
epi-	on, upon	epicardium, epidermis, epidural, episclera, epistaxis
erythr(o)-	denotes a red colour	erythrocyte
ex-	out of, away from	excision, exophthalmos
exo-	denotes something as 'outside' another	exoskeleton
extra-	outside	extradural haematoma
faci(o)-	of or pertaining to the face	facioplegic
fibr(o)	fibre	fibroblast
fore-	before or ahead	forehead
fossa	a hollow or depressed area; trench or channel	fossa ovalis
front-	of or pertaining to the forehead	frontonasal
galact(o)-	milk	galactorrhoea
gastr(o)-	of or pertaining to the stomach	gastric bypass
-genic	formative, pertaining to producing	cardiogenic shock
gingiv-	of or pertaining to the gums	gingivitis
glauc(o)-	denoting a grey or bluish-grey colour	glaucoma
gloss(o)-, glott(o)-	of or pertaining to the tongue	glossology
gluco-	sweet	glucocorticoid

Prefix or suffix	Meaning	Example(s)
glyc(o)-	sugar	glycolysis
-gnosis	knowledge	diagnosis, prognosis
gon(o)-	seed, semen; also, reproductive	gonorrhoea
-gram, -gramme	record or picture	angiogram
-graph	instrument used to record data or picture	electrocardiograph
-graphy	process of recording	angiography
gyn(aec)o-	woman	gynaecomastia
haemangi(o)-	blood vessels	haemangioma
haemat(o)-,haem-	of or pertaining to blood	haematology
halluc-	to wander in mind	hallucinosis
hemi-	one-half	cerebral hemisphere
hepat- (hepatic-)	of or pertaining to the liver	hepatology
heter(o)-	denotes something as 'the other' (of two), as an addition, or different	heterogeneous
hist(o)-, histio-	tissue	histology
home(o)-	similar	homeopathy
hom(o)-	denotes something as 'the same' as another or common	homosexuality
hydr(o)-	water	hydrophobe
hyper-	denotes something as 'extreme' or 'beyond normal'	hypertension
hyp(o)-	denotes something as 'below normal'	hypovolaemia
hyster(o)-	of or pertaining to the womb, the uterus	hysterectomy, hysteria
iatr(o)-	of or pertaining to medicine, or a physician	iatrogenic
-iatry	denotes a field in medicine of a certain body component	podiatry, psychiatry
-ics	organised knowledge, treatment	obstetrics
ileo-	ileum	ileocaecal valve
infra-	below	infrahyoid muscles
inter-	between, among	interarticular ligament
intra-	within	intramural
ipsi-	same	ipsilateral hemiparesis
ischio-	of or pertaining to the ischium, the hip joint	ischioanal fossa

Prefix or suffix	Meaning	Example(s)
-ismus	spasm, contraction	hemiballismus
iso-	denoting something as being 'equal'	isotonic
-ist	one who specialises in	pathologist
-itis	inflammation	tonsillitis
-ium	structure, tissue	pericardium
juxta- (iuxta-)	near to, alongside or next to	juxtaglomerular apparatus
karyo-	nucleus	eukaryote
kerat(o)-	cornea (eye or skin)	keratoscope
kin(e)-, kin(o)-, kinesi(o)-	movement	kinesthaesia
kyph(o)-	humped	kyphoscoliosis
labi(o)-	of or pertaining to the lip	labiodental
lacrim(o)-	tear	lacrimal canaliculi
lact(i)-, lact(o)	milk	lactation
lapar(o)-	of or pertaining to the abdomen wall, flank	laparotomy
laryng(o)-	of or pertaining to the larynx, the lower throat cavity where the voice box is	larynx
latero-	lateral	lateral pectoral nerve
-lepsis, -lepsy	attack, seizure	epilepsy, narcolepsy
lept(o)-	light, slender	leptomeningeal
leuc(o)-, leuk(o)-	denoting a white colour	leukocyte
lingu(a)-, lingu(o)-	of or pertaining to the tongue	linguistics
lip(o)-	fat	liposuction
lith(o)-	stone, calculus	lithotripsy
-logist	denotes someone who studies a certain field	oncologist, pathologist
log(o)-	speech	logopaedics
-logy	denotes the academic study or practice of a certain field	haematology, urology
lymph(o)-	lymph	lymphoedema
lys(o)-, -lytic	dissolution	lysosome
-lysis	destruction, separation	paralysis

Prefix or suffix	Meaning	Example(s)
macr(o)-	large, long	macrophage
-malacia	softening	osteomalacia
mammill(o)-	of or pertaining to the nipple	mammillitis
mamm(o)-	of or pertaining to the breast	mammogram
manu-	of or pertaining to the hand	manufacture
mast(o)-	of or pertaining to the breast	mastectomy
meg(a)-, megal(o)-, -megaly	enlargement, million	splenomegaly, megameter
melan(o)-	black colour	melanin
mening(o)-	membrane	meningitis
meta-	after, behind	metacarpus
-meter	instrument used to measure or count	sphygmomanometer
metr(o)-	pertaining to conditions of the uterus	metrorrhagia
-metry	process of measuring	optometry
micro-	denoting something as small, or relating to smallness	microscope
milli-	thousandth	millilitre
mon(o)-	single	infectious mononucleosis
morph(o)-	form, shape	morphology
muscul(o)-	muscle	musculoskeletal system
my(o)-	of or relating to muscle	myoblast
myc(o)-	fungus	onychomycosis
myel(o)-	of or relating to bone marrow or spinal cord	myeloblast
myri-	ten thousand	myriad
myring(o)-	eardrum	myringotomy
narc(o)-	numb, sleep	narcolepsy
nas(o)-	of or pertaining to the nose	nasal
necr(o)-	death	necrosis, necrotising fasciitis
neo-	new	neoplasm
nephr(o)-	of or pertaining to the kidney	nephrology
neur(i)-, neur(o)-	of or pertaining to nerves and the nervous system	neurofibromatosis

Prefix or suffix	Meaning	Example(s)
normo-	normal	normocapnia
ocul(o)-	of or pertaining to the eye	oculist
odont(o)-	of or pertaining to teeth	orthodontist
odyn(o)-	pain	stomatodynia
-oesophageal, oesophag(o)-	gullet	gastro-oesophageal reflux
-oid	resemblance to	sarcoidosis
-ole	small or little	arteriole
olig(o)-	denoting something as 'having little, having few'	oliguria
-oma (*sing.*), -omata (*pl.*)	tumour, mass, collection	sarcoma, teratoma
onco-	tumour, bulk, volume	oncology
onych(o)-	of or pertaining to the nail (of a finger or toe)	onychophagy
oo-	of or pertaining to an egg, a woman's egg, the ovum	oogenesis
oophor(o)-	of or pertaining to the woman's ovary	oophorectomy
ophthalm(o)-	of or pertaining to the eye	ophthalmology
optic(o)-	of or relating to chemical properties of the eye	opticochemical
orchi(o)-, orchid(o)-, orch(o)-	testis	orchiectomy, orchidectomy
-osis	a condition, disease or increase	ichthyosis, psychosis, osteoporosis
osseo-	bony	osseous
ossi-	bone	peripheral ossifying fibroma
ost(e)-, oste(o)-	bone	osteoporosis
ot(o)-	of or pertaining to the ear	otology
ovo-, ovi-, ov-	of or pertaining to the eggs, the ovum	ovogenesis
pachy-	thick	pachyderma
paed-, paedo-	of or pertaining to the child	paediatrics
palpebr-	of or pertaining to the eyelid (uncommon as a root)	palpebra
pan-, pant(o)-	denoting something as 'complete' or containing 'everything'	panophobia, panopticon

Prefix or suffix	Meaning	Example(s)
papill-	of or pertaining to the nipple (of the chest/breast)	papillitis
papul(o)-	indicates papulosity, a small elevation or swelling in the skin, a pimple, swelling	papulation
para-	alongside of, abnormal	paracyesis
-paresis	slight paralysis	hemiparesis
parvo-	small	parvovirus
path(o)-	disease	pathology
-pathy	denotes (with a negative sense) a disease, or disorder	sociopathy, neuropathy
pector-	breast	pectoralgia, pectoriloquy, pectorophony
ped-, -ped-, -pes	of or pertaining to the foot; -footed	pedoscope
pelv(i)-, pelv(o)-	hip bone	pelvis
-penia	deficiency	osteopenia
-pepsia	denotes something relating to digestion, or the digestive tract	dyspepsia
peri-	denoting something with a position 'surrounding' or 'around' another	periodontal
-pexy	fixation	nephropexy
phaco-	lens-shaped	phacolysis, phacometer, phacoscotoma
-phage, -phagia	forms terms denoting conditions relating to eating or ingestion	sarcophagia
-phago-	eating, devouring	phagocyte
-phagy	forms nouns that denotes 'feeding on' the first element or part of the word	haematophagy
pharmaco-	drug, medication	pharmacology
pharyng(o)-	of or pertaining to the pharynx, the upper throat cavity	pharyngitis, pharyngoscopy
phleb(o)-	of or pertaining to the (blood) veins, a vein	phlebography, phlebotomy
-phobia	exaggerated fear, sensitivity	arachnophobia
phon(o)-	sound	phonograph, symphony
phot(o)-	of or pertaining to light	photopathy
phren(i)-, phren(o)-, phrenico	the mind	phrenic nerve, schizophrenia

Prefix or suffix	Meaning	Example(s)
-plasia	formation, development	achondroplasia
-plasty	surgical repair, reconstruction	rhinoplasty
-plegia	paralysis	paraplegia
pleio-	more, excessive, multiple	pleiomorphism
pleur(o)-, pleur(a)	of or pertaining to the ribs	pleurogenous
-plexy	stroke or seizure	cataplexy
pneumat(o)-	air, lung	pneumatocele
pneum(o)-	of or pertaining to the lungs	pneumonocyte, pneumonia
-poiesis	production	haematopoiesis
poly-	denotes a 'plurality' of something	polymyositis
post-	denotes something as 'after' or 'behind' another	post-operation, post-mortem
pre-	denotes something as 'before' another (in [physical] position or time)	premature birth
presby(o)-	old age	presbyopia
prim-	denotes something as 'first' or 'most important'	primary
proct(o)-	anus, rectum	proctology
prot(o)-	denotes something as 'first' or 'most important'	protoneuron
pseud(o)-	denotes something false or fake	pseudoephedrine
psor-	itching	psoriasis
psych(e)-, psych(o)	of or pertaining to the mind	psychology, psychiatry
-ptosis	falling, drooping, downward placement, prolapse	apoptosis, nephroptosis
-ptysis	(a spitting), spitting, haemoptysis, the spitting of blood derived from the lungs or bronchial tubes	haemoptysis
pulmon-, pulmo-	of or relating to the lungs	pulmonary
pyel(o)-	pelvis	pyelonephritis
py(o)-	pus	pyometra
pyr(o)-	fever	antipyretic
quadr(i)-	four	quadriceps
radio-	radiation	radiowave

Prefix or suffix	Meaning	Example(s)
ren(o)-	of or pertaining to the kidney	renal
retro-	backward, behind	retroversion, retroverted
rhin(o)-	of or pertaining to the nose	rhinoplasty
rhod(o)-	denoting a rose-red colour	rhodophyte
-rrhage	burst forth	haemorrhage
-rrhagia	rapid flow of blood	menorrhagia
-rrhaphy	surgical suturing	nephrorrhaphy
-rrhexis	rupture	karyorrhexis
-rrhoea	flowing, discharge	diarrhoea
-rupt	break or burst	erupt, interrupt
salping(o)-	of or pertaining to tubes, e.g. Fallopian tubes	salpingectomy, salpingopharyngeus muscle
sangui-,sanguine-	of or pertaining to blood	exsanguination
sarco-	muscular, flesh-like	sarcoma
scler(o)-	hard	scleroderma
-sclerosis	hardening	atherosclerosis, multiple sclerosis
scoli(o)-	twisted	scoliosis
-scope	instrument for viewing	stethoscope
-scopy	use of instrument for viewing	endoscopy
semi-	one-half, partly	semiconscious
sial(o)-	saliva, salivary gland	sialagogue
sigmoid(o)-	sigmoid, S-shaped curvature	sigmoid colon
sinistr(o)-	left, left side	sinistrocardia
sinus-	of or pertaining to the sinus	sinusitis
somat(o)-, somatico-	body, bodily	somatic
-spadias	slit, fissure	hypospadias, epispadias
spasmo-	spasm	spasmodic dysphonia
sperma(to)-, spermo-	semen, spermatozoa	spermatogenesis
splen(o)-	spleen	splenectomy
spondyl(o)-	of or pertaining to the spine, the vertebra	spondylitis

Prefix or suffix	Meaning	Example(s)
squamos(o)-	denoting something as 'full of scales' or 'scaly'	squamous cell
-stalsis	contraction	peristalsis
-stasis	stopping, standing	cytostasis, homeostasis
-staxis	dripping, trickling	epistaxis
sten(o)-	denoting something as 'narrow in shape' or pertaining to narrowness	stenography
-stenosis	abnormal narrowing in a blood vessel or other tubular organ or structure	restenosis, stenosis
stomat(o)-	of or pertaining to the mouth	stomatogastric, stomatognathic system
-stomy	creation of an opening	colostomy
sub-	beneath	subcutaneous tissue
super-	in excess, above, superior	superior vena cava
supra-	above, excessive	supraorbital vein
tachy-	denoting something as fast, irregularly fast	tachycardia
-tension, -tensive	pressure	hypertension
tetan-	rigid, tense	tetanus
thec-	case, sheath	intrathecal
therap-	treatment	hydrotherapy, therapeutic
therm(o)-	heat	thermometer
thorac(i)-, thorac(o)-,thoracico-	of or pertaining to the upper chest, chest; the area above the breast and under the neck	thorax
thromb(o)-	of or relating to a blood clot, clotting of blood	thrombus, thrombocytopenia
thyr(o)-	thyroid	thyrocele
thym-	emotions	dysthymia
-tome	cutting instrument	osteotome
-tomy	act of cutting; incising, incision	gastrotomy
tono-	tone, tension, pressure	tonometer
-tony	tension	
top(o)-	place, topical	topical anaesthetic

Prefix or suffix	Meaning	Example(s)
tort(i)-	twisted	torticollis
tox(i)-, tox(o)-, toxic(o)-	toxin, poison	toxoplasmosis
trache(a)-	trachea	tracheotomy
trachel(o)-	of or pertaining to the neck	tracheloplasty
trans-	denoting something as moving or situated 'across' or 'through'	transfusion
tri-	three	triangle
trich(i)-, trichia, trich(o)-	of or pertaining to hair, hair-like structure	trichocyst
-tripsy	crushing	lithotripsy
-trophy	nourishment, development	pseudohypertrophy
tympan(o)-	eardrum	tympanocentesis
-ula, -ule	small	nodule
ultra-	beyond, excessive	ultrasound
un(i)-	one	unilateral hearing loss
ur(o)-	of or pertaining to urine, the urinary system; (specifically) pertaining to the physiological chemistry of urine	urology
uter(o)-	of or pertaining to the uterus or womb	uterus
vagin-	of or pertaining to the vagina	vagina
varic(o)-	swollen or twisted vein	varicose
vasculo-	blood vessel	vasculotoxicity
vas(o)-	duct, blood vessel	vasoconstriction
ven-	of or pertaining to the (blood) veins, a vein (used in terms pertaining to the vascular system)	vein, venospasm
ventricul(o)-	of or pertaining to the ventricles; any hollow region inside an organ	cardiac ventriculography
ventr(o)-	of or pertaining to the belly; the stomach cavities	ventrodorsal
-version	turning	anteversion, retroversion
vesic(o)-	of or pertaining to the bladder	vesical arteries
viscer(o)-	of or pertaining to the internal organs, the viscera	viscera

Prefix or suffix	Meaning	Example(s)
xanth(o)-	denoting a yellow colour, an abnormally yellow colour	xanthopathy
xen(o)-	foreign, different	xenograft
xer(o)-	dry, desert-like	xerostomia
zo(o)-	animal, animal life	zoology
zym(o)-	fermentation	enzyme, lysozyme

How to use your textbook

Features contained within your textbook

Learning outcome boxes give a summary of the topics covered in a chapter.

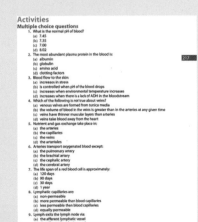

Learning outcomes

After reading this chapter you will be able to:

- Describe the levels of organisation of a body
- Describe the characteristics of life
- Understand and be able to explain an atom and how it relates to molecules
- Describe and understand the ways in which atoms can bind together
- Describe elements and their characteristics
- Understand how to read chemical equations
- Describe the pH scale and its importance to life
- List the differences between organic and inorganic substances
- List the various ways in which we measure things

Your textbook is full of **illustrations and tables**.

Figure 2.2 Structure of a cell. Source: Peate and Nair (2011). Reproduced with permission of John Wiley & Sons.

Table 2.1 Cellular compartments and their functions

Self-assessment review questions help you test yourself after each chapter.

Activities

Multiple choice questions

The website icon indicates that you can find accompanying resources on the book's companion websites.

About the companion websites

Don't forget to visit the student and instructor companion websites for this book:

www.wileyfundamentalseries.com/anatomy

On this companion website, students will find valuable material designed to enhance their learning, including:

- Case studies
- Glossary terms
- Interactive multiple choice questions
- Interactive true/false questions
- Flashcards
- Links to further reading
- Matching items questions

Scan this QR code to visit the student companion website:

www.wiley.com/go/instructor/anatomy

On this companion website, instructors will find valuable material designed to enhance their teaching, including:

- PowerPoint slides to be used as a complete slide set: including slides with explanatory text combined with figures from the book to cover the main topics for each chapter
- An image bank of all the figures and tables from the book, to download as PowerPoint slides

Scan this QR code to visit the instructor companion website:

Chapter 1

Basic scientific principles of physiology

Peter S Vickers

Test your prior knowledge

- What is the difference between anatomy and physiology?
- Why is the process of osmosis essential for the functioning of the human body?
- What is an electrolyte?
- What is the process of external respiration in humans?
- Define homeostasis.

Learning outcomes

After reading this chapter you will be able to:

- Describe the levels of organisation of a body
- Describe the characteristics of life
- Understand and be able to explain an atom and how it relates to molecules
- Describe and understand the ways in which atoms can bind together
- Describe elements and their characteristics
- Understand how to read chemical equations
- Describe the pH scale and its importance to life
- List the differences between organic and inorganic substances
- List the various ways in which we measure things

Fundamentals of Anatomy and Physiology: For Nursing and Healthcare Students, Second Edition. Edited by Ian Peate and Muralitharan Nair.
© 2017 John Wiley & Sons, Ltd. Published 2017 by John Wiley & Sons, Ltd.
Student companion website: www.wileyfundamentalseries.com/anatomy
Instructor companion website: www.wiley.com/go/instructor/anatomy

Introduction

Learning about the physiology of the body is very much like learning a foreign language – there are new vocabulary, grammar and concepts to learn and understand. This first chapter introduces you to this new language so that you can then use your knowledge to understand the physiology of the different parts of the body that are discussed in all the other chapters of this book.

First of all there are two terms to learn and understand:

- **anatomy**, the study of structure;
- **physiology**, the study of function.

However, structure is always related to function because the structure determines the function, which in turn determines how the body/organ, and so on, is structured – the two are interdependent.

Levels of organisation

The body is a very complex organism that consists of many components, starting with the smallest of them – the atom – and concluding with the organism itself (Figure 1.1). Starting from the smallest component and working towards the largest, the body is organised in the following way:

- The atom – for example, hydrogen, carbon.
- The molecule – for example, water, glucose.
- The macromolecule (large molecule) – for example, protein, DNA.
- The organelle (found in the cell) – for example, nucleus, mitochondrion.
- The tissues – for example, bone, muscle.
- The organs – for example, heart, kidney.
- The organ system – for example, skeletal, cardiovascular, respiratory, renal.
- The organism – for example, mouse, dog, elephant, and, of course, humans.

Characteristics of life

All living organisms have certain characteristics in common. Although these characteristics may differ from organism to organism, they are all important for the maintenance of life. These characteristics are:

- **Reproduction** – at both the micro- and the macrolevel, reproduction is an essential process. At the macrolevel is the reproduction of the organism, and at the microlevel is the reproduction of new cells to maintain the efficiency and growth of the organism.
- **Growth** – essential for the growth and development of an organism.
- **Movement** – changes in position as well as motion are parts of movement. This characteristic is essential to allow the organism to seek out nutrition, partners for reproduction, escape from predators, and so on
- **Respiration** – external respiration is important for obtaining oxygen and releasing carbon dioxide (or obtaining carbon dioxide and releasing oxygen if a green plant), while internal respiration releases energy from foods.

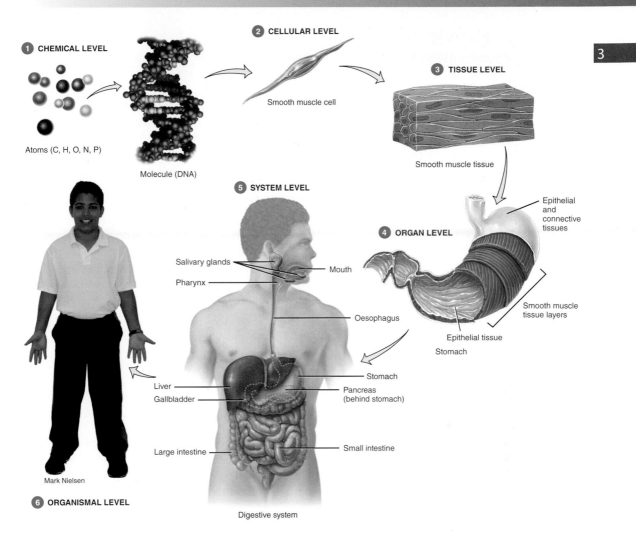

Figure 1.1 Levels of organisation of the body. *Source*: Tortora and Derrickson (2014). Reproduced with permission of John Wiley & Sons.

- **Responsiveness** – organisms need to be able to respond to changes in the environment, for example, or to other stimuli such as predator danger.
- **Digestion** – this is the breakdown of food substances, so that the organism can produce the energy necessary for its life.
- **Absorption** – the movement of substances, such as digested food, through membranes and into body fluids, including blood and lymph, which then carry the substances to the parts of the organism requiring them.
- **Circulation** – the movement of substances through the body in the body fluids.
- **Assimilation** – the changing of absorbed substances into different substances, which can then be utilised by the tissues of the body.
- **Excretion** – the removal of waste substances from the body, either because they are of no use to the body or because they are harmful to the body.

Bodily requirements

There are five essential requirements that all organisms, including humans, require:

1. **Water**
   - Water is the most abundant substance found in the body. At birth, up to 78% of a baby's body is composed of water, at 1 year of age this has dropped to 65%. In adult males the figure has dropped to 60% and in adult females the figure is 55% (females have more fat than males as a percentage of their body, which accounts for the difference, although a fat adult male would also have a lower percentage than a thin adult male).
   - Water is required for the various metabolic processes that are necessary for an organism's survival.
   - Water is necessary to transport essential substances around the organism.
   - Water helps to regulate body temperature – a human operates within a very narrow temperature range and has an inability to cope with large temperature changes within the body. If body temperature exceeds this range – either below or above – then death will occur. Sweating is an example of water helping to reduce a high temperature – it cools the body surface as it evaporates (evaporative cooling).

2. **Food**
   - Food supplies the energy for the organism to fulfil all the essential characteristics mentioned above.
   - It also supplies the raw materials for these characteristics – particularly growth.

3. **Oxygen**
   - Oxygen forms 20% of air and is used in the release of energy from the assimilated nutrients.

4. **Heat**
   - Heat is a form of energy that partly controls the rate at which metabolic reactions occur.

5. **Pressure**
   - There are two types of pressure that are required by an organism:
     - atmospheric pressure, which is important in the process of breathing;
     - hydrostatic pressure, which keeps the blood flowing through the body.

Atoms

It is now time to consider the smallest building block of the body (indeed of all matter), namely the atom. The word 'atom' comes from a Greek word which means 'incapable of being divided'. However, we now know that an atom consists of electrons, neutrons and protons.

The atom, as can be seen from Figure 1.2, is made up of even smaller matter, namely:

- protons
- neutrons
- electrons.

Protons carry a positive electrical charge and electrons carry a negative electrical charge, while the neutron, as its name implies, carries no electrical charge (it is neutral).

As can be seen from Figure 1.3, electrons move rapidly around the nucleus of the atom, which itself is made up of protons and neutrons. The electrons of an atom are bound to the nucleus by electromagnetic force.

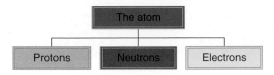

Figure 1.2 The atom.

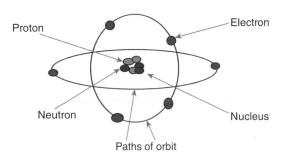

Figure 1.3 Schematic diagram of an atom.

Although there are many different types of atoms, they always have the same make-up – just different numbers of paths of orbit, **electrons, neutrons** and **protons** – and the same characteristics, while atoms of different elements (e.g. iron, carbon, sodium) have different numbers of electrons, protons and neutrons. For example:

- The nucleus is always central.
- The inner shell (path of orbit) always has a maximum of two electrons.
- The second shell can have a maximum of eight electrons.
- The third shell can have a maximum of 18 electrons, and so on.
- Of importance is the valence shell. This is the outermost shell of an atom and determines how the atom behaves in chemical reactions with other atoms. This can have a maximum of eight electrons (known as the octet rule). These **valence electrons** can participate in the formation of a **chemical bond**. See 'Covalent bonds' section.

Atomic number

All atoms are designated a number, known as the atomic number, and the atomic number of an atom is the same as the number of protons in that atom. Consequently, the atomic number of a carbon atom, which has six protons, is 6, while the sodium atom has 11 protons and therefore its atomic number is 11, and a chlorine atom has 17 protons and so has an atomic number of 17.

Carbon atom

Carbon, a very important atom for life forms because we are all carbon-based entities, will demonstrate the make-up of an actual atom.

As you can see from Figure 1.4, carbon has six electrons orbiting the nucleus, which is made up of six protons and six neutrons. Therefore, it has the same number of electrons, protons and neutrons. This is unusual, because while it is normal to have the same number of electrons and protons, usually the number of neutrons differs from the numbers of electrons and protons in an atom.

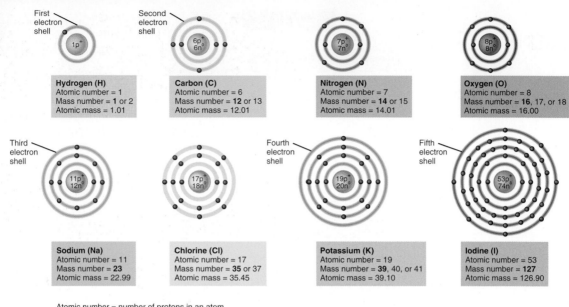

Atomic number = number of protons in an atom
Mass number = number of protons and neutrons in an atom (emboldening indicates most common isotope)
Atomic mass = average mass of all stable atoms of a given element in daltons

Figure 1.4   The carbon atom. *Source*: Tortora and Derrickson (2014). Reproduced with permission of John Wiley & Sons.

A basic principle of the atom is that the number of electrons is equal to the number of protons in each atom, and this is all to do with electricity. As mentioned above, protons carry a positive electrical charge, electrons carry a negative electrical charge and neutrons carry a neutral charge (i.e. they carry no charge), and the aim of all atoms is to remain electrically stable (electrically neutral). Therefore, as neutrons carry no electrical charge, it is important that electrons and protons are equal in number to maintain the stability/neutrality.

Thus, as the carbon atom carries six electrons, six protons and six neutrons, the electrical charges of the electrons and protons cancel one another out. As a consequence, overall, the atom is neutrally charged and it is said to be in a state of equilibrium.

Molecules

This need for the atom to be in equilibrium is the driving force behind the combining of atoms to make molecules (the next stage in the building of life forms). A molecule is the smallest particle of an element or compound that exists independently. It contains atoms that have bonded together. For example, sodium chloride (NaCl) is a molecule containing one atom of sodium (also known as natrium, hence the symbol Na) which has bonded to one atom of chlorine (symbol Cl). Similarly, the molecule H_2O is made up of two atoms of hydrogen (H) bonded to one atom of oxygen (O). H_2O is better known as water.

Chemical bonds

A chemical bond is the way in which atoms bind to one another by the atoms attaining a lower energy state through losing, gaining or sharing their outer shell electrons with other atoms.

A chemical bond is the 'attractive' force that holds atoms together. This interaction results in the formation of atoms or ions that are in a lower energy state than the original atoms.

The formation of chemical bonds also results in the release of energy previously contained in the atoms, as shown in the formula

$$atom + atom \rightarrow atom—atom + energy$$

The combining power of atoms is known as **valence**. Because the only shell that is important in bonding is the outermost shell, this shell is known as the valence shell (Marieb, 2014).

There are several types of chemical bonds that occur between atoms, namely:

- ionic bonds
- covalent bonds
- polar bonds/hydrogen bonds.

Ionic bonding of atoms

Atoms always prefer to be in a state of electrical equilibrium. However, sometimes an atom that has a stable structure may lose an electron, in which case it becomes unstable. For example, a sodium (Na) atom is an atom that may lose an electron, and in this case, in order to become stable again, it must connect with an atom that can accept an electron – for example, chlorine (Cl). So, consequently, when sodium atoms and chlorine atoms are mixed together, one electron of each sodium atom will move to an equivalent atom of chlorine – as depicted in Figure 1.5 – thus forming the molecule sodium chloride (NaCl), also known as common salt. This is known as **ionic bonding**, because **ions** are involved.

Ions

An ion is an atom or a molecule in which the total number of electrons is not equal to the total number of protons – hence the atom or molecule has a net positive or negative electrical charge. It is no longer in an electrically neutral state. In the example above, sodium and chlorine have positive and negative electrical charges respectively due to the interchange of electrons, so they are now ions, and we depict them with a small positive or minus sign, as in the examples below:

- Na^+ (sodium positive)
- Cl^- (chlorine negative).

However, we can write the resultant sodium chloride molecule as NaCl because the positive (+) and the negative (−) have attracted each other and cancelled out the electrical charges, leaving us with a molecule that has a neutral electrical charge.

- Ions that carry a positive electrical charge are known as **cations**
- Ions that carry a negative electrical charge are known as **anions**.

To summarise, an ionic bond is a bond that is formed between ions, some of which are positively charged and some of which are negatively charged. These atoms are known as ions and are attracted to, and stabilise, each other, but they neither transfer nor share electrons between themselves. Consequently, this can be seen more as an interaction between atoms rather than as a bond between them (Fisher and Arnold, 2012).

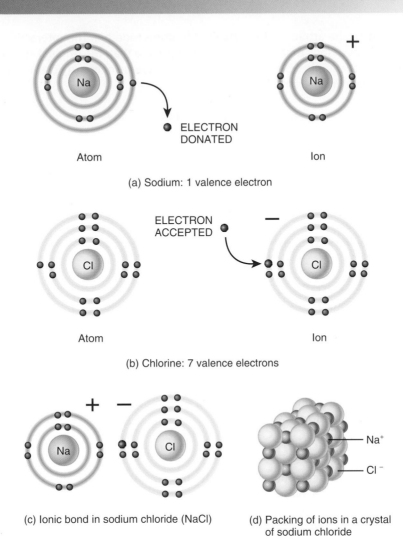

(a) Sodium: 1 valence electron

(b) Chlorine: 7 valence electrons

(c) Ionic bond in sodium chloride (NaCl)

(d) Packing of ions in a crystal of sodium chloride

Figure 1.5 (a–d) Ionic bonding of a sodium and a chlorine atom to form a sodium chloride molecule. *Source*: Tortora and Derrickson (2014). Reproduced with permission of John Wiley & Sons.

Covalent bonds

Unlike ionic bonding, covalent bonding does involve the sharing of valence electrons with compatible adjacent electrons. In this way, none of the atoms involved in this type of bonding actually loses or gains electrons. Instead, electrons are shared between them so that each of the atoms will have a complete valence shell (i.e. outermost shell) for at least part of the time (Marieb, 2014).

Covalent bonding occurs when two atoms are close to one another and so an overlapping of the outer shell electrons occurs. Following this overlapping, each outer shell becomes attracted to the nucleus of the other atom (Figure 1.6). This type of bonding does not require positive and negative electrical charges as ionic bonding does.

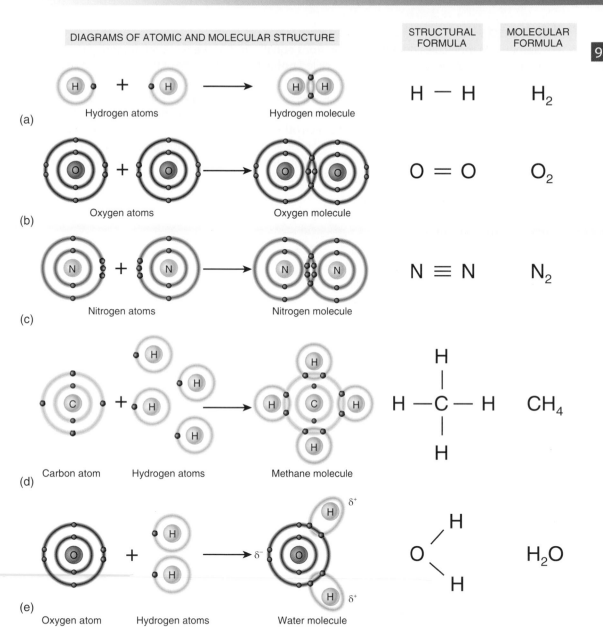

DIAGRAMS OF ATOMIC AND MOLECULAR STRUCTURE   STRUCTURAL FORMULA   MOLECULAR FORMULA

(a) Hydrogen atoms → Hydrogen molecule $H - H$ H_2

(b) Oxygen atoms → Oxygen molecule $O = O$ O_2

(c) Nitrogen atoms → Nitrogen molecule $N \equiv N$ N_2

(d) Carbon atom   Hydrogen atoms → Methane molecule $H - C - H$ (with H above and H below) CH_4

(e) Oxygen atom   Hydrogen atoms → Water molecule O with H and H H_2O

Figure 1.6   (a–e) Covalent bond. *Source*: Tortora and Derrickson (2014). Reproduced with permission of John Wiley & Sons.

There are three types of covalent bonding, depending upon the number of electrons that are shared between the bonded atoms:

1. single covalent bonds (one electron from each atom is shared in the outermost shell, e.g. hydrogen molecule);
2. double covalent bonds (two electrons from each atom are shared, e.g. oxygen molecule);
3. triple covalent bonds (three electrons from each atom are shared, e.g. nitrogen molecule).

Polar bonds

Sometimes molecules do not share electrons equally and so there is a separation of the electrical charge into positive or negative. This is called **polarity**, and because of this separation of electrical charge there is an additional weak bond. However, note that this bond is *not* between **atoms**, but is between the **molecules** themselves. Just as with ionic bonding, this polar bonding comes about because of the electrical rule that **opposites attract**. Thus, the small opposing charges from different polar molecules can be attracted to each other. Polar bonding only occurs with molecules that contain the atom hydrogen – so a polar bond is also known as a **hydrogen bond** (see Figure 1.7).

The fact that polar molecules can bond (albeit only weakly) is very important in determining the structure and function of physiologically active substances such as

- enzymes
- antibodies
- genetic molecules
- pharmacological agents (drugs).

Electrolytes

A further development of bonding is the production of electrolytes. Electrolytes are substances that move to oppositely charged electrodes in fluids. They occur in the following way: if molecules that are bonded together ionically (see 'Ionic bonding of atoms' section) are dissolved in water within the body cells, then they undergo a process where the ions separate; that is, they become dissociated. These ions are now known as electrolytes.

However, this does not apply to molecules that are produced by other types of bonding (e.g. covalent bonding). Molecules that are produced as a result of other types of bonding are called non-electrolytes, and these include most organic compounds, such as glucose, urea and creatinine.

Electrolytes are particularly important for three things within the body:

1. Many are essential minerals.
2. They control the process of osmosis.
3. They help to maintain the acid–base balance, which is necessary for normal cellular activity.

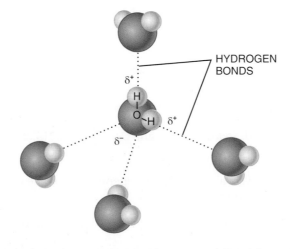

Figure 1.7 Hydrogen bonds and water. *Source*: Tortora and Derrickson (2014). Reproduced with permission of John Wiley & Sons.

Elements

A chemical element is a pure chemical substance that cannot be broken down into anything simpler by chemical means. Each element consists of just one type of atom, which is distinguished by its atomic number (which in turn is determined by the number of protons in the nucleus of an atom – see earlier). If the number of protons in the nucleus of an atom changes, then we have a new element, not the original one. This differs from the case with electrons, the number of which can change but the atom remains basically the same – and it is now an **ion**. Some common examples of elements found in the body include

- iron
- hydrogen
- carbon
- nitrogen
- oxygen
- calcium
- potassium
- sodium
- chlorine
- sulphur
- phosphorus.

As of February 2015, a total of 118 elements have been confirmed; however, only the first 98 are known to occur naturally on Earth. These elements are usually presented as a **periodic table**. All chemical matter consists of these elements, although new elements of higher atomic number are discovered from time to time – but only as a result of artificial nuclear reactions, and so are not found in the body.

There are three classes of elements:

1. metals (e.g. iron – symbol 'Fe' from ferrum)
2. non-metals (e.g. oxygen – symbol 'O')
3. metalloids (e.g. arsenic – symbol 'As').

These three classes of elements all have certain characteristics that define them:

Metals	Non-metals	Metalloids
They conduct heat and electricity	They are poor conductors of heat and electricity	They are neither metals nor non-metals – they are sometimes referred to as semi metals
They donate electrons (to other atoms to make molecules)	They accept electrons (from donor atoms)	They tend to have the physical properties of metals while having the chemical properties of both metals and non-metals depending upon their oxidation state. However, they are not relevant to biochemistry, so will not be discussed in this book
At normal temperatures they are all solids – with the exception of mercury (symbol 'Hg')	They may exist as a solid, a liquid or a gas	

Usually metals bond with non-metals (i.e. electron donors with electron acceptors). The following are some examples of elements important for the body that are metals and non-metals:

Metals	Non-metals
Calcium (Ca)	Chlorine (Cl)
Potassium (K)	Nitrogen (N)
Sodium (Na)	Oxygen (O)
	Carbon (C)
	Sulphur (S)
	Phosphorus (P)

As well as sodium chloride – NaCl (met previously in this chapter) – some other important compounds that a nurse will need to know about include:

- sodium bicarbonate – $NaHCO_3$
- potassium chloride – KCl.

An interesting element is hydrogen (H), because hydrogen actually has properties of both metals and non-metals. As a consequence, water (H_2O) is an example of a substance that, although made up of two gases – oxygen (one atom) and hydrogen (two atoms) – becomes a liquid once these gases have bonded together.

Properties of elements

All substances have certain individual properties, particularly in the way that they react (i.e. behave):

- *physical properties* – these include such characteristics as colour, density, boiling point, melting point, solubility, hardness, and so on;
- *chemical properties* – these include whether or not a substance is a metal or non-metal (or even metalloid), whether it reacts with an acid or an alkaline substance, or whether it dissolves in water or alcohol.

Compounds

A 'compound' is a pure substance that is made up of two or more elements chemically bonded together. The properties of a compound are totally different from the individual properties of the elements that are bonded together to make that compound. In addition, compounds can be broken down chemically, while elements cannot. Examples of compounds include:

- water (H_2O)
- salt (NaCl)
- carbon dioxide (CO_2).

Note that when the symbol for an atom has a small lower number after it, then that denotes there are that number of that particular atom in the molecule. So, water (H_2O) is made up of two atoms of hydrogen and one atom of oxygen, while carbon dioxide (CO_2) consists of one atom of carbon and two atoms of oxygen. This will be discussed again later in this chapter.

Chemical equations/chemical reactions

Any mention of chemical equations and most non-chemists/non-scientists immediately start to panic and quickly turn the page. Not to worry, however, because if anyone is capable of doing simple addition sums, then they are capable of working through chemical equations. Everyone has worked through simple mathematical equations, such as

- $1+1=2$
- $2+2=4$
- $4+4=8$
- $1+1+2+2+2=8$
- $1+1+2+2+2=4+3+1$

and so on.

Chemical equations work on the same basic principles. When a chemical reaction occurs (which is portrayed as an equation), then a new substance is formed. This is called the **product** (as with a mathematical equation). However, in a chemical equation, this new substance (product) will have different properties from the individual substances involved in the reaction (called the reactants).

As discussed above, when atoms are combined they form elements or molecules, and symbols are used to describe this process. This look at chemical equations will start with a very simple example, namely the production of water (Figure 1.8).

As mentioned previously, two atoms of hydrogen (H) combined with one atom of oxygen (O) produce one molecule of water (H_2O). The chemical equation for this process is

$$H+H+O \rightarrow H_2O$$
$$hydrogen+hydrogen+oxygen \rightarrow water$$

In this equation (of a chemical reaction) there are two atoms of hydrogen and one atom of oxygen on the left-hand side, and there are two atoms of hydrogen and one atom of oxygen on the right-hand side. However, on the right, because of a chemical reaction, the same three atoms of gas have created water – a liquid.

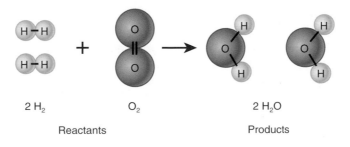

$2\ H_2$ O_2 $2\ H_2O$

Reactants   Products

Figure 1.8 Pictorial depiction of the chemical equation (reaction) producing water. *Source*: Tortora and Derrickson (2014). Reproduced with permission of John Wiley & Sons.

Thus, a chemical equation is just a shorthand way of describing a chemical reaction. Note that the equals sign in a mathematical equation is replaced by an arrow, meaning 'leads to', in a chemical equation. Basically, all chemical equations are as simple as this. There may be more reactants and products, but there are similar basic principles involved in chemical equations as in mathematical equations.

A very important basic principle is that when chemical reactions occur, the amount of each substance must be the same after the reaction has occurred as was present before the reaction. The two sides of a chemical reaction (and therefore a chemical equation) – the reactants and the products – must balance. In other words, no atoms/molecules are lost in a chemical reaction, they are just organised differently. Another thing to be aware of with chemical reactions is that although the numbers of atoms are the same before and after the reaction, during a chemical reaction, something extra is usually produced every time – namely, heat. This is known as an exothermic reaction, which is a process/reaction that gives out energy in the form of heat.

In a chemical equation, the reactants and the product may be separated by a single arrow ($\rightarrow$) as in the earlier example of H_2O. This indicates that the reaction occurs only in one direction, namely in the direction that the arrow is pointing.

Sometimes the reactants and product may be separated by two arrows – one above the other and pointing in different directions ($\rightleftarrows$). This indicates that the chemical reaction can be reversed.

If the reactants and the products are separated by an equals sign '=' (which is a symbol used in mathematics to indicate a state of equality), instead of single or double arrows, this indicates that a state of chemical equilibrium exists.

Another important principle to be aware of, as regards chemical reactions and equations, is that a chemical equation has to be consistent. The elements cannot be changed into other elements by chemical means.

If electrical charges are involved (as occurs with the involvement of ions), the net charge on both sides of the equation must be equal – that is, they must balance.

So, to summarise, all equations must balance (i.e. the number of reactants and their electrical charges must equal the number of products and their electrical charges). However, balancing a chemical equation (and thus a reaction) may require the altering of the quantity of molecules.

Here is a more complicated chemical reaction/equation, but the principles will still hold for this:

$$Zn + 2HCl \rightarrow ZnCl_2 + H_2$$
zinc + hydrogen chloride $\rightarrow$ zinc chloride + hydrogen

Note: mention has been made previously in this chapter of the principle that, when using the chemical symbols of substances (elements, compounds, molecules, etc.), if a small number comes after an atom as in H_2O, then that number applies to the atom immediately before it. In other words H_2O is composed of two atoms of hydrogen and one atom of oxygen. However, if an atom or molecule is preceded by a large number, then that applies to everything immediately afterwards until another mathematical symbol (e.g. +, $\rightarrow$) occurs. For example, 2HCl means that there are two atoms of hydrogen and two atoms of chlorine bonded together to make two molecules of hydrogen chloride.

In this chemical reaction/equation, two molecules of hydrogen chloride (in the form of two ions of chloride, Cl^-, and two ions of hydrogen, H^+) along with one atom of zinc have been changed to one molecule of zinc chloride ($ZnCl_2$) and one molecule of hydrogen (H_2). So, even though the original atoms have now been combined differently following the chemical reaction, the balance between the two sides of the equation in terms of numbers and types of atoms and electrical charge has not been altered.

With this even more complicated chemical reaction/equation, it is a good idea to take some time and work out just what is going on here before reading on:

$$HCl + NaHCO_3 \rightleftarrows NaCl + H_2CO_3$$

hydrochloric acid + sodium bicarbonate $\rightleftarrows$ sodium chloride + carbonic acid

Also in this reaction, H_2CO_3 can be broken down further:

$$H_2CO_3 \rightleftarrows CO_2 + H_2O$$

The reactants on the left-hand side are duplicated on the right-hand side (the products) but in different combinations. Note the double arrow – what does this mean?

The presence of the double-headed arrow means that the equation is capable of being reversed, so that the products become the reactants, and the reactants the products. Note that sodium bicarbonate ($NaHCO_3$) is made up of one atom each of sodium, hydrogen and carbon and three atoms of oxygen, while carbonic acid (H_2CO_3) is composed of two atoms of hydrogen, one atom of carbon and three atoms of oxygen. Counting the numbers and types of each atom on both sides demonstrates again that nothing is added and nothing deleted when the reaction takes place – everything is just rearranged in such a way that elements that can be used by the body are produced (along with any waste elements, which are then excreted).

This is the end of the section on chemical equations, and as can be seen, if someone can do simple arithmetic, then they can understand and work with chemical equations (remembering that the equations are a depiction of chemical reactions that are taking place within the body all the time).

Acids and bases (pH)

This section may initially appear complicated, but it is important to understand **pH** values, along with alkalinity and acidity, as our bodies (indeed our very lives) depend upon the relationship between acidity and alkalinity.

- An **acid** is any substance that donates hydrogen ions (H^+) into a solution.
- An **alkali** (also known as a **soluble base**) is any substance that donates hydroxyl ions (OH^-) into a solution or accepts H^+ ions from a solution.

The more OH^- ions that have been donated or H^+ ions accepted, the greater the alkalinity of a substance; conversely, the greater the number of H^+ ions that are released, the more acidic is the solution. Obviously, whenever the numbers of H^+ and OH^- ions are the same, then a **neutral** solution exists.

The chemical equation for the ionisation of water is shown as

$$H_2O \rightleftarrows H^+ + OH^-$$

In other words, water contains hydrogen and hydroxyl ions, and in one litre of pure water, 10^{-14} mol (**moles**) of water are dissociated into H^+ ions and OH^- ions. If there are 10^{-7} mol of H^+ ions and 10^{-7} mol of OH^- ions in one litre, then they are balanced and the water is neutral (neither acidic nor alkaline).

- Note that a **mole** in chemistry is a unit of amount of substance (it is a unit of measurement for chemicals) and is defined as the mass of substance that contains as many elements (atoms, molecules, etc.) as there are atoms in 12 g of carbon-12 (International Bureau of Weights and Measures, 2006).

  The concept of a mole in chemistry is quite complicated, but it is only necessary in this chapter to use it in relation to acid–base balance.

- The concept of 10^{-14} is an arithmetic one and denotes a very small number: $10^{-14} = 0.00000000000001$ of a mole.

- In biochemistry, **dissociation** is the separation of a substance into two or more simpler substances – such as a molecule into atoms or ions – by the action of heat or a chemical process. This process is usually reversible.

The properties of water are such that the minimum concentration of H^+ ions and OH^- ions is 10^{-14} mol L^{-1} (moles per litre), while the maximum concentration of H^+ ions and OH^- ions is 1 mol L^{-1} or 1.00 mol L^{-1}. Thus, the dissociation properties of water restrict the concentration of H^+ ions and OH^- ions to the range of 10^{-14} to 100 mol L^{-1}.

A scale of acidity and alkalinity has been devised that uses this range of 10^{-14} to 100 mol L^{-1} of H^+ and OH^- ions – known as the **pH scale** (see Figures 1.9 and 1.10). Consequently, the addition of H+ ions to pure water results in a proportionate decrease of OH^- ions from the initial concentration of 10^{-7} mol L^{-1}. Thus, an H^+ ion concentration of 10^{-8} mol L^{-1} results in an OH^- concentration of 10^{-6} mol L^{-1}. In this way, the combined totals of H^+ and OH^- molecules will always equal 10^{-14}. The pH scale represents the powers of 10 of H^+ ions from 10^{-14} to 10^0, but for convenience the scale uses positive numbers, so the scale is from pH 14 to pH 0.

At pH 7 an equal number of H^+ ions and OH^- ions occurs, while solutions with a pH that is lower than 7 are **acids** and those with a pH that is greater than 7 are **bases/alkaline**. The further away from a pH of 7 a solution becomes the more acidic or alkaline it is.

The pH scale is a logarithmic scale so consequently each whole pH value below 7 is 10 times more acidic than the next highest value. For example, a solution with a pH 3 value is 10 times more acidic than a solution with a pH 4 value. In addition, it is 100 times (i.e. 10×10) more acidic than solution with a pH 5, and 1000 times (i.e. $10 \times 10 \times 10$) more acidic than a solution that has a

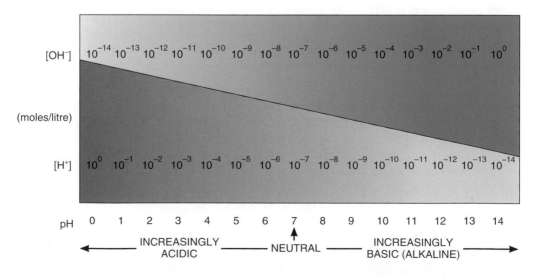

Figure 1.9 The pH scale. *Source*: Tortora and Derrickson (2014). Reproduced with permission of John Wiley & Sons.

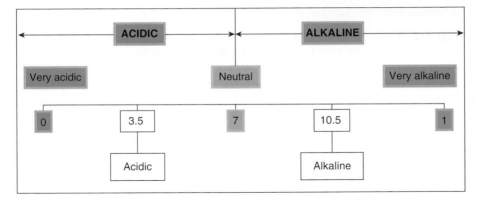

Figure 1.10   Simplified diagram of a pH scale.

pH value of 7 (i.e. a neutral solution). Exactly the same applies to pH values that are above 7 (i.e. alkaline solutions), in that each is 10 times more alkaline than the next lowest value. For example, a solution with a pH of 10 is 10 times more alkaline than one with a pH of 9, 100 times (10×10) more alkaline than a solution with a pH of 8, and so on.

This last concept of logarithmic values and pH is very important for us, as can be seen in the next section, which looks at pH values and blood.

Blood and pH values

In blood, the physiologically normal pH range is 7.35–7.45; that is, it is slightly alkaline. However, a blood pH lower than 7.35 is considered to be acidic, whereas a pH greater than 7.45 is alkaline, and when either of these events occurs it can have a serious effect on the body, as is discussed in other chapters within this book. The reason is that because the scale is a logarithm, then just a small change in pH indicates a very significant alteration in H^+ concentration. Every change in one pH unit represents a 10-fold change in H^+ ion concentration. Thus, an alteration of pH from pH 7.4 to pH 7.3 results in a doubling of the H^+ ion concentration. In other words:

- pH 8 contains 10^{-8} mol L^{-1} or 10 nmol L^{-1} (nanomoles per litre) of H^+
- pH 7 contains 10^{-7} mol L^{-1} or 100 nmol L^{-1} of H^+
- pH 6 contains 10^{-6} mol L^{-1} or 1000 nmol L^{-1} of H^+

and so on.

Homeostasis

Homeostasis is the body's attempt to maintain a stable internal environment by achieving some sort of balance. The body is normally able to achieve a relatively stable internal environment even though the external environment is constantly changing – from cold to hot, or from dry to wet, and so on. The body uses various homeostatic mechanisms to monitor and maintain a dynamic state of equilibrium within the body – that is, a balance in which the internal environment conditions can react to external environmental conditions by changing within quite narrow limits.

The homeostatic mechanisms include:

- **receptors** – the body has receptors that sense external and internal environmental changes and provide information on the changes to the control centre;
- **control centre** – the control centre determines what a particular value (e.g. pH value or blood pressure) should be and sends out a message to the effectors;
- **effectors** – once they have received the information from the control centre, the effectors cause responses to take place within the body's internal environment that hopefully will produce the changes that will enable the internal environment to return to normal values.

Organic and inorganic substances

All substances are classed either as organic or inorganic depending upon their molecules.

- **Organic** molecules:
  - contain carbon (C) and hydrogen (H);
  - are usually larger than inorganic molecules;
  - dissolve in water and organic liquids;
  - as a group include carbohydrates (sugars), proteins, lipids (fats) and nucleic acids (part of DNA) – see Chapter 3, Genetics.

- **Inorganic** molecules:

  - as a group include water (H_2O) and carbon dioxide (CO_2) and inorganic salts. It is true that H_2O and CO_2 do contain carbon atoms, but only in such small quantities that they are, at the moment, still classified as inorganic – although there is a lot of discussion around this within the scientific community
  - are usually smaller than organic molecules;
  - usually dissolve in water or they react with water and release ions;
  - as a group include water (H_2O) carbon dioxide (CO_2) and inorganic salts.

Examples of organic substances

Carbohydrates

Monosaccharides (one of the group of sugars known as carbohydrates) provide energy to cells as well as supplying the materials that allow for the building of the various structures of the cell (see Chapter 2). They contain carbon (C), hydrogen (H) and oxygen (O) and their structure has the chemical formula $C_6H_{12}O_6$. There are three types of carbohydrates:

- monosaccharides – glucose and fructose;
- disaccharides – sucrose, lactose;
- polysaccharides – glycogen, cellulose.

Fats (lipids)

Fats are lipids (known as triglycerides) and are soluble in organic solvents. They are mainly used to provide energy. Like carbohydrates, they consist of carbon (C), hydrogen (H) and oxygen (O), but because the numbers and proportions of these molecules are different from the carbohydrates, they have different properties. The chemical formula for stearin (one type of lipid) is $C_{57}H_{110}O_6$. Lipids can be either saturated or unsaturated. One important group of lipids is the steroid group, which is used to synthesise (produce/construct) hormones. Cholesterol is an important member of the steroid group of lipids.

Proteins

Proteins are built up from amino acids – this will be discussed in Chapter 3. Proteins are very important as they provide the structural material for the body, as well as being an energy source. They also help to form many other substances, including hormones, receptors, enzymes and antibodies.

Examples of inorganic substances

Water (H_2O)

As mentioned above, water is the most abundant compound found in all living material and is a major component of all body fluids. It has an important role to play in most metabolic reactions as well as in transporting chemicals around the body. Water can both absorb and transport heat, so it plays a crucial role in maintaining body temperature.

Oxygen (O_2)

Oxygen is necessary for survival. It is used by the organelles of the nucleus to release energy from nutrients (see Chapter 2).

Units of measurement

To conclude this chapter, which introduces certain bioscientific concepts and prepares the reader for the remaining chapters, just some brief notes about units of measurement. This is an important section because the ability to identify and understand units of measurement will enhance the understanding of the complex human organism.

A unit is a standardised, descriptive word that specifies the dimension of a number. Traditionally there have been seven properties of matter that have been measured independently of each other, namely:

- **time** – measures the duration that something occurs;
- **length** – measures the length of an object;
- **mass** – measures the mass (commonly taken to be the weight) of an object;
- **current** – measures the amount of electric current that passes through an object;
- **temperature** – measures how hot or cold an object is;
- **amount** – measures the amount of a substance that is present;
- **luminous intensity** – measures the brightness of an object.

Originally, each country/society had its own units of measurement. In the UK, for example, there were such units as furlongs, miles, poles, gallons, quarts, bushels, pecks, and so on. This made it difficult for people, particularly scientists, from other countries to work with each other, so several years ago an international system of units was agreed upon by most major countries (however, a notable exception to this agreement is the USA). This new agreed system became known as the Système International d'Unités (or SI units for short). It is a system of units that relates present scientific knowledge to a unified system of units. Tables 1.1, 1.2, 1.3, 1.4, 1.5, 1.6 and 1.7 give the SI units, unit prefixes and some Imperial unit equivalents that will be useful as reference while working through this book.

Table 1.1   The fundamental SI units

Quantity	Name	Symbol
Length	metre	m
Mass	kilogram	kg
Time	second	s
Current	ampere	A
Temperature	Kelvin	K
Amount of substance	mole	mol
Luminous intensity	candela	cd

Table 1.2   Other common SI units

Physical quantity	Name	Symbol
Force	Newton	N
Energy	joule	J
Pressure	pascal	Pa
Potential difference	volt	V
Frequency	hertz	Hz
Volume	litre	L

Table 1.3   Multiples of SI units

Prefix	Symbol	Meaning	Scientific notation
tera	T	one million million	10^{12}
giga	G	one thousand million	10^{9}
mega	M	one million	10^{6}
kilo	k	one thousand	10^{3}
hecto	h	one hundred	10^{2}
deca	da	ten	10^{1}
deci	d	one tenth	10^{-1}
centi	c	one hundredth	10^{-2}
milli	m	one thousandth	10^{-3}
micro	μ	one millionth	10^{-6}
nano	n	one thousandth of a millionth	10^{-9}
pico	p	one millionth of a millionth	10^{-12}
femto	f	one thousandth of a pico	10^{-15}
atto	a	one millionth of a pico	10^{-18}

Table 1.4 Measures of weight

1 kg = 1000 g
1 g = 1000 mg
1 mg = 10^{-3} g
1 µg = 10^{-6} g
1 pound = 0.454 kg/454 g
1 ounce = 28.35 g
25 g = 0.9 ounce
1 ounce = 8 dram

Table 1.5 Measures of volume

1 L = 1000 mL
100 mL = 1 dL
1 mL = 1000 µL
1 UK gallon = 4.5 L
1 pint = 568 mL
1 fluid ounce = 28.42 mL
1 teaspoon = 5 mL
1 tablespoon = 15 mL

Table 1.6 Measures of length

1 m = 10^{-3} km
1 cm = 10^{-2} m
1 mm = 10^{-3} m
1 m = 39.37 inches
1 mile = 1.6 km
1 yard = 0.9 m
1 foot = 0.3 m
1 inch = 25.4 mm

Table 1.7 Measures of energy

1 calorie = 4.184 J
100 calories = 1 dietary Calorie or kilocalorie
1 dietary Calorie = 4184 J or 4.184 kJ
1000 Calorie = 4184 kJ
1 kJ = 0.238 Calories

Conclusion

This concludes this introduction to the very basics of the biochemistry of physiology. As you can now appreciate, biochemistry and physiology are really quite complicated – but also very interesting, and indeed exciting. After all, as you work through this book, you are learning about yourself – how your body works and functions – both in good times (when you are fit and healthy) and in bad times (when you are sick or have had an accident). Everyone is interested in how they function and what happens when they eat and drink, or exercise, or go to the toilet, and so on – not just you, but also your patients. So this is important knowledge for you to have when you are talking to patients. This first chapter is just the beginning of a journey – think of it as a map to help you to complete this journey. This journey is one of self-knowledge and awareness that will lead you to your ultimate goal – a good knowledge of the human body and its functioning. Good luck.

Glossary

Acid   A chemical substance with a low **pH**. The opposite of an **alkaline** substance.

Acid–base balance   The relationship between an **acidic** environment and an **alkaline** one. This is essential for maintaining our good health. See **pH**.

Alkali   A chemical substance with a high **pH**. The opposite of an **acidic** substance.

Anatomy   The study of the structures of the body.

Antibody   Antibodies are proteins that can recognise and attach to infectious agents in the body, and so provoke an immune response to these infectious agents.

Atomic number   Relates to the number of **protons** to be found in any one **atom**.

Atoms   The base of all life, atoms are extremely minute and consist of different numbers of protons, neutron and electrons.

Base   Another name for an **alkaline** substance.

Bonds   The joining together of various substances, particularly atoms and molecules. See **chemical bond**, **covalent bonds**, **ionic bonds**, and **polar bonds**.

Chemical bond   The 'attractive' force that holds **atoms** together.

Chemical reaction   A process in which chemical substances are transformed into something completely different. This is usually depicted in a chemical equation.

Compounds   A pure substance that is made up of two or more **elements** that are **chemically bonded** together.

Covalent bonds   Bonds between **atoms** caused by the sharing of **electrons** between the **atoms**.

Electrolyte   Substance that is able to move to opposite electrically charged electrodes in fluids.

Electrons   The parts of an **atom** that carry a negative electrical charge. See **neutrons** and **protons**.

Elements   A pure chemical substance which cannot be broken down into anything simpler by chemical means (e.g. iron, hydrogen).

Enzymes   Proteins that are produced by cells and can cause very rapid biochemical reactions in the body.

Homeostasis   The name given to processes in which both negative and positive controls are given over variables; they usually involve negative feedback, and the aim is to maintain a stable internal environment.

Inorganic substances   Substances that do not contain carbon **molecules** (e.g. water).

Ionic bonds   Bonding that takes place when atoms lose or gain **electrons**. This alters the electrical charge of the **atoms**.

Ions   Ions are **atom**s that are no longer in a stable state (i.e. they are no longer electrically neutral but are either positively or negatively electrically charged).

Mole   The unit of measurement for the amount of a substance.

Molecules   The smallest part of an **element** or **compound** that can exist on its own (e.g. sodium chloride).

Neutral substance   A chemical substance that is neither **acidic** nor **alkaline**.

Neutron   The parts of an **atom** that carry a neutral electrical charge (i.e. they have no electrical charge). See **electrons** and **protons**.

Organelle   Structural and functional parts of a cell.

Organic substances   Substances that contain carbon **molecules** (e.g. carbohydrates, lipids (fats) and proteins).

Osmosis   The movement of water across a semi permeable membrane from an area of low solute concentration to an area of high solute concentration; this allows for equilibrium of solute and water density on both sides of the semi permeable membrane.

pH   A measure of the acidity or alkalinity of a solution. See **acid–base balance**.

Physiology   The study of the way in which the body structures function.

Polar bonds   Polar bonds occur when atoms of different electronegativities form a bond. Consequently, the **molecules** that are then formed also carry a weak negative electrical charge, which allows molecules to **ionically bond**, just like **atom**s. They are also known as hydrogen bonds because hydrogen molecules have to be present for polar bonding to exist. Examples of such **molecules** include hydrochloric acid and water.

Product (chemical reactions)   The new substance formed following a **chemical reaction**.

Protons   The parts of an **atom** that carry a positive electrical charge. See **electrons** and **neutrons**.

Reactant (chemical reactions)   The individual substances involved in a **chemical reaction**.

Shell (of an atom)   The name that is given to the orbits of **electrons** moving around the nucleus (containing **protons** and **neutrons**) of an **atom**.

Valency   A measure of the combining power of **atoms**.

References

Fisher, J. and Arnold, J.R.P. (2012) *BIOS Instant Notes in Chemistry for Beginners*. London: BIOS Scientific Publishers.

International Bureau of Weights and Measures (2006) *The International System of Units (SI)*, 8th edn. Paris: BIPM (updated 2014).

Marieb, E.N. (2014) *Essentials of Human Anatomy and Physiology*, 11th edn. Harlow: Pearson Education.

Tortora, G.J. and Derrickson, B.H. (2014) *Principles of Anatomy and Physiology*, 14th edn. Hoboken, NJ: John Wiley & Sons.

Activities
Multiple choice questions

1. The characteristics of life include:
   (a) digestion, excretion, irritation
   (b) absorption, bleeding, circulation
   (c) excretion, perspiration, reproduction
   (d) intelligence, growth, responsiveness

2. There are five essential requirements for all organisms. These are:
   (a) carbon dioxide, water, mouths, rectums, oxygen
   (b) oxygen, pressure, heat, water, food
   (c) food, low temperatures, carbon dioxide, oxygen, pressure
   (d) pressure, spatial awareness, sight, water, food

3. Protons possess:
   (a) a stable electrical charge
   (b) no electrical charge
   (c) a negative electrical charge
   (d) a positive electrical charge

4. Which of the following is not a type of chemical bond?
   (a) polar
   (b) equatorial
   (c) ionic
   (d) covalent

5. There are three classes of elements, namely:
   (a) metals, non-metals, metalloids
   (b) metals, oxidants, electrons
   (c) carbons, non-metals, metalloids
   (d) metalloids, non-metals, atomic

6. Which of the following are organic substances?
   (a) carbohydrates, proteins, lipids
   (b) carbohydrates, water, oxygen
   (c) water, proteins, lipids
   (d) lipids, oxygen, proteins

7. Homeostasis is:
   (a) the effective use of receptors
   (b) a measurement of acidity in the body
   (c) the body's attempt to maintain a stable environment
   (d) a combination of physical properties

8. A molecule of water is a combination of which atoms:
   (a) 1×hydrogen, 1×oxygen, 1×carbon atoms
   (b) 2×oxygen, 1×carbon atoms
   (c) 2×oxygen, 1×hydrogen atoms
   (d) 1×oxygen, 2×hydrogen atoms
9. In biochemistry, a 'mole' is a unit of:
   (a) intensity
   (b) luminosity
   (c) pH values
   (d) substance
10. Water is a requirement for the body in order to help:
    (a) release energy
    (b) regulate body temperature
    (c) provide energy
    (d) keep blood flowing through the body

True or false

1. An ion is an atom that is in an electrically neutral state.
2. Molecules are combinations of atoms.
3. Polar bonds occur between molecules.
4. Many electrolytes are essential minerals.
5. Reactions with an acid or alkaline substance are physical properties of elements.
6. Salt is not a compound.
7. There are always more atoms and molecules present following a chemical reaction.
8. Organic substances contain carbon and hydrogen.
9. Lipids are examples of inorganic substances.
10. Proteins are built up from amino acids and provide the structural material for the body.

Label the diagram 1

Label the diagram using the following list of words:

Proton, Neutron, Paths of orbit, Nucleus, Electron

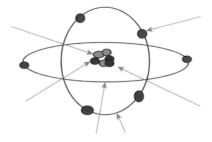

Fill in the blanks 1

Using words from the following list, fill in the missing blanks:

body   effectors   environmental   external   feelers   homeostatic   internal   mechanisms
messages physical   pressure   problems   receptors   response   stable   stimuli type   unstable

Homeostasis is the body's attempts to maintain a _____ internal environment. To do this, it has to be able to change in response to both _____ (e.g. environmental temperature) and internal _____ (e.g. blood pressure) changes. Various _____ are utilised by the body to maintain homeostasis, including _____ to sense external and internal _____ changes. Receptors then send out messages to the _____ control centre, which determines the particular value – for example, the correct temperature or blood _____ required for the essential functioning of the body. This then sends a _____ to the body's _____, which, in turn, cause the body's _____ environment to counteract the effects of the various stimuli/changes.

Word search 1

Find the words listed in the following grid.

A	C	O	Z	E	J	I	R	O	N	K	P	A
N	A	J	O	Z	Y	O	F	Q	I	U	R	N
A	T	O	M	I	P	N	E	U	T	R	O	N
T	O	J	M	O	R	T	I	O	N	B	T	L
O	C	H	E	R	L	S	N	T	R	H	O	E
M	A	Y	B	G	S	E	D	A	H	A	N	Y
Y	E	D	A	A	H	T	C	Q	O	J	E	K
E	N	R	Y	N	E	X	T	U	R	N	I	P
P	R	O	T	E	I	N	S	A	L	T	C	H
S	I	G	P	L	I	P	I	D	F	E	V	L
U	V	E	B	L	Y	I	F	R	U	K	L	O
Z	E	N	Y	E	L	E	M	E	N	T	O	X
E	S	S	T	I	M	A	B	L	E	Q	U	E

Anatomy, Atom, Carbon, Element, Hydrogen, Ion, Iron, Lipid, Molecule, Neutron, Organelle, Protein, Proton

Test your learning

1. What is the importance of respiration for the body?
2. Why is water essential for all organisms, including humans?

3. How is the atomic number of an atom calculated?
4. What is an ion, and what is its importance for us?
5. Make a list of some of the common elements found in the body.
6. Explain what is happening in the chemical reaction as depicted by this chemical equation:

$$C_6H_{12}O_6 + 6O_2 \rightarrow 6CO_2 + 6H_2O + ATP \; (\text{cellular energy})$$

7. Discuss the importance of the pH of blood.
8. Discuss the importance of carbohydrates to the body.

Find out more

1. Look at a copy of the periodic table of elements and mark off the ones you have come across in this chapter and that are important for humans.
2. Many electrolytes are essential minerals for the body. Find out which these are.
3. Find out about, and make notes on, the process of osmosis and its importance for human functioning and health.
4. Discuss the acid–base balance and its importance for maintaining good health – and, indeed, for life itself.
5. Discuss what is happening in these two equations – you will need to have access to chemical abbreviations to help you understand the symbols:

$$N_2 + 3H_2 \rightarrow 2NH_3$$

$$H_2CO_3 \rightarrow H^+ + HCO_3^-$$

6. Find out the normal range of human pH and then discuss why it is important for the nurse to alert medical staff if a patient's pH is found to be outside the normal range.
7. Find out more about the importance of homeostasis to health.
8. Lipids/fats can be either saturated on unsaturated – find out from the foodstuffs that you normally eat which of them contain either or both of these types of lipids and their role(s) in healthy nutrition.
9. Take one day, and on that day look at your breakfast, lunch and tea/dinner (as well as snacks, etc.) and try to find out the contents of them all in terms of carbohydrates, lipids and proteins.
10. How can a nurse help to provide a healthy diet for their patients while they are in hospital and/or the community?

Fill in the blanks 2

Using words from the following list fill in the missing blanks:

atom   chemical   electrical   electron   electrons   equal   to   greater   than   ion
less   than   minus   molecule   negative   neutron   organ   organelle   physical
plus   positive   protein   protons

An _____ is an atom or _____ in which the total number of _____ is not _____ _____ the total number of protons. Hence the _____ or molecule has a net _____ or negative _____ charge.

Word search 2

Find the following words below in the grid, and then write something about each of them:

Alkali, Atom, Calcium, Covalent, Fats, Hydrogen, Ion, Mass, Mercury, Metal, Organ, pH, Physiology, Polar Bonds, Sodium

P	O	L	A	R	B	O	N	D	S	U	Z	K
P	H	R	E	M	O	Z	I	A	X	Y	N	X
S	A	Y	G	O	N	I	L	A	K	L	A	V
T	M	A	S	S	T	T	Q	U	E	R	G	H
C	H	R	M	I	G	M	E	R	C	U	R	Y
A	O	V	O	U	O	H	Z	W	R	D	O	D
L	O	V	T	X	E	L	E	I	P	U	S	R
C	S	I	A	O	R	S	O	D	I	U	M	O
I	N	F	V	L	T	I	O	G	L	X	A	G
U	Q	A	Y	Z	E	I	N	L	Y	A	Z	E
M	E	T	A	L	X	N	Z	A	S	I	O	N
P	W	S	R	E	A	C	T	I	O	N	G	H
Q	U	E	R	T	Y	U	I	O	P	L	K	J

Label the diagram 2

Fill in the missing words in the three lower boxes.

THE ATOM

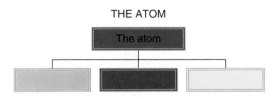

Chapter 2

Cells, cellular compartments, transport systems, fluid movement between compartments

Muralitharan Nair

Test your prior knowledge

- Draw and label the structures of a human cell.
- What is the function of cytoplasm?
- List the functions of the cell membrane.
- Where would you find the extracellular compartment in a cell?
- Describe the functions and regulatory mechanisms that maintain water and electrolyte balance in the body.

Learning outcomes

After reading this chapter you will be able to:

- Outline the structure and function of the plasma membrane
- Describe the functions of the organelles
- Explain the cellular transport system
- Identify the fluid compartments of the body
- List the major electrolytes of the extracellular and intracellular compartments of the body

Fundamentals of Anatomy and Physiology: For Nursing and Healthcare Students, Second Edition. Edited by Ian Peate and Muralitharan Nair.
© 2017 John Wiley & Sons, Ltd. Published 2017 by John Wiley & Sons, Ltd.
Student companion website: www.wileyfundamentalseries.com/anatomy
Instructor companion website: www.wiley.com/go/instructor/anatomy

Introduction

Cells are the structural and functional units of all living organisms. Some organisms, such as bacteria, are unicellular, consisting of a single cell. Other organisms, such as humans, are multicellular, indicating that humans are made up of many cells (see Figure 2.1). They are the smallest independent units of life with different parts (see Figure 2.2) that perform their own function (see Table 2.1). For the cells to survive some fundamental chemical activities occur within the cell. Some of these activities include cellular growth, metabolism and reproduction. Each cell is an amazing unit of life; it can take in nutrients, convert these nutrients into energy, carry out specialised functions and reproduce as necessary. Most amazingly, each cell stores its own set of instructions for carrying out each of these activities.

Substances such as water, electrolytes and nutrients move in and out of a cell utilising a transport system. There is constant movement of fluid and electrolytes between the intracellular and extracellular compartments. The movement of fluid and electrolytes ensures that the cells receive a constant supply of electrolytes, such as sodium, chloride, potassium, magnesium, phosphates, bicarbonate and calcium, for cellular function. The cell consists of four basic parts:

- cell membrane
- cytoplasm
- nucleus
- nucleoplasm.

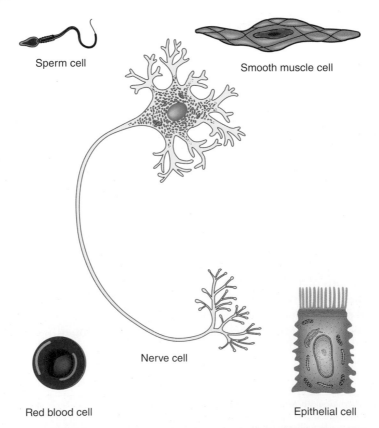

Sperm cell

Smooth muscle cell

Nerve cell

Red blood cell

Epithelial cell

Figure 2.1   Examples of some cells of the human body. *Source*: Tortora and Derrickson (2009). Reproduced with permission of John Wiley & Sons.

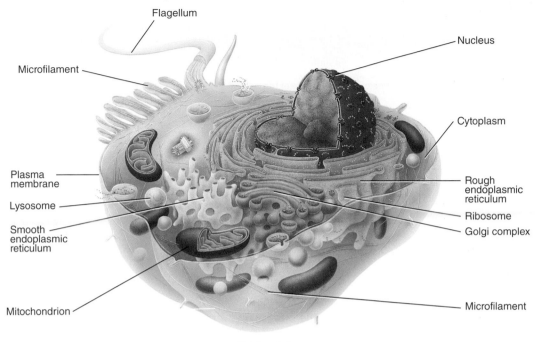

Sectional view

Figure 2.2   Structure of a cell. *Source*: Nair and Peate (2009). Reproduced with permission of John Wiley & Sons.

Table 2.1   Cellular compartments and their functions

Components	Functions
Centrioles	Cellular reproduction
Chromatin	Contains genetic information
Cilia (pleural)	Moves fluid or particles over the surface of the cell
Cytoplasm	Fluid portion that supports organelles
Cytoskeleton	Provides support and site for specific enzymes
Endoplasmic reticulum (rough and smooth)	Many functions, including site for protein transportation, modification of drugs and synthesis of lipids and steroids
Glycogen granules	Stores for glycogen
Golgi complex	Packages proteins for secretion
Intermediate filament	Helps to determine the shape of the cell
Lysosomes	Break down and digest harmful substances – in normal cells, some of the synthesised proteins may be faulty; lysosymes are responsible for their removal
Microfilaments	Provide structural support and cell movement
Microtubules	They also provide conducting channels through which various substances can move through the cytoplasm; provide shape and support for cells

(Continued)

Table 2.1   (*Continued*)

Components	Functions
Microvilli	Increase cell surface; site for secretion, absorption and cellular adhesion
Mitochondria	Energy-producing site of the cell; mitochondria are self-replicating
Nucleolus	Site for the formation of ribosomes
Nucleus	Contains genetic information
Peroxisomes	Carry out metabolic reactions; site for the destruction of hydrogen peroxide; protect the cell from harmful substances, such as alcohol and formaldehyde
Plasma membrane	Regulates substances in and out of a cell
Ribosomes	Sites for protein synthesis
Secretory vesicles	Secrete hormones, neurotransmitters

Cell membrane

Like all other cellular membranes, the plasma membrane consists of both lipids and proteins. The fundamental structure of the membrane is the phospholipid bilayer, which forms a stable barrier between two aqueous compartments. In the case of the plasma membrane, these compartments are the inside and the outside of the cell. Proteins embedded within the phospholipid bilayer carry out the specific functions of the plasma membrane, including selective transport of molecules and cell–cell recognition.

The cell membrane is a thin membrane that forms the outermost layer of a cell, and it is also called the plasma membrane. This membrane ensures the boundary and integrity of the cell and that its contents are separated from the surrounding environment. The cell membrane contains a variety of biological molecules, mainly proteins and lipids, which are involved in many cellular functions, such as cellular communication and cellular transport. The cell membrane is made up of a double layer (bilayer) of phospholipid (fatty) molecules with protein molecules interspersed between them (see Figure 2.3). The cell membrane can vary from 7.5 to 10 nm (nanometres) in thickness (Jenkins and Tortora, 2013).

The phospholipid bilayer consists of a polar 'head' end, which is hydrophilic (water loving), and fatty acid 'tails', which are hydrophobic (water hating). The hydrophilic heads are situated on the outer and inner surfaces of the cell, while the hydrophobic areas point into the cell membrane (see Figure 2.3) as they are 'water-hating' ends. These phospholipid molecules are arranged as a bilayer with the heads facing outwards. This means that the bilayer is self-sealing. It is the central part of the plasma membrane, consisting of hydrophobic 'tails', that makes the cell membrane impermeable to water-soluble molecules, and so prevents the passage of these molecules into and out of the cell (Marieb and Hoehn, 2013). However, substances need to enter and leave the cells for the cells to survive and function; these are provided by special proteins, such as integral and peripheral membrane proteins (see Figure 2.3).

The integral transmembrane proteins are attached to the cell membrane and they can form channels that allow for the transportation of materials into and out of the cell. Examples of integral transmembrane proteins include voltage-gated ion channels, such as those that transport potassium ions in and out of cells, certain types of T cell receptors, the insulin receptor, and many other receptors and neurotransmitters. On the other hand, peripheral membrane proteins are

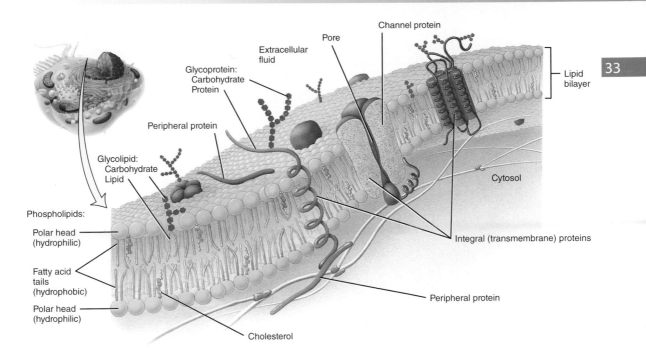

Figure 2.3   Cell membrane. *Source*: Tortora and Derrickson (2009). Reproduced with permission of John Wiley & Sons.

proteins that adhere temporarily to the cell membrane with which they are associated. Peripheral membrane proteins may interact with other proteins or directly with the lipid bilayer.

Functions of the cell membrane

Cell membranes serve several important functions:

- They are selective semi permeable membranes, which means that some molecules can diffuse across the lipid bilayer but others cannot. Small hydrophobic molecules and gases like oxygen and carbon dioxide cross membranes rapidly. Small polar molecules, such as water and ethanol, can also pass through membranes, but they do so more slowly. On the other hand, cell membranes restrict diffusion of highly charged molecules, such as ions, and large molecules, such as sugars and amino acids. The passage of these molecules relies on specific transport proteins embedded in the membrane.
- Membrane transport proteins are specific and selective for the molecules they move, and they often use energy to catalyse passage. Also, these proteins transport some nutrients against the concentration gradient, which requires additional energy. The ability to maintain concentration gradients and sometimes move materials against them is vital to cell health and maintenance. Thanks to membrane barriers and transport proteins, the cell can accumulate nutrients in higher concentrations than exist in the environment and, conversely, get rid of waste products (Figure 2.4).
- Other transmembrane proteins have communication-related jobs. These proteins bind signals, such as hormones or immune mediators, to their extracellular portions. Binding causes a conformational change in the protein that transmits a signal to intracellular

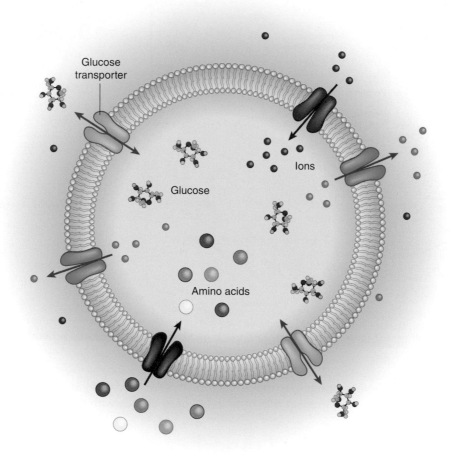

Figure 2.4   Selective transport system. *Source*: O'Connor and Adams (2010). Reproduced with permission of Nature Publishing Group.

messenger molecules. Like transport proteins, receptor proteins are specific and selective for the molecules they bind (Figure 2.5).

Some of the proteins embedded in a cell membrane provide structural support to the cell, while others are enzymes where chemical reactions occur. Some membrane proteins regulate water-soluble substances through pores in the cell membrane; others are receptors where hormones and other substances such as neurotransmitters act. Other important cell membrane proteins are glycoproteins, which play an important role in cell–cell recognition. An example of glycoproteins is mucins, which are secreted in the mucus of the digestive and respiratory tracts.

Cellular fluid compartments

The two principal body fluid compartments are intracellular and extracellular. The intracellular compartment is the space inside a cell and the fluid inside the cell is called intracellular fluid (ICF). The extracellular compartment is found outside the cell and the fluid outside the cell is called extracellular fluid (ECF). However, the extracellular compartment is further divided into

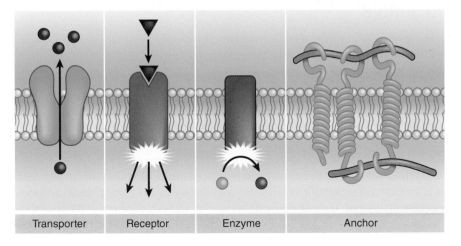

Figure 2.5   Action of transmembrane proteins. *Source*: O'Connor and Adams (2010). Reproduced with permission of Nature Publishing Group.

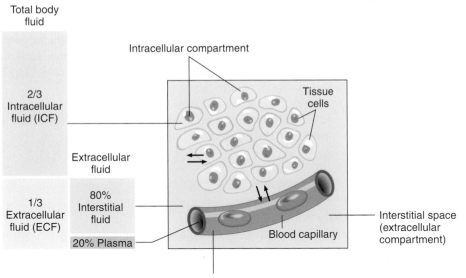

Figure 2.6   Fluid compartments. *Source*: Nair and Peate (2009). Reproduced with permission of John Wiley & Sons.

the interstitial and the intravascular compartments. Two-thirds of body fluid is found inside the cell and one-third of the fluid outside the cell. The interstitial compartment contains 80% of the ECF, and 20% is in the intravascular compartment as plasma (Figure 2.6).

Intracellular fluid

- The ICF is primarily a solution of potassium and organic anions, proteins, and so on.
- The cell membranes and cellular metabolism control the constituents of this ICF.
- ICF is not consistent in the body. It represents a collection of fluids from all the different cells.

Extracellular fluid

- The ECF primarily consists of NaCl and $NaHCO_3$ solution.
- The ECF is further subdivided into three compartments:

  - Interstitial fluid (ISF) consists of all the bits of fluid that lie in the interstices of all body tissues. This is also a 'virtual' fluid (i.e. it exists in many separate small bits but is spoken about as though it is a pool of fluid of uniform composition in the one location). The ISF bathes all the cells in the body and is the link between the ICF and the intravascular compartment. Oxygen, nutrients, wastes and chemical messengers all pass through the ISF. ISF has the compositional characteristics of ECF (as mentioned above), but in addition it is distinguished by its usually low protein concentration (in comparison with plasma). Lymph is considered as a part of the ISF. The lymphatic system returns protein and excess ISF to the circulation. Lymph is more easily obtained for analysis than other parts of the ISF.
  - Plasma is the only major fluid compartment that exists as a real fluid collection all in one location. It differs from ISF in its much higher protein content and its high bulk flow (transport function). Blood contains suspended red and white cells, so plasma has been called the 'ISF of the blood'. The fluid compartment called the blood volume is interesting in that it is a composite compartment containing ECF (plasma) and ICF (red cell water).
  - Transcellular fluid is a small compartment that represents all those body fluids that are formed from the transport activities of cells. It is contained within epithelial-lined spaces. It includes cerebrospinal fluid, gastrointestinal tract fluids, bladder urine, aqueous humour and joint fluid. It is important because of the specialised functions involved. The fluid fluxes involved with gastrointestinal tract fluids can be quite significant.
  - The fluid of bone and dense connective tissue is significant because it contains about 15% of the total body water. This fluid is mobilised only very slowly, and this lessens its importance when considering the effects of acute fluid interventions.

Snapshot

Loss of fluid and electrolytes through burns

Boon Sew, a 48-year-old male, was brought in by ambulance to the emergency department after being rescued from his burning house. He was asleep at night when a spark from the family fireplace started a fire, leaving him trapped in his bedroom. By the time the fire rescue team arrived, he had suffered severe burns and excessive smoke inhalation.

On arrival to the emergency department, he was unconscious. He had second-degree burns over 5% of his body and third-degree burns over 20% of his body – both covering his thoracic and abdominal regions and his right elbow. His vital signs were quite unstable: blood pressure was 53/35 mmHg; heart rate was 200 beats/min; and respiratory rate was 38 breaths/min. He was deteriorating from circulatory failure. Two intravenous lines were inserted and fluids and electrolytes were administered through each. His vital signs stabilised and he was admitted to the intensive care unit.

Boon Sew regained consciousness the following day and was able to respond verbally. Once his condition was stable and he was able to respond to treatment, he was transferred to the ward where he continued to make a good recovery. He was then discharged into the community after making a full recovery.

Fluid movement between compartments

The movement of fluid between the intracellular and the extracellular compartments is primarily controlled by two forces:

- *hydrostatic pressure* – the pressure exerted by the fluid;
- *osmotic pressure* – the pressure that must be exerted on a solution to prevent the passage of water into it across a selective permeable membrane.

Furthermore, the movement of fluid is dependent on solutes dissolved within the fluid; changes in the concentration of solutes will affect fluid movement between compartments. Similarly, changes in fluid volume will also affect fluid movement between compartments. An example of fluid and solute movement that occurs in the body is when blood pressure (hydrostatic pressure) forces fluid and solutes from the arterial end of the capillaries into the ISF space (see Figure 2.7). Fluid and solutes return to the capillaries at the venous end as a result of the osmotic pressure. Fluid also enters the lymphatic capillaries from the interstitial space as a result of the osmotic pressure in the lymphatic vessels.

The movement of fluid between the intracellular and extracellular compartments is the result of hydrostatic and osmotic pressures. In a normal state of health, the hydrostatic pressure in the intracellular compartment and the interstitial space is in balance and therefore the fluid movement is minimal. However, changes in the osmotic pressure either in the intracellular or extracellular compartments can affect fluid movement. As the capillary barrier is readily permeable to ions, the osmotic pressure within the capillary is principally determined by plasma proteins that are relatively impermeable. Therefore, instead of speaking of 'osmotic' pressure, this pressure is referred to as the 'oncotic' pressure or 'colloid osmotic' pressure because it is generated by colloids. Albumin generates about 70% of the oncotic pressure. This pressure is typically 25–30 mmHg. The oncotic pressure increases along the length of

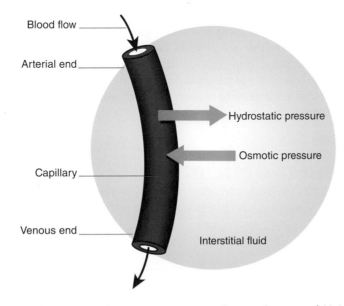

Figure 2.7   Capillary hydrostatic and osmotic pressures. *Source*: Peate and Nair (2011). Reproduced with permission of John Wiley & Sons.

the capillary, particularly in capillaries having high net filtration (e.g. in renal glomerular capillaries), because the filtering fluid leaves behind proteins, leading to an increase in protein concentration.

Composition of body fluid

The body fluid is composed of water and dissolved substances such as electrolytes (sodium, potassium and chloride), gases (oxygen and carbon dioxide), nutrients, enzymes and hormones. The total body water constitutes 60% of the total body weight, and water plays an important part in cellular function (LeMone *et al.*, 2011). Water is essential for the body as:

- It acts as a lubricant, which makes swallowing easy.
- It is also the major component of the body's transport systems. The blood transports nutrients, oxygen, glucose and fats to various tissues and cells. Also, the waste products of cellular metabolism are removed, such as lactic acid and carbon dioxide. Via the urine, a number of waste products are transported out of the body; for example, urea, phosphates, sulfites, minerals, ketones from fat metabolism and nitrogenous waste from protein breakdown.
- It is needed for regulation of body temperature at 37 °C. When body temperature starts to rise, blood vessels near the surface of the skin dilate to release some of the heat; the reverse happens when body temperature starts to drop. Also, when body temperature rises, sweat glands secrete sweat, which is 99% water. As the sweat evaporates, heat is removed from the body.
- It provides an optimum medium for the cells to function.
- There are chemical reactions in the body which require water. A synthesis reaction involves the joining of two molecules by the removal of a water molecule, and a hydrolysis reaction involves a molecule being split into two smaller molecules with the addition of water.
- It breaks down food particles in the digestive system.
- It provides lubrication for the joints as it is a component of synovial fluid. It is also a component of tears, which lubricate the eyes, and of saliva to provide lubrication to food, which aids chewing, swallowing and digestion of food. It also has protective roles, washing away particles that get into the eyes, providing cushioning against shock for the eyes and the spinal cord. It is also a component of amniotic fluid, which provides protection for the foetus during pregnancy.

Effects of water deficiency

Deficiency of water in the body can affect various functions, and in severe conditions it might also lead to death. Some of the problems associated with water deficiency include:

- low blood pressure
- increased clotting of blood
- kidney dysfunction, leading to renal failure
- severe constipation
- multisystem failure
- proneness to infection
- electrolyte imbalance.

Medicines management

Diuretics

Diuretics increase urine excretion of both water and electrolytes, and are commonly called 'water tablets'. In general, they inhibit electrolyte reabsorption from the lumen of the nephron, increasing osmolarity and enhancing water excretion. Diuretics have different clinical uses depending on their sites and mechanisms of action. The sub-classes of diuretics include:

- Thiazides (e.g. bendroflumethiazide, hydrochlorothiazide, and the thiazide-like diuretic indapamide) are used mainly in low doses in the treatment of hypertension, but also, in the case of metolazone, in combination with loop diuretics to treat severe heart failure.
- Loop diuretics (e.g. furosemide, bumetanide, torasemide) are widely used for the symptomatic treatment of heart failure and fluid retention in chronic kidney disease.
- Potassium-sparing diuretics (e.g. amiloride, triamterene) are weak diuretics, whereas spironolactone and eplerenone are used in the treatment of hypertension, oedema of liver failure, and heart failure.
- Osmotic diuretics (mannitol) are used in a hospital setting for the treatment of cerebral oedema.
- Carbonic anhydrase inhibitors (acetazolamide) are used for the prophylaxis of mountain sickness (unlicensed indication) and glaucoma.

Common problems are:

- potassium loss when non-potassium-sparing diuretics are used;
- metabolic disturbances;
- hypotension;
- renal failure – at high doses, diuretics may cause a pre-renal uraemia.

See Rull (2013).

Variation in body fluid content

Neonates contain more water than adults: 75–80% water with proportionately more ECF than adults. At birth, the amount of ISF is proportionally three times larger than in an adult. By the age of 12 months this has decreased to 60%, which is the adult value. Total body water as a percentage of total body weight decreases progressively with increasing age. By the age of 60 years, total body water may decrease to only 50% of total body weight in males, mostly due to an increase in adipose tissue.

Clinical considerations

Dehydration

Dehydration may be caused by restricted water intake, excessive water loss or both. The most common cause of dehydration is failure to drink liquids. The deprivation of water is far more serious than the deprivation of food. The average person loses approximately 2.5% of total body water per day (approximately 1200 mL) in urine, in expired air, by insensible perspiration and from the gastrointestinal tract. If, in addition to this loss, the loss through perspiration is greatly increased,

(Continued)

dehydration may result in shock and death within only a few hours. When swallowing is difficult in extremely ill patients, or when people cannot respond to a sense of thirst because of age or illness or dulling of consciousness, the failure to compensate for the daily loss of body water will result rapidly in dehydration and its consequences. Large volumes of water also may be lost from the body by vomiting or diarrhoea.

The symptoms of dehydration depend in part on the cause and in part on whether there is associated salt deprivation. When loss of water is disproportionately greater than loss of electrolytes (salt), the osmotic pressure of the ECFs becomes higher than in the cells. Since water passes from a region of lower osmotic pressure to a region of higher osmotic pressure, water flows out of the cells into the ECF, tending to lower its osmotic pressure and increase its volume toward normal. As a result of the flow of water out of the cells, they become dehydrated. This results in the thirst that always accompanies 'pure' water depletion.

Transport systems

Cells utilise two processes to move substances in and out of the cell: the passive and active transport systems. When molecules pass in and out of a cell membrane without the use of cellular energy it is called a passive transport system. This includes:

- simple diffusion
- facilitated diffusion
- osmosis
- filtration.

On the other hand, an active transport system requires energy to move substances in and out of a cell. The active transport systems include:

- active transport with the utilisation of adenosine triphosphate (ATP)
- endocytosis
- exocytosis.

Simple diffusion

The term simple diffusion refers to a process whereby a substance passes through a membrane without the aid of an intermediary, such as an integral membrane protein (Figure 2.8). Water, oxygen, carbon dioxide, ethanol and urea are examples of molecules that readily cross cell membranes by simple diffusion. They pass either directly through the lipid bilayer or through pores created by certain integral membrane proteins. Small non-polar molecules can diffuse directly through the plasma membrane. One example of simple diffusion is the exchange of respiratory gases between the cells of the alveolar sac and the blood in the lungs. The rate of diffusion depends on several factors, and they are:

- gases diffuse rapidly and liquids diffuse more slowly;
- at high temperature, the rate of diffusion is much faster;
- smaller molecules, such as glycerol, will diffuse much faster than larger molecules, like fatty acids;
- surface area of the cell membrane over which the molecule can work;
- solubility of the molecule;
- concentration gradient.

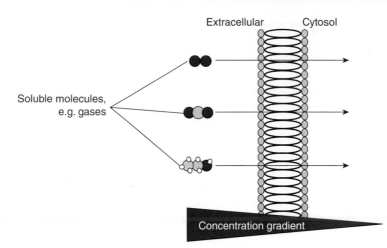

Figure 2.8 Simple diffusion. *Source*: Nair and Peate (2009). Reproduced with permission of John Wiley & Sons.

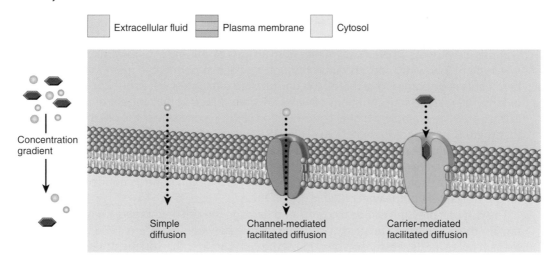

Figure 2.9 Facilitated diffusion. *Source*: Tortora and Derrikson (2009). Reproduced with permission of John Wiley & Sons.

Facilitated diffusion

Facilitated diffusion (facilitated transport) is a process of passive transport (diffusion) via which molecules diffuse across cell membranes, with the help of transport proteins. Small uncharged molecules can easily diffuse across cell membranes. However, due to the hydrophobic nature of the lipids that make up cell membranes, water-soluble molecules, and ions cannot do so; instead, they are helped across by transport proteins. Larger molecules, such as amino acids, cannot pass the cell membrane and therefore they use a process called facilitated diffusion to go through the cell membrane (see Figure 2.9). No direct cellular energy is used in this process. Glucose, sodium and chloride ions are just a few examples of molecules and ions that must efficiently get across the plasma membrane. Their transport must therefore be 'facilitated' by proteins that span the cell membrane and provide a passageway for these substances. Like simple diffusion, facilitated diffusion transport substances from an area of high concentration to an area of low concentration.

Clinical considerations

Administration of intravenous fluids

Administration of excess fluid may cause several problems after surgery. The resulting increased demands on cardiac function, due to an excessive shift to the right on the Starling myocardial performance curve, may potentially increase postoperative cardiac morbidity. Fluid accumulation in the lungs may predispose patients to pneumonia and respiratory failure. The excretory demands of the kidney are increased, and the resulting diuresis may lead to urinary retention mediated by the inhibitory effects of anaesthetics and analgesics on bladder function. Gastrointestinal motility may be inhibited, prolonging postoperative ileus. Excess fluid may decrease tissue oxygenation with implications for wound (anastomotic) healing. Finally, coagulation may be enhanced with crystalloids, which may predispose patients to postoperative thrombosis.

Nurses need to be aware of these complications when administering prescribed intravenous fluid to patients. They should ensure that the fluid is running on time. Monitor the patient's observations regularly and check for signs such as breathlessness, tachycardia and peripheral cyanosis.

See Holte *et al.* (2002).

Osmosis

Osmosis is a process where water moves from an area of volume of high water concentration to a volume of low water concentration through a selective permeable membrane. A selectively permeable membrane is one that allows unrestricted passage of water, but not solute molecules or ions. The relative concentrations of water are determined in the amount of solutes dissolved in the water. For example, a higher concentration of salt on one side of the cell membrane means that there is less space for water molecules. Water then will move from the side where there is the greater number of water molecules through the cell membrane to the other side of the cell where there are fewer water molecules. This is known as osmotic pressure. The higher the concentration of the solute on one side of the membrane, the higher the osmotic pressure available for the movement of the water (Colbert *et al.*, 2012).

The osmotic pressure can be too great and damage the cell membrane; therefore, it is important for the cell to have a relatively constant pressure between the internal and external environment. If the osmotic pressure on one side of the cell is greater than on the other side, changes to the cell could take place resulting in cell damage. A red blood cell placed in a solution with a lower concentration of solute will undergo haemolysis, and if placed in a fluid with a high concentration of solutes the red blood cell will crenate (see Figure 2.10). On the other hand, if the

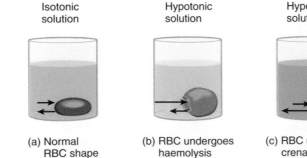

| Isotonic solution | Hypotonic solution | Hypertonic solution |

(a) Normal RBC shape

(b) RBC undergoes haemolysis

(c) RBC undergoes crenation

Figure 2.10   (a–c) Effect of solute concentration on a red blood cell. *Source*: Tortora and Derrikson (2009). Reproduced with permission of John Wiley & Sons.

red blood cell is placed in a solution with a relatively constant osmotic pressure between the internal and external environment, the red blood cell does not undergo any changes. The net movement of water in and out of the cell is minimal.

Filtration

Filtration is a process where small substances are forced through a semipermeable membrane with the aid of hydrostatic pressure. One example of filtration within the human body is at the capillary end of the blood vessels. With the aid of blood pressure, fluid and solutes are forced out of the single-layered cells of the capillaries into the ISF space. Large molecules, such as proteins and red blood cells, remain in the capillaries. Another example of filtration that occurs in the human body takes place in the kidneys. Blood pressure forces water and dissolved waste products, such as urea and uric acid, into the kidney tubules during the formation of urine (see Chapter 10).

Active transport system

The main difference between the active and passive transport systems is that the active transport system utilises cellular energy to move substances through a semipermeable membrane. The energy is obtained by splitting ATP into adenosine diphosphate (ADP) and phosphate (see Figure 2.11). Examples of active transport processes are active transport, endocytosis and exocytosis.

Active transport

An active process is one in which substances move against a concentration gradient from an area of lower to higher concentration. The cell must expend energy that is released by splitting ATP into ADP and phosphate. ATP is a compound of a base, a sugar, and three phosphate groups (triphosphate). These phosphate groups are held together by high-energy bonds, which when broken release a high level of energy. Once one of these phosphate bonds has been broken and a phosphate group has been released, that compound now has only two phosphate groups (diphosphate) and there is now also a spare phosphate group. This, in turn, will join up with another adenosine diphosphate group, so forming another molecule of ATP (with energy stored in the phosphate bonds), and the whole process continues recurring (Marieb, 2012).

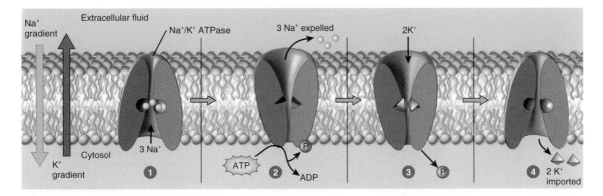

Figure 2.11   Active transport system. *Source*: Tortora and Derrikson (2009). Reproduced with permission of John Wiley & Sons.

In the human body, the four main active transport systems considered when discussing cellular energy include:

- sodium–potassium pump – sodium and potassium concentration gradients are generated to produce electrical energy;
- calcium pump – calcium ions essential for muscle contraction are transported into muscle cells;
- sodium-linked co-transport – glucose and amino acids are actively transported into the cells and at the same time sodium moves passively via the co-transporter;
- hydrogen-linked co-transporter – glucose is actively transported into the cell and at the same time hydrogen ions move into the cell via the co-transporter.

Endocytosis

Endocytosis is the process by which cells take in molecules such as proteins from outside the cell by engulfing them with their cell membranes. It is used by all cells of the body because most substances important to them are polar and consist of big molecules, and thus cannot pass through the hydrophobic plasma membrane. During endocytosis the cell membrane plays a part to form a fold and a new intracellular pod is formed containing the substance. There are three types endocytosis.

- Pinocytosis ('cell drinking'; see Figure 2.12):
  - the drop engulfed is relatively small;
  - it occurs in almost all cells;
  - it occurs continuously.

- Phagocytosis ('cell eating'; see Figure 2.12):
  - particulate matter (e.g. bacteria) from the ECF is ingested;
  - the endosome is very large and is called a phagosome or vacuole;

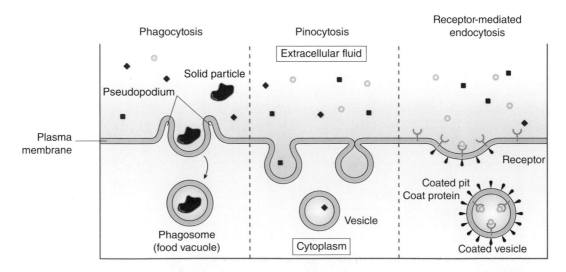

Figure 2.12   Pinocytosis, phagocytosis and receptor-mediated endocytosis. *Source*: Peate and Nair (2011). Reproduced with permission of John Wiley & Sons.

- occurs only in certain specialised cells (e.g. neutrophils, macrophages);
- occurs sporadically.

- Receptor-mediated endocytosis (see Figure 2.12):

- specific receptors bind to large molecules in the ECF;
- the substance bound to the receptor is called a ligand.

Exocytosis

Exocytosis is a process for moving items from the cytoplasm of the cell to the outside. The intracellular vesicle with its ingested substances fuses with the cell membrane to get rid of the unwanted substance from the cell (see Figure 2.13). This process is also utilised by nerve cells to release chemical messengers into the synapse of a neurone. Gland cells release proteins by exocytosis. Gland cells are an organ or group of specialised cells in the body that produces and secretes a specific substance, such as a hormone.

Many cells in the body use exocytosis to release enzymes or other proteins that act in other areas of the body, or to release molecules that help cells communicate with one another. For instance, clusters of α- and β-cells in the islets of Langerhans in the pancreas secrete the hormones glucagon and insulin respectively. These enzymes regulate glucose levels throughout the body. As the level of glucose rises in the blood, the β-cells are stimulated to produce and secrete more insulin by exocytosis. When insulin binds to liver or muscle, it stimulates uptake of glucose by those cells. Exocytosis from other cells in the pancreas also releases digestive enzymes into the gut.

Cells also communicate with each other, through exocytosis, more directly through the products that they secrete. For instance, a neurone cell relays an electrical pulse through the use of neurotransmitters. The neurotransmitters are stored in vesicles and lie next to the cytoplasmic face of the plasma membrane. When the appropriate signal is given, the vesicles holding the neurotransmitters must make contact with the plasma membrane and secrete their contents into the synaptic junction, the space between two neurones, for the other neurone to receive those neurotransmitters.

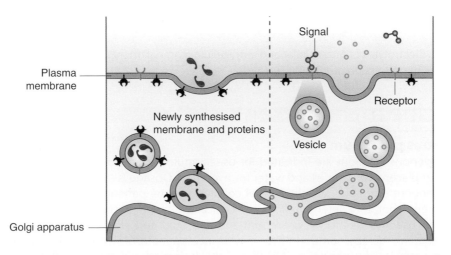

Figure 2.13   Exocytosis. *Source*: Nair and Peate (2009). Reproduced with permission of John Wiley & Sons.

Electrolytes

Chemically, electrolytes are substances that become ions in solution and acquire the capacity to conduct electricity. Electrolytes are present in the human body, and the balance of the electrolytes in our bodies is essential for normal function of our cells and our organs.

Fluid balance is linked to electrolyte balance. Electrolytes are chemical compounds that dissociate in water to form charged particles called ions (LeMone *et al.*, 2011). They include potassium (K^+), sodium (Na^+), chloride (Cl^-), magnesium (Mg^{2+}) and hydrogen phosphate (HPO_4^{2-}). Electrolytes are either positively or negatively charged. Positively charged ions are called cations (e.g. Na^+ and K^+) and negatively charged ions are called anions (e.g. Cl^- and HCO_3^-). Remember that an anion and a cation will combine to form a compound; for example, potassium (K^+) and chloride (Cl^-) will combine to form potassium chloride (KCl). The composition of electrolytes differs between the intracellular and the extracellular compartments (see Figure 2.14).

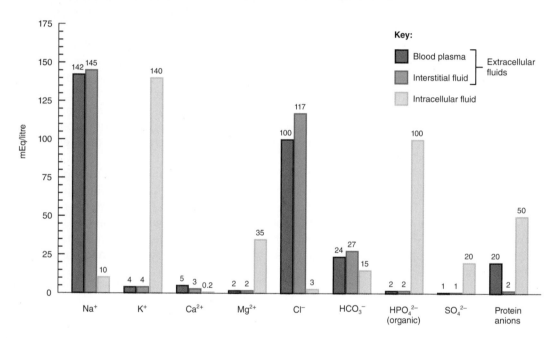

Figure 2.14   Electrolytes of intracellular and extracellular compartments. *Source*: Nair and Peate (2009). Reproduced with permission of John Wiley & Sons.

Medicine management

Intravenous potassium

These intravenous solutions are indicated for use in adults and paediatric patients as sources of electrolyte replacement, calories and water for hydration. Dosage is to be directed by a physician and is dependent upon age, weight, clinical condition of the patient and laboratory determinations. Frequent laboratory determinations and clinical evaluation are essential to monitor changes in blood glucose and electrolyte concentrations, and fluid and electrolyte balance during prolonged parenteral therapy. Some additives may be incompatible. Always consult with a pharmacist for the compatibility of the additives. Mix thoroughly before administering the fluid.

Functions of electrolytes

Electrolytes are compounds that dissociate into ions when placed in liquid, thus enabling the liquid to conduct electric current. Electrolytes are salts and minerals, such as sodium, potassium, chloride and bicarbonate, that are found in the blood. They can conduct electrical impulses in the body. Electrolytes have numerous functions in the body. They:

- regulate fluid movement between compartments;
- regulate hydrogen ion concentration for normal cellular function;
- play a vital role in membrane potentials and action potentials;
- are essential for neuronal function.

To function normally, the body must be able to maintain the levels of electrolytes within very narrow limits. These limits are controlled by hormones. The body maintains the levels of electrolytes in each compartment (cells, tissues, organs) by moving electrolytes into or out of cells based upon the signals provided by the hormones. If the balance of electrolytes is disturbed, disorders can develop. An imbalance of electrolytes can occur if a person:

- uses certain drugs, especially long-term use of laxatives and/or diuretics;
- becomes dehydrated as a result of profuse sweating, vomiting, chronic diarrhoea, very poor nutrition, and so on;
- has certain heart, liver or kidney disorders;
- is given intravenous fluids in inappropriate amounts.

Loss of electrolytes can have serious consequences for the body. In severe dehydration, the loss of electrolytes can result in circulatory problems such as tachycardia (rapid heartbeat) and problems with the nervous system, such as loss of consciousness and shock. See Table 2.2 for a summary of electrolytes and their functions.

Table 2.2   Principal electrolytes and their functions

Electrolytes	Normal values in ECF (mmol L^{-1})	Function	Main distribution
Sodium (Na^+)	135–145	Important cation in generation of action potentials. Plays an important role in fluid and electrolyte balance. Increases plasma membrane permeability. Helps promote skeletal muscle function. Stimulates conduction of nerve impulses. Maintains blood volume.	Main cation of the ECF
Potassium (K^+)	3.5–5	Important cation in establishing resting membrane potential. Regulates acid–base balance. Maintains ICF volume. Helps promote skeletal muscle function. Helps promote the transmission of nerve impulses.	Main cation of the ICF
Calcium (Ca^{2+})	135–145	Important clotting factor. Plays a part in neurotransmitter release in neurones. Maintains muscle tone and excitability of nervous and muscle tissue. Promotes transmission of nerve impulses. Assists in the absorption of vitamin B_{12}.	Mainly found in the ECF
Magnesium (Mg^{2+})	0.5–1.0	Helps to maintain normal nerve and muscle function; maintains regular heart rate, regulates blood glucose and blood pressure. Essential for protein synthesis.	Mainly distributed in the ICF

(Continued)

Table 2.2 (*Continued*)

Electrolytes	Normal values in ECF (mmol L^{-1})	Function	Main distribution
Chloride (Cl$^-$)	98–117	Maintains a balance of anions in different fluid compartments. Combines with hydrogen in gastric mucosal glands to form hydrochloric acid. Helps to maintain fluid balance by regulating osmotic pressure.	Main anion of the ECF
Bicarbonate (HCO$_3^-$)	24–31	Main buffer of hydrogen ions in plasma. Maintains a balance between cations and anions of ICF and ECF.	Mainly distributed in the ECF
Hydrogen phosphate (HPO$_4^{2-}$)	0.8–1.1	Essential for the digestion of proteins, carbohydrates and fats and absorption of calcium. Essential for bone formation.	Mainly found in the ICF
Sulphate (SO$_4^{2-}$)	0.5	Involved in detoxification of phenols, alcohols and amines.	Mainly found in the ICF

Clinical considerations

Water and electrolyte balance

In clinical practice, fluid and electrolyte therapy is undertaken either to provide maintenance requirements or to replace serious losses or deficits. Body losses of water and/or electrolytes can result from a number of causes, including vomiting, diarrhoea, profuse sweating, fever, chronic renal failure, diuretic therapy, surgery and others. The type of therapy undertaken (i.e. oral or parenteral) and the content of the fluid administered depend on a patient's specific requirements.

For example, a patient taking diuretics may simply require a daily oral potassium supplement along with adequate intake of water. An athlete may require rehydration with or without added electrolytes. Hospitalised patients commonly receive parenteral maintenance therapy of fluids and electrolytes to support ordinary metabolic function. In severe cases of deficit, a patient may require the prompt and substantial intravenous replacement of fluids and electrolytes to restore acute volume losses resulting from surgery, trauma, burns or shock.

Snapshot

Hyponatraemia

Meria presented to the emergency department with severe hyponatraemia. According to her daughter, the patient was falling and was having difficulty with her motor function. She was unable to walk and her speech was difficult to understand. Despite these symptoms, she was also noted to be conversing with her daughter in the room.

The patient had been having 'flu-like symptoms' for the previous 2 weeks and had been vomiting for the previous 4 days. She complained of abdominal pain on one occasion during the emergency doctor's assessment. The doctor carried out a blood test for urea and electrolytes. The result showed that her sodium level was 100 mmol L^{-1}. During the assessment, Meria informed that she has been taking large amounts of water to flush her system from toxins.

(*Continued*)

She was then commenced on hypertonic normal saline solution. A series of blood tests was carried out at intervals to check her urea and electrolytes.

- By 10:20 that morning, the patient's sodium had risen to 107 mmol L^{-1}.
- At 11:40, repeat labs were carried out. Results reported at 12:20 showed that the sodium level had risen to 114 mmol L^{-1}.
- By 15:00, the patient's sodium level was 120 mmol L^{-1} and it gradually returned to normal values.

Over the course of her stay in the hospital, Meria continued to make a steady recovery and was discharged following dietary assessment and advice from the dietician.

See American College of Emergency Physicians (n.d.).

Snapshot

Acute calcium pyrophosphate arthritis

It is normal for calcium crystals to be found in parts of the body such as the bones and teeth, but when they occur in and around the joints they can sometimes cause sudden (acute) attacks of painful inflammation. The main crystals that cause problems are calcium pyrophosphate (CPP) crystals and apatite crystals, and the problems they cause are referred to collectively as calcium crystal diseases. In many cases these crystals occur in otherwise normal cartilage or tendons without causing any symptoms at all. If the crystals are embedded deep in the tissues they do not usually affect the way the tissues work. However, crystals can cause attacks of painful inflammation if they become loose from:

- the cartilage into the joint cavity (Figure 2.15);
- a tendon into the surrounding soft tissues (Figure 2.16).

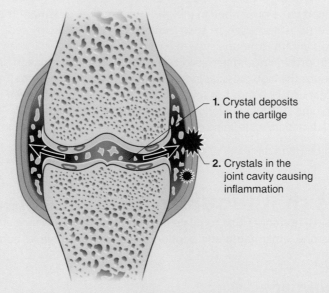

1. Crystal deposits in the cartilge

2. Crystals in the joint cavity causing inflammation

Figure 2.15   Crystals in the joint cavity. *Source*: Adapted from www.arthritisresearchuk.org.

(*Continued*)

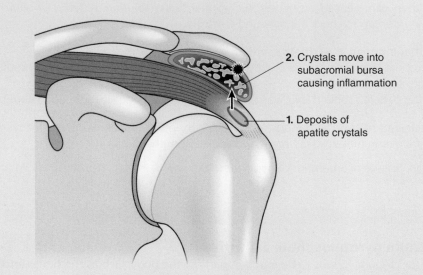

2. Crystals move into subacromial bursa causing inflammation

1. Deposits of apatite crystals

Figure 2.16   Crystals in the tissue. *Source*: Adapted from www.arthritisresearchuk.org.

This movement of crystals is called crystal shedding, and the inflammation occurs because the crystals are exposed to the body's immune system. When CPP crystals shed into the joint cavity this is called acute CPP arthritis. The crystals cause inflammation in the lining of the joint, resulting in pain and swelling in the joint. The condition was previously known as 'pseudogout', meaning 'false gout' because the inflammation resembles gout (a condition caused by urate crystals).

The treatment includes non-steroidal anti-inflammatory drugs, such as ibuprofen, naproxen or diclofenac, which can help to ease the pain of an acute attack. For the intense pain of an acute attack, these will need to be prescribed at a high dose. Another treatment that is sometimes used is colchicine. This drug is also used to treat acute gout and works by reducing the interaction between the crystals and the immune system.

Removal of fluid from the joint and steroid injection to treat the inflammation may be carried out. This can very quickly reduce the high pressure in the joint that is causing the extreme pain. This is a quick, simple procedure that usually brings fast relief. Usually, once the fluid has been drawn out the doctor will inject a small volume (1–2 mL) of a long-acting steroid into the joint through the same needle. This helps to reduce inflammation in the lining of the joint and prevent the build-up of more fluid.

See Arthritis Research UK (n.d.).

Hormones that regulate fluid and electrolytes

The four principal hormones that regulate fluid and electrolyte balance are antidiuretic hormone (ADH), aldosterone, atrial natriuretic peptide (ANP) and parathyroid hormone (Thibodeau and Patton, 2011).

Antidiuretic hormone

ADH is a peptide hormone, and its main role is to regulate fluid balance in the body. This hormone is produced in the hypothalamus by neurones called osmoreceptors, and the hormone is stored by the posterior pituitary gland. Osmoreceptors are sensitive to plasma osmolality and a decrease in blood volume. The target organs for ADH are the kidneys. ADH acts on the distal convoluted tubule and the collecting ducts, making the tubules more permeable to water and thus increasing reabsorption of water. This occurs through insertion of additional water channels (aquaporin-2s) into the apical membrane of the tubules and collecting duct epithelial cells. The aquaporins allow water to pass out of the nephron (at the distal convoluted tubules and the conducting tubules) and into the cells, increasing the amount of water reabsorbed from the filtrate. Therefore, when a person is lacking fluid, as in dehydration, more ADH is released, thus increasing water reabsorption and resulting in less fluid loss. The secretion of ADH is decreased by a drop in plasma osmotic pressure, increased ECF volume and increased alcohol intake. ADH is also known as vasopressin because it causes constriction of arterioles, thus raising blood pressure.

Medicines management

Diabetes insipidus – vasopressin (antidiuretic hormone)

Diabetes insipidus is a rare disorder where the system used by the body to regulate its water levels becomes disrupted. Diabetes insipidus is caused by problems with a hormone called ADH, also known as vasopressin. Desmopressin is a manufactured version of ADH, and is more powerful than the ADH naturally produced by the body. It works just like natural ADH, stopping the kidneys producing urine when the level of water in the body is low. Desmopressin can be taken as a nasal spray or in tablet form.

Desmopressin is very safe to use. There are few side effects, but they can include:

- headache
- stomach pain
- feeling sick
- blocked or runny nose
- nosebleeds.

If you take too much desmopressin or drink too much fluid while taking it, it can cause your body to retain too much water. This can result in:

- headaches
- dizziness
- feeling bloated
- hyponatraemia (a dangerously low level of sodium (salt) in the blood).

See NHS Choices (2014).

Aldosterone

Aldosterone is a steroid hormone produced by the adrenal glands, which are situated on top of each kidney. The adrenal gland is divided into the cortex and the medulla. The cortex produces the steroid hormone aldosterone. Aldosterone regulates electrolyte and fluid balance by increasing the reabsorption of sodium and water and the release of potassium in the kidneys. This increases blood volume and therefore increases blood pressure. Aldosterone stimulates H^+ secretion by intercalated cells in the collecting duct, regulating plasma bicarbonate (HCO_3^-) levels, thus maintaining acid–base and electrolyte balance. The main target areas for aldosterone are the kidney tubules and the collecting duct epithelial cells.

Atrial natriuretic peptide

ANP, atrial natriuretic factor, atrial natriuretic hormone or atriopeptin is a powerful vasodilator and a polypeptide hormone secreted by heart muscle cells (myocytes). The myocytes produce, store and release ANP in response to atrial stretch. It is involved in the homeostatic control of body water, sodium, potassium and fat (adipose tissue). It is released by muscle cells in the upper chambers (atria) of the heart (atrial myocytes), in response to high blood pressure. ANP acts to reduce the water, sodium and adipose loads on the circulatory system, thereby reducing blood pressure. ANP stimulates vasodilatation, increases glomerular filtration and salt and water excretion, and blocks the release and/or actions of several hormones, including angiotensin II, aldosterone and vasopressin. ANP levels are commonly elevated in situations of excessive fluid volume or hypertension, and the hormone plays an important role in regulating fluid and electrolyte balance.

Parathyroid hormone

Parathyroid hormone regulates serum calcium levels through its effects on bone, kidney and intestine via the kidney. Although the four parathyroid glands are quite small, they have a very rich blood supply. This suits them well since they are required to monitor the calcium level in the blood 24 h a day. As the blood filters through the parathyroid glands, they detect the amount of calcium present in the blood and react by making more or less parathyroid hormone. When the calcium level in the blood is too low, the cells of the parathyroid sense it and make more parathyroid hormone. Once the parathyroid hormone is released into the blood, it circulates to act in a number of places to increase the amount of calcium in the blood (like removing calcium from bones). When the calcium level in the blood is too high, the cells of the parathyroids make less parathyroid hormone (or stop making it altogether), thereby allowing calcium levels to decrease. This feedback mechanism runs constantly, thereby maintaining calcium (and parathyroid hormone) in a very narrow 'normal' range. In a normal person with normal parathyroid glands, their parathyroid glands will turn on and off dozens of times per day, in an attempt to keep the calcium level in the normal range so the brain and muscles function properly.

Conclusion

Cells are the basic living structures of the body, and they contain special proteins that perform specific functions to maintain homeostasis within the cell. All cells have four basic parts: cytoplasm, plasma membrane, nucleus and nucleolus. Although the cell membrane is in a constant state of flux, it allows substances into and out of the cell. The nucleus is the place where genetic information is stored. The cells utilise various transport systems to move nutrients, oxygen, electrolytes, water and hormones into the cell and waste products of cellular metabolism, such as carbon dioxide, urea and uric acid, out of the cell. Electrolytes and hormones play a vital role in maintaining homeostasis. Many hormones, such ADH, aldosterone and atrial natriuretic hormone, help to regulate fluid balance and maintain homeostasis.

Body fluids consist of the water of the body and substances dissolved in it. Water is the main component of the human body, and, in any individual, the body water content stays remarkably constant from day to day. There is constant movement of fluid between compartments. There are two main body fluid compartments; inside and outside the cells (intracellular and extracellular). The extracellular compartment is divisible into (a) the plasma, which is ECF within the blood vessels; (b) the ISF, which is ECF outside the blood vessels and separated from plasma by the walls of the capillaries; and (c) transcellular fluids, which are fluids with specialised functions.

They include synovial fluid (which lubricates joints), cerebrospinal fluid (which cushions and nurtures the brain), and the aqueous and vitreous humours of the eyes (which maintain the shape of the eyeball and the integrity of structures within it). The transcellular fluids are separated from the plasma by a cellular membrane, which takes part in their formation, in addition to the capillary wall.

Glossary

Active transport   The process in which substances move against a concentration gradient by utilising cellular energy.

Adenosine diphosphate   ADP is the end product that results when ATP loses one of its phosphate groups located at the end of the molecule.

Adenosine triphosphate   Compound that is necessary for cellular energy.

Chemical reactions   Reactions that involve molecules, in which they are formed, changed or broken down.

Compartments   Spaces.

Cytoplasm   Fluid found inside the cell.

Diffusion   The most common form of passive transport of materials, it is the ability for gases, liquids and solutes to disperse randomly and to occupy any space available, so that there is an equal distribution.

Electrolytes   Substances that dissociate in water to form ions.

Endocytosis   Processes by which cells ingest foodstuffs and infectious microorganisms.

Extracellular   Space found outside the cell.

Exocytosis   The system of transporting material out of cells.

Facilitated diffusion   Diffusion with the aid of a transport protein.

Hydrophilic   Water loving.

Hydrophobic   Water hating.

Hypertonic   Solution that has large amounts of solutes dissolved in it.

Hypotonic   Solution that has a low concentration of solutes.

Interstitial   Space between cells.

Intracellular   Space inside the cell.

Organelles   Structural and functional parts of a cell.

Osmosis   Movement of water through a selectively permeable membrane so that concentrations of substances in water are the same on either side of the membrane.

Osmotic pressure   The pressure that must be exerted on a solution.

Passive transport   The process by which substances move on their own down a concentration gradient without utilising cellular energy.

Plasma membrane   Outer layer of the cell.

Transport protein   Small molecules that help in the movement of ions across a cell membrane.

References

American College of Emergency Physicians (n.d.) *Hyponatremia case review*. http://www.acep.org/Clinical-Practice-Management/Hyponatremia-Case-Review/ (accessed 12 November 2015).

Arthritis Research UK (n.d.) *What are calcium crystal diseases?* http://www.arthritisresearchuk.org/arthritis-information/conditions/calcium-crystal-diseases/what-is-pseudogout.aspx (accessed 12 November 2015).

Colbert, B.J., Ankney J. and Lee, K.T. (2012) *Anatomy and Physiology for Health Professionals: An Interactive Journey*, 2nd edn. Upper Saddle River, NJ: Pearson Prentice Hall.

Holte, K., Sharrock, N.E. and Kehlet, H. (2002) Pathophysiology and clinical implications of perioperative fluid excess. *British Journal of Anaesthesia* **89**: 622–632.

Jenkins, G. and Tortora, G.J. (2013) *Anatomy and Physiology: From Science to Life*, 3rd edn. Hoboken, NJ: John Wiley & Sons, Inc.

LeMone, P., Burke, K. and Bauldaoff, G. (2011) *Medical–Surgical Nursing: Critical Thinking in Client Care*, 5th edn. Upper Saddle River, NJ: Pearson Education.

Marieb, E.N. (2012) *Human Anatomy and Physiology*, 9th edn. San Francisco, CA: Pearson.

Marieb, E.N. and Hoehn, K. (2013) *Human Anatomy and Physiology*, 9th edn. San Francisco, CA: Pearson Benjamin Cummings.

Nair, M. and Peate, I. (2009) *Fundamentals of Applied Pathophysiology: An Essential Guide for Nursing Students*. Oxford: John Wiley & Sons, Ltd.

NHS Choices (2014) *Diabetes Insipidus – Treatment*. http://www.nhs.uk/Conditions/Diabetes-insipidus/Pages/Treatment.aspx (accessed 12 November 2015).

O'Connor, C.M. and Adams, J.U. (2010) *Essentials of Cell Biology*. Cambridge, MA: NPG Education, 2010. www.nature.com/scitable/topicpage/cell-membranes-14052567.

Peate, I. and Nair, M. (2011) *Fundamentals of Anatomy and Physiology for Student Nurses*. Chichester: John Wiley & Sons, Ltd.

Rull, G. (2013) *Diuretics*. http://www.patient.co.uk/doctor/diuretics (accessed 12 November 2015).

Thibodeau, G.A. and Patton, K.T. (2011) *Anatomy and Physiology*, 8th edn. St Louis, MO: Elsevier Mosby.

Tortora, G.J. and Derrickson, B.H. (2009) *Principles of Anatomy and Physiology*, 12th edn. Hoboken, NJ: John Wiley & Sons, Inc.

Further reading

Hyperkalemia

Lederer, E., Nayak, V., Alsauskas, Z.C. and Mackelaite, L. (2015) *Hyperkalemia Treatment and Management*. http://emedicine.medscape.com/article/240903-treatment (accessed 12 November 2015).

This is a Medical News site where you will be able to find out more about various diseases and medical conditions.

Diabetes insipidus

NHS Choices (2014) *Introduction*. http://www.nhs.uk/conditions/diabetes-insipidus/Pages/Introduction.aspx (accessed 12 November 2015).

Useful NHS website for up-to-date information on diseases you may come across in practice.

Activities

Multiple choice questions

1. Red blood cells placed in pure water would:
   - (a) crenate and die
   - (b) swell and burst
   - (c) remain the same
   - (d) swell initially and then return to normal size once equilibrium is reached
2. Cell membrane is:
   - (a) a double layer of protein enclosing the plasma

(b) single-layer cell
(c) membrane composed of carbohydrate
(d) the phospholipid layer surrounding the cell

3. Which of the following is true of diffusion?
   (a) the rate of diffusion is dependent on temperature
   (b) the diffusion is greater when the concentration gradient is greater
   (c) the molecular weight of the molecule does not affect diffusion
   (d) diffusion is greater when the body temperature is low

4. In a cell, calcium ions are stored in:
   (a) the nucleus
   (b) the Golgi apparatus
   (c) the mitochondria
   (d) in both smooth and rough endoplasmic reticulum

5. Which of the following is *not* a subcellular structure?
   (a) intercellular material
   (b) cytoplasm
   (c) membranes
   (d) organelles

6. Which of the following transport systems requires energy?
   (a) simple diffusion
   (b) osmosis
   (c) sodium and potassium pump
   (d) facilitated diffusion

7. Phospholipids:
   (a) contain only polar tails
   (b) are hydrophilic and hydrophobic
   (c) contain only non-polar tails
   (d) have their tails directed to the outside

8. Mitochondria:
   (a) contain some of the genes to replicate themselves
   (b) synthesise proteins for use outside the cell
   (c) have the same shape all the time
   (d) are single-membrane structures involved in the breakdown of carbohydrate

9. Fluid moves through a process called:
   (a) osmosis
   (b) diffusion
   (c) mitosis
   (d) exocytosis

10. Cells in a hypertonic solution will:
    (a) crenate and die
    (b) swell and burst
    (c) will remain the same
    (d) both a and b

True or false

1. Diffusion occurs from areas of lesser concentration to greater concentration.
2. Facilitated diffusion does not require energy.
3. Interstitial compartment is part of the extracellular compartment.
4. Mitochondria contain their own genetic material.

5. The cell membrane contains large amounts of cholesterol.
6. Potassium is the principal extracellular ion.
7. Chlorides are negatively charged.
8. Hyponatraemia indicates high sodium levels.
9. 0.9% normal saline is a hypertonic solution.
10. ADH is produced in the pituitary gland.

Label the diagram 1

Label the diagram using the following list of words:

Flagellum, Microfilament, Plasma membrane, Lysosome, Smooth endoplasmic reticulum, Mitochondrion, Sectional view, Nucleus, Cytoplasm, Rough endoplasmic reticulum, Ribosome, Golgi complex, Microfilament

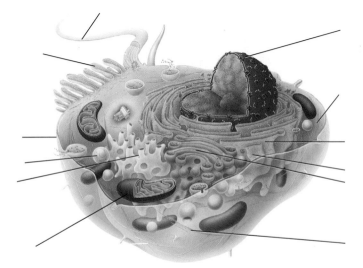

Label the diagram 2

Label the diagram using the following list of words:

Phagocytosis, Solid particle, Pseudopodium, Phagosome (food vacuole), Pinocytosis, Vesicle, Receptor-mediated endocytosis, Coated pit, Receptor, Coat protein, Coated vesicle, Plasma membrane, Extracellular fluid, Cytoplasm

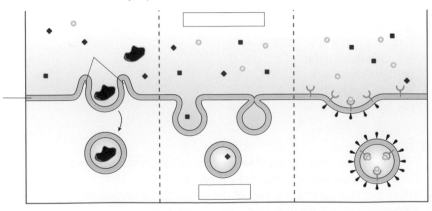

Circle the word or term

Relating to cellular organelles, circle the word or term that does not belong in the following groups:

1.	Centrioles	Lysosomes	Peroxisomes	Enzymatic breakdown
2.	Centrioles	Cilia	Mitochondria	Flagella
3.	Nucleus	Nucleolus	Lysosomes	DNA
4.	Ribosomes	Rough ER	Protein synthesis	Smooth ER
5.	Microtubules	Cilia	Intermediate filaments	Cytoskeleton

Word search

Find the words listed in the following grid.

M	R	S	I	S	O	T	Y	C	O	D	N	E	P	K
R	A	L	U	L	L	E	C	A	R	T	N	I	O	Y
S	I	S	O	M	S	O	P	S	F	Q	Y	U	T	J
H	E	E	X	T	R	A	C	E	L	L	U	L	A	R
R	Y	T	C	J	T	W	A	D	G	H	T	O	S	D
E	N	D	A	I	T	M	U	I	D	O	S	N	S	A
X	C	O	R	R	N	S	E	M	O	S	O	B	I	R
O	H	O	I	O	D	O	M	J	G	S	Q	U	U	X
C	L	L	C	S	P	Y	T	E	W	E	J	P	M	B
Y	O	C	N	Q	U	H	H	O	M	A	A	Y	M	R
T	R	D	S	T	A	F	O	O	P	B	T	C	R	E
O	I	J	O	Y	S	T	F	B	B	Y	R	E	B	M
S	D	F	Z	Y	S	J	B	I	I	R	H	A	R	M
I	E	A	S	U	Z	C	E	A	D	C	A	S	N	Z
S	E	L	E	C	T	R	O	L	Y	T	E	C	V	E

Water, Osmosis, Diffusion, Membrane, Ribosomes, Extracellular, Fats, Carbohydrate, Hydrophobic, Intracellular, Electrolyte, Hypotonic, Exocytosis, Endocytosis, Sodium, Potassium, Chloride

Find out more

1. What are organelles and their functions?
2. What are the factors affecting diffusion.
3. Discuss the effects of low potassium level on the cardiovascular system.
4. What do you understand by the term 'third fluid space'? Do they play any role in fluid balance?

5. Explain the term 'ascites'. What are the causes of 'ascites'?
6. Explain the nurse's role when adding potassium to an intravenous infusion bag.
7. Explain what happens to fluid in the fluid compartments when a person is
   (a) dehydrated
   (b) overhydrated.
8. What do you understand by the term secondary active transport?
9. What is the role of mitochondria in a cell?
10. In an active transport system, where do the cells get their energy from?

Chemical symbols

For the following electrolytes write the correct chemical symbols:

Potassium _____
Sodium _____
Bicarbonate _____
Chloride _____
Organic phosphate _____
Sulphate _____
Calcium _____

Fill in the blanks 1

Fill in the blanks using the correct words from the list below:

Plasma is the only _____ compartment that exists as a real fluid collection all in one location. It differs from _____ in its much _____ content and its high _____ (transport function). Blood contains suspended _____ cells so _____ has been called the _____ of the blood. The fluid compartment called the _____ is interesting in that it is a composite compartment containing _____ (plasma) and _____ (red cell fluid).

blood volume, bulk flow, extracellular fluid, higher protein, interstitial fluid (ISF), intracellular fluid, ISF, major fluid, plasma, red and white

Fill in the blanks 2

Fill in the blanks using the correct words from the list below:

_____ are vital to one's _____ and _____. They are _____ and _____ charged particles (ions) that are formed when mineral or other salts dissolve and separate (dissociate) in water. Since electrolytes carry a _____, they can conduct _____ in water, which itself in its pure form is a _____ of electricity. This characteristic of electrolytes is important because the current enables electrolytes to _____ how and where fluids are distributed throughout the _____, which includes keeping water from floating freely across _____.

body, cell membranes, charge, electrical current, electrolytes, health, negatively, poor conductor, positively, regulate, survival

Conditions

The following is a list of conditions that are associated with the subjects discussed in this chapter. Take some time and write notes about each of the conditions. You may make the notes taken from text books or other resources (e.g. people you work with in a clinical area) or you may make the notes as a result of people you have cared for. If you are making notes about people you have cared for you must ensure that you adhere to the rules of confidentiality.

Water intoxication	
Pulmonary oedema	
Nausea and vomiting	
Acidosis	
Alkalosis	

Chapter 3

Genetics

Peter S Vickers

Test your prior knowledge

- What are the four bases that are found in DNA and what is their role in the double helix?
- If we have a DNA base sequence of ACATGGCTA, what would the corresponding RNA bases be?
- What is happening during the interphase stage of mitosis?
- What do we mean by Mendelian inheritance?
- What is the difference between autosomal recessive inheritance and autosomal dominant inheritance?

Learning outcomes

After reading this chapter you will be able to:

- Understand what a gene is and its importance to our health
- Describe the double helix, including the bases
- Know the difference between DNA and RNA, and their roles in genetics
- Describe the anatomy and functions of a chromosome
- Understand and describe protein synthesis
- Explain cell division
- Understand Mendelian genetics and how it relates to gene transfer from parents to children
- Explain the three modes of inheritance: dominant, recessive and X-linked

Fundamentals of Anatomy and Physiology: For Nursing and Healthcare Students, Second Edition. Edited by Ian Peate and Muralitharan Nair.
© 2017 John Wiley & Sons, Ltd. Published 2017 by John Wiley & Sons, Ltd.
Student companion website: www.wileyfundamentalseries.com/anatomy
Instructor companion website: www.wiley.com/go/instructor/anatomy

Anatomical map

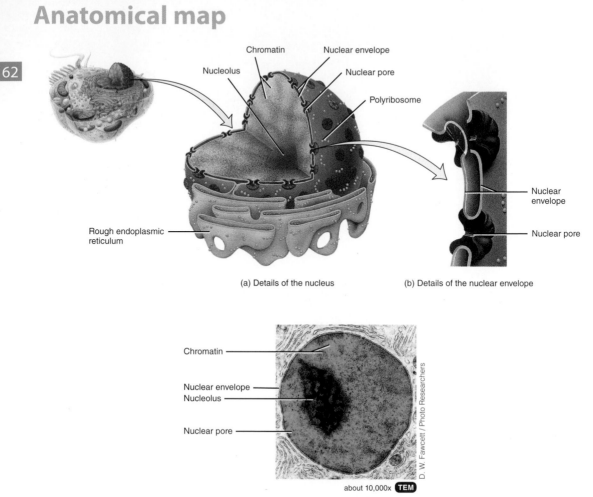

(a) Details of the nucleus

(b) Details of the nuclear envelope

about 10,000x **TEM**

(c) Transverse section of the nucleus

Figure 3.1   (a–c) The cell nucleus. *Source*: Tortora and Derrickson (2014). Reproduced with permission of John Wiley & Sons.

Introduction

Genetics is a very important and endlessly fascinating subject, because we are the sum total of our genes, and many health problems are linked to genes. This chapter will explore the nature of our genes and their importance to us.

To begin at the beginning, genes are sections of deoxyribonucleic acid (DNA) that are carried within our **chromosomes**, and our genes contain particular sets of instructions related to our

- growth
- development
- reproduction
- functioning
- ageing

among many others.

Basically, we cannot function without our genes, and our genes make us what we are – human for a start. We inherit all our genes from our parents, who in turn inherited theirs from their parents. Our grandparents inherited theirs from their parents, and so on.

A few technical terms have already been mentioned, so we can begin by defining them. This will help in the understanding of this chapter.

DNA	deoxyribonucleic acid – part of the double helix/chromosome
RNA	ribonucleic acid, transcribed from DNA
mRNA/tRNA	messenger RNA/transfer RNA – both of these work together with **ribosomes** to produce proteins from **amino acids** that have been coded for by the DNA/gene.

So, **DNA**, the essential ingredient of heredity, makes all the basic units of hereditary material – the genes. The capacity of DNA to replicate itself constitutes the basis of all hereditary transmission and it provides our genetic code by acting as a template for the synthesis of mRNA.

RNA and **mRNA** determine the **amino acid** composition of proteins, which in turn determines the functions of those proteins and hence the function of any particular cell.

Each chromosome, a complicated strand of DNA and protein, is made up of two **chromatids** joined by a **centromere**. Each nucleated cell in our body contains, within its genes, all the genetic material to make an entire human being. Normally, a human has 46 chromosomes (23 pairs) in each nucleated cell – 22 pairs of autosomes, and either two X chromosomes (female) or one X chromosome and one Y chromosome (male). The exception to this is the cells involved in reproduction (the gametes – ovum from the mother and spermatozoa from the father), which just have one copy of each chromosome (i.e. 23 chromosomes). However, some people have more than 46 chromosomes (e.g. people with Down syndrome have 47 chromosomes, with three copies of chromosome 21 – a condition known as trisomy 21), while others have fewer. For example, people with Turner syndrome, also known as 45,X, have 45 chromosomes, because they often have only one X chromosome – which mainly comes from the mother (Crespi, 2008).

The double helix

The **double helix** was famously discovered in the 1950s by two Cambridge scientists, James Watson and Francis Crick, who were awarded a Nobel Prize for their work (although due regard must be paid to Rosalind Franklin who led the way with X-ray crystallography of genes, and who unfortunately died before she could be considered for the Nobel Prize). So what exactly is the double helix and why is it important? Well, first of all, look at the drawing of part of the double helix in Figure 3.2.

The double helix is made up of two strands of DNA, and it is a spiral molecule, resembling a ladder, with rungs built up of pairs of **bases**. To be more precise, our genetic information is encoded in a linear sequence of chemical subunits, called **nucleotides**.

Nucleotides

Nucleotides consist of three molecules:

- **deoxyribose** – a five-carbon cyclic sugar;
- **phosphate** – an inorganic, negatively charged molecule;
- **base** – a nitrogen–carbon ring structure.

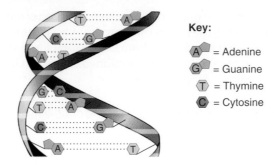

Figure 3.2 A pictorial representation of a portion of the double helix. *Source*: Tortora and Derrickson (2009). Reproduced with permission of John Wiley & Sons.

The biochemistry of DNA can become quite complex, but it will be easier to understand if you remember that the double helix is like a ladder and consists of two parallel **deoxyribose–phosphate** supports (known as **strands** – so they are really deoxyribose–phosphate strands) along with a series of **bases** that make up the rungs of the ladder.

But what are the bases? The bases are simply those elements of the double helix that carry the genetic code and determine such things as what we look like and how we function.

These bases are arranged in different sequences along the deoxyribose–phosphate supports of the ladder-like double helix, and it is these different sequences that determine the actual type of gene produced.

Bases

DNA contains four bases:

- **adenine** (A)
- **thymine** (T)
- **guanine** (G)
- **cytosine** (C).

It is the order in which the bases appear along the length of the DNA molecule that provides the variation, which in turn leads to the production of different genes.

However, just as important in this respect is the order of the pairs of bases. Look again at the drawing of the double helix in Figure 3.2; each deoxyribose–phosphate strand carries different bases. However, because there are two parallel supports, the bases join together and make the molecule stable. Imagine climbing a ladder where the rungs were all cut and separated in the middle – it would not be very stable, would it? Well, it is the same with the DNA molecule.

However, these bases do not pair haphazardly. Each base is very particular as to which other base it will pair with, and there is a golden rule for you to remember.

Golden rule

- **Adenine** always pairs with **thymine**.
- **Guanine** always pairs with **cytosine**.

So, if one half of the DNA has a base sequence AGGCAGTGC then the opposite side of the DNA will have a complementary base sequence TCCGTCACG.

It is important to remember this fact, just as it is also very important that you understand two more facts:

- The bases are joined by means of hydrogen/polar bonding (see Chapter 1).
- The individual bases are connected to the deoxyribose of the strand (or support of the ladder) by means of covalent bonds (see Chapter 1).

The reason why this is important is that, as discussed in Chapter 1, hydrogen bonds are not as strong as covalent bonds and so can separate more easily. The importance of this biochemical fact will become apparent when we discuss DNA replication and protein synthesis (Jorde *et al.*, 2009).

Chromosomes

First of all, look again at the previous brief discussion of chromosomes to be found near the beginning of this chapter. In actual fact, the chromosome does not consist of just DNA. Instead, the nuclear DNA (also known as **nucleic acid**) of eukaryotes is combined with protein molecules known as **histones**. Note that a eukaryote is any organism whose cells contain a nucleus and other organelles enclosed within membranes (see Chapter 2 for more about the cell).

The DNA and histones together make up the **nucleosomes** contained within the cell nucleus. This nucleic acid–histone complex is known as **chromatin**.

Now we run into a problem: if we unravelled all the nucleic acid from every cell in a human adult body it would stretch to the Moon and back about 8000 times. So how do we manage to package that number of DNA and histone molecules into our rather small bodies? The answer, of course, is that we have to fold them so that they fit into each cell of the body – just like having to fold clothes to ensure that they fit into a suitcase when going on holiday. And just as clothes often will only fit in the suitcase if they are neatly folded, the same applies to the chromatin in our cells. It cannot just be pushed in haphazardly – it would never fit and there would be a great possibility of things going wrong.

So, in order to fit within our cells, the chromosomes twist on one another, then twist into loops, before finally assuming the shape that is commonly recognised as a chromosome – the X shape which is easily seen in a human cell (Figure 3.3) (Jorde *et al.*, 2009).

Let us look in more detail at **chromosomes**. Each chromosome is made up of two **chromatids** joined by a **centromere**. Looking at Figure 3.3, you can see that one half of the chromosome is a **chromatid**, and where they join near the top of the X, that is the centromere.

In most humans, each nucleated cell (i.e. each cell with a nucleus) within the body has 46 chromosomes, arranged in 23 pairs (Figure 3.4). Of those 23 pairs, one pair determines the gender of the person.

- Females have a matched **homologous** (means 'the same') pair of X chromosomes.
- Males have an unmatched **heterologous** (means 'different') pair – one X and one Y chromosome.
- The remaining 22 pairs of chromosomes are known as **autosomes**. In biology the word 'some' means body, so autosome means 'self body'. Thus, '**autosome**' can be defined as the chromosomes that determine physical/body characteristics – in other words, all the characteristics of a person that are not connected with gender.

The position a gene occupies on a chromosome is called a **locus**, and there are different **loci** for colour, height, hair, and so on ('loci' is the plural of 'locus'). Think of the locus as the address of that particular gene on Chromosome Street – just like your address signifies that that is where you live.

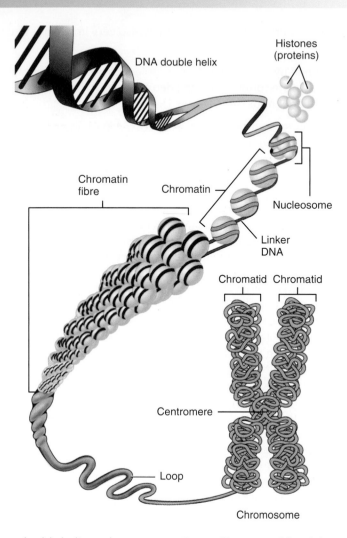

Figure 3.3 DNA from double helix to chromosome. *Source*: Tortora and Derrickson (2009). Reproduced with permission of John Wiley & Sons.

Genes that occupy corresponding loci are called **alleles**. So, the gene for the same characteristic on each of the two chromatids is an **allele**. Alleles are found at the same place in each of the two corresponding chromatids, and an allele determines an alternative form of the same characteristic. Remembering that one of your chromatids comes from your mother and the other corresponding chromatid comes from your father may be of help in understanding this. As an example, think of the colour of eyes. There is one particular gene that determines eye colour and it is found at the same place on each of the two chromatids of one chromosome. One gene will come from the father and the other from the mother. If parents of a child have different coloured eyes from each other, perhaps the mother has green eyes and the father brown eyes, then the child may have green or brown eyes, depending upon factors that will be discussed later in this chapter.

So each of these particular genes at that same point (or locus) on each chromatid determines eye colour. This applies to every one of a person's characteristics. A person with a pair of identical alleles for a particular gene locus is said to be **homozygous** for that gene, while someone with a dissimilar pair is said to be **heterozygous** for that gene.

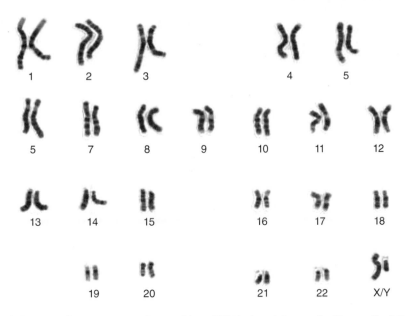

Figure 3.4   Male human chromosomes. *Source*: Lister Hill National Center for Biomedical Communications (2015). Reproduced with permission from US National Library of Medicine.

Just a couple of new things about genes – namely, some genes are **recessive** and some genes are **dominant**.

- A **dominant gene** (or **genotype**, i.e. type of gene) is one that exerts its effect and is physically manifested (the **phenotype**) when it is present on only one of the chromosomes.
- A **recessive** gene (**genotype**) has to be present on both chromosomes in order to manifest itself physically (**phenotype**).

This will be explained more fully later in this chapter, but it is very important because of the significance that it has in hereditary disorders.

From DNA to proteins

As explained earlier in this chapter, nucleic acids are components of DNA and they have two major functions:

- the direction of all protein synthesis (i.e. the production of protein);
- the accurate transmission of this information from one generation to the next (from parents to their children), and from one cell to its daughter cells.

Protein synthesis

Synthesis simply means 'production'; hence, the production of protein from raw materials. All the genetic instructions for making proteins are found in DNA, but in order to synthesise these proteins the genetic information encoded in the DNA has first to be translated.

The first thing that happens in this process is that the DNA has to separate to allow for all of the genetic information in a region of DNA to be copied onto RNA (Figure 3.5).

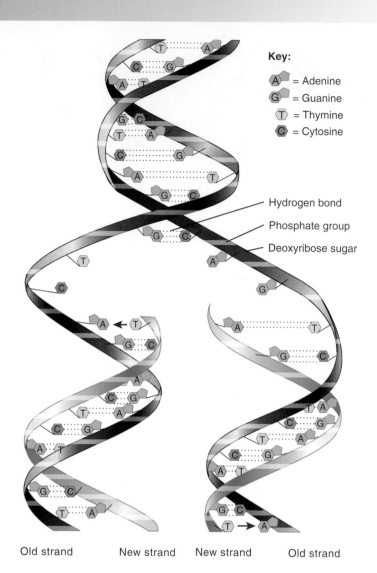

Key:

A = Adenine
G = Guanine
T = Thymine
C = Cytosine

Hydrogen bond
Phosphate group
Deoxyribose sugar

Old strand   New strand   New strand   Old strand

Figure 3.5   The separation of DNA. *Source*: Tortora and Derrickson (2009). Reproduced with permission of John Wiley & Sons.

Then, through a complex series of reactions, the information contained in RNA is translated into a corresponding specific sequence of amino acids in a newly produced protein molecule.

So we will look at this process in more detail. To make it easier to understand, we will break the process into two sections: **transcription** and **translation**.

Transcription

In transcription, the DNA has to be transcribed into RNA because our bodies cannot work with DNA as it stands. By using a specific portion of the cell's DNA as a template, the genetic information stored in the sequence of bases of DNA is rewritten so that the same information appears in the bases of RNA. To do this, the two strands of the DNA have to separate, and the bases that are attached to each strand then pair up with bases that are attached to strands of RNA. As with the two strands of DNA, the bases of DNA can only join up with a specific base of RNA (think back to the **Golden rule**).

- As with DNA, guanine can only join up with cytosine in RNA.
- But while the thymine in DNA can only join to adenine in the RNA, there is no thymine in RNA.
- So, adenine joins to a new base called uracil (U) in mRNA.

DNA	mRNA
guanine (G)–cytosine (C)	
cytosine (C)–guanine (G)	
thymine (T)–adenine (A)	
adenine (A)–uracil (U)	

For example, if **DNA** has a base sequence AGGCAGTGC, then **mRNA** will have a complementary base sequence UCCGUCACG.

Figure 3.5 demonstrates the way in which the DNA separates and makes more DNA. This same process occurs during transcription, except the new strand with its bases is RNA rather than DNA.

Question: In the DNA sequence **TGACTACAG**, what should the RNA bases be?
Answer: **ACUGAUGUC**

So, in the process of transcription, DNA acts as a template for mRNA. However, in addition to serving as the template for the synthesis of mRNA, DNA also synthesises two other kinds of RNA – rRNA and tRNA:

- **rRNA** (ribosomal RNA) – rRNA, together with the ribosomal proteins, makes up the **ribosomes**.
- **tRNA** (transfer RNA) – this is responsible for matching the code of the mRNA with **amino acids**.

Once prepared and ready, mRNA, rRNA and tRNA leave the nucleus of the cell and in the cytoplasm of the cell commence the next step in protein synthesis, namely **translation**.

Translation

Translation allows us to make sense of what we have before us. In genetics, translation is the process by which information in the bases of mRNA is used to specify the amino acid of a protein (proteins are composed of amino acids). This involves all three types of RNA, as well as ribosomal proteins.

The key steps are shown in the next section.

Key steps in protein synthesis

The key steps of protein synthesis (the production of proteins from DNA) are shown in Figures 3.6 and 3.7.

- In the cytoplasm, a small ribosomal subunit (see Chapter 2) binds to one end of the mRNA molecule.
- There are a total of 20 different amino acids in the cytoplasm that may take part in protein synthesis.
- The amino acid comes from the food that we eat, and is then taken up by the cells.
- For each amino acid there is a different small tRNA strand of just three bases (known as a **triplet**).

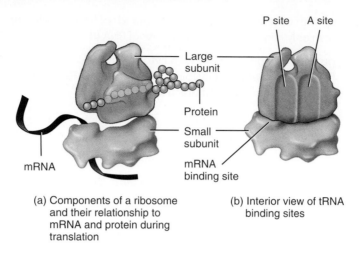

P site   A site

Large
subunit

Protein

Small
subunit

mRNA

mRNA
binding site

(a) Components of a ribosome
and their relationship to
mRNA and protein during
translation

(b) Interior view of tRNA
binding sites

Figure 3.6   (a, b) The mRNA becomes associated with a small ribosomal subunit. *Source*: Tortora and Derrickson (2009). Reproduced with permission of John Wiley & Sons.

Now follow the rest of this description of translation along with Figure 3.5:

- A tRNA triplet picks up the selected amino acid.
- This triplet is known as an **anticodon**.
- One end of the tRNA **anticodon** couples with a specific amino acid – it has receptors on it that only allow it to couple with that particular type of amino acid.
- The other end of the tRNA **anticodon** has a specific sequence of bases.
- That tRNA **anticodon** then seeks out the corresponding three bases on the mRNA strand that is bound to the small ribosomal subunit.
- These three bases are known as a **codon**.
- By means of base pairing, the **anticodon** of the specific tRNA molecule recognises the corresponding **codon** of the mRNA strand and attaches to it. For example, if the **anticodon** is **UAC**, then the mRNA **codon** is **AUG**.
- In the process of attaching itself to the mRNA codon, the tRNA anticodon brings the specific amino acid with it.
- Remember that this base pairing of **codon** and **anticodon** only occurs when the mRNA is attached to a ribosome.
- Once the first tRNA **anticodon** attaches to the mRNA strand, the ribosome moves along the mRNA strand and the second tRNA **anticodon**, along with its specific amino acid, moves into position.
- The two amino acids that are attached to the two tRNA **anticodons** (which in turn are paired to the mRNA **codons**) are joined by a peptide bond.
- The larger ribosomal subunit contains the enzymes that organise the joining of the amino acids together.
- Once this has happened, the first tRNA **anticodon** detaches itself from the mRNA strand and then goes back into the body of the cell to pick up another molecule of its specific amino acid.
- Meanwhile, the ribosome continues to move along the strand of mRNA.

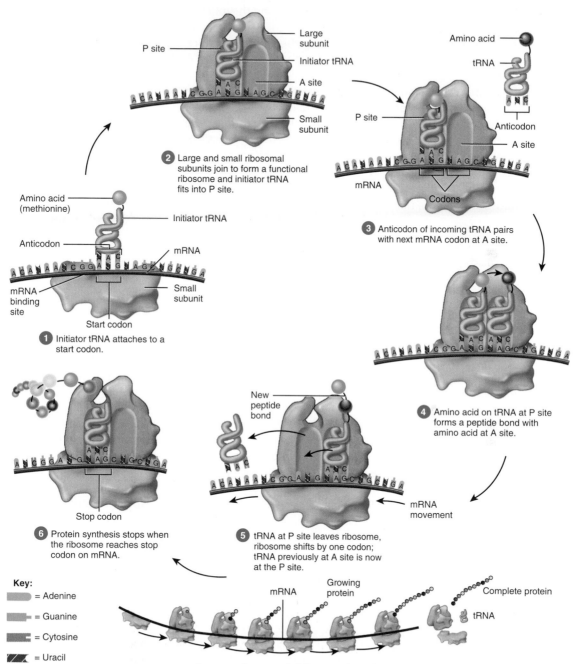

Figure 3.7 Summary of the movement of the ribosome along mRNA. *Source*: Tortora and Derrickson (2009). Reproduced with permission of John Wiley & Sons.

- The smaller ribosomal subunit then moves along the mRNA strand and the process continues in the same way.
- As more amino acids are detached by their tRNAs and are brought into line, one by one, peptide bonds are formed between them and so the protein becomes progressively larger.
- This process is continued until the protein specified by the mRNA strand (which was initially specified by the genes on the DNA strand) is complete – in other words, the correct number of amino acids have been joined together in the correct order.
- Once the specified protein is completed, further synthesis of amino acids/protein is stopped by a special **codon** known as a **termination codon**, a combination of three bases that signals the end of the protein synthesis process for that particular protein.
- When the **termination codon** occurs, the assembled new protein is released from the ribosome, and the ribosome separates again into its two discrete component subunits.

Although this process of protein synthesis has probably taken a long time to work through, the process is actually very quick. In fact, protein synthesis progresses at the rate of about 15 amino acids per second.

Summary of protein synthesis

- As each ribosome moves along the mRNA strand it 'reads' the information coded in the mRNA and synthesises a protein according to that information.
- The ribosome synthesises the protein by translating the codon sequence into an amino acid sequence.
- As the ribosome moves along the mRNA, and before it completes translation of the first gene into protein, another ribosome may attach to the beginning of the mRNA strand and begin translation of the same strand to form a second copy of the protein. So, several ribosomes moving simultaneously in tandem along the same mRNA molecule permit the translation of a single mRNA strand into several identical proteins almost simultaneously.
- Thus, we can now define a **gene** as a group of nucleotides on a DNA molecule that serves as the master mould for manufacturing a specific protein.
- Genes average about 1000 pairs of nucleotides, which appear in a specific sequence on the DNA molecule.
- No two genes have exactly the same sequence of nucleotides, and this is the key to heredity.

Remember now that (Jorde *et al.*, 2009):

- The base sequence of the gene determines the sequence of bases in the mRNA.
- The sequence of the bases in the mRNA determines the order and types of amino acids that will form the protein (Figure 3.8).
- Each gene is responsible for making a particular protein, and the process is in the order shown in Figure 3.8.

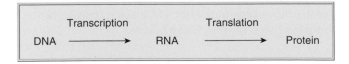

Figure 3.8   Brief summary of protein synthesis.

New therapies for genetic disorders

Three-parent babies!

This is a very new procedure that is aimed at preventing the passing of severe mitochondrial disorders to new generations. As you will know from Chapter 2, mitochondria are organelles found in cells that act as the energy-producing sites of the cell (but not in the nucleus). However, if they mutate they can pass on very serious, often fatal, diseases to the offspring of the mother with the problem mitochondria. These include muscle wastage, nerve damage, loss of sight and heart failure.

The problem is that in the egg only the mother's mitochondria are present, as sperm does not have them. Consequently, if there are faulty genes in the mitochondria, which is then passed into the developing foetus, then there is no possibility of their effects being ameliorated by the father's mitochondria.

Approximately 1 in 4000 women are clinically affected or are at risk for the development of a mitochondrial mutation, and the increased energy requirements of pregnancy may well be the factor that causes mitochondrial disease to be present for the first time.

In January 2015, the UK became the first country to allow what have become known as 'three-parent babies'. Basically, the mother's egg is fertilised *in vitro* by the father, but then the nucleus containing the DNA (a combination of maternal and paternal DNA) is removed from the egg and placed in an egg belonging to a donor. This egg has already had the nucleus containing the DNA removed, and so the new fertilised nucleus is transplanted into the egg in its place, and inserted into the mother who, with the father, has supplied the DNA. Thus, in effect, the resulting child will have three biological parents – their mother and father who supplied the DNA, and the woman who supplied the mitochondria and other organelles. The child will, genetically, still belong to the mother and father and will be an amalgam of them genetically and physically, because only the DNA in the nucleus is concerned with the phenotype of a person, not the mitochondria. Thus, the child, and, if a girl, her descendants, will not carry the mitochondrial mutation to future generations, while the child will still look like their biological parents - hence the three parents.

However, there are still concerns about this procedure. The first concern is about the ethics of this, particularly surrounding the fact that this procedure would be the first to introduce genetic changes that will be passed on not only to the intended child, but to any children that individual goes on to have in the future. The second concern is a physiological/health concern. Depending on where the cell is within the body, there may be from one to hundreds of mitochondria present within that cell. For example, a cell forming part of the brain will need large amounts of energy to function properly and will need many more mitochondria than will, for example, a fat cell. Interestingly, red blood cells are the only cells not to contain any mitochondria at all.

Turning now to the role of the mitochondria in our cells, as mentioned above, and in Chapter 2, we know that the mitochondria supply the energy for the cell to be able to function. However, we now know that the mitochondria do more than that, and are, in fact, an essential part of the whole cell. In the process of producing energy, mitochondria create many by-products, including reactive oxygen and nitrogen species, which then pass into the nucleus and commence a signalling role, which may possibly affect DNA. At the moment we are still trying to find out more concerning the overall importance of mitochondria to the entire cell, and hence to the body as a whole. So it is possible that the mitochondria do play a role in the development of the embryo. Unfortunately, this technique has only been tested on rhesus monkeys, so there is no guarantee that there will be the same results in humans.

The transference of genes

This section discusses how genetic information is transferred from cells to new cells, and also from parents to children. The first thing to do is to look at how cells pass on genetic information to new cells.

In order for the body to grow, and also for the replacement of body cells that have died, our cells must be able to reproduce themselves, but in order for genetic information not to be lost, they must be able to reproduce themselves accurately. They do this by cloning themselves.

In some prokaryotic organisms this occurs by binary fission, whereby the nucleus in a single cell becomes elongated and then divides to form two nuclei in the same cell, each of which carries identical genetic information. The cytoplasm then divides in the middle between the two nuclei, and so two identical daughter cells result, each with its own nucleus and other essential organelles.

However, humans, being much more complicated, have eukaryotic cells, which divide by means of cell division, whereby the division of the nucleus occurs first of all, after which the division of cytoplasm (known as cytokinesis) takes place. After this division, the new cells will grow until they reach a stage when the process can be repeated.

Within this process of cell division, the process of transference of genes (or reproduction of cells carrying genetic information) is divided into two stages: **mitosis** and **meiosis**.

Mitosis

This section commences by looking at the way that cells reproduce, particularly how they reproduce their genetic material.

In humans, cell reproduction takes place using a complex process called **mitosis**, in which the number of chromosomes in the daughter cells has to be the same as in the original parent cell.

In the figures below, only a few of the chromosomes are depicted in order to improve the clarity of the figures.

Mitosis can be divided into four stages:

- prophase
- metaphase
- anaphase
- telophase.

Before and after it has divided, the cell enters a stage known as **interphase** until the time comes for the next cell reproduction.

Interphase

Mitosis begins with **interphase**. This was often thought to be a resting period for the cell, but we now know that the cell is actually very busy during this period getting ready for replication. If we look at the **cell cycle** and suppose that one full cycle represents 24 hours, then the actual process of replication (**mitosis**) would only last for about one of those 24 hours (Figure 3.9). During the rest of the time the cell is undertaking DNA synthesis (i.e. producing DNA). During this period of interphase the cell has to produce two of everything, not just DNA, but all the other organelles in the cell (see Chapter 2), such as the mitochondria. In addition, the cell has to go through the process of obtaining and digesting nutrition so that it has the raw materials for this duplication and also for the energy that will power the various functions of the cell.

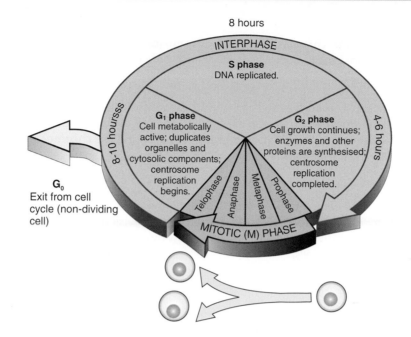

Figure 3.9 The cell cycle. *Source*: Tortora and Derrickson (2009). Reproduced with permission of John Wiley & Sons.

During interphase, the chromosomes in the nucleus are very difficult to see because they are in the form of long threads. They need to be in this state to make it easier for them to be duplicated. During the process of duplication, the cells have to ensure that there will be sufficient and accurate genetic material for each of the two 'daughter cells'. The strands of DNA separate and reattach to new strands of DNA. Because of the selectivity of the bases as to which other base they are able to join in this process, an exact replication of the DNA occurs (Figure 3.5).

In addition, extra cell **organelles** are manufactured or produced by the replication of existing **organelles**. Also during interphase, the cell builds up a store of energy, which is required for the process of division.

Prophase

The first stage after interphase is prophase. During prophase, the **chromosomes** become shorter, fatter and more visible. Each chromosome now consists of two **chromatids**, each containing the same genetic information (in other words, the DNA has exactly replicated itself during interphase). These two **chromatids** are joined together at an area known as the **centromere**. The two **centrosomes** move to opposite ends of the cell (the **poles**) and are joined together by the **nuclear spindle**, which stretches from end to end (or pole to pole) of the cell. The centre of the cell is now called the **equator**. Finally, the **nucleolus** and **nuclear membrane** disappear, leaving the **chromosomes** within the cytoplasm.

Metaphase

During metaphase, the 46 **chromosomes** (two of each of the 23 **chromosomes**) each consisting of two **chromatids** move to the **equator** of the **nuclear spindle**, and here they become attached to the **spindle fibres**.

Anaphase

During anaphase, the **chromatids** in each **chromosome** are separated, and one **chromatid** from each **chromosome** then moves towards each **pole** of the **spindle**.

Telophase

There are now 46 c**hromatids** at each pole, and these will form the **chromosomes** of the daughter cells. The **cell membrane** constricts in the centre of the cell, dividing it into two cells. The **nuclear spindle** disappears, and a **nuclear membrane** forms around the **chromosomes** in each of the daughter cells. The **chromosome**s become long and thread-like again.

Cell division

Cell division is now complete (Figure 3.10) and the daughter cells themselves enter the interphase stage in order to prepare for their replication and division.

This process of cell division explains how we grow by producing new cells as well as replacing old, damaged and dead cells.

Meiosis

Whereas mitosis is concerned with the reproduction of individual cells, meiosis is concerned with the development of whole organisms (e.g. human beings).

The reproduction of a human being depends upon the fusion of reproductive cells (known as **gametes**) from each of the parents. These **gametes** are:

- **spermatozoa** (sperm) from the male;
- **ova** (eggs) from the female.

Each cell of the human body contains 23 pairs of **chromosomes** (i.e. 46 in total). It is very important that during the process of human reproduction the cell formed when the gametes fuse has the correct number of chromosomes for a human being (23 pairs). Therefore, each gamete must possess only 23 single chromosomes, because when gametes fuse during reproduction all their chromosomes remain intact in the new life form. If each gamete had a full complement of 46 chromosomes, then the resulting fused cell would possess 92 chromosomes – or four copies of each chromosome rather than the two that a human cell should possess. From then on, each succeeding generation would have double the number of chromosomes, so that after several generations humans would have cells that possess millions and millions of copies of the 23 chromosomes. To stop this happening, the gametes only possess one copy of each chromosome, so that the resulting fused cell has 46 chromosomes, like the parents.

Now you have two new terms to learn and understand: **diploid** and **haploid** cells.

- **Diploid cell:** a cell with a full complement of 46 chromosomes (i.e. 23 pairs).
- **Haploid cell:** a cell with only half that number of chromosomes (i.e. 23 single chromosomes).

Gametes are therefore haploid cells, because they only possess one copy of each chromosome, while all other cells of the body are diploid cells.

Gametes actually develop from cells with 46 chromosomes, and it is through the process of **meiosis** that they end up with just 23 chromosomes. In effect, in **meiosis** the cells actually divide twice, without the replication of DNA occurring again before the second division.

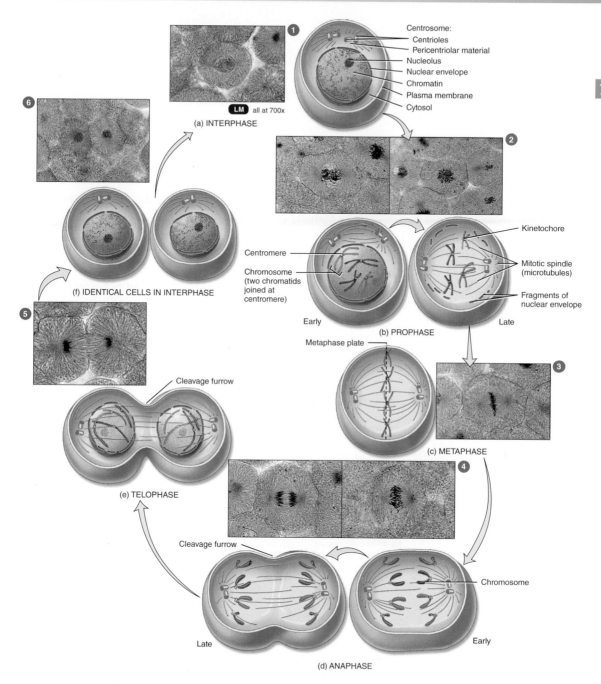

Figure 3.10 (a–f) Mitosis. *Source*: Tortora and Derrickson (2009). Reproduced with permission of John Wiley & Sons.

For descriptive purposes, **meiosis** can be divided into eight stages (not the four of **mitosis**), but rather two **meiotic** divisions each with four stages. However, they do have the same names, but are given the number I or II. As with **mitosis**, these stages are continuous with one another.

- First meiotic stage:
  - prophase I
  - metaphase I
  - anaphase I
  - telophase I.

- Second meiotic stage:
  - prophase II
  - metaphase II
  - anaphase II
  - telophase II.

However, there are differences between what happens during the process of **mitosis** and what happens during meiosis, as well as many similarities.

First meiotic division

Prophase I

Prophase I is similar to the stage of prophase in **mitosis.** However, instead of being scattered randomly, the **chromosomes** (consisting of two **chromatids**) are arranged in 23 pairs. For example, the two chromosome 1s will pair up, as will the two chromosome 2s, and so on. Each pair of chromosomes is called a **bivalent**. Within each pair of chromosomes, genetic material may be exchanged between the two chromosomes, and it is these exchanges that are partly responsible for the differences between children of the same parents. This process is called **gene crossover** (Figure 3.11).

The important point to remember about meiosis is that the DNA is not replicated during the first meiotic division.

Metaphase I

As in mitosis, the chromosomes become arranged on the spindles at the equator. However, they remain in pairs.

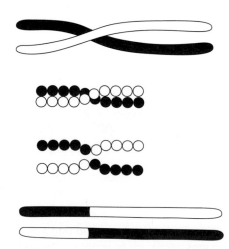

Figure 3.11   Gene crossover.

Anaphase I

One chromosome from each pair moves to each pole, so that there are now 23 chromosomes at each end of the spindle.

Telophase I

The cell membrane now divides the cell into two halves, as in mitosis. Each daughter cell now has half the number of chromosomes that each parent cell had (Jorde *et al.*, 2009).

Second meiotic division

During the second meiotic division, both of the cells produced by the first meiotic division now divide again.

Prophase II, **metaphase II**, **anaphase II** and **telophase II** are all similar to their equivalent stage in **mitosis**, with the exception that the chromosomes are not replicated, before **prophase II**, so there are only 23 single chromosomes in each of the granddaughter cells. That way, when the gametes fuse during reproduction, there are still only 23 pairs of chromosomes per human cell, rather than the 46 pairs if the chromosomes had replicated during the **first meiotic division**.

Of the 23 pairs of chromosomes, 22 pairs are **autosomal** and two **chromosomes** (i.e. one pair) are the sex chromosomes. Remember, **autosomal** means 'of the self body' (auto = self; somatic = of the body). In other words, autosomal chromosomes are concerned with the body. On the other hand, the sex chromosomes determine the gender of a person. Male sex chromosomes are designated by the letter Y, and female chromosomes are designated by the letter X. A male will carry the chromosomes XY (an X chromosome from the mother and a Y chromosome from the father), while a female will carry the chromosomes XX (an X chromosome from both the father and the mother).

Mendelian genetics

So far this chapter has examined the biology of genetics, and now it is going to look at the role of genetics in inheritance. This is very important because, as stated previously, what we are is designated to a large extent by our genetic make-up – which is inherited from our parents. The caveat 'to a large extent' is because as well as being a product of our genes we are also a product of our environment – time, space, relationships, education, and so on.

So how do we inherit our genes from our parents? To understand this we have to return to the 1860s. In Brno (which is now a large town in the Czech Republic but was then a small, sleepy town in Bohemia) there was a monastery, and in that monastery there lived and worked a monk with a very inquiring mind. His name was **Gregor Mendel** and he worked in the monastery gardens where he put his mind to good use trying to perfect the ideal pea. As part of this work, he experimented with cross-breeding. Now, at that time, cross-breeding went on everywhere – on farms and in gardens; and of course, we humans cross-breed as well. However, what was different about Mendel was that not only did he experiment with cross-breeding different peas, but he also made notes on his experiments and observations. He introduced three novel approaches to the study of cross-breeding – at least novel for his time, because no one else was doing this. Not only did he observe, but he experimented and observed. Having observed and experimented he then used statistics. He ensured that the original parental stocks, from which his crosses were derived, were pure breeding stocks (the use of statistics was not at that time fully part of the tradition of biology).

The phenomena that Mendel discovered/observed were statistical in form: the now famous ratios made sense only in the context of counting large numbers of specimens and calculating averages. However, the methods for evaluating statistical data in a scientific way did not exist then and were not to be developed for a further 30 years or so. It was only much later that the validity of such an approach could be accepted.

In 1866, Mendel wrote and published a paper on his experiments, and the response from the scientific community to this paper was deafening in its silence – his observations and theories were completely ignored until their 'rediscovery' in the early 1900s.

In addition, Mendel's work was carried out not in one of the main centres of science, but at the periphery and it was obscurely published. In science, as in the rest of life, who expresses an idea and where they work affects its reception. This is as true today as it was in 1866. But, without a doubt, the science of inheritance is based upon what Mendel discovered all those years ago.

So, what did Mendel discover? Well he demonstrated that members of a pair of alleles separate clearly during meiosis (remember that alleles are different sequences of genetic material occupying the same gene **locus** or place on the DNA, but on different chromosomes).

Remember also that we all have a pair of genes (alleles) at each locus, but because of the process of **meiosis** (discussed above) we can only pass one of those genes to our child.

Figure 3.12 makes things clearer. In this figure, at the same locus on a chromosome, the father has the two alleles Aa and the mother has the two alleles Bb. When they reproduce, the father can pass either **gene A** or **gene a** (both are at the same locus and are therefore alleles) and the mother can pass on either **gene B** or **gene b** (again both at the same locus). However, each child can only inherit one of **gene A** or **gene a** from the father and one of **gene B** or **gene b** from the mother.

What the child cannot do is inherit both **gene A** and **gene a** or **gene B** and **gene b**. Only one allele from each parent can be inherited by a child. This is known as **Mendel's first law.**

What are the statistical chances of a child inheriting any one of those sets of genes from the parents **AB**, **Ab**, **aB**, **ab**? The answer is 1 in 4 (or 1:4). In other words, there is a 25% chance that any child will inherit one of those pairs of genes from his parents.

So, that brings us to Mendel's second law, which asserts that members of different pairs of alleles sort independently of each other during gametogenesis (the production of gametes), and each member of a pair of alleles may occur randomly with either member of another pair of alleles. Note that **gametogenesis** is the production of haploid sex cells, which each carry one half the genetic make-up of the parents.

This now brings us to the concept of dominant and recessive genes. This has a great bearing on many health disorders that we may encounter, as well as determining such characteristics as eye colour, hair colour, and so on.

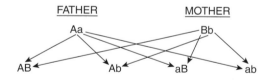

Figure 3.12   Genetic inheritance.

Dominant genes and recessive genes

At each locus, the two **alleles** (genes) can be either **dominant** or **recessive**. A **dominant** gene is an allele that will be reflected in the phenotype (the physical manifestation) no matter what the other allele does. By contrast, a **recessive** gene is one that will only appear in the phenotype if the corresponding allele is also recessive and has the same characteristic as the first allele.

Note that in genetic representations dominant genes are usually given capital letters, while recessive genes are usually given lower-case letters – but not always. Therefore, in the figures above and below, one gene is dominant and one is recessive.

Look again at Figure 3.12. Suppose parents had four children and they all had different genotypes (genetic make-up), so that they each were represented by one of the pairs of genes. How many of the offspring would carry at least one **dominant** gene, and how many would carry only **recessive** genes at this locus?

The answer is that three of the four children (75%) would carry at least one **dominant** gene, and one of the four children (25%) would carry both **recessive** genes. Of course, all four children may inherit the same pair of genes at this locus, or maybe two will inherit the same genes. **Mendel's first law** is relevant only in saying that there is a 1-in-4 chance at each pregnancy that the children will carry a certain genotype.

Another example: a man with red hair marries a woman with brown hair. As time goes by, they have several children, all of whom have brown hair. Which is the dominant gene for hair colour and who carries it?

The gene for brown hair carried by the mother is the dominant gene in this instance. Their offspring all marry partners with brown hair, but some of their offspring have red hair, like their maternal grandfather. How can this be explained?

There are two possible explanations:

- Some of the children carry the red hair recessive gene from their father and their partners also carry a recessive red hair gene – this is most likely.
- The father was not the genetic father of those children.

Autosomal dominant inheritance and ill health

If the dominant gene of one of the parents is one that causes a medical disorder, for example Huntington's disease or neurofibromatosis, what is the risk of any child of those parents having the disease?

The answer is 50% or a 1-in-2 risk of a child having an **autosomal dominant disorder**.

Why is this? Look at Figure 3.12, and assume that the father (genes **A** and **a**) carries the mutant gene on gene **A**. As a dominant gene is always expressed in the phenotype, then statistically there will be a 50% chance of any child having the disease, because the child could inherit gene **a** from the father rather than **gene A**. Of course, any child who carries gene **A** will have a 100% chance of having the disease; there will be no escaping it.

Autosomal recessive inheritance and ill health

Autosomal recessive diseases occur when both parents are carrying the same defect on a recessive gene at the same locus. Both parents have to carry the defective gene otherwise the child cannot be affected by the disease.

In autosomal recessive diseases, if the child (or parent) only carried the defect on one gene, then he (or she) is a carrier of that disease and can pass on that defective gene to his (or her) children. They in turn could pass it on to their children, who, if they inherit it, would also be carriers, and this situation could continue through many generations until the carrier has children with someone who is also a carrier of that mutant gene. There is then a risk of their children being either a carrier or having the disorder.

So, then, what are the risks of:

- A child being a carrier of the recessive gene?
- A child having the disease caused by this mutated/abnormal gene?

Medicines management

Gene replacement therapy

Gene therapy is one way in which genetic disorders can be treated, or at least ameliorated, by

- replacing the mutated or malfunctioning gene;
- manipulating or turning off the gene that is causing the disease;
- stimulating other bodily functions to fight the disease.

The most common form of gene therapy is by replacing a malfunctioning or missing gene with a healthy one. There have been many attempts in the past to cure diseases with gene therapy. In the late 1990s, attempts were made to treat cystic fibrosis, but these attempts failed. However, in the early 2000s, in France, gene replacement therapy was successful with a particular type of immune deficiency: adenosine deaminase deficiency severe combined immunodeficiency. However, gene therapy poses a risk of potentially serious complications, in the first place due to the method that is used to insert the 'new' corrective genes, namely by inserting them inside viruses which are then inserted into the body. These can identify certain cells as well as transmit the genetic material into the cells containing a malfunctioned or missed gene. For that reason, modified viruses are used as vectors or carriers of the healthy genes. This method of insertion of healthy genes may not seem problematic at first glance, but it can cause potentially serious complications – and indeed, as in the early originally successful transplants, two children contracted leukaemia as a result of the virus inserting the corrective genes into the wrong place in the genome. However, these days, this problem has been largely eliminated, and gene replacement for this and other primary immunodeficiencies is regularly carried out in specialist centres.

However, other problems could arise; for example, the inserted virus could be perceived as a foreign invader by the immune system so that the immune system would then release antibodies to destroy the virus, which could lead to organ failure. Also, the use of viruses as vectors could risk a viral dispersion, so causing other diseases to develop, including cancer. However, so far, in the case of children with specific severe primary immunodeficiencies, this has not been a problem, but it is an ever-present risk. On the other hand, most other treatments for these diseases are not particularly successful, so risks and benefits have to be very carefully weighed up by medical staff and, more importantly, by parents. Like every advance, once there has been such success, however small scale it may be, it then spurs on other researchers, doctors, and so on to explore this procedure for other genetic conditions.

To work this out, look again at Figure 3.12. In this case, the lower-case letters **a** and **b** represent the abnormal recessive gene. As can be seen, both parents carry this abnormal gene; for example, for **cystic fibrosis** – this is a well-known disease that is inherited as an autosomal recessive disorder.

If the two recessive genes (**a** or **b**) that code for cystic fibrosis are carried by the parents, then the chances at each pregnancy of

- having an affected child are 1 in 4 (or 25%);
- having a child who is a carrier are 2 in 4 (or 50%);
- having a child who is neither affected nor a carrier is 1 in 4 (or 25%).

Why is this? Look at Figure 3.12 again.

- Only one child has two affected genes (**a** and **b**), and because both affected genes have to be present in order for the disease to appear, this is one child out of four, or 25%.
- Only one child does not have an affected gene (**a** and **b**), and so the disease cannot occur; neither can the child be a carrier, because there is no affected gene to be carried, so this is one child out of four, or 25%.
- Two children have an affected gene (either **a** or **b**), but they also have an unaffected dominant gene (**A** or **B**).

Whenever there is a dominant gene, the affected recessive gene cannot be expressed in the phenotype (physically) as the dominant gene blocks the action of the affected recessive gene. So, there are two children out of four that lead to the carrier state (or 50%). However, always remember that children who are carriers can pass on the affected gene to their children.

It is important to remember that these odds occur for each pregnancy, so you could have four children and have:

- one affected
- two carriers and one unaffected
- four carriers, three affected and one carrier
- and so on.

Remember that the odds are the same for each child born to those parents (LeMone *et al.*, 2015).

Clinical considerations

Genetic counselling

Generally, the clinical application of genetics in health is, at the moment, the responsibility of doctors and scientists. However, there is one extremely important aspect of genetics in ill health that is within the nurse's scope of practice, and that is genetic counselling.

A genetic counsellor has to provide information, offer support to the patient and family, as well as being able to attempt to deal with a patient's and family's specific questions and concerns. The inclusion of the family is very important when dealing with genetic illnesses because, particularly if the illness is an inherited one, that has ramifications for the family as a whole. However, if requested, the patient will be seen separately from the family – and indeed, the family may wish to have individual consultations with the genetic counsellor as they may have questions that are particularly relevant to them.

For a consultation, a genetics counsellor will need

- knowledge of genetics and genetic diseases;
- knowledge of the variety of treatments available for genetic diseases;
- empathy and respect for the patient and family;
- time and patience;
- a box of tissues.

(Continued)

During a consultation, the genetics counsellor will

- Start to build up a rapport and trust with the patient and family members.
- Explain in terms appropriate for the patient/family complex medical and scientific information.
- Help the patient/family to make informed and independent decisions concerning the present and future implications of the genetic illness.
- Give the patient/family the time to start to come to terms with the information they have received, and help them by repetition and innovative explanations until they have absorbed and understood the situation.
- Respect the patient's/family member's individual beliefs and feelings and not attempt to impose their own feelings and beliefs on the situation.
- Not tell anyone what they should do; for example, advise a couple not to have children, end a pregnancy, undergo testing for a genetic disorder or have specific treatment.
- Maintain privacy and confidentiality at all times.
- Be truthful as to potential consequences, but emphasise any positives over negatives. For example, if a couple are found to carry an autosomal recessive gene, explain that there is a 1-in-4 chance that any children will be affected and a 2-in-4 chance that any children will be a carrier of the disease, but then tell them that this means that, in fact, there is a 3-in-4 chance that any children will not have the genetic disease. Also, it is important to stress that these odds apply to every pregnancy, so a couple could have four children and all be affected, or they could have four children and none of them be affected.
- Allow the patient/family members time to go away and think about the information and its potential ramifications, and arrange for them to be seen again in the near future, as well as be available to answer queries as and when they crop up.

Most hospitals now have specialist genetics counsellors, but they can only see the patients and families every now and then. This is where the nurse on the ward or in the clinic comes into their own. Patients and families with health problems with a genetic underpinning will always want to discuss it with people they know and trust when they need to, not by appointment. Consequently, the nurse, as well, as the genetics counsellor, needs to have a knowledge of the conditions and their treatments and outcomes. This is especially so when it comes to genetic inheritance medical problems. As their nurse, it is important to give them the time (and hopefully some of the answers), support and honesty that they are asking for and require. Much of what the genetics counsellor has discussed with the patient/family needs to be repeated and reinforced during the long days that patients and families spend in hospital – and, perhaps more importantly, during the long, quiet nights when concerns and fears come to the fore. At the end of the day, as a nurse you need to use your knowledge and skills (physical, psychosocial and empathetic) to help them to come to terms with their diagnosis and prognosis, whether that be good or bad.

Morbidity and mortality of dominant versus recessive disorders

Autosomal dominant disorders are generally less severe than recessive disorders because if someone carries the affected gene they would have that disorder, whereas with autosomal recessive disorders a person can be a carrier but not have the disease.

If autosomal dominant disorders were as severe and fatal as autosomal recessive disorders, then the disease would die out as all the people with an affected autosomal dominant gene would normally die before being old enough to pass it on to their offspring.

An exception is Huntington's disease, which is a fatal autosomal dominant disorder, but it survives because the symptoms do not usually become apparent until the person with it is in their 30s, by which time they could have passed on the affected gene to their children.

X-linked recessive disorders

As well as autosomal inheritance, we can also inherit disorders via the sex chromosomes. The main role of these chromosomes is to determine the gender of the baby:

- **XX = girl**
- **XY = boy**.

First of all, look at the possibilities of having a boy or a girl when you decide to have a baby. From Figure 3.13, it can be seen that the chances for each pregnancy of a boy or a girl are 50%.

Some disorders are only passed on via the X chromosome. Examples are X-linked haemophilia and Duchenne muscular dystrophy. With these disorders, only boys are affected and only girls are carriers but are unaffected.

If we consider that the lower-case **x** is the affected gene for haemophilia, then what is going to happen?

- The first child is a girl who does not carry the affected gene, but two normal genes, so she is neither a carrier nor affected.
- The second child carries a normal X and a Y, so he is a boy who does not carry the abnormal gene. Consequently, he is neither a carrier nor affected.
- The third child is a girl who carries the abnormal gene, but the action of that gene is blocked by the other normal X gene, so she is not affected, but is a carrier.
- The fourth child is a boy who carries an abnormal X gene and a normal Y gene. Unfortunately, the Y gene is unable to block the action of the abnormal gene, so he is a carrier and is also affected.

Consequently, we can say that there is a chance that:

- one out of two girls (50%) will be a carrier;
- one out of two boys (50%) will be affected.

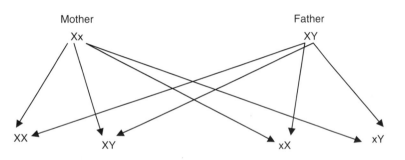

Figure 3.13   X-linked inheritance.

Medicines management

Bone marrow transplants

One of the problems with trying to treat gene disorders is that, unfortunately, only the symptoms can be treated, not the underlying genetic disease. A major reason for this is a lack of knowledge of the underlying causes of genetic disorders by researchers and medical staff. As a consequence, most genetic disorders cannot be cured unfortunately, so treatment at the moment can realistically only be concerned with managing the symptoms. However, one therapy with some success is bone marrow transplantation (BMT).

BMT is the only known treatment for a variety of genetic diseases, mainly inborn errors of metabolism/storage diseases. These diseases are caused by a deficiency of a specific substance in the body, usually a protein, which results in the accumulation of toxic chemicals inside the cells.

These successfully treated storage diseases include:

- Hurler's mucopolysaccharidosis – also known as MPS I
- adrenoleukodystrophy
- metachromatic leukodystrophy
- Krabbe's disease
- Niemann–Pick.

There have been other successful treatments, but too few have been evaluated to know whether or not BMT will be helpful.

However, there have been more than 300 patients with Hurler's disease treated by BMT, and in many cases the donors have been human leukocyte antigen (HLA)-matched siblings (a complete HLA match for the essential antigens – see Chapter 16. These transplants do require conditioning regimens, including high doses of chemotherapy, which can, in itself, cause problems, and even death. Those successfully transplanted do have less risk of organ damage. However, as yet, we do not know too much about the long-term effects of this treatment on growth and skeletal development. Of greatest significance is the effect on the central nervous system. Results have, though, shown that any prior brain damage will not be reversed, although long-term studies appear to show that further nervous system degeneration is reduced or even prevented.

Spontaneous mutation

Now to briefly mention another way in which an unusual or abnormal gene can occur in someone and cause genetic disorders. This is known as **spontaneous mutation**. Because of the great speed and precision needed at each replication of DNA of the germ cells, or of protein synthesis, it is possible for mistakes to occur, and in this way genetic mutations arise. There is no way of predicting or preventing this; the first anyone will know about it is when it is manifested as a disease.

Finally, there are also the problems of chemical and trauma mutations – mutations due to outside occurrences that can cause disease due to their effects on various genes.

Conclusion

This completes the chapter on basic genetics. Although genetics may appear complicated, it is a very important subject because our genes make us what we are, but also they can leave us susceptible to certain diseases and have a say in how we respond to treatment for diseases, and how we live our lives, work, develop relationships, and indeed survive in the world.

Glossary

Adenine   One of the four nitrogen–carbon bases of **DNA**.

Allele   The place on the **chromosomes** where **genes** which code for the same function are to be found.

Amino acid   Amino acids, which are coded for by **genes**, can be considered as the building blocks of proteins.

Anaphase   The stage in cell division where the **chromosome** separates and moves to the **poles** of the cells.

Anticodon   A **triplet** of **bases** on **tRNA** encoding for **amino acids** that join with other **triplets** (or anticodons) to produce the appropriate proteins.

Autosome   The name given to **chromosomes** that are not one of the two sex **chromosomes**.

Autosomal dominant disorder   A medical disorder caused by a faulty **dominant gene** inherited from one of the parents.

Autosomal recessive disorder   A medical disorder caused by the same fault on **recessive genes** inherited from both parents.

Base   Part of the **double helix**, bases are the code that will eventually lead to the formation of protein.

Bivalent   A pair of associated **homologous chromosomes** formed after replication of the **chromosomes**, with each replicated **chromosome** consisting of two **chromatids**.

Cell cycle   The process by which a cell prepares for, and undertakes, cell growth and division.

Chromatid   One half of a **chromosome**.

Centromere   The point at which two **chromatids** become attached to form a **chromosome**.

Centrosome   An **organelle** found in **eukaryotic** cells and which is the main place where cell microtubules are organised. It is particularly important because it regulates cell division.

Chromosome   Mixture of **DNA** and protein – contains our genetic make-up.

Codon   A triplet of **bases** on **mRNA** that encodes for a particular **amino acid**.

Cytosine   One of the four nitrogen–carbon bases of **DNA**.

Deoxyribose   A major part of **DNA**, deoxyribose is derived from a sugar known as ribose but has lost an atom of oxygen – which leads to its name.

Diploid cell   A cell that contains two sets of identical **chromosomes**. See **haploid cell**.

DNA   Deoxyribonucleic acid – part of the **double helix**.

Dominant gene   A **gene** that can exert its effects on the body on its own. In other words, it dominates the **recessive gene** at the same **locus**.

Double helix   Two strands of **DNA** joined together in a spiral formation.

Equator of the cell   The centre of the cell during cell division.

Gamete   A reproductive cell; for example, **spermatozoon** or **ovum**.

Gametogenesis   The production of **gametes**.

Gene   A unit of **heredity** in a living organism.

Gene crossover   The process at the commencement of **meiosis** whereby genetic material may be transferred between **chromosomes**.

Genotype   The genotype of a person is their genetic make-up. See **phenotype**.

Guanine   One of the four nitrogen–carbon bases of **DNA**.

Haploid cell   A cell that contains just one set of **chromosomes.** See **diploid cell.**

Heredity   The passing down of **genes** from generation to generation.

Heterologous   'Different', as opposed to **homologous**, which means 'the same'.

Heterozygous   A pair of dissimilar **alleles** for a particular **gene locus**. See **homozygous**.

Histone   **Proteins** found in cell nuclei, which package and order the **DNA** into **nucleosomes** – so making it possible for the **chromosomes** to be fitted into a cell without becoming tangled.

Homologous   'Same' – see **heterologous**.

Homozygous   A pair of identical **alleles** for a particular **gene locus**. See **heterozygous**.

Interphase   The longest stage of the **cell cycle**, during which the cell is growing and preparing for replication.

Locus   A **gene's** position on a **chromosome**.

Meiosis   Concerned with the development of whole organisms and is a process in which **diploid cells** become **haploid cells**, so ensuring that the correct number of **chromosomes** are passed to the offspring.

Mendelian genetics   The genetics of inheritance (named after Gregor Mendel).

Mendel's first law   Only one **allele** from each parent can be inherited by their child.

Mendel's second law   During **gametogenesi**s, members of different pairs of **alleles** are randomly sorted independently of each other.

Metaphase   The stage in the **cell cycle** when the **chromosomes** move to the **equator** of the cell preparatory to separating.

Mitosis   The process by which **chromosomes** are accurately reproduced in cells during cell division.

mRNA   Messenger ribonucleic acid; it is important in the production of proteins from **amino acids**.

Nucleic acid   A mixture of phosphoric acid, sugars, and organic **bases**, nucleic acids direct the course of protein synthesis (or production), so regulating all cell activities. **DNA** and **RNA** are nucleic acids.

Nucleosome   The basic unit of **DNA** once it is packaged in a cell's nucleus; it consists of a segment of **DNA** wound around a **histone**.

Nucleotide   The name for the parts of **DNA** consisting of sugar (deoxyribose) and one of the four bases (**adenine, thymine, guanine** and **cytosine**). In other words, it is the basis of our **genes**.

Ova   Female reproductive cells (also known as eggs).

Phenotype   The phenotype is the expressed features of a person, and is derived from the interaction of the **genotype** of a person with the environment.

Phosphate   An inorganic molecule forming part of the **double helix**.

Poles of the cell   The ends of a cell during the stages of cell division.

Prophase   The first stage of cell division where **chromosomes** fold together and become more visible.

Recessive gene   A recessive gene requires another recessive gene at the same **locus** before it can have an effect on the body. In other words, it is not **dominant** over another **gene** at the same **locus**.

Ribosomes   Small, bead-like structures in a cell that, along with **RNA**, are involved in making proteins from **amino acids** (see Chapter 2).

RNA   Ribonucleic acid – **transcribed** from **DNA**.

Spermatozoa   Male reproductive cells.

Spontaneous mutation disorder   A medical disorder caused by a new fault that has developed on a **gene**; that is, neither of the parents carries that faulty **gene**.

Strand   The long parts of the **double helix**, consisting of **deoxyribose** and **phosphate**.

Telophase   The stage in cell division where the cell actually divides and forms two identical daughter cells.

Termination codon   A **triplet** of **bases** that stops the synthesis of **amino acids** once the specified protein of that sequence has been produced.

Thymine   One of the four nitrogen–carbon bases of **DNA**.

Transcription   The process by which something with which we cannot work is changed into something that we can. In genetics, this is the changing of **DNA** into **RNA**.

Translation   The process that allows us to make sense of what we have in front of us. In genetics, translation is the process by which information in the bases of **mRNA** is used to specify the **amino acid** of a protein.

Triplet   Sequences of three **RNA bases** that code for different amino acids.

tRNA   Transfer ribonucleic acid; it is important in the production of proteins from **amino acids**.

X-linked recessive disease   A medical disorder caused by a fault on the X **gene** (one of the sex genes). Only females are carriers and only males can have these disorders.

References

Crespi, B. (2008) Turner syndrome and the evolution of human sexual dimorphism. *Evolutionary Applications* **1**(3): 449–461.

Jorde, L.B., Carey, J.C., Bamshad, M.J. and White, R.L. (2009) *Medical Genetics*, 4th edn. St Louis, MO: Mosby.

LeMone, P., Burke, K., Bauldoff, G. and Gubrud, P. (2015) *Medical–Surgical Nursing: Critical Thinking in Client Care*, 6th edn. Upper Saddle River, NJ: Pearson Prentice Hall.

Lister Hill National Center for Biomedical Communications (2010) *Genetics Home Reference: Your Guide to Understanding Genetic Conditions*. Bethesda, MD: NIH; p. 17. http://ghr.nlm.nih.gov/handbook.pdf (accessed 18 November 2015).

Tortora, G.J. and Derrickson, B.H. (2009) *Principles of Anatomy and Physiology*, 12th edn. Hoboken, NJ: John Wiley & Sons, Inc.

Tortora, G.J. and Derrickson, B.H. (2014) *Principles of Anatomy and Physiology*, 14th edn. Hoboken, NJ: John Wiley & Sons.

Further reading

Bartels, D. (2010) *Genetic Counseling: Ethical Challenges and Consequences*. Piscataway, NJ: Transaction Publishers.

Fletcher, H. and Hickey, I. (2012) *BIOS Instant Notes in Genetics*, 4th edn. Abingdon: Taylor & Francis.

Jones, S. and Van Loon, B. (2014) *Introducing Genetics: A Graphic Guide*. London: Icon Books Ltd.

Robinson, T.R. (2010) *Genetics for Dummies*. Chichester: John Wiley & Sons, Ltd.

Skirton, H. and Patch, C. (2013) *Genetics for Healthcare Professionals*. New York: Garland Science.

Vipond, K. (2013) *Genetics: A Guide for Students and Practitioners of Nursing and Health Care*, revised edn. Banbury: Scion Publishing Ltd.

Activities

Multiple choice questions

1. With regard to DNA bases, cytosine in the DNA joins with:
   - (a) guanine
   - (b) uracil
   - (c) adenine
   - (d) thymine

2. Nucleotides consist of three components; these are:
   - (a) base, helix, amino acid
   - (b) helix, deoxyribose, base
   - (c) phosphate, base, deoxyribose
   - (d) ribonucleic acid, deoxyribose, helix

3. Normally, humans have:
   - (a) 44 chromosomes
   - (b) 46 chromosomes
   - (c) 47 chromosomes
   - (d) 45 chromosomes

4. The position that a gene occupies on a chromosome is known as:
   - (a) the allele
   - (b) the locus
   - (c) the autosome
   - (d) the histone

5. Protein synthesis is the process of:
   - (a) protein breakdown
   - (b) protein encoding
   - (c) protein translation
   - (d) protein production

6. If DNA has a base sequence of GCGTATGA, then the corresponding sequence of mRNA will be:
   - (a) TATCGCTG
   - (b) CGCAUACU
   - (c) AUAGCGCU
   - (d) UCUAUAUC

7. During protein synthesis, which of the following are sequentially attached to tRNA triplets?
   - (a) ribosomal proteins
   - (b) codons
   - (c) nucleotides
   - (d) amino acids

8. The four stages of mitosis take place in which of the following orders?
   - (a) metaphase, prophase, telophase, anaphase
   - (b) prophase, anaphase, telophase, metaphase
   - (c) prophase, metaphase, anaphase, telophase
   - (d) anaphase, telophase, prophase, metaphase

9. The period between the actual process of cell and nuclear replication within cells is known as:
   (a) protophase
   (b) interphase
   (c) rephrase
   (d) organophase

10. In Mendelian genetics, Mendel's first law states that:
    (a) alleles are different sequences of genetic material occupying the same locus
    (b) humans have 46 chromosomes
    (c) only one allele from each parent can be inherited by a child
    (d) different pairs of alleles sort independently of each other

True or false

1. Genes are sections of RNA carried within our chromosomes.
2. Deoxyribonucleic acid is a major component of our DNA.
3. DNA consists of deoxyribose, phosphate and base.
4. Each chromosome consists of two centromeres joined by a chromatid.
5. In the double helix, the bases are joined together by hydrogen bonding.
6. During protein synthesis, the synthesis of amino acids/protein is stopped at the correct point by an anticodon.
7. Huntington's disease is an example of X-linked inheritance.
8. Autosomal dominant disorders are generally more severe than autosomal recessive disorders.
9. Duchene muscular dystrophy is an example of X-linked inheritance.
10. In autosomal dominant disorders, statistically, there is a 25% chance of having an affected child.

Label the diagram 1

Label the diagram using the following list of words:

Nucleus, DNA, Nuclear pore, RNA, Plasma membrane, Cytoplasm, RNA, Ribosome, Protein

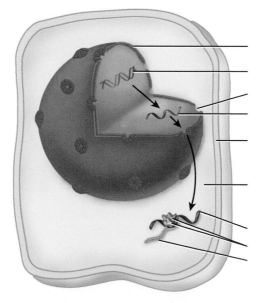

Source: Tortora and Derrickson (2014). Reproduced with permission of John Wiley & Sons.

Label the diagram 2

Label the diagram using the following list of words:

Transcription, Translation, DNA, RNA, Protein

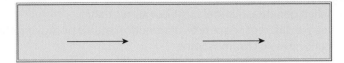

Test your learning

1. Describe DNA, RNA, chromosome.
2. Explain how the chromosome is organised so that it can fit in a cell.
3. Explain dominant and recessive genes.
4. List the bases of DNA and their corresponding RNA bases.
5. Describe in your own words the process of protein synthesis.
6. List the stages of mitosis and meiosis.
7. Explain the importance of gene crossover during meiosis.
8. Discuss autosomal dominant and autosomal recessive genes in relation to ill health.

Fill in the blanks

Fill in the blanks using the correct words from the list:

During protein synthesis all the _____ instructions for making proteins are found in _____. The first stage of protein production involves the _____ of this information into _____, which, in turn, is _____ into a corresponding sequence of _____ that join together to form _____ molecules.

amino acids, DNA, genetic, protein, RNA, transcription, translated

Word search

Find the following words within the grid:

Amino acid, Anaphase, Carrier, Cell, DNA, Mendel, Mitosis, Protein, Recessive, RNA, Tears, Telophase, Translation

D	Y	N	A	S	T	P	O	B	J	E	C	T
T	N	U	X	V	Z	R	U	Q	M	N	V	E
L	R	A	M	I	N	O	A	C	I	D	W	L
P	R	A	E	D	I	T	R	O	T	O	R	O
N	T	Z	N	C	O	E	T	G	O	S	T	P
P	L	Y	D	S	N	I	E	V	S	C	I	H
T	W	Y	E	Y	L	N	R	G	I	O	R	A
C	E	L	L	T	E	A	R	S	S	P	E	S
N	H	Y	C	O	D	A	T	E	A	E	I	E
P	G	R	E	C	E	S	S	I	V	E	R	N
L	N	V	N	T	V	S	O	Z	O	X	R	G
A	Q	U	A	E	S	A	H	P	A	N	A	T
V	L	P	R	T	Y	O	I	Y	J	W	C	Y

Conditions

The following is a list of common genetic conditions. Take some time and write notes about each of the conditions. You may make the notes taken from text books or other resources (e.g. people you work with in a clinical area), or you may make the notes as a result of people you have cared for. If you are making notes about people you have cared for you must ensure that you adhere to the rules of confidentiality.

Motor neurone disease	
Prader–Willi syndrome	
Alzheimer disease, type 2	
Neurofibromatosis	
Down syndrome	
Turner syndrome	

Chapter 4

Tissue

Anthony Wheeldon

Test your prior knowledge

- List the four main types of body tissue.
- What are the main functions of epithelial tissue?
- Name the four types of connective tissue.
- Which types of muscle are involuntary?
- What are the main steps of tissue repair?

Learning outcomes

After reading this chapter you will be able to:

- Describe the characteristics of epithelial tissue
- List the classifications of epithelial tissue
- Discuss the functions of connective tissue
- List the classifications of connective tissue
- Describe the process of tissue repair

Fundamentals of Anatomy and Physiology: For Nursing and Healthcare Students, Second Edition. Edited by Ian Peate and Muralitharan Nair.
© 2017 John Wiley & Sons, Ltd. Published 2017 by John Wiley & Sons, Ltd.
Student companion website: www.wileyfundamentalseries.com/anatomy
Instructor companion website: www.wiley.com/go/instructor/anatomy

Introduction

The human body consists of around 50 trillion to 106 trillion individual structural working units called cells (Marieb and Hoehn, 2008). Cells work together to ensure that homeostasis is maintained. Cells come in many different shapes, sizes and life spans; however, they can be categorised depending on their structure and functions. A group of cells that have a similar structure and function are called tissue, and within the human body there are four distinct types of tissue. Cells that provide a covering for organs and structures, for example, are referred to as epithelial tissue, whereas cells that provide support for structures are called connective tissue. Cells that govern body movement are muscle tissue, and cells that help control homeostasis are nervous tissue. Most organs of the body contain a selection of all four tissue types. The heart, for example, contains muscle tissue, is controlled by nervous tissue, lined by epithelial tissue and supported by connective tissue. Tissue also has the capacity to repair itself. This chapter examines all four types of tissue and the process of tissue repair.

Epithelial tissue

Epithelial tissue is essentially a sheet of cells that covers an area of the body. Epithelial tissue covers or lines body surfaces (i.e. skin), or it lines the walls and the organs within body cavities. The major role of epithelial tissue is as an interface; indeed, nearly all the substances absorbed or secreted by the body must pass through epithelial tissue. Broadly speaking, epithelial tissue has six main functions:

- absorption
- protection
- excretion
- secretion
- filtration
- sensory reception.

Not all epithelial tissue carries out all six functions. In many areas of the body epithelial tissue specialises in just one or two functions. Epithelial tissue in the digestive system, for example, specialises in absorption of nutrients, whereas epithelial tissue within skin provides a protective layer.

Epithelial tissue cells are closely bonded together in continuous sheets, which have an apical and a basal surface. The apical surface faces outwards, towards the exterior of the organ it covers. Apical surfaces can be smooth, but most have hair-like extensions called microvilli. Microvilli dramatically increase the surface area of the epithelial tissue and therefore increase its ability for absorption and secretion. Some areas, within the respiratory tract for example, possess larger hair-like extensions called cilia, which are also capable of propelling substances. Lying close to the basal surface is a thin sheet of glycoproteins that acts as a selective filter, governing which substances can enter epithelial tissue. Epithelial tissue is innervated by neurones, but it has no blood supply as such. Rather than being served by a network of capillaries, epithelial tissue receives a supply of nutrients from nearby blood vessels. Owing to its protective role, epithelial tissue needs to endure a great deal of abrasion and environmental damage, and epithelial cells need to be very hardy and tough. This hardiness is generated by their ability to divide and regenerate rapidly, resulting in the swift replacement of damaged epithelial cells. However, this regenerative capacity is reliant upon a plentiful supply of nutrients.

Epithelial tissue can be categorised into the following three distinct types:

- simple
- stratified
- glandular.

Simple epithelium consists of a single layer of cells bound into a continuous sheet. Stratified epithelium is also arranged into a continuous sheet but is thicker with numerous layers of cells. Glandular epithelium forms the glands of the body.

All epithelial cells have six sides; indeed, under a microscope a cross-section of epithelial tissue looks like a honeycomb. Epithelial cells can be subdivided further into the following three different six-sided shapes:

- cuboidal
- columnar
- squamous.

As their names suggest, cuboidal and columnar epithelial cells are square and tall respectively, whereas squamous epithelial cells are rather flat and scaly (see Figure 4.1). When examining the many different types of epithelial cell it is easy to work out its size and shape by its name. For instance, simple squamous epithelium is thin, flat and scale-like.

Simple epithelium

Because simple epithelia consist of a single cellular layer it specialises in absorption, secretion and filtration rather than protection.

Simple squamous epithelium is quite often very permeable and is found where the diffusion of nutrients is essential. Capillary walls, the alveoli of the lungs and the glomeruli in the kidneys

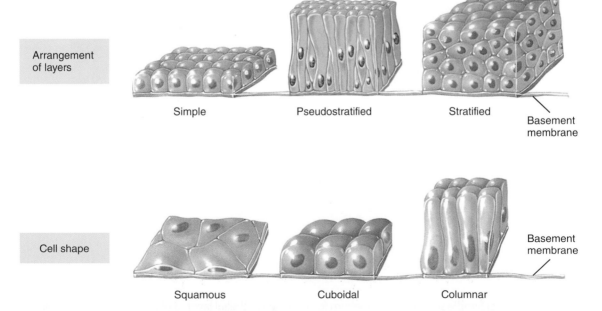

Figure 4.1 Epithelial tissue is classified by shape and depth. *Source*: Tortora and Derrickson (2009). Reproduced with permission of John Wiley & Sons.

are all lined with simple squamous epithelium, which facilitates the rapid diffusion of nutrients. Simple squamous epithelium is also found within the heart and blood and lymph vessels. Simple squamous epithelium found within the heart and blood and lymph vessels is called endothelium (see Figure 4.2).

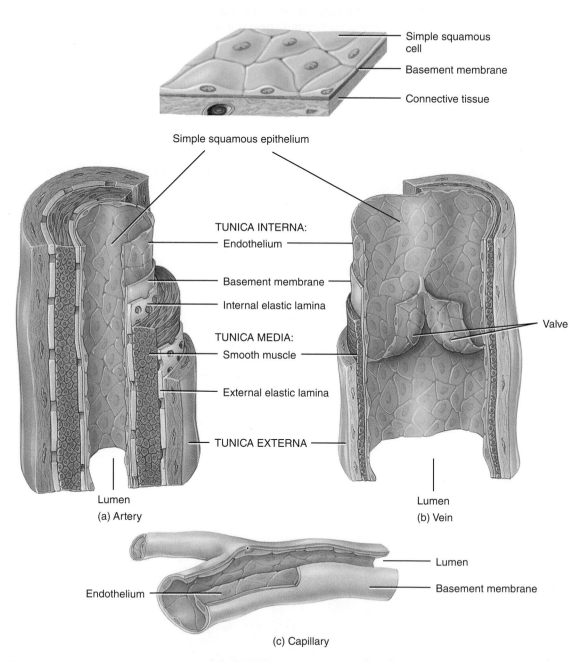

Simple squamous cell

Basement membrane

Connective tissue

Simple squamous epithelium

TUNICA INTERNA:
Endothelium

Basement membrane

Internal elastic lamina

TUNICA MEDIA:
Smooth muscle

External elastic lamina

TUNICA EXTERNA

Valve

Lumen

(a) Artery

Lumen

(b) Vein

Lumen

Endothelium

Basement membrane

(c) Capillary

Figure 4.2 (a–c) Simple squamous epithelium forms the endothelial layer of blood vessels. *Source*: Tortora and Derrickson (2009). Reproduced with permission of John Wiley & Sons.

Simple cuboidal epithelium specialises in secretion as well as absorption. Simple cuboidal epithelium is found in the lining of the ovaries, the kidney tubules and the ducts of smaller glands. It also forms part of the secretory portions of glands such as the thyroid and pancreas (see Figure 4.3).

Simple columnar epithelium can be ciliated or non-ciliated. As its name suggests, ciliated simple columnar epithelium has cilia on its apical surface. It is found in areas of the body where movement of fluids, mucus or other substances is required. Ciliated simple columnar epithelial tissue, for example, lines the passageways of the central nervous system and helps propel cerebrospinal fluid. It also lines the Fallopian tubes and helps move oocytes recently expelled from the ovaries (see Figure 4.4). A common location for non-ciliated simple columnar epithelium is the lining of the digestive tract from the stomach to the rectum (see Figure 4.5). Non-ciliated simple columnar epithelium performs two broad functions. Some possess microvilli, greatly increasing their surface area for absorption; others specialise in the secretion of mucus. Such cells are referred to as goblet cells owing to their cup-like shape. Simple columnar epithelial cells are generally of equal size. However, in some instances simple columnar epithelial cells vary in height, with only the tallest reaching the apical surface. This gives the illusion that the tissue has

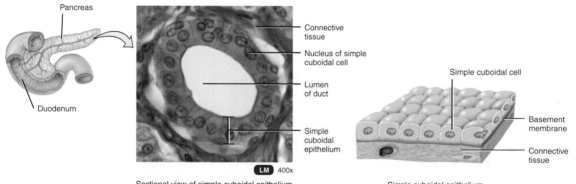

Sectional view of simple cuboidal epithelium of intralobular duct of pancreas

Simple cuboidal epithelium

Figure 4.3 Simple cuboid epithelium forms part of the secretory portion of the pancreas. *Source*: Tortora and Derrickson (2009). Reproduced with permission of John Wiley & Sons.

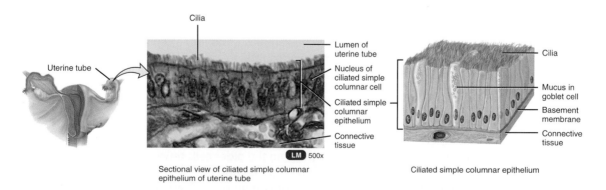

Sectional view of ciliated simple columnar epithelium of uterine tube

Ciliated simple columnar epithelium

Figure 4.4 Ciliated simple columnar epithelium lines the Fallopian tubes. *Source:* Tortora and Derrickson (2009). Reproduced with permission of John Wiley & Sons.

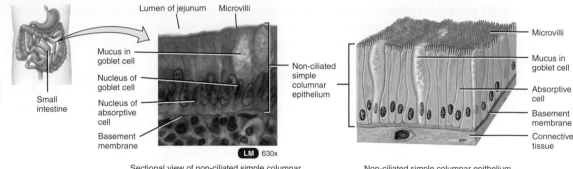

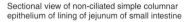

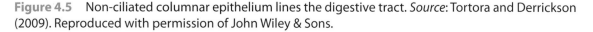

Sectional view of non-ciliated simple columnar
epithelium of lining of jejunum of small intestine

Non-ciliated simple columnar epithelium

Figure 4.5 Non-ciliated columnar epithelium lines the digestive tract. *Source*: Tortora and Derrickson (2009). Reproduced with permission of John Wiley & Sons.

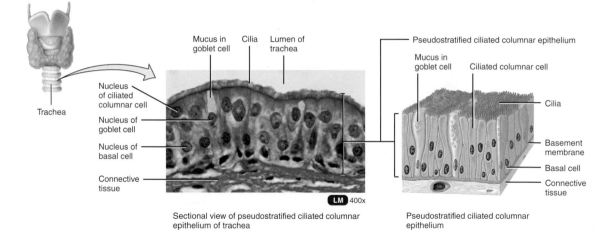

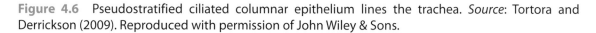

Sectional view of pseudostratified ciliated columnar
epithelium of trachea

Pseudostratified ciliated columnar
epithelium

Figure 4.6 Pseudostratified ciliated columnar epithelium lines the trachea. *Source*: Tortora and Derrickson (2009). Reproduced with permission of John Wiley & Sons.

many layers, like stratified epithelium. Such examples of columnar epithelial tissue are called **pseudostratified columnar epithelium**. Pseudostratified columnar epithelium is found within the lining of the male reproductive system; however, the most common location is the lining of the respiratory tract (see Figure 4.6).

Stratified epithelium

Unlike simple epithelia, stratified epithelia have many layers. The cells regenerate from below, with new cells dividing on the basal layer pushing the older cells towards the surface. As stratified epithelium is thicker, its principal function is protection.

Stratified squamous epithelium is the most common stratified epithelium and forms the external part of skin (see Chapter 17). Stratified squamous epithelial tissue is keratinised, toughened by the presence of keratin, a special tough fibrous protein. Non-keratinised stratified

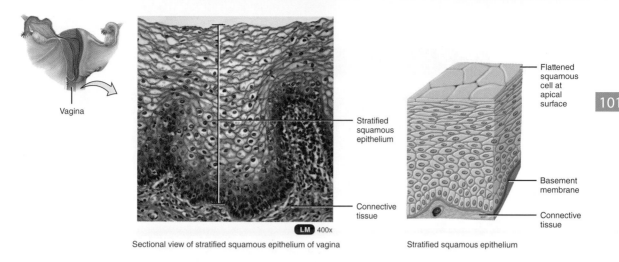

Vagina

Stratified squamous epithelium

Connective tissue

Flattened squamous cell at apical surface

Basement membrane

Connective tissue

LM 400x

Sectional view of stratified squamous epithelium of vagina

Stratified squamous epithelium

Figure 4.7 Non-keratinised stratified squamous epithelial tissue lines the vagina. *Source*: Tortora and Derrickson (2009). Reproduced with permission of John Wiley & Sons.

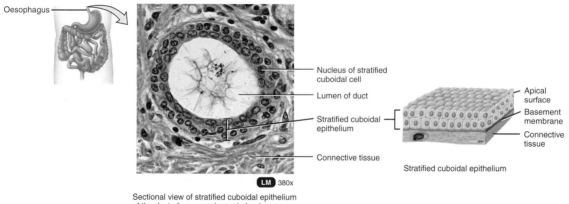

Oesophagus

Nucleus of stratified cuboidal cell

Lumen of duct

Stratified cuboidal epithelium

Connective tissue

Apical surface

Basement membrane

Connective tissue

LM 380x

Sectional view of stratified cuboidal epithelium of the duct of an oesophageal gland

Stratified cuboidal epithelium

Figure 4.8 Cuboidal epithelial tissue is found in the oesophagus. *Source*: Tortora and Derrickson (2009). Reproduced with permission of John Wiley & Sons.

squamous epithelial tissue lines wet areas of the body – the mouth, the tongue and the vagina for example (see Figure 4.7). Only the outer layers of stratified squamous epithelium are actually squamous in shape; the basal layers may be cuboidal or columnar.

Stratified cuboidal epithelium is found in the oesophagus, sweat glands and in the male urethra (see Figure 4.8). **Stratified columnar epithelium**, however, is quite rare. Small amounts can be found in the male urethra and in the ducts of some glands. Another common example of stratified epithelium is **transitional epithelium**, which may have both squamous and cuboidal cells in its apical surface. The basal surface may contain both cuboidal and columnar cells. Transitional epithelium can withstand a great deal of stretch and is found in organs such as the bladder, which is subject to considerable distension (see Figure 4.9).

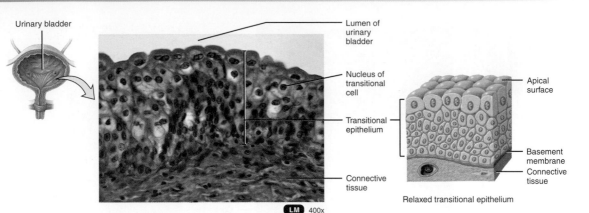

Sectional view of transitional epithelium of urinary bladder in relaxed state

Figure 4.9   Transitional epithelium lines the bladder and allows for distension. *Source*: Tortora and Derrickson (2009). Reproduced with permission of John Wiley & Sons.

Glandular epithelia

The glands of the body are formed by glandular epithelia. All glands are classified as *endocrine* or *exocrine*. Glands that secrete their products internally are called endocrine glands. Endocrine glands release hormones, regulatory chemicals for use elsewhere in the body (see Chapter 15). Exocrine glands release their products onto the surface of epithelial tissue. Exocrine glands are either *unicellular* or *multicellular*. Unicellular exocrine glands consist of a single cell type and the main example is the goblet cell, which releases a glycoprotein called mucin. Once dissolved in water mucin forms mucus, which lubricates and protects surfaces. Multicellular exocrine glands are far more complex, coming in several shapes and sizes. Some exocrine glands are simple and consist of a single branched duct, whereas others are more complex with multibranched ducts (see Figure 4.10). However, they all contain two distinct areas: an epithelial duct and secretory cells (acinus). Exocrine glands that are tubular in shape can be found within the digestive system and stomach. Other exocrine glands are spherical and referred to as alveolar or acinar. The oil glands within skin and mammary glands are two examples of spherical- or acinar-shaped exocrine glands. Glands that are both tubular and acinar are referred to as tubulacinar. The salivary glands, for example, are tubulacinar.

Connective tissue

Connective tissue is the most abundant tissue in the human body. Its main functions are to bind tissues together, reinforcement, insulation, protection and support. All epithelial tissue is reinforced by the connective tissue base it rests upon (see Figure 4.11). There are four types of connective tissue:

- connective tissue proper
- cartilage
- bone
- liquid connective tissue.

Connective tissue is not present on body surfaces and, unlike epithelial tissue, is highly vascular and receives a rich blood supply.

103

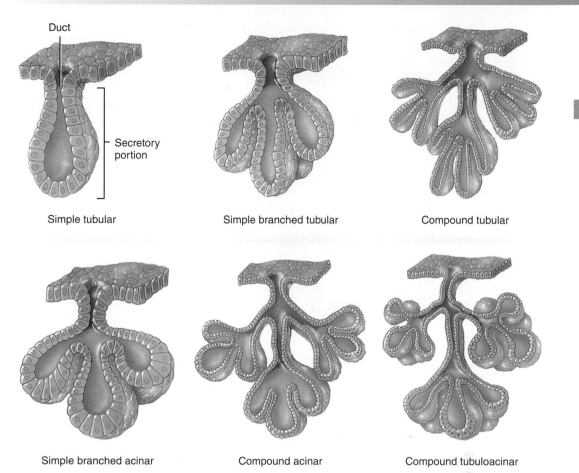

Figure 4.10 Exocrine glands classified by shape, with examples of location. *Source*: Tortora and Derrickson (2009). Reproduced with permission of John Wiley & Sons.

The following types of cell are present in connective tissue

- adipocytes
- primary blast cells
- macrophages
- plasma cells
- mast cells
- leucocytes (white blood cells).

Adipocytes are fat cells. Within connective tissue adipocytes store triglycerides (fats). Primary blast cells continually secrete ground substance and produce mature connective tissue cells. Each type of connective tissue contains its own unique primary blast cells (see Table 4.1). Macrophages, plasma cells and white blood cells form part of the body's immune system. Their functions are as follows:

- Macrophages engulf invading substances and plasma cells produce antibodies.
- White blood cells are not normally found in significant numbers within connective tissue; however, they do migrate into connective tissue during inflammation.
- Mast cells produce histamine, which promotes vasodilatation during the body's inflammatory response.

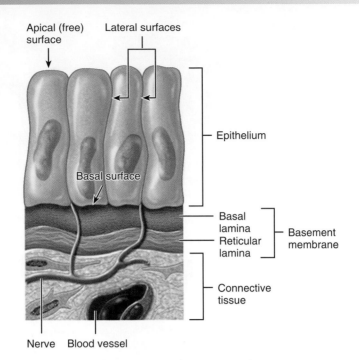

Figure 4.11 Connective tissue reinforces epithelial tissue. *Source*: Tortora and Derrickson (2009). Reproduced with permission of John Wiley & Sons.

Table 4.1 The major primary blast cells and their connective tissue type

Connective tissue type	Primary blast cell	Connective tissue cell
Connective tissue proper	Fibroblast	Fibrocyte
Cartilage	Chondroblast	Chondrocyte
Bone	Osteoblast	Osteocyte

Connective tissue cells are surrounded by a collection of substances referred to as the extracellular matrix. The function of the extracellular matrix is to ensure that connective tissue can bear weight and withstand tension, abuse and abrasion. As a result, connective tissue can cope with stresses and strains other tissues would not be able to tolerate. The two main elements of extracellular matrix are:

- ground substance
- fibres.

Ground substance: This consists of interstitial fluid, cell adhesion proteins and glycoaminoglycans. Cell adhesion proteins act as connective glue, keeping the tissue cells together. Glycoaminoglycans trap water and ensure ground substance has a jelly-like constitution. The higher the amount of glycoaminoglycans present the harder the ground substance will be.

Fibres: There are three types of fibre found within extracellular matrix:

- collagen
- elastic
- reticular.

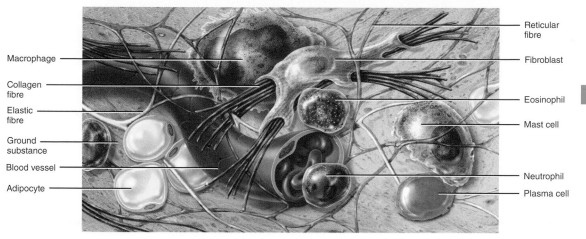

Macrophage

Collagen
fibre

Elastic
fibre

Ground
substance

Blood vessel

Adipocyte

Reticular
fibre

Fibroblast

Eosinophil

Mast cell

Neutrophil

Plasma cell

Figure 4.12 Constituents of connective tissue. *Source*: Tortora and Derrickson (2009). Reproduced with permission of John Wiley & Sons.

Collagen fibres are the most abundant fibre found within the extracellular matrix and are essentially the protein collagen. Collagen is very tough; indeed, collagen fibres are stronger than similar-sized steel fibres (Marieb and Hoehn, 2008). **Reticular fibres** are much thinner but also contain bundles of collagen. They provide support and strength and are found in greater numbers in soft organs such as the spleen and lymph nodes. **Elastic fibres** contain the rubber-like protein called elastin, which facilitates stretch and recoil. Elastic fibres are found in greater numbers in tissue that has to endure stretch, such as skin and blood vessel walls (see Figure 4.12).

Connective tissue proper

Aside from cartilage, bone and blood, all connective tissue belongs to this class. Connective tissue proper is subdivided further into

- loose connective tissue
- dense connective tissue.

Loose connective tissue contains fewer fibres than dense connective tissue (see Table 4.2).

Loose connective tissue

There are three types of loose connective tissue:

- areolar
- adipose
- reticular.

Areolar is the most abundant loose connective tissue. It contains all three fibres (collagen, elastic and reticular) and its primary functions are support, elasticity and strength. Areolar tissue is combined with adipose tissue to form the subcutaneous layer, which connects skin with other tissues and organs.

Adipose tissue contains adipocytes, whose primary function is to store triglycerides (fat). The primary functions of adipose tissue are to provide insulation, protection and an energy store.

Table 4.2   Types of connective tissue proper, their main constituents, functions and locations

Connective tissue	Main constituent	Functions	Main locations
Loose areolar	Collagen, elastic, reticular fibres	Strength Elasticity Support	Subcutaneous layer beneath skin
Loose adipose	Adipocytes	Insulation Protection Energy store	Subcutaneous layer beneath skin Tissue surrounding heart and kidneys Padding around joints
Loose reticular	Reticular fibres Reticular cells	Support Filtration	Liver Spleen Lymph nodes
Dense regular	Collagen fibres in parallel	Strength Support	Tendons Ligaments
Dense irregular	Collagen fibres arranged randomly	Strength	Skin Heart Tissue surrounding bone Tissue surrounding cartilage
Dense elastic	Elastic fibres	Stretch	Lung tissue Arteries

Reticular tissue only contains reticular fibres. Its main function is to form a protective framework or stroma that surrounds the liver, spleen and lymph nodes. Within the spleen, reticular connective tissue can also filter blood, assisting with the removal of old blood cells.

Dense connective tissue

Dense connective tissue contains more collagen or elastic fibres. Dense connective tissue that is made primarily from collagen is said to be either **regular** or **irregular** depending on the organisation of the collagen fibres. Dense regular connective tissue contains collagen fibres that are arranged in parallel rows. It has a silvery appearance and is both tough and pliable. Dense, irregular connective tissue is found in ligaments and tendons. Its collagen fibres are randomly arranged but closely knitted together. Dense irregular tissue can withstand pressure and pulling forces and is found in skin and the heart as well as the membranes that surround cartilage and bone. Dense elastic connective tissue consists of elastic fibres. Dense elastic connective tissue is found in areas of the body that have to withstand great amounts of stretch, such as arteries and lung tissue.

Cartilage

Cartilage contains a compact network of collagen fibres and is stronger than both loose and dense connective tissue. It has the ability to return to its original shape after stress and movement. Its strength and resilience are provided by a gel-like substance called **chondroitin sulphate**, which is found in cartilage ground substance. Cartilage is surrounded by a layer of dense irregular tissue called **perichondrium**. Perichondrium is the only area of cartilage that is served by blood and nervous tissue. There are three types of cartilage:

- hyaline
- fibrocartilage
- elastic.

Hyaline cartilage is the most common cartilage in the human body. It mainly comprises collagen fibres with cartilage cells, with chondrocytes accounting for around 10% of its volume. The collagen fibres are so fine they are almost invisible, giving hyaline cartilage a bluish appearance. Because hyaline cartilage is both strong and flexible it can act as a shock absorber, reducing friction around joints. Hyaline cartilage is also found in the rib cage and airways.

Elastic cartilage is almost identical to hyaline cartilage. The major difference between hyaline and elastic cartilage is the greater presence of elastic fibres. Elastic cartilage can withstand greater movement and bending and is found in areas of the body where stretchability is required, the outer ear for example.

Fibrocartilage is the strongest of the three cartilages. Its strength is provided by rows of chondrocytes and collagen. Because it can withstand great pressure it is found where hyaline cartilage meets tendons or ligaments, between the discs of the vertebrae for example (see Figure 4.13).

Bone

Along with cartilage, bones make up the human skeletal frame. Bone is similar to cartilage but contains even greater amounts of collagen. For this reason bone is harder and more rigid, facilitating greater protection and support for body structures. However, unlike cartilage, bone receives a rich supply of blood. Bone also stores fat and plays an important role in the production of blood cells. A more detailed examination of bones can be found in Chapter 5.

Liquid connective tissue

Connective tissue that has a liquid extracellular matrix includes:

- blood
- lymph.

Blood and lymph are said to be atypical connective tissues because, strictly speaking, they do not connect tissues or provide mechanical support. The extracellular matrix of blood is plasma. Blood cells include erythrocytes, leucocytes and platelets. Blood and plasma perform many important functions. For a detailed explanation of blood, see Chapter 7. Lymph has a clear extracellular matrix very similar to plasma. The primary function of lymph is defence against invading pathogens. A more detailed exploration of lymph can be found in Chapter 16.

Membranes

Membranes are sheets of tissue that cover or line areas of the human body. Structurally, membranes consist of an epithelial tissue layer that is bound to a basement layer of connective tissue. There are four major types of membrane:

- cutaneous
- mucous
- serous
- synovial.

Cutaneous membranes

The principal example of a cutaneous membrane is skin. It consists of an outer stratified squamous epithelial layer, which sits on top of a thick layer of dense irregular connective tissue. Chapter 17 is dedicated to the functions and structure of skin.

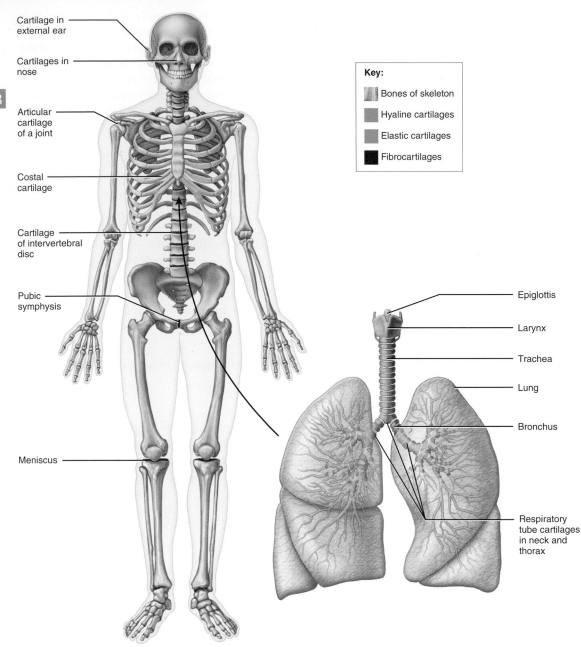

Figure 4.13   Where cartilage is found within the body. *Source*: Jenkins *et al*. (2007). Reproduced with permission of John Wiley & Sons.

Mucous membranes

Mucous membranes line the external surfaces of body cavities. Examples include hollow organs of the digestive tract, the respiratory system and the renal system. All mucous membranes are wet or moist, but not all secrete lubricating mucus. The mucous membranes of the renal system, for example, are wet due to the presence of urine. Most mucous membranes contain stratified squamous or simple columnar epithelium supported by a layer of connective tissue referred to as **lamina propria**.

Serous membranes

Serous membranes or a *serosa* cover internal body cavities. They consist of areolar connective tissue that is covered by a special kind of simple squamous epithelium called **mesothelium**. Mesothelium secretes a watery substance referred to as serous fluid, which allows organs to slide against one another with ease. Serous membranes consist of an outer or **parietal** layer and an inner or **visceral** layer. The largest example is the peritoneum, which lines the organs of the abdominopelvic cavity. The protective lining of the lungs, the parietal and visceral pleura, provides another example of an important serous membrane. The parietal and visceral pleura glide over one another when the thorax expands on inspiration.

Synovial membranes

Unlike serous, mucous and cutaneous membranes, synovial membranes do not contain any epithelial tissue. Synovial membranes are mainly found in moving joints and consist of areolar connective tissue, adipocytes, and elastic and collagen fibres. They secrete synovial fluid, which bathes, nourishes and lubricates the joints. Synovial fluid also contains macrophages, which destroy invading microbes and remove debris from the joint cavity. Synovial membranes are also found in cushion-like sacs in the hands and feet that ease the movement of tendons (see Figure 4.14).

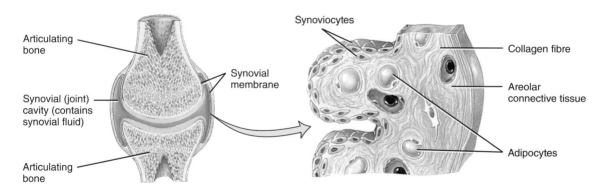

Figure 4.14 Synovial membranes fill joint cavities. *Source*: Tortora and Derrickson (2009). Reproduced with permission of John Wiley & Sons.

Clinical considerations

Peritonitis

Peritonitis is the inflammation of the peritoneum, the serous membrane that lines both the digestive organs and the wall of the abdominopelvic cavity. The causes of peritonitis are either **chemical** or **bacterial**. Chemical peritonitis results from damage to neighbouring structures; that is, a piercing wound or ulcer that leaks digestive juices into the peritoneum. Bacterial peritonitis results from the direct contamination of the peritoneum; that is, a burst appendix or perforated bowel. If left unaddressed, chemical peritonitis will lead to bacterial peritonitis.

Peritonitis is an acute medical emergency and is associated with high mortality. Survival rates have increased since the use of prophylactic antibiotics (Lawrence *et al.*, 2003; Gould, 2014).

Clinical considerations

Pneumothorax

A pneumothorax or collapsed lung occurs when air accumulates in the pleural cavity, the small space between the visceral and parietal pleura. It most often occurs as the result of trauma but can also occur in chronic lung disease. In a small number of cases the pleura separate spontaneously due to a congenital defect. In small pneumothoraces the lungs will reinflate over time, but large pneumothoraces are potentially life threatening. Chest drains are often inserted to remove the air from the pleura and allow the lungs to reinflate (Ryan, 2005; Sullivan, 2008).

Muscle tissue

Muscle tissue contains long muscle fibres whose primary function is to generate force. Muscle tissue is found where there is a need for movement and maintenance of posture. Muscle is classified in three ways:

- skeletal
- smooth
- cardiac.

Skeletal muscle is found adjacent to the skeleton and its function is twofold: the movement of the skeleton and the maintenance of body posture. The structure of the muscle fibres within skeletal muscle gives a striped or **striated** appearance. Skeletal muscle is also voluntary, meaning its movement can be controlled by conscious control (see Figure 4.15).

(a)

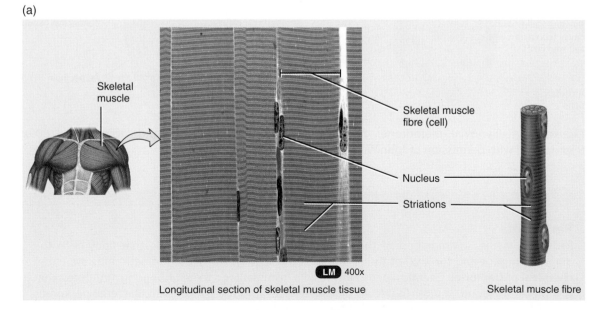

Skeletal muscle

Skeletal muscle fibre (cell)

Nucleus

Striations

LM 400x

Longitudinal section of skeletal muscle tissue

Skeletal muscle fibre

Figure 4.15   The major muscle types with examples of their location: (a) skeletal muscle; (b) cardiac muscle; (c) smooth muscle. *Source*: Tortora and Derrickson (2009). Reproduced with permission of John Wiley & Sons.

(b)

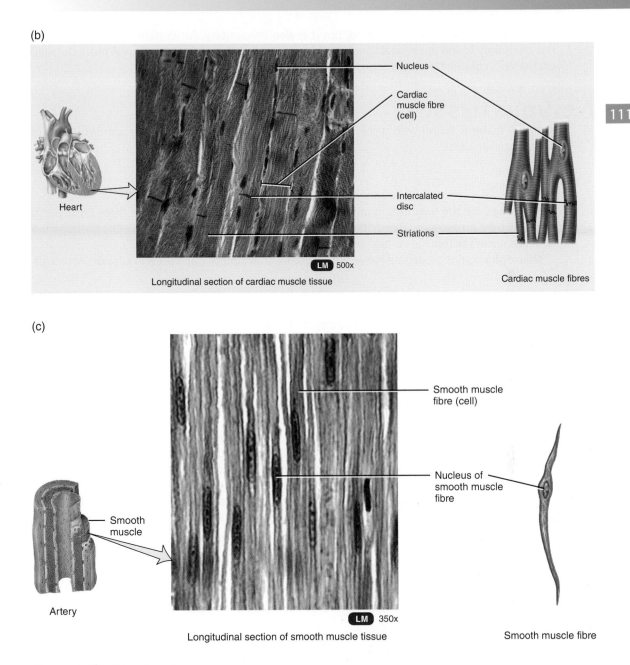

LM 500x

Longitudinal section of cardiac muscle tissue

Cardiac muscle fibres

(c)

Longitudinal section of smooth muscle tissue

LM 350x

Smooth muscle fibre

Figure 4.15 (*Continued*)

Smooth muscle, on the other hand, is both involuntary and **non-striated**. Smooth muscle is found in hollow internal structures where fluid or solid substances need to be propelled from one area to another. Smooth muscle is found in blood vessels, where blood is propelled through the vascular system, and the gastrointestinal tract, where chyme is moved from the stomach through the intestines towards the rectum.

Cardiac muscle muscle is striated, but it is also involuntary. As its name suggests, cardiac muscle is only found in the heart and provides the driving force of contraction. A more detailed examination of muscle can be found in Chapter 6.

Nervous tissue

Nervous tissue is found within the nervous system (see Chapter 13). There are two types of nervous tissue cells:

- neurones
- neuroglia.

Neurones are the functioning unit of the nervous system. They consist of three basic parts: the cell body, an axon and dendrites (see Figure 4.16). Their primary function is the propagation of nerve signals within the central and peripheral nervous systems.

Neuroglia do not propagate nerve signals; rather, they nourish, protect and support neurones.

Tissue repair

Tissue repair occurs in order to replace cells that are damaged, worn out or dead. Each of the four tissue types has the capacity to regenerate and replace cells injured by trauma, disease or other events. However, the tissue types have differing success rates. Because epithelial cells have to withstand large amounts of wear and tear they have great capacity for renewal. Epithelial tissue often contains immature cells called stem cells, which can divide and replace lost cells easily. Most connective tissue also has great capacity for renewal; however, owing to the lack of blood supply, cartilage can take a long time to heal.

Muscle and nervous tissue by comparison have poor regeneration properties. Skeletal muscle and smooth muscle fibres divide very slowly, and mitosis does not occur in cardiac muscle tissue. Stem cells migrate from blood to the heart where they divide and produce a small number of new cardiac muscle fibres. Nervous tissue does not normally undergo mitosis to replace damaged neurones.

Tissue repair involves the proliferation of new cells, which stem from cell division in the parenchyma (tissue cells/organ cells) or from the stroma (supporting connective tissue). The replenishing

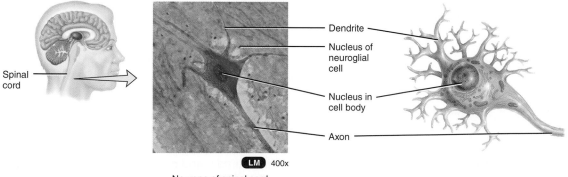

Spinal cord

Dendrite

Nucleus of neuroglial cell

Nucleus in cell body

Axon

LM 400x

Neurone of spinal cord

Figure 4.16   An example of nervous tissue. Source: Tortora and Derrickson (2009). Reproduced with permission of John Wiley & Sons.

of tissue by parenchymal and stroma cells is called **regeneration**. If parenchymal cells are solely responsible for tissue repair, then a near-perfect regeneration may occur. If fibroblasts from stroma are involved in tissue repair, new connective tissue is generated to replace the damaged tissue. This new connective tissue, primarily consisting of collagen, is referred to as **scar tissue**. The process of scar tissue generation is called **fibrosis**. Unlike cells regenerated from parenchymal cells, scar tissue cells are not designed to perform the original functions of the damaged cells. Therefore, any organ or structure with scar tissue will have impaired function.

In open or large wounds **granulation** occurs. Granulation describes the formation of granulation tissue, which covers the healing tissue and secretes bacterial fluid. During this process both parenchymal and stromal cells are active in the repair. Fibroblasts provide new collagen tissue to strengthen the area, and new blood capillaries sprout new buds and bring the necessary nutrients to the area.

Clinical considerations

Diabetic foot ulcers

Between 12 and 25% of diabetic patients develop leg and foot ulcers. This is because diabetes can cause macroangiopathy, which obstructs blood flow in large arteries. The slower flow of blood through the arteries in legs results in the development of leg and foot ulcers. Diabetic patients also experience lengthy recovery times from leg and foot injuries. The lack of blood flow also reduces the tissue's ability to fight off infection. Diabetic patients are therefore at increased risk of developing gangrene and amputation (Cavanagh *et al.*, 2005; Gould, 2014).

Conclusion

All human cells can be categorised into four classifications: epithelial tissue, connective tissue, muscle tissue and nervous tissue. Epithelial tissue covers or lines structures and organs. It specialises in absorption, secretion, protection, excretion, filtration and sensory reception. Almost every substance that passes in and out of the body travels through epithelial tissue. Connective tissue not only connects tissues, it also protects, supports and insulates them. Connective tissue is dense and strong; examples include cartilage and bone. Muscle tissue provides movement and posture, whereas nervous tissue forms the major part of the nervous system. Tissue has the ability to regenerate and renew itself; however, epithelial and connective tissues have a greater capacity for repair than other tissues.

Glossary

Abdominopelvic cavity   Body cavity that encompasses the abdominal and pelvic cavities. The abdominal cavity contains the stomach, intestines, spleen, liver and other associated digestive organs. The pelvic cavity contains the bladder and some reproductive organs.

Apical surface   Surface of body organ that faces outwards, towards the surface.

Avascular   Structure that does not contain blood vessels.

Basal surface   Surface that forms the base of a body organ.

113

Cartilage   Strong form of connective tissue that contains a dense network of collagen and elastic fibres.

Chyme   A fluid substance consisting of partially digested food and digestive enzymes, which is found travelling through the digestive tract.

Connective tissue   Tissue that binds, reinforces, insulates, protects and supports structures.

Diffusion   The movement of particles from areas of high concentration to low concentration.

Endocrine gland   Glands that release hormones.

Epithelial tissue   Tissue that lines or covers body surfaces.

Exocrine glands   Glands that secrete their products externally (i.e. mucus, sweat).

Extracellular matrix   A collection of largely non-living substances that separate the living cells of connective tissue.

Gland   A structure that manufactures a product (e.g. hormones, mucus, sweat).

Glycoproteins   Special proteins that contain simple sugar chains. Glycoproteins play an important role in cell-to-cell communication.

Hormones   Regulatory chemicals released by endocrine glands for use elsewhere in the body (e.g. thyroxine, insulin).

Innervated (innervate)   Stimulated by nerve cells.

Interstitial fluid   The fluid that bathes cells.

Keratin   A special tough fibrous protein found in skin.

Lymph nodes   Small lymphatic structures that filter lymphatic fluid.

Macrophages   White blood cells that specialise in the destruction and consumption of invading pathogens.

Membrane   A sheet of tissue that covers or lines an area of the body.

Mitosis   The division and replication of cells.

Neuroglia   Cells of the nervous system that support and nourish neurones.

Neurone   A nerve fibre.

Parenchyma   The cells that constitute the function part of an organ.

Prophylactic antibiotics   Antibiotics prescribed to prevent infection.

Oocytes   Female reproductive cell.

Spleen   Large lymph organ, responsible for production of lymphocytes, immune response and the cleansing of blood.

Stroma   The internal framework of an organ.

Subcutaneous   Underneath the skin.

Vertebrae   The disc-shaped bones that make up the spinal column.

References

Cavanagh, P.R., Lipsky, B.A., Bradbury, A.W. and Botek, G. (2005) Treatment for diabetic foot ulcers. *Lancet* **366**: 1725–1735.

Gould, B.E. (2014) *Pathophysiology for the Health Professions*, 5th edn. Philadelphia, PA: Saunders Elsevier.

Jenkins, G.W., Kemnitz, C.P. and Tortora, G.J. (2007) *Anatomy and Physiology from Science to Life*. Hoboken, NJ: John Wiley & Sons, Inc.

Lawrence, K.R., Adra, M. and Schwaitzberg, S.D. (2003) An overview of the pathophysiology and treatment of secondary peritonitis. *Formulary* **38**: 102–111.

Marieb, E. and Hoehn, K. (2008) *Human Anatomy and Physiology*, 8th edn. San Francisco, CA: Pearson Benjamin Cummings.

Ryan, B. (2005) Pneumothorax assessment and diagnostic testing. *Journal of Cardiovascular Nursing* **20**(4): 251–253.

Sullivan, B. (2008) Nursing management of patients with a chest drain. *British Journal of Nursing* **17**(6): 388–393.

Tortora, G.J. and Derrickson, B.H. (2009) *Principles of Anatomy and Physiology*, 12th edn. Hoboken, NJ: John Wiley & Sons, Inc.

Activities

Multiple choice questions

1. Which of the following epithelial tissues has a single layer of square-shaped cells?
   - (a) pseudostratified columnar epithelium
   - (b) ciliated simple columnar epithelium
   - (c) simple cuboidal epithelium
   - (d) stratified cuboidal epithelium

2. Which of the following is not a function of simple epithelium?
   - (a) protection
   - (b) secretion
   - (c) absorption
   - (d) filtration

3. What is the primary function of transitional epithelium?
   - (a) absorption
   - (b) stretch
   - (c) secretion
   - (d) protection

4. Which fibres ensure that connective tissue is strong and tough?
   - (a) collagen fibres
   - (b) reticular fibres
   - (c) elastic fibres
   - (d) plasma fibres

5. Which of the following connective tissues stores triglycerides?
   - (a) areolar tissue
   - (b) adipose tissue
   - (c) dense regular connective tissue
   - (d) reticular tissue

6. Which of the following statements on cartilage is true?
   - (a) fibrocartilage is found within the ears
   - (b) elastic cartilage is almost identical to fibrocartilage

(c) hyaline cartilage is the most abundant in the human body
(d) the weakest cartilage tissue is fibrocartilage cartilage
7. Blood is an example of _____ connective tissue.
   (a) liquid
   (b) loose

   (c) avascular
   (d) dense
8. Which of the following areas does not contain mucous membranes?
   (a) the urinary tract
   (b) the respiratory system
   (c) the pericardium
   (d) the digestive tract
9. Smooth muscle is both:
   (a) involuntary and striated
   (b) involuntary and non-striated
   (c) voluntary and striated
   (d) voluntary and non-striated
10. Scar tissue is generated by:
   (a) fibroblasts
   (b) osteoblasts
   (c) stem cells
   (d) parenchymal cells

True or false

1. Simple epithelial consists of a single layer of cells.
2. Simple squamous epithelial tissue provides tough protection.
3. Cuboidal cells are flat and scaly in appearance.
4. Transitional epithelium may have both cuboidal and columnar cells in its apical surface.
5. The glands of the body are formed by glandular epithelium.
6. Connective tissue is the most abundant tissue in the human body.
7. There are five types of loose connective tissue.
8. Elastic cartilage is the most common cartilage in the human body.
9. Skin is a good example of a cutaneous membrane.
10. Skeletal muscle is both striated and voluntary.

Label the diagram 1

Label the diagram using the following list of words:

Arrangement of layers, Simple, Pseudostratified, Stratified, Basement membrane, Cell shape, Squamous, Cuboidal, Columnar, Basement membrane

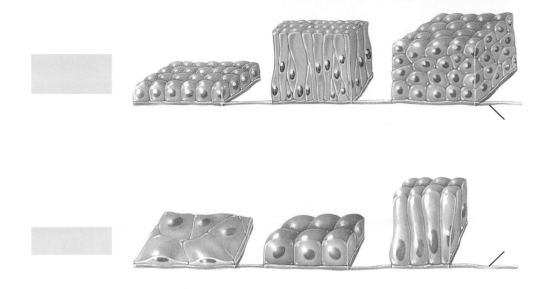

Label the diagram 2

Label the diagram using the following list of words:

Duct, Secretory portion, Simple tubular, Simple branched tubular, Compound tubular, Simple branched acinar, Compound acinar, Compound tubuloacinar

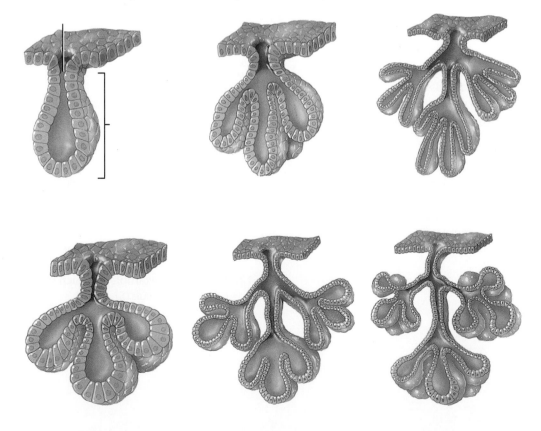

Crossword

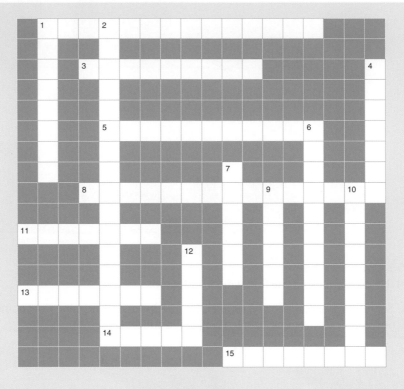

Across:

1. Epithelial tissue that consists of a single layer of square-shaped cells (6, 8).
3. Type of loose connective tissue (9).
5. Bone cells (11).
8. Forms a substantial part of the extracellular matrix (6, 9).
11. Type of dense connective tissue (7).
13. Most abundant type of cartilage (7).
14. _____ connective tissue can be regular, or irregular (5).
15. Major constituent of bone (8).

Down:

1. Type of muscle (8).
2. Word that describes single-layered epithelial tissue that contains different shaped cells (16).
4. Fat tissue (7).
6. Word used to describe multilayered epithelial tissue (10).
7. _____ membranes have wet or moist surfaces (6).
9. _____ membranes cover organs that lie within a cavity (6).
10. Type of connective tissue that is avascular (9).
12. Areolar is an example of which type of connective tissue (5).

Word search

A	C	N	Q	C	E	R	D	O	O	L	B	T	E	Y
P	O	O	O	I	A	D	I	P	O	S	E	L	U	B
L	N	I	L	K	J	R	H	G	F	D	C	S	O	E
M	N	T	N	L	B	V	T	C	X	S	Z	N	A	L
Q	E	P	W	E	A	R	T	I	U	Y	E	U	I	A
R	C	R	J	K	L	G	E	M	L	P	O	M	E	S
A	T	O	H	G	F	N	E	D	S	A	U	A	N	T
L	I	S	B	V	I	C	S	N	X	I	G	Z	A	I
U	V	B	N	L	M	E	A	Q	L	Q	W	E	R	C
D	E	A	A	I	R	S	U	E	U	Y	T	R	B	E
N	O	Y	P	B	U	L	H	K	J	A	H	G	M	F
A	H	B	I	O	V	T	C	X	Z	A	M	S	E	D
L	N	F	R	M	I	Q	W	E	R	T	Y	O	M	U
G	L	E	P	P	A	R	E	O	L	A	R	O	U	I
J	S	H	E	G	L	A	D	I	O	B	U	C	F	S

Absorption, Squamous, Epithelium, Cuboidal, Glandular, Connective, Cartilage, Bone, Blood, Collagen, Fibres, Elastic, Areolar, Adipose, Hyaline, Membrane, Serous, Muscle

Fill in the blanks

Muscle tissue contains _____ muscle fibres whose primary function is to generate _____. It is found where there is a need for _____ and _____. _____ muscle is found adjacent to the skeleton and is said to be _____ or stripy in appearance and _____ in action. _____ muscle, on the other hand, is _____ and _____. As its name suggests, _____ muscle is only found in the heart and provides the driving force of _____.

smooth, voluntary, movement, skeletal, contraction, long, striated, force, involuntary, cardiac, maintenance of posture, non-striated

Find out more

1. One function of epithelial tissue is sensory perception – explore what this term means.
2. What do you understand by the term cilia and what is their role in airway clearance?
3. Simple cuboidal epithelium is found in the ovaries and the tubules of the kidneys, what is the function of simple cuboidal epithelium in these organs?
4. Stratified cuboidal epithelium is found within the oesophagus and sweat glands, what is the function of stratified cuboidal epithelium in these organs?

5. Discuss the differences between endocrine and exocrine glands.
6. Investigate the function of adipose tissue and explore its use as an energy store.
7. Explore the medical and nursing care of patients with cartilage injuries.
8. What would the key nursing care interventions be when caring for a patient undergoing a blood transfusion?
9. Discuss the role of the nurse and healthcare team in the care of a patient with peritonitis.
10. What is the role of the nurse and other healthcare professionals in the prevention of wound infection?

Chapter 5

The skeletal system

Ian Peate

Test your prior knowledge

- Why is calcium an important mineral in respect to bone?
- What do you understand by the skeletal system?
- What are the functions of the skeletal system?
- Why do babies have more bones than adults?
- What makes bones so strong?
- How does spongy bone differ from compact bone?
- Compare the appendicular and axial skeletons.
- What are the regions of the vertebral column?
- How many bones make up the cranium?
- What is synovial fluid and where is it found?

Learning outcomes

After reading this chapter you will be able to:

- Discuss the function of the skeletal system
- Describe the divisions of the skeleton
- List the four general bone categories
- Discuss bone composition
- Describe the various joints
- Understand the organisation of bone based on shape

Fundamentals of Anatomy and Physiology: For Nursing and Healthcare Students, Second Edition. Edited by Ian Peate and Muralitharan Nair.
© 2017 John Wiley & Sons, Ltd. Published 2017 by John Wiley & Sons, Ltd.
Student companion website: www.wileyfundamentalseries.com/anatomy
Instructor companion website: www.wiley.com/go/instructor/anatomy

Body map

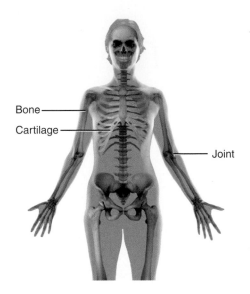

Bone

Cartilage

Joint

Introduction

Despite what seems to be a solid, dry, inert material, bone is in fact a complex living organism that is being recreated constantly; bone is metabolically active. As old bone dies new bone is being rebuilt. There are a number of complex activities occurring as bone is destroyed and reformed. Bones are therefore living organs that are made up of a number of different tissues, and this includes bone tissue.

The human skeleton, in contrast to other skeletons, is built to move erect as opposed to walking on all fours. The skeleton provides us with shape and the power to move, but it cannot do this in isolation. It needs many other systems of the body for it to function properly – for example, the nervous system and the muscles and for the body to move in its various and complex ways (the spine, for example, allows us to twist and bend); this is attributed to the joints and their ability to articulate.

Like a house, the human body needs a framework, but the framework for the body is not made of wood and steel as is the case with the house. The skeletal system is made up of bones, ligaments and tendons. The human skeleton is built to take the hard knocks of life. It is an engineering wonder; for its weight, bone is nearly as strong as steel.

The skeleton produces blood cells. The bones also act as storage areas for minerals, vital for blood clotting, nerve function and contraction of muscles. The bones begin to form *in utero* and continue to grow into adulthood. Bones develop from cartilage, so infants are born with large amounts of cartilage as well as having more bones than adults. As the child ages, the bones usually fuse together and the child ends up with the normal adult number of bones. The bones of babies are soft, but as more minerals are deposited they become harder – this is known as ossification.

The axial and appendicular skeleton

There are 206 named bones in the adult human skeleton. For classification purposes the skeleton is divided into two parts: the axial skeleton and the appendicular skeleton. Both have their own purposes.

Table 5.1 The bones of the axial skeleton

Structure	Number of bones
Skull	
Cranium	8
Face	14
Total	**22**
Hyoid	1
Auditory ossicles (bones)	6
Vertebral column	26
Thorax	
Sternum	1
Ribs	24
Total	**25**
Total number of bones in the axial skeleton	**80**

The axial skeleton

The axial skeleton forms the central axis of the body and consists of 80 bones. This part of the skeleton supports the head (including the bones in the ear), neck and the torso (this is also referred to as the trunk). It consists of the skull, the vertebral column, the ribs and the sternum. The 80 bones in the axial skeleton are noted in Table 5.1.

The appendicular skeleton

The bones of the appendicular skeleton are those bones of the upper and lower extremities – the arms and the legs as well as the bones that attach them to the axial skeleton. There are 126 bones in the appendicular skeleton, and these bones are shown in Table 5.2.

See Figure 5.1 depicting the human skeleton.

Bone and its functions

The skeletal system – and this includes the bones of the skeleton, the ligaments, cartilage and connective tissues that provide stability or attach the bones – has a number of key functions:

1. provides support
2. enables movement
3. stores minerals and lipids
4. protects the body
5. produces blood cells.

Support

Apart from bone and cartilage, all body tissue is soft, and without the skeleton the body would be jelly-like and would not be able to stand up. The way the bones are arranged provides the body with its shape/form. The skeletal system provides structural support for the body, providing a bony framework for the attachment of soft tissues and organs.

Table 5.2   The bones of the appendicular skeleton

Structure	Number of bones
Pectoral girdle	
Clavicle	2
Scapula	2
Total	**4**
Upper limbs	
Humerus	2
Ulna	3
Radius	4
Carpals	16
Metacarpals	10
Phalanges	28
Total	**60**
Pelvic girdle	
Pelvic bone	2
Lower limbs	
Femur	2
Patella	2
Fibula	3
Tibia	3
Tarsals	14
Metatarsals	10
Phalanges	28
Total	**60**
Total number of bones in the appendicular skeleton	**126**
Total number of bones in the adult human skeleton	**206**

Snapshot

Bone scan

Radionuclide scans can detect abnormalities such as fractures, bone infections, arthritis, rickets and tumours that have metastasised, and other diseases.

A bone scan involves the intravenous injection into a peripheral vein of a very small amount of radioactive material (radiotracer). The substance travels through the bloodstream to the bones and organs. As it decays, it emits a small amount of gamma radiation that is detected by a camera (gamma camera) that slowly scans the body. When the tracer has collected in the target organ the area is scanned.

To evaluate metastatic bone disease, images are taken after a 3- to 4-h delay. The scanning aspect of the test lasts approximately 1 h. The scanner's camera moves above and around the person, and the person may be required to change positions.

Prior to the test the person is required to remove jewelry and other metal objects and to wear a hospital gown. The patient should inform the doctor or radiographer if they are or may be pregnant. The person should not take any medicine with bismuth in it for 4 days before the test.

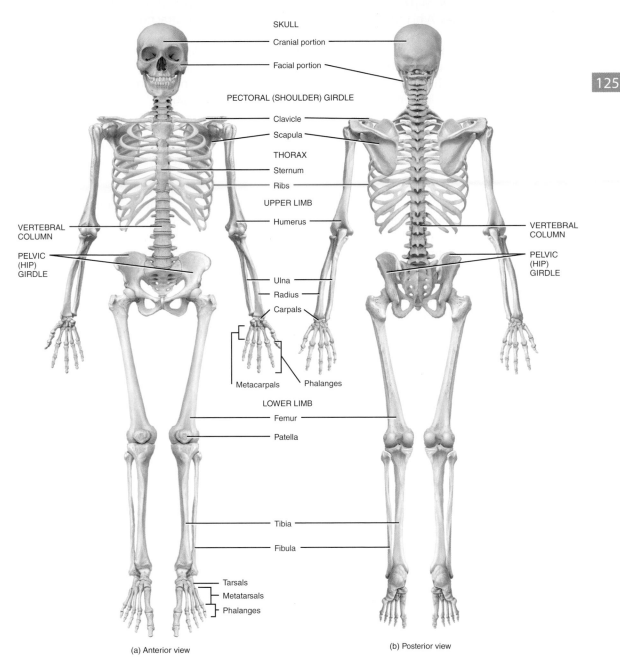

Figure 5.1 The human skeleton (a) anterior view, (b) posterior view. Axial skeleton blue and appendicular skeleton white. *Source*: Tortora and Derrickson (2009). Reproduced with permission of John Wiley & Sons.

Movement

The skeleton allows and enables movement. The bones act as levers, providing the transmission of muscular forces. A number of bones can (through leverage, contracting and pulling) change the extent and direction of the forces generated by skeletal muscles, through the work of the tendons and the ligaments. These movements can be very intricate, such as the ability to write, the ability to thread a needle (the coordination of fine movement), to gross movement, such as the ability to change body posture. The skeleton with the interaction of muscles permits breathing to occur. Movement becomes possible through articulation.

Clinical considerations

Gout

This is an acute inflammatory joint disease, an arthritis, resulting in an acute inflammatory state and tissue damage. The condition is very painful.

Gout is a disorder of metabolism where uric acid or urate accumulates in blood and tissues; when supersaturated urate salts precipitate they form needle-like crystals, occurring in cool, peripheral joints of the metatarsophalangeal joint of the big toe.

The condition can be classified into primary or secondary gout subject to the cause of hyperuricaemia, occurring mainly in men aged 30–60 years who present with acute attacks. It is often associated with osteoarthritis in the older person.

Gout affects the upper and lower limbs and can present with painful, tophaceous deposits (there may be discharge) in Heberden's and Bouchard's nodes.

The majority of people (about 90%) with gout develop excess urate as a result of an inability to excrete adequate amounts of uric acid in the urine.

Overproduction of uric acid occurs in disorders that cause high cell turnover, releasing purines. Cell death caused by chemotherapy can raise uric acid levels, as can excessive exercise and obesity. Causes of secondary gout as a result of underexcretion of uric acid include renal insufficiency, starvation or dehydration, some drugs and long-term abuse of alcohol (beer and spirits).

There are a number of comorbid conditions related to a higher incidence of gout; for example, hypertension, diabetes mellitus, renal insufficiency, hypertriglyceridaemia, hypercholesterolaemia, obesity and anaemia. Foods rich in purines (anchovies, sardines, sweetbreads, kidney, liver and meat extracts) and consumption of fructose-rich foods and beverages are associated with an increased risk of gout.

Storage

The bones are capable of storing essential minerals such as calcium, magnesium and phosphorus; calcium is the most abundant mineral in the human body. The bone also has the ability to release stored minerals in response to the body's demands; for example, when the amount of calcium in the blood is high (a high concentration) the calcium can be deposited in the bones. When calcium in the blood is low or it decreases, the bones give up calcium into the bloodstream. This ability to provide an internal homeostasis is regulated by hormones. Lipids are also stored in the yellow marrow of some bones; lipids are stored or released depending on the body's needs when providing energy.

Protection

Bone, a rigid structure, protects most of the soft tissues of the body and the internal organs; for example, the skull protects the brain, the sternum and ribs protect the lungs and heart, the spinal cord is protected by the vertebrae, the orbit protects the eyes and the periosteum protects the red bone marrow. The pelvis shields and protects the delicate internal abdominal digestive and reproductive organs.

Snapshot

Pathological fracture: Ann Di Silvestro

Ann is a 72-year-old lady who was diagnosed with osteoporosis 8 years ago; she has remained fit and healthy since diagnosis and has no other significant medical history. Ann was playing bowls with a group of her friends recently and when assuming an upright position from bowling suddenly experienced excruciating pain in her left hip; she was unable to bear weight. A paramedic was called and noted shortening in the left leg and external rotation of the limb. It was assumed at this point that Ann had sustained a left intertrochanteric hip fracture; she was transferred to hospital.

A pathological fracture occurs when a bone breaks in an area that is weakened by another disease process (in Ann's case this was osteoporosis). Causes of weakened bone include tumours, infection and some inherited bone disorders. There are many diseases and conditions that can lead to a pathological fracture.

A pathological fracture usually occurs when people are carrying out normal activities (Ann was playing bowls); they may be doing very routine activities when their bone suddenly fractures. The reason for this is the underlying disease process weakens the bone to the point where the bone is unable to perform its normal function.

In treating Ann, both the fracture and the underlying process had to be considered in order for her treatment to be safe and effective. In Ann's case her fracture required the same treatment as a normal fracture. The underlying osteoporosis was also reassessed and her treatment plan amended.

Production

There are some bones in the body that produce red and white blood cells; this is known as haematopoiesis. Haematopoiesis mainly occurs in red bone marrow. The red bone marrow fills the internal cavity of most bones; yellow bone marrow can also be found in some bones, but this is made up mainly of fat.

Clinical considerations

Red bone marrow

Understanding the role and function of bone marrow can aid the nurse helping people being cared for who may experience any condition affecting the bone marrow or its production.

Bone marrow is a spongy material that fills the bones. There are two types: yellow and red. Red bone marrow contains cells called stems cells; these are early blood cells. In the healthy person these blood cells grow and divide, providing the basis for the formation of new blood cells. Red bone marrow is only found in certain bones, for example, the pelvis, the sternum, the ends of the thigh and arm bones.

(Continued)

Some cancer drugs act on the bone marrow by slowing down the production of blood cells by killing them off as they grow and divide. Hence, some cancer treatment drugs – chemotherapy (and some biological therapies) – have the potential to help and to harm.

When white blood cells (the cells primarily responsible for fighting infection), for example, are killed off, this means the person may be at risk of developing an infection. When the red cells are killed off (these are the cells that have a key role to play in transporting oxygen around the body) a person may experience anaemia. The platelets, the cells responsible for helping the blood to clot, are also formed within the red bone marrow. A disruption in the production of platelets can also have health and well-being implications for the person being cared for. The person may bruise easily, bleed more than they usually do, even from small cuts or grazes when shaving for example, and experience nose bleeds (epistaxis).

When caring for a person who has problems with the bone marrow, for example, those with cancer, the nurse must be aware of the issues discussed above in order to provide safe and effective care.

Bone formation and growth (ossification)

The strength of bone comes from the protein matrix, which provides it with resilience and elasticity. This allows bone to give a little as it is comes under pressure. Within the bone are a number of minerals that have been deposited there; these add to the strength of bone, protecting it and supporting it as pressure and force are applied. It is important to understand how bone develops, as this can help understand its strengths and boundaries.

By the end of the third month of pregnancy the skeleton of a foetus is completely formed (Rizzo, 2006). Most of the skeleton at this stage is primarily cartilage; the formation of bone takes place as the pregnancy develops. The process of bone formation is known as ossification. Bone formation takes place during various phases of a person's life. Tortora and Derrickson (2012) discuss four principal situations in a person's life when bone formation occurs (see Table 5.3).

Embryonic formation

As the foetus develops, an embryonic skeleton is forming; at first this appears as mesenchyme, which is shaped similar to bones and in the sites where ossification will take place. Bone formation at this stage goes through a number of stages and changes. Hyaline cartilage develops from the mesenchyme. Osteoblasts converge on the cartilage and then the process of ossification begins.

Table 5.3   Bone formation throughout a person's life

Stage	Activity
1	The initial formation of bone *in utero* in the foetus
2	The growth of bones during infancy, childhood and adolescence
3	The replacement of old bone with new bone (bone remodelling) – this occurs throughout an individual's life
4	The repair of fractures that can occur throughout a person's life

Source: Adapted from Tortora and Derrickson (2013). Reproduced with permission of John Wiley & Sons.

Intramembranous ossification

The mesenchymal cells at the site of ossification – the ossification centre – cluster together and differentiate at first into osteogenic cells and then into osteoblasts. The extracellular matrix of bones is secreted by the osteoblasts. Secretion of extracellular matrix ceases and the cells, now known as osteocytes, sit within the lacunae. These cells have narrow cytoplasmic processes that extend into the canaliculi radiating in many different directions. After a few days the extracellular matrix calcifies (hardens) as a result of calcium and other minerals being deposited.

When the bone and the extracellular matrix form, these develop into trabeculae; the trabeculae fuse with one another and spongy bone is formed. Angiogenesis (blood vessel formation) occurs between the trabecular spaces. Red bone marrow is formed as the connective tissue within the trabeculae differentiates, and periosteum is formed as mesenchyme condenses along with the formation of trabeculae. Spongy bone remains in the centre despite a thin layer of compact bone forming on the surface of the spongy bones. The process outlined here is known as intramembranous ossification. Figure 5.2 provides an illustration of intramembranous ossification.

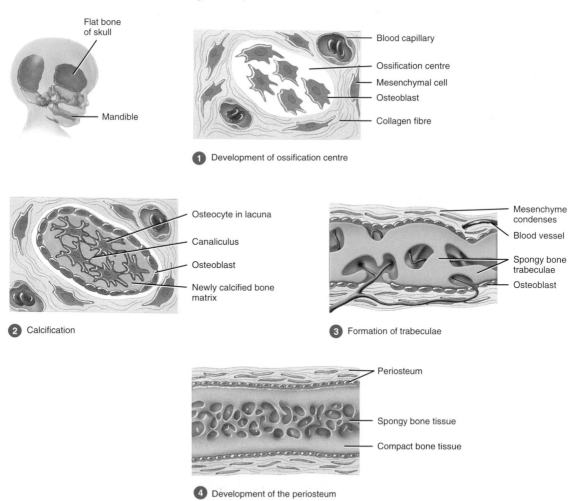

Figure 5.2   Intramembranous ossification. *Source*: Tortora and Derrickson (2009). Reproduced with permission of John Wiley & Sons.

Endochondral ossification

Cartilage that is replaced by bone is called endochondral ossification; the majority of bones in the body are formed in this way. Mesenchymal cells crowd together at the site where bone is going to form and they take on the shape of the future bone and develop into chondroblasts. These chondroblasts secrete the extracellular matrix and produce a cartilage model that is made up of hyaline cartilage. The perichondrium – a membrane – develops around the cartilage model.

As the chondroblasts become buried deep into the cartilage matrix they change and become chondrocytes. As growth continues through cell division the chondrocytes also grow and the extracellular matrix starts to calcify. The chondrocytes also start to die as they are unable to receive nutrients through the extracellular matrix; as death occurs, lacunae form and merge into small cavities.

A nutrient artery enters the perichondrium and the matrix that is calcifying; ossification occurs inwardly from the external surface of the bone. This activity encourages osteogenic bone cell production within the perichondrium to become (through differentiation) osteoblasts. The formation of bone is called periosteum; towards the centre the blood vessels grow, and eventually bone replaces most of the cartilage.

The bone marrow is developed as the primary ossification centre grows towards the ends of the bone; here, osteoblasts break down some of the newly formed spongy bone. As this action continues it produces a cavity, the medullary cavity (bone marrow), in the shaft of the bone (called the diaphysis).

Secondary ossification centres frequently develop prior to or just after birth when the blood vessels enter the epiphyses. Bone formation in secondary ossification is similar to that in primary ossification; however, there are no medullary cavities left. In secondary ossification the process occurs outwardly from the centre of the epiphysis towards the surface of the bone.

The articular cartilage and the epiphyseal plates are formed from the hyaline cartilage that covers the epiphyses. Before a person reaches adulthood, hyaline cartilage remains between the diaphysis and epiphysis. Figure 5.3 provides an illustration depicting endochondral ossification.

Bone length and thickness

As the person grows (e.g. during infancy, childhood and adolescence), long bones grow in length and thickness. This longitudinal growth and expansion of thickness continues until the person is usually 15 years of age in girls and 16 years of age in boys.

The chondrocytes present in the epiphyseal plate are constantly dividing, and this activity is related to the length of bone growth. As adolescence ends, the formation of new cells decreases, and between the ages of 18 and 25 years this activity ceases altogether.

Growth of bone (thickness) occurs as the cells in the perichondrium differentiate into osteoblasts; the osteoblasts then develop into osteocytes. Lamella are added to the bone surface, and osteons (the basic units of structure of the adult compact bone) are formed. Osteoblastic and osteoclastic activity occurs, and the result is an enlarged medullary cavity and thicker bone is formed.

Bone remodelling

As adolescence ends between the ages of 18 and 25 years, formation of new cells occurs and bone continually renews itself through bone remodelling. This happens when ongoing replace-ment of old bone is renewed by new bone. Remodelling takes place at different rates in different parts of the body. When bones reach their adult shapes the old bones are being repeatedly demolished and new bone is formed in its place; this clearly demonstrates that bone is a living, metabolising organ.

130

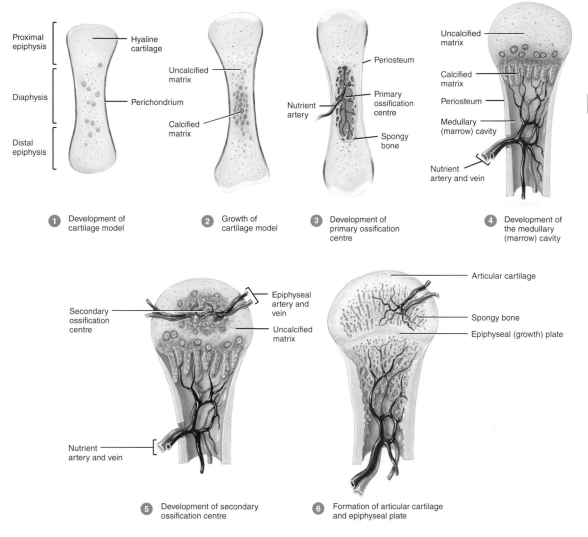

Figure 5.3 Endochondral ossification of the tibia. *Source*: Tortora and Derrickson (2009). Reproduced with permission of John Wiley & Sons.

Snapshot

Osteomyelitis: Vijay

Vijay Palmar, a 27-year-old accountant, plays squash; in a rather clumsy clash with one of the walls of the squash court he sustained a traumatic injury.

Osteomyelitis is a bone infection that can occur spontaneously or, in Vijay's case, following trauma or surgery on bones and joints. Implant-related bone infections, occurring after joint prosthesis (hip, knee, shoulder, ankle, etc.) or osteosynthesis (plates, screws, nails implant for fractures or osteotomies) are one of the most challenging complications in orthopaedic and trauma surgery, the condition often requires complex treatment in specialised centres.

(Continued)

Signs and symptoms of osteomyelitis include

- pyrexia or chills
- lethargy
- pain associated with the area of the infection
- swelling, warmth and redness over the area of the infection.

However, sometimes osteomyelitis causes no signs and symptoms or has signs and symptoms that may be difficult to distinguish from other problems. Owing to the structure of bone, this makes this infection a challenge, and often it will require surgical procedure(s) to remove the diseased or dead bone (osteonecrosis) and prolonged antibiotic therapy, for 6 weeks or more.

A fine balance must exist between the breakdown and build-up of bone: if bone is built up too quickly, then an abnormally thick and heavy bone will be formed. Weak bone, as a result of too much calcium or bone tissue loss, can result in bone that breaks easily.

Clinical considerations

Osteoarthritis

As a person ages, the action of bone breakdown and bone build-up continues. As well as breakdown and rebuilding, the bone also thickens and bone mass increases. Damage to joints, the tissues surrounding the joints and the bones themselves can also occur as the ageing process occurs.

The condition osteoarthritis is a degenerative non-inflammatory condition. It is more common in those people aged over 50 years; however, younger people can also be affected by this condition, and women suffer with osteoarthritis more than men do.

The joints are characteristically affected: damage appears to the cartilage, bony growths occur at the ends of the bones and around the joints, and synovitis can occur (inflammation of the tissues around the joints).

The impact of osteoarthritis will differ from person to person; the care of those with osteoarthritis will depend on the assessment of individual needs. There is no cure for osteoarthritis, but there are many interventions that can be implemented to help improve the health and well-being of the person being cared for.

A multidisciplinary approach to care is required, be this in a hospital setting or in the person's own home. Adjustments to lifestyle, for example, an increase in exercise and the modification of footwear can help. The administration of medicines to control pain and inflammation can also help the person carry out their activities of living in a more effective way, promoting independence.

Bone fractures

Tucker (2011) defines a fracture as the breakage of bone due either to an injury or disease. There are a number of types of fracture, including:

1. simple
2. compound
3. comminuted
4. greenstick (incomplete).

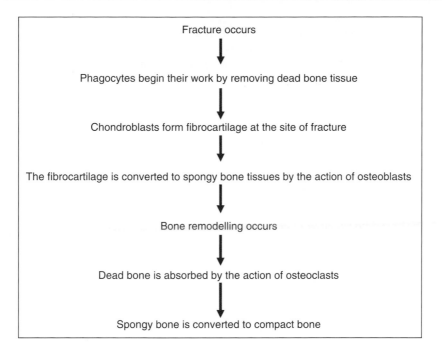

Fracture occurs

Phagocytes begin their work by removing dead bone tissue

Chondroblasts form fibrocartilage at the site of fracture

The fibrocartilage is converted to spongy bone tissues by the action of osteoblasts

Bone remodelling occurs

Dead bone is absorbed by the action of osteoclasts

Spongy bone is converted to compact bone

Figure 5.4   The stages a broken bone goes through for repair to occur.

The repair of a bone that has been broken (fractured) goes through a number of stages (see Figure 5.4). Although bone has a rich blood supply, healing can sometimes take many months. The break in the bone will interfere with the blood supply to the bone temporarily, and this will result in a delay in healing.

As a fracture occurs, phagocytes remove any dead bone tissues. Osteocytes will proliferate when a break in bone occurs as the fracture stimulates production. The bone will heal gradually as calcium and phosphorus (needed to strengthen and harden new bone) is deposited and bone cells slowly grow and duplicate. McRae (2006) suggests that full bone healing can take months to take place.

Bone has the capacity to regenerate and heal itself; the action of osteoblasts and osteoclasts produces new cells and removes those cells that have died. Tortora and Grabowski (2009) suggest that the balance of calcium is an essential requirement in bone growth and repair; this is affected by the level of vitamin D in the body as well as renal and intestinal functioning, parathyroid gland functioning and the ability of the adrenal glands to work effectively.

Medicines management

Arthrotec
Arthrotec is a drug that contains a combination of two drugs: diclofenac and misoprostol. Diclofenac is a non-steroidal anti-inflammatory drug (NSAID) and works by reducing hormones that cause inflammation and pain in the body. Misoprostol, the other ingredient, reduces stomach acid and replaces protective substances in the stomach that are reduced by NSAIDs. NSAIDs have a propensity to cause gastric bleeding.

(Continued)

This drug is used to treat skeletal conditions such as osteoarthritis and rheumatoid arthritis and is given to those people who may be at high risk for developing gastric or intestinal ulcers.

Arthrotec should not be used in those who are pregnant as misoprostol may cause birth defects, miscarriage, premature labour or uterine rupture. Those who have active gastric or intestinal bleeding should not use Arthrotec. The diclofenac used in this drug can increase the risk of fatal heart attack or stroke; this risk is increased if the medication is used long term or if the person has heart disease.

Prior to administering this medicine the nurse must determine if the person is allergic to diclofenac or misoprostol, or if there is an active gastric or intestinal bleed. The drug should not be given until after a detailed medical history has been taken as it is contraindicated in some conditions.

Administer Arthrotec with food or milk to lessen stomach upset. Do not crush or break the medicine; the drug should be swallowed whole and not chewed. If the person is taking the medication long term, then frequent blood tests will be needed.

Bone structure and blood supply (histology)

There are a number of factors that will impinge upon bone growth, and therefore its structure (see Table 5.4).

Medicines management

Hyaluronan injections

Normal synovial fluid contains large amounts of hyaluronic acid, permitting the joint fluid to be slippery. Synthetic hyaluronates may be injected into the knee in order to treat arthritis. Once the injection has been given, pain relief occurs within days and may last for several months. The medication is usually injected in the knee; however, use in other joints is being considered, such as the shoulder, ankle and elbow.

It is usual for a course of three to five injections to be given, each separated by 1–3 weeks. The first two injections may be given close together, and the period between those remaining is extended. Repeat courses may be recommended.

This type of medication is only usually used for those people with osteoarthritis who cannot take NSAIDs or who have used them but do not achieve adequate pain relief when using them. People awaiting joint surgery may benefit from these injections.

The drug has very few side-effects: there may be some people who may experience a slight allergic reaction, it may cause temporary pain and swelling in the joint after the injection and there is a small risk of infection. If the patient develops severe joint pain after an injection, the nurse should advise them to call the hospital or clinic where the injection occurred.

An alternative to hyaluronan injections is a steroid injection into the joint. Steroid injections have anti-inflammatory as opposed to lubricating properties.

All of the factors cited in Table 5.4 are required for bone growth, and an alteration in any of them will impact on bone structure as well as a number of other bodily functions.

Table 5.4 Some factors that impact on bone structure

Factor	Comment
Vitamins	A, C, D, K and B$_{12}$. There are a number of sources of these vitamins, and their roles and functions vary. Too high amounts can be toxic and too low amounts can, for example, stunt growth.
Hormones	Human growth hormone (hGH), insulin-like growth factors (IGFs), oestrogens, androgens and thyroid hormones. Some of these hormones are produced in the pituitary gland; hence, any condition affecting this gland could result in problems related to bone formation and structure. IGFs are produced by the liver in response to hGH. Oestrogen (the sex hormone produced in the ovaries) and androgens (the sex hormone produced in the testes): if these hormones are not released there are potential complications associated with a number of body functions, including bone.
Minerals	Calcium, phosphorus, magnesium and fluoride. Calcium is a mineral that becomes available to the rest of the body when remodelling occurs. The amount of calcium in the bloodstream must be within precise limits otherwise serious problems can occur; the heart may stop if there is too much circulating calcium.
Exercise	All exercise is beneficial to the body, but weight-bearing exercise is particularly important for the stimulation of bone growth, particularly those exercises that place stress on the bones. When placed under stress, bone tissue becomes stronger as remodelling occurs; without this stress the bone will weaken and demineralisation occurs.

Source: Adapted from Tortora and Derrickson (2009) and Rizzo (2006). Reproduced with permission of John Wiley & Sons.

Blood supply

Blood supply to the bone comes via three routes:

- the Haversian canals
- the Volkmann canals
- the vessels.

The Haversian canals are minute channels that are laid down parallel to the axis of the bone and are the passages for arterioles; they allow for the efficient metabolism of bone cells. These are central canals that contain blood vessels, nerves and lymphatic vessels. The canals are surrounded by lamellae that are made up of rings of hard, calcified extracellular matrix. Lying between the lamellae are the lacunae, which contain the osteocytes, and radiating in all directions are the canaliculi filled with extracellular fluid. These various interconnecting structures provide nutrients and oxygen to the bones as well as provide a route for waste to be removed.

The periosteum provides the route for the blood vessels, nerves and lymphatic vessels to penetrate the compact bones through the Volkmann canals. These blood vessels, lymph vessels and nerves connect with those of the bone marrow, periosteum and Haversian canals. The fluid present in the Volkmann canals bathes the osteocytes, bringing in oxygen and removing waste (including carbon dioxide), helping to keep the osteocytes alive and healthy (Rizzo, 2006). Figure 5.5 provides an illustration of the Haversian system in compact bone and trabeculae in spongy bone.

Organisation of bone based on shape

There are, according to Rizzo (2006), five categories that individual bones of the body can be divided into:

- long
- short

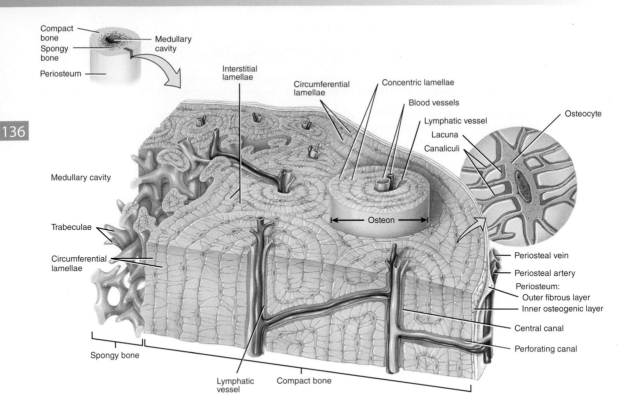

Figure 5.5 The Haversian system in compact bones and trabeculae in spongy bone. *Source*: Tortora and Derrickson (2009). Reproduced with permission of John Wiley & Sons.

- flat
- irregular
- sesamoid.

Long bones

Some examples of long bones are the humerus, clavicle, radius, ulna, femur, tibia and fibula. The metacarpals, metatarsals and phalanges are also classed as long bones (despite their shortness) as the length of these bones exceeds their width. They allow movement, particularly in the limbs (e.g. the femur and the humerus).

Long bones consist of a diaphysis composed primarily of compact bone and a metaphysis that is composed mainly of cancellous or spongy bone. There are two extremities that are separated from the metaphysis called the epiphyses; the separating line is called the epiphyseal line. The diaphysis is thickest towards the middle of the bone. There is a reason for this: it is where most strain on the bone occurs. The long bone has a slight curve to it – this also aids strength – distributing weight. The interior of the shaft contains the bone marrow (the medullary cavity). Figure 5.6 shows a long bone.

Short bones

These bones are usually grouped in pairs; they are strong and compact. Often they are found in parts of the body where little movement is needed. Examples of short bones include the carpal bones of the wrist and the tarsal bones of the foot (see Figure 5.7).

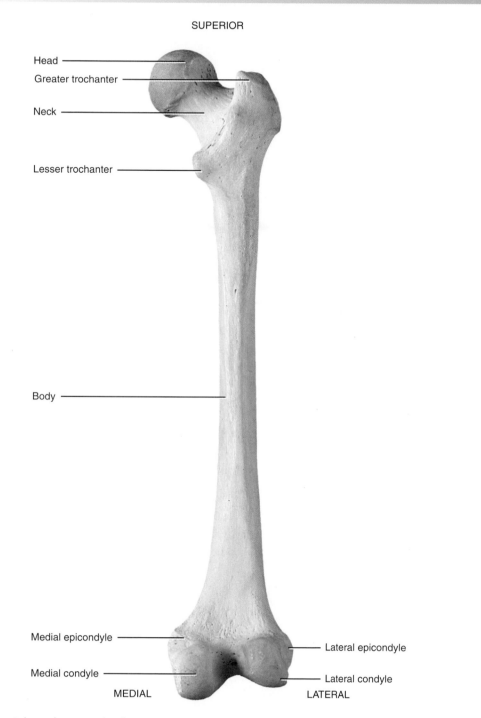

SUPERIOR

Head

Greater trochanter

Neck

Lesser trochanter

Body

Medial epicondyle

Lateral epicondyle

Medial condyle

Lateral condyle

MEDIAL

LATERAL

Figure 5.6 A long bone – the femur. *Source*: Tortora (2008). Reproduced with permission of John Wiley & Sons.

138

LATERAL   POSTERIOR   MEDIAL

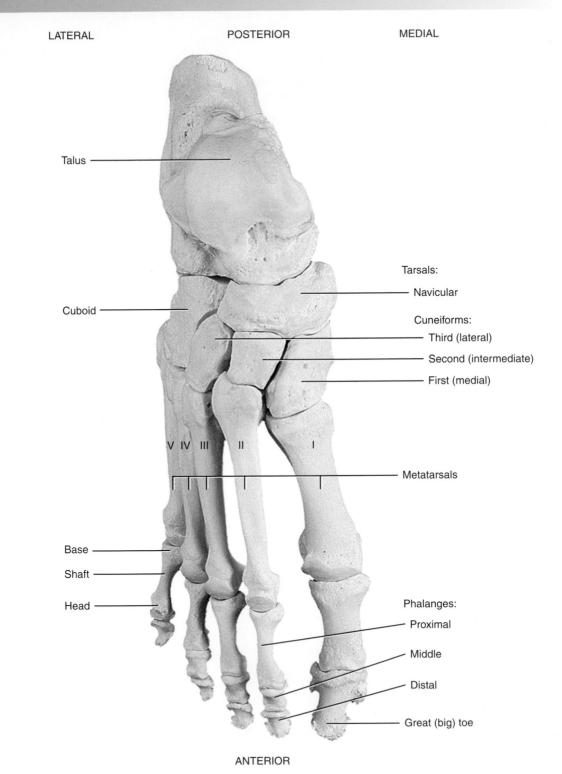

Talus

Tarsals:

Navicular

Cuboid

Cuneiforms:

Third (lateral)

Second (intermediate)

First (medial)

V IV III   II   I

Metatarsals

Base

Shaft

Head

Phalanges:

Proximal

Middle

Distal

Great (big) toe

ANTERIOR

Figure 5.7   The tarsal bones – short bones. *Source*: Tortora (2008). Reproduced with permission of John Wiley & Sons.

Short bones are not just shorter versions of long bones, they do not have a long axis and are irregular in shape. They have a thin layer of compact tissue over a predominantly spongy or cancellous bone.

Flat bones

These are thin bones that are found where there is a need for muscle attachment or for protection of soft or important aspects of the body. Their broad flat surface allows for extensive muscle attachment. Examples of flat bones are the sternum, ribs, scapula, some bones of the skull and some bones of the pelvis (see Figure 5.8). These bones are often curved and are made up of compact tissues enclosing a layer of cancellous bone.

Irregular bones

These bones do not fit into the categories described above as they have a number of different characteristics. As the name suggests, they are irregular, different and peculiar. These bones consist of spongy bone that is enclosed by thin layers of compact bones. These bones include the vertebrae, coccyx, sphenoid, zygomatic and the ossicles of the ear (see Figure 5.9).

Sesamoid bones

The patella is a sesamoid bone, although some of the bones of the wrist or ankle could be classed as sesamoid. Sesamoid bones are bones within tendons; they are small and round, and assist in the functioning of muscles. Figure 5.10 shows the patella.

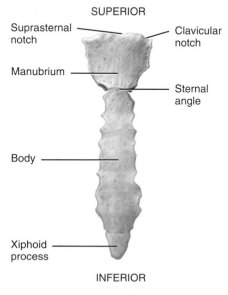

SUPERIOR

Suprasternal notch — — Clavicular notch

Manubrium —

— Sternal angle

Body —

Xiphoid process —

INFERIOR

Anterior view of sternum

Figure 5.8   A flat bone – the sternum. *Source*: Tortora and Derrickson (2009). Reproduced with permission of John Wiley & Sons.

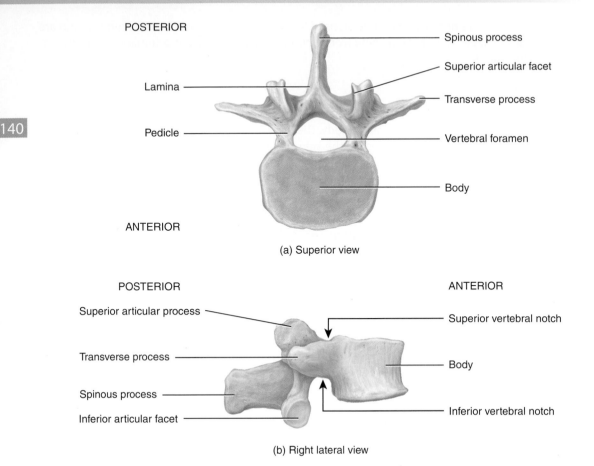

POSTERIOR

Spinous process

Superior articular facet

Lamina

Transverse process

Pedicle

Vertebral foramen

Body

ANTERIOR

(a) Superior view

POSTERIOR   ANTERIOR

Superior articular process

Superior vertebral notch

Transverse process

Body

Spinous process

Inferior articular facet

Inferior vertebral notch

(b) Right lateral view

Figure 5.9 (a, b) The vertebrae – an irregular bone. *Source*: Tortora and Derrickson (2009). Reproduced with permission of John Wiley & Sons.

Joints

A joint is the point at which two or more bones meet. Joints are sometimes also called articulations. There are a number of ways of classifying joints; for example:

- fibrous
- cartilaginous
- synovial.

Fibrous joints

These joints are also called synarthrodial joints and are held together by only a ligament, a dense irregular tissue that is made up of collagen-rich fibres. There is no synovial cavity in this type of joint. Examples of synarthrodial joints are where the teeth are held to their bony sockets; other examples include both the radioulnar and tibiofibular joints.

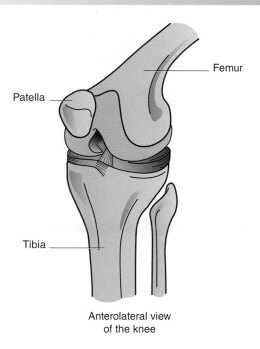

Femur

Patella

Tibia

Anterolateral view
of the knee

Figure 5.10   The patella – a sesamoid bone. *Source*: Peate and Nair (2009). Reproduced with permission of John Wiley & Sons.

Cartilaginous joints

These joints are also called synchondroses and symphyses (singular symphysis). They occur where the connection between the articulating bones is made up of cartilage with no synovial cavity; for example, the joints occurring between vertebrae in the spine.

The synchondroses are temporary joints and are only present in children until the end of puberty, by which stage the hyaline cartilage converts to bone; for example, the epiphyseal plates of long bones. Symphysis joints are permanent cartilagenous joints that have an intervening pad of fibrocartilage; for example, the symphysis pubis.

Synovial joints

Synovial joints, also called diarthrosis joints, are by far the most common classification of joint within the human body. They are extremely movable joints with a synovial cavity and all have an articular capsule enclosing the whole joint, a synovial membrane (the inner layer of the capsule) that produces synovial fluid (a lubricating solution) and cartilage known as hyaline cartilage, which pads the ends of the articulating bones.

Synovial fluid is a thin film that is usually viscous, clear or yellowish. This fluid helps to prevent friction by providing the joint with lubrication, supplying nutrients and removing waste products. If the joint becomes immobile for a period of time the fluid becomes gel-like, returning to its normal viscous consistency when the joint begins to move again.

There are six types of synovial joints, and these are classified by the shape of the joint and the movement available (see Table 5.5).

Table 5.5   Six types of joint

Type of joint	Movement at joint	Examples	Structure
Hinge	A convex portion of one bone fits into a concave portion of another bone. The movement reflects the hinge and bracket movement of a household hinge and bracket; movement is limited to flexion and extension. The joint produces an open and closing motion. These joints are uniaxial.	Elbow Knee	
Pivot	A rounded part of one bone fits into the groove of another bone. These joints will only permit movement of one bone around another – uniaxial movement.	Radius and ulna The atlas and the axis	
Ball and socket	The spherical end of one bone fits into a concave socket of another bone; hence, ball and socket. Movement occurs through flexion, extension and adduction. This is triaxial joint.	Hip Shoulder	

142

Type of joint	Movement at joint	Examples	Structure
Saddle	Similar to condyloid joints, but these joints permit greater movement. Allows flexion, extension and adduction. The joint is classed as triaxial.	The carpometacarpal joints of the thumb	
Condyloid	Where an oval surface of one bone fits into a concavity of another bone. Allows flexion, extension and adduction. This is a biaxial joint.	The radiocarpal and metacarpophalangeal joints of the hand	
Gliding	These joints have a flat or slightly curved surface, permitting gliding movements. The joints are bound by ligaments, and movement in all directions is restricted. The joint moves back and forth and side to side.	Intertarsal and intercarpal joints of the hands and feet	

Medicines management

Medicine containers

People with skeletal conditions such as arthritis may struggle to open medicine containers, particularly those that have childproof tops on. This can cause frustration when the person is trying to get to the medicines that have been prescribed to relieve their pain, and this then causes additional pain.

A discussion with the pharmacist or occupational therapist may be needed to ensure that those who need their medication can access it with ease and at the same time ensure a safe environment. There are also several commercial products available to help people grip and open containers; these often come with a rubber non-slip coating on the grip points, so that the person's hand does not slide.

Conclusion

All activities that people perform are related to movement; for example, verbal communication, moving the mouth (jaw) to speak, requires the skeleton. The skeleton and the bones of the body are required in order to perform in the best possible way. When gases are exchanged during breathing, mobility is required for this life-sustaining activity to occur. The intact skeletal system permits these activities to occur. Mobility is an essential activity of living.

The human skeleton is a living organism that is constantly metabolising. The skeletal system links very closely to muscles; muscles provide leverage and movements, and the skeleton provides the framework. The long bones are responsible for the production of erythrocytes (haemopoiesis); production (or failure to produce erythrocytes) can have an impact on the person's health and well-being. The nervous system is closely related to the skeletal system, as muscles require a nerve impulse to contract; this then results in skeletal movement. The digestive system enables food to be broken down to such a level that the nutrients can be used for bone production. Hormones produced by the kidneys help to stimulate the production of bone marrow in the long bones.

The skeletal system is essential for life, providing support and protection of the internal organs. The bones store and, when needed, release calcium, a mineral that is essential to ensure safe bodily functioning.

Glossary

Abduction   Movement away from the body's midline.

Adduction   Movement towards the body's midline.

Anatomy   The study of body structures and their relation to other structures in the body.

Artery   A blood vessel that carries blood away from the heart.

Articulation   Sometimes called a joint, where bones meet.

Ball-and-socket joint   A synovial joint in which the rounded surface of one bone fits within the cup-shaped depression of the socket of the other bone.

Calcification   Deposition of mineral salts in a framework formed by collagen fibres in which tissue hardens.

Cancellous   A type of structure as seen in spongy bone tissue; resembles a latticework structure.

Cartilage   Strong, tough material on the bone ends that helps to distribute the load within the joint; the slippery surface allows smooth movement between the bones; a type of connective tissue.

Cartilaginous joint   A joint where the bones are held together tightly by cartilage; little movement occurs in this joint. This joint does not have a synovial cavity.

Collagen   A protein that makes up most of the connective tissue.

Condyloid joint   A synovial joint that allows one oval-shaped bone to fit into an elliptical cavity of another.

Diaphysis   The shaft of a long bone.

Epiphysis   The end of long bone.

Fibrous joint   A type of joint that allows little or no movement.

Flexion   Movement where there is a decrease in the angle between two bones.

Fracture   A break in a bone.

Gliding joint   A synovial joint whose articulating surfaces are usually flat, allowing only side-to-side or back-and-forth movement.

Haemopoiesis   The formation and development of blood cells in the bone marrow after birth.

Histology   The microscopic study of tissue.

Homeostasis   A state whereby the body's internal environment remains relatively constant within physiological limits.

Hormone   The secretion of endocrine cells that have the ability to alter the physiological activity of target cells in the body.

Insulin-like growth factor (IGF)   Produced by the liver and other tissues, this is a small protein that is produced in response to hGH.

In utero   Within the uterus.

Kinesiology   The study of movement of the body.

Lacuna   A small, hollow space found in the bones where osteocytes lie.

Lamellae   Rings of hard, calcified matrix found in compact bones.

Ligaments   Tough fibrous bands of connective tissue that hold two bones together in a joint.

Macrophage   Cells that engulf and then digest cellular debris and pathogens.

Marrow   A sponge-like material found in the cavities of some bones.

Mesenchyme   Embryonic connective tissue from which nearly all other connective tissue arises.

Metaphysis   The aspect of a long bone that lies between the diaphysis and the epiphysis.

Ossification   The formation of bone; sometimes called osteogenesis.

Osseous   Bony.

Ossicle   A small bone of the middle ear – the malleus, the incus, the stapes.

Osteoblasts   Cells that arise from osteogenic cells; these cells participate in bone formation.

Osteoclasts   Large cells that are associated with absorption and removal of bone.

Osteocytes   Mature bone cells.

Osteon   The basic unit of structure in adult compact bone.

Osteophytes   Overgrowth of new bone around the side of osteoarthritic joints; also known as spur growth.

Periosteum   Membrane covering bone consisting of osteogenic cells, connective tissue and osteoblasts. This is vital for bone growth, repair and nutrition.

Pivot joint   A joint where a rounded or conical-shaped surface of a bone articulates with a ring formed partly by another bone or ligament.

Remodelling   Replacement of old bone by new.

Resorption   Absorption of what has been excreted.

Saddle joint   A synovial joint articulates the surface of a saddle-shaped bone on the other bone that is said to be shaped like the legs of the rider.

Spongy (cancellous) bone tissue   Bone tissue comprised of an irregular latticework of thin plates of bone known as trabeculae. Some bones are filled with red bone marrow, and these are found in short, flat and irregular bones as well as the epiphyses of long bones.

Synovial cavity   The space between the articulating bones of a synovial cavity, filled with synovial fluid.

Synovial fluid   A clear pale, yellow, viscid fluid. It lubricates joints.

Trabeculae   A network of irregular latticework of thin plates of spongy bones.

References

McRae, R. (2006) *Pocket Book of Orthopaedics and Fractures*, 2nd edn. Edinburgh: Churchill Livingstone.

Rizzo, D.C. (2006) *Delmar's Fundamentals of Anatomy and Physiology*, 2nd edn. New York: Thompson.

Tortora, G.J. and Derrickson, B. (2009) *Principles of Anatomy and Physiology*, 12th edn. Hoboken, NJ: John Wiley & Sons, Inc.

Tortora, G.J. and Derrickson, B. (2013) *Essentials of Anatomy and Physiology*, 9th edn. New York: John Wiley & Sons, Inc.

Tortora, G.J. and Grabowski, S.R. (2009) *Principles of Anatomy and Physiology*, 11th edn. New York: John Wiley & Sons, Inc.

Tortora, G.J. (2008) *A Brief Atlas of the Human Skeleton, Surface Anatomy and Selected Medical Images*. New York: John Wiley & Sons, Inc.

Tucker, L. (2011) *An Introductory Guide to Anatomy and Physiology*, 4th edn. London: EMS Publishing.

Further reading

Arthritis Research UK

www.arthritisresearchuk.org

This organisation works with patients and healthcare professionals to take the pain away from those living with all forms of arthritis, helping them to remain active. They fund high quality research, educate healthcare professionals and provide information to those with arthritis and their carers.

National Osteoporosis Foundation UK

https://www.nos.org.uk

The National Osteoporosis Society is a UK-wide charity dedicated to improving the diagnosis, prevention and treatment of osteoporosis and fragility fractures. The National Osteoporosis Society UK Allied Health Professional Network has been developed to provide support and professional development to allied health professionals who are specialists working in the field of osteoporosis and/or fragility fractures in the UK.

Sarcoma UK

http://sarcoma.org.uk

Sarcoma UK is the only UK cancer charity that focuses on all types of sarcoma. Sarcomas are rare cancers developing in the muscle, bone, nerves, cartilage, tendons, blood vessels and the fatty and fibrous tissues.

Activities
Multiple choice questions

1. What is an osteophyte?
   - (a) a bone cell
   - (b) a small bony outgrowth
   - (c) a bone cancer cell
   - (d) a lymph cell
2. Where would you find the medial malleolus?
   - (a) the hip
   - (b) in the thoracic cavity
   - (c) the lower end of tibia
   - (d) the cranium
3. What is another name for the clavicle?
   - (a) the rib
   - (b) the breastbone
   - (c) the collarbone
   - (d) the pelvis
4. What does the term kinesiology mean?
   - (a) the study of light
   - (b) the study of brain
   - (c) the study of art
   - (d) the study of movement of the body
5. A joint that allows free movement is known as:
   - (a) diarthrosis
   - (b) haemathrosis
   - (c) synarthrosis
   - (d) amphiarthroses
6. The jaw bone is:
   - (a) the calcaneus
   - (b) the maxilla
   - (c) the ischium
   - (d) the mandible
7. A joint such as the elbow joint that only moves in one plane is known as:
   - (a) a hinge joint
   - (b) a socket joint
   - (c) an arthritic joint
   - (d) a saddle joint

8. Bone is covered by a protective tissue membrane called:
   (a) the lacunae
   (b) the diaphysis
   (c) the peritoneum
   (d) the periosteum
9. The skull and ribs are part of:
   (a) the appendicular skeleton
   (b) the external skeleton
   (c) the axial skeleton
   (d) the internal skeleton
10. The ribs are attached to:
    (a) the cervical vertebrae
    (b) the thoracic vertebrae
    (c) the lumbar vertebrae
    (d) the skull

True or false

1. The skeleton is a living organism.
2. There are more bones in adults than in babies.
3. Bone stores and releases calcium.
4. The ribs protect the pancreas.
5. Yellow bone marrow produces red blood cells.
6. There is no difference between the weight and size of male and female bones.
7. The patella is located in the humerus.
8. Osteoblasts forms new bone.
9. Replacement of old bone by new is called remodelling.
10. The axial skeleton has more bones than the appendicular skeleton.

Label the diagram 1

Label the diagram using the following list of words:

Head, Greater trochanter, Neck, Lesser trochanter, Body, Medial epicondyle, Medial condyle, Lateral epicondyle, Lateral condyle

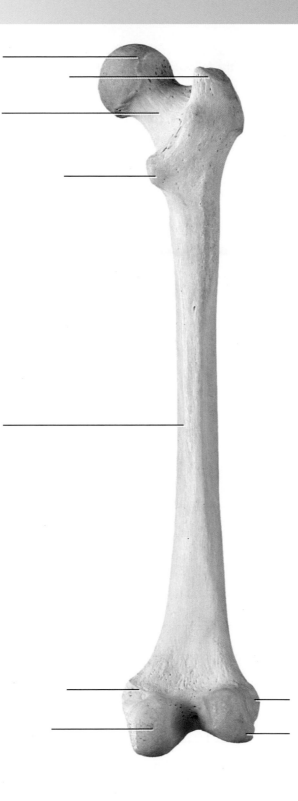

Label the diagram 2

Label the diagram using the following list of words:

Femur, Tibia, Patella

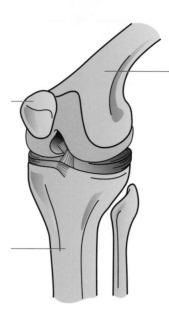

Word search

In the following there are 15 words that you will have seen in this chapter. Can you find them all?

O	P	C	H	T	S	A	L	B	O	E	T	S	O	W	J
N	E	A	R	B	E	T	R	E	V	R	F	I	T	O	I
O	L	T	D	I	O	M	H	T	E	O	P	P	I	P	E
T	A	A	K	L	U	C	O	B	O	N	E	N	O	A	R
E	S	L	I	N	S	Y	S	R	S	C	T	Y	D	T	U
L	R	F	R	C	R	O	O	S	S	E	O	U	S	E	T
E	A	E	P	I	P	H	Y	S	E	A	L	A	N	L	U
K	T	I	B	I	A	B	M	L	O	M	A	X	E	L	S
S	O	S	T	E	O	C	L	A	S	T	N	D	I	A	O

Osteoblast, Vertebrae, Skeleton, Sternum, Rib, Epiphyseal, Ulna, Osteoclast, Patella, Suture, Osseous, Bone, Ethmoid, Joint, Tibia

Fill in the blanks

The _____ is the _____ and _____ bone of the _____ arm. The head of the humerus is _____ and _____ to the rest of the bone by the anatomic _____. The upper aspect of the bone has two prominences: the _____ and _____ tubercles. The ulna is _____ than the radius. The bones of the wrists are called the _____; they are arranged in _____ rows of four each. The palms of the hands are made up of the _____ _____ bones. Metatarsals are small _____ bones; they each have a _____ and a _____. The thumb has only a _____ and _____ phalanx.

151

carpals, distal, five, greater, head, humerus, joined, largest, lesser, long, longer, longest, metatarsal, neck, proximal, rounded, shaft, two, upper

Match the bone to the shape

1. Irregular bone
2. Long bone
3. Flat bone
4. Short bone

    A. Sternum
    B. Zygomatic
    C. Metacarpal
    D. Hyoid
    E. Tarsal
    F. Femur
    G. Ethmoid
    H. Scapula

Find out more

1. Why do healthy bones require exercise?
2. Describe the composition of bone.
3. How does the skeletal system help to maintain homeostasis?
4. In bone remodelling how do osteoblasts and osteoclasts work together?
5. What happens to bone as we age?
6. What is synovial fluid?
7. Describe the healing that occurs after a fracture has been sustained.
8. Discuss intramembranous ossification.
9. What factors are essential for bone remodelling?
10. Where in the body are the two sesamoid bones and what are they called?

Conditions

The following is a list of conditions that are associated with the skeletal system. Take some time and write notes about each of the conditions. You may make the notes taken from text books or other resources (e.g. people you work with in a clinical area), or you may make the notes as a result of people you have cared for. If you are making notes about people you have cared for you must ensure that you adhere to the rules of confidentiality.

Fractured neck of femur

Osteoarthritis

Osteoporosis

Gout

Osteomyelitis

Osteosarcoma

Chapter 6

The muscular system

Janet G Migliozzi

Test your prior knowledge

- List the functions of the muscular system.
- Name the different types of muscles found in the human body.
- Describe the energy sources that enable muscles to contract.
- List the stages involved in muscle contraction.
- List the different types of body movement.

Learning outcomes

After reading this chapter you will be able to:

- Describe the structure and functions of the muscular system
- Describe the different types of muscles in the human body
- Name the major muscles of the body and their functions
- Describe how a muscle contracts
- Describe the energy sources that muscles use

Fundamentals of Anatomy and Physiology: For Nursing and Healthcare Students, Second Edition. Edited by Ian Peate and Muralitharan Nair.
© 2017 John Wiley & Sons, Ltd. Published 2017 by John Wiley & Sons, Ltd.
Student companion website: www.wileyfundamentalseries.com/anatomy
Instructor companion website: www.wiley.com/go/instructor/anatomy

Body map

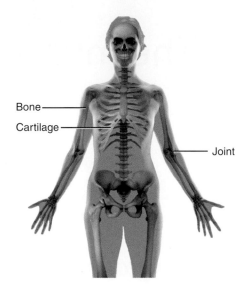

Bone
Cartilage
Joint

Introduction

All physical function of the body involves muscular activity, and as muscles are responsible for all body movement they can be considered the 'machines' of the body (Marieb, 2013). This chapter will discuss the structure and function of the muscular system.

Types of muscle tissue

The body contains three types of muscle tissue: smooth, cardiac and skeletal. Table 6.1 provides a summary of the different types of muscle tissue.

Smooth or visceral muscle

Smooth or visceral muscle is located in the walls of hollow internal organs and blood vessels of the body; for example, the small intestine, blood vessels (arteries, arterioles, venules and veins), bronchioles of the respiratory tract, urinary bladder and ureters, uterus and Fallopian tubes, but not the heart. Smooth muscle fibres have a single nucleus, are usually arranged in parallel lines

Table 6.1   Different types of muscle tissue

Skeletal muscle	Smooth muscle	Cardiac muscle
Attached to bones or the skin (facial muscles only)	Found in the walls of hollow visceral organs and blood vessels	Located in the walls of the heart
Single, long cylindrical cells	Single, narrow, rod-shaped cells	Branching chains of cells
Striated, multinucleated cells	Non-striated, uninucleated cells	Non-striated, uninucleated cells
Under voluntary control	Involuntary control	Involuntary control

and are not striated. Smooth muscles are involuntary, do not fatigue easily and are controlled by the medulla oblongata in the brain, which is responsible for controlling involuntary action throughout the body. Smooth muscle is discussed in more detail in Chapter 9.

Cardiac

Cardiac muscle, found only in the heart, is also a form of involuntary muscle and forms the walls of the heart. Its main function is to propel blood into the circulation by making the right atrium contract. Cardiac muscles also have a single nucleus, are striated, branched and tubular. Cardiac muscle is discussed in more detail in Chapter 8.

Skeletal

The skeletal muscles make up the muscular system of the body (composed of over 600 muscles) and account for 40–50% of the body weight in an adult. The skeletal muscles are the only voluntary muscles of the body (i.e. are consciously controlled) and are the muscles involved in moving bones and generating external movement. Skeletal muscle is also referred to as striped or striated muscle because of the banded patterns of the cells seen under the microscope.

The rest of this chapter will focus on skeletal muscle only as both smooth and cardiac muscle are discussed in more detail elsewhere.

Functions of the muscular system

The muscular system plays four important roles in the body:

- maintains posture
- produces movement
- stabilises joints
- protection
- generates heat.

Maintenance of body posture

Despite the continuous downward pull of gravity, the body is able to maintain an erect or seated posture because of the continuous tiny adjustments that the skeletal muscles make.

Production of movement

The body's ability to mobilise is a result of skeletal muscle activity and muscle contraction, as when muscles contract they pull on the tendons and bones of the skeleton to produce movement.

Stabilisation of joints

Muscle tendons play a vital role in stabilising and reinforcing the joints of the body. During movement the skeletal muscles pull on bones which stabilise the joints of the skeleton.

Protection and control of internal tissue structures/organs

Skeletal muscle plays an important role in protecting the internal organs as the visceral organs and internal tissues contained within the abdominal cavity are protected by layers of skeletal tissue within the abdominal wall and floor of the pelvic cavity. Similarly, the orifices contained within the digestive and urinary tracts are encircled by skeletal muscle, and this allows for voluntary control over swallowing, urination and defaecation (Martini and Bartholomew, 2012).

Generation of heat

Heat generation is vital in maintaining normal body temperature, and skeletal muscles, which account for 40% of the body's mass, are the muscle type mostly responsible for the body's heat generation. During muscle contraction, adenosine triphosphate (ATP) is used to release the needed energy, with nearly three-quarters of its energy escaping as heat.

Composition of skeletal muscle tissue

As muscles contain other types of tissues, such as blood vessels and connective and nervous tissue, they are considered to be organs (Logenbaker, 2013). Each cell in skeletal muscle tissue is known as a single muscle fibre, which, owing to its large size, contains hundreds of nuclei (i.e. are multinucleate). A skeletal muscle consists of individual muscle fibres that are markedly different from a 'typical' cell (not least by their size) bundled into fascicles and surrounded by three layers of connective tissue.

Gross anatomy of skeletal muscles

Muscle is separated from skin by the hypodermis, which consists of adipose tissue (which provides insulation and protects the muscle from physical damage) and a dense, broad band of connective tissue known as fascia, which supports and surrounds muscle tissue and provides a

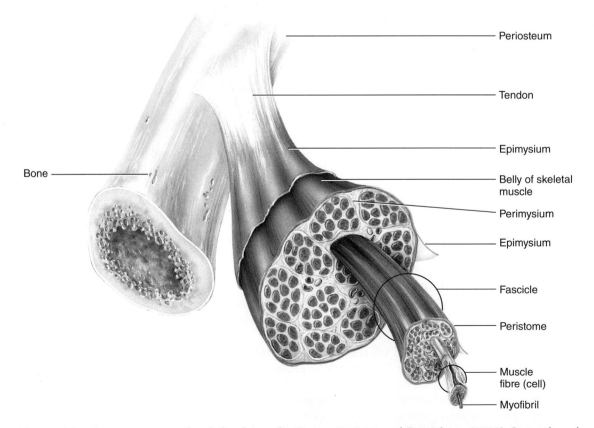

Figure 6.1   Gross anatomy of a skeletal muscle. *Source*: Tortora and Derrickson (2009). Reproduced with permission of John Wiley & Sons.

pathway for nerves and the lymphatic and blood vessels to enter and exit a muscle. Extending from the fascia are three layers of connective tissue that also play a role in supporting and protecting the muscle and are necessary to ensure that the force of contraction from each muscle cell is transmitted to its points of attachment to the skeleton (see Figure 6.1). These include:

- the **epimysium**, which is wrapped around the entire muscle;
- the **perimysium**, which surrounds bundles of muscle fibres known as fascicles;
- the **endomysium**, which is wrapped around each individual muscle cell.

The epimysium, perimysium and endomysium blend into either strong, cord-like tendons or into sheet-like aponeuroses that attach muscles indirectly to bones, cartilages or connective tissue (Marieb, 2013).

Clinical considerations

Intramuscular injection

An intramuscular (IM) injection is given directly into a selected muscle, and while there are several sites on the body that are suitable for IM injections, the most common areas used are:

- the deltoid muscle of the upper arm;
- the vastus lateralis muscle, which forms part of the quadriceps muscle group of the upper leg;
- the gluteus medius (ventrogluteal site) muscle, which runs beneath the gluteus maximus from the ilium to the femur.

IM injections are used for the delivery of certain drugs that (for various reasons) cannot be given via an oral, intravenous or subcutaneous route. The IM route enables a large amount (up to 5 mL) of drug to be introduced at one time, minimises tissue irritation and provides a faster route than subcutaneous/intradermal injections.

Microanatomy of skeletal muscle fibre

When examined microscopically, skeletal muscle cells appear cylindrical in shape, have a distinctive banded appearance of alternate light and dark stripes and lie parallel to each other (see Figure 6.2). Table 6.2 provides a summary of the cellular components of a muscle fibre.

The sarcolemma and transverse tubules

Each muscle fibre is covered by a plasma membrane called the sarcolemma and cylindrical structures called myofibrils that are suspended inside the muscle fibre in a matrix called the sarcoplasm (cytoplasm), which extends along the entire length of the muscle fibre. The surface of the sarcolemma is scattered with openings that lead into a network of narrow tubules called transverse or 'T' tubules that are filled with extracellular fluid and form passageways though the muscle fibre (Martini and Bartholomew, 2012).

The sarcoplasm

The sarcoplasm contains multiple mitochondria, which produce large amounts of ATP during muscle contraction (Tortora and Derrickson, 2012) and it is here that the T tubules make contact with a membrane known as the sarcoplasmic reticulum (SR). The SR stores calcium ions (essential for muscle contraction) in structures called cisternae and myoglobin (a reddish-brown pigment that is similar to haemoglobin), which stores oxygen until needed to generate ATP.

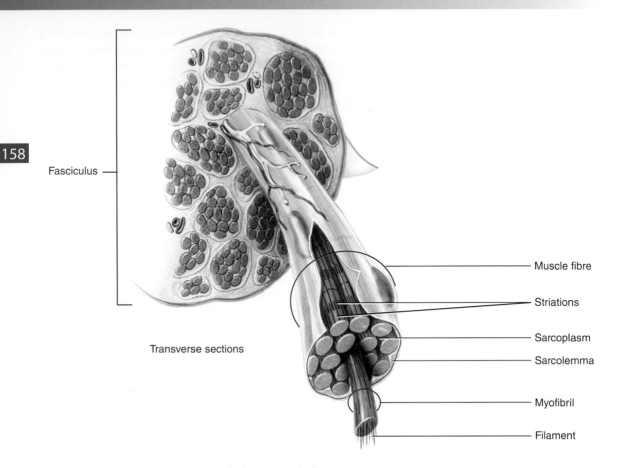

Fasciculus

Transverse sections

Muscle fibre

Striations

Sarcoplasm

Sarcolemma

Myofibril

Filament

Figure 6.2 Diagram showing a skeletal muscle fibre.

Table 6.2 Cellular components of a muscle fibre

Name	Function
Sarcolemma	Plasma membrane of a muscle fibre that forms T tubules
Sarcoplasm	Cytoplasm of the muscle fibre that contains myofibrils
Myofibril	Consists of bundles of myofilament and plays a key role in muscle contraction
Myofilament	Consists of thick and thin filaments that give muscle tissue its striated appearance and plays a role in muscle contraction
Myoglobin	A reddish-brown pigment (gives muscle tissue its dark-red colour) that stores oxygen for muscle contraction
T tubule	Fluid-filled tubular structure that releases calcium from the sarcoplasmic reticulum
Sarcoplasmic reticulum	Storage site for calcium ions

The myofibrils

Myofibrils (which are bundles of myofilaments) are thread-like structures that are found in abundance in the sarcoplasm. The myofibrils play a key role in the muscle contraction mechanism and contain two types of protein filaments: thick filaments composed of myosin and thin filaments composed of actin and two other proteins, tropomyosin and troponin. These filaments form compartments know as sarcomeres, which are the basic functional units of striated muscle fibres (Tortora and Derrickson, 2012), and each myofibril contains approximately 10,000 sarcomeres arranged end to end. The sarcomeres are separated from each other by dense zig-zagging protein-based structures called Z discs.

The sarcomeres

Extending across each of the thick filaments found within the sarcomere is a dark area known as the A band in the centre of which is a narrow H zone. On either side of the A band there is a lighter coloured area consisting of thin filaments called the I band. The alternating A and I bands give skeletal muscles their striated (striped) appearance.

Snapshot

Muscular dystrophy

Muscular dystrophy is a broad term applied to an inherited group of disorders that destroy the muscles by causing muscle fibres to degenerate, shrink in size and eventually die. The muscle fibres that die are replaced with fat and connective tissue.

The most common form of the disease is Duchenne's muscular dystrophy, which is inherited via a flawed gene carried by the mother and results in a lack of protein called dystrophin that plays a part in the structure and function of muscle fibres. The lack of dystrophin causes calcium to leak into muscle fibres and activate an enzyme that causes the muscle fibre to dissolve.

The condition occurs predominantly in males and manifests itself between the ages of 2 and 6 years. The disease is progressive, and most sufferers are wheelchair bound by the age of 12 years and do not live beyond young adulthood (Marieb, 2013). While treatment in the form of injections of immature muscle cells that produce dystrophin provides some relief (Longenbaker, 2013), there is no known cure.

Types of muscle fibres

Three types of muscle fibres are found in skeletal muscles and are found in varying proportions throughout the body:

- **Slow oxidative fibres** are small, dark-red fibres (due to containing large amounts of myoglobin) that generate ATP by aerobic respiration, make up approximately 50% of skeletal muscle and are capable of slow, prolonged contractions and are not easily fatigued.
- **Fast oxidative–glycolytic fibres** are medium, dark-red fibres that also generate ATP by aerobic respiration, but owing to their high glycogen content are also able to generate ATP by anaerobic glycolysis. Fast oxidative–glycolytic fibres are able to contract and relax more quickly than slow oxidative fibres.
- **Fast glycolytic fibres** are large white fibres (low myoglobin content) that generate ATP mainly by anaerobic glycolysis and provide the most rapid and powerful muscle contractions, but they fatigue easily.

Blood supply

Skeletal muscles have a very extensive blood supply and receive a total of 1 L of blood each minute, which equates to 20% of the resting cardiac output. This increases to 15–20 L min^{-1} when exercising intensively. As a general rule, each skeletal muscle is supplied by an artery and one or two veins, and each muscle fibre is in close contact with a network of microscopic capillaries within the endomysium.

Snapshot

Acute compartment syndrome

In the limbs the connections between the muscle fibres and the skeleton are robust; consequently, muscles are commonly isolated in dense collagen-based compartments. These compartments are where the blood vessels and nerves that supply a specific muscle enter.

When an injury to a limb occurs, if the resulting oedema that normally occurs develops within a compartment where there is little room for tissue expansion, the interstitial pressure increases. As pressure within the compartment is higher than that within the capillaries, blood flow, and hence tissue perfusion, slows and may ultimately stop (Harris and Hobson, 2015). This can result in tissue ischaemia and muscle death, with the resultant contents of the affected muscle fibres potentially entering the bloodstream (rhabdomyolysis). Common causes of compartment syndrome include limb fractures, crush injuries, vascular compromise and drug overdoses involving heroin or cocaine.

Skeletal muscle contraction and relaxation

The ability of skeletal muscle to contract is controlled by the body's nervous system, and each muscle fibre is controlled by a motor neurone (nerve cell), which may stimulate a few muscle cells or several hundred depending on the particular muscle and the work it does (Marieb, 2013). Skeletal muscle contracts in response to stimulation by an electrical signal (muscle action potential) delivered by the motor neurone, which is found halfway along the muscle cell, where it terminates at the neuromuscular junction. Here, the muscle fibre membrane is specialised to form a motor end plate.

Although a muscle fibre normally has a single motor end plate, the densely branched motor neurone axons (see Figure 6.3) mean that one motor neurone axon can connect and control

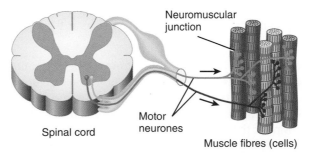

Figure 6.3 Motor unit. *Source*: Tortora and Derrickson (2009). Reproduced with permission of John Wiley & Sons.

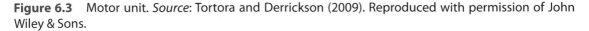

many muscle fibres. The motor neurone and the muscle fibres it controls are known as a motor unit.

When a nerve impulse reaches the axon terminals, the neurotransmitter acetylcholine (ACh) that stimulates skeletal muscle is released into the synaptic cleft, which is a small gap that separates the membrane of the nerve cell from the membrane of the muscle fibre (Shier *et al.*, 2012). The synaptic cleft and motor end plate contain acetylcholinesterase (AChE), which breaks down molecules of ACh. The release of ACh results in changes to the sarcolemma that trigger the contraction of the muscle fibre.

Snapshot

Botulism

Botulism can arise from the consumption of contaminated or smoked food and is caused by ingestion of spores from the bacterium *Clostridium botulinum*, which is commonly found in soil and water. One of the toxins released from the bacterium prevents the release of ACh at the synaptic terminals of muscle cells and prevents an action potential in the sarcolemma from occurring. If not treated quickly this can result in potentially fatal muscular paralysis. Treatment is with an anti-toxin and the use of mechanical ventilation if the respiratory system is affected (Public Health England, 2014).

Skeletal muscle fibres are stimulated by neurones that control the production of an action potential (electrical impulse) in the sarcolemma by:

- **The release of ACh** – an action potential travels along a motor neurone until it reaches the synaptic terminal where vesicles contained within the synaptic terminal release ACh into the synaptic cleft between the motor neurone and the motor end plate.
- **The binding of ACh at the motor end plate** – the ACh molecules diffuse across the synaptic cleft and bind to ACh receptors on the sarcolemma. This changes the permeability of the membrane and allows sodium ions (Na^+) into the sarcoplasm, which triggers the production of a muscle action potential in the sarcolemma.
- **The conduction of action potentials by the sarcolemma** – the action potential spreads across the entire surface of the sarcolemma and then travels down the transverse tubules to the cisternae which encircle the sarcomeres of the muscle fibre. As a result of the action potential travelling across it, the cisternae releases significant amounts of calcium ions (Ca^{2+}) which leads to the initiation of a muscle contraction. Each nerve impulse normally results in one muscle action potential and stages 2 and 3 are repeated if more ACh is released by another nerve impulse.
- **Muscle relaxation** – action potential generation ceases as ACh is broken down by **AChE** and the concentration of calcium ions in the sarcoplasm declines. Once calcium ions return to normal resting levels, muscle contraction will end and muscle relaxation occurs.

Figure 6.4 provides a summary of the steps involved in skeletal muscle contraction and relaxation.

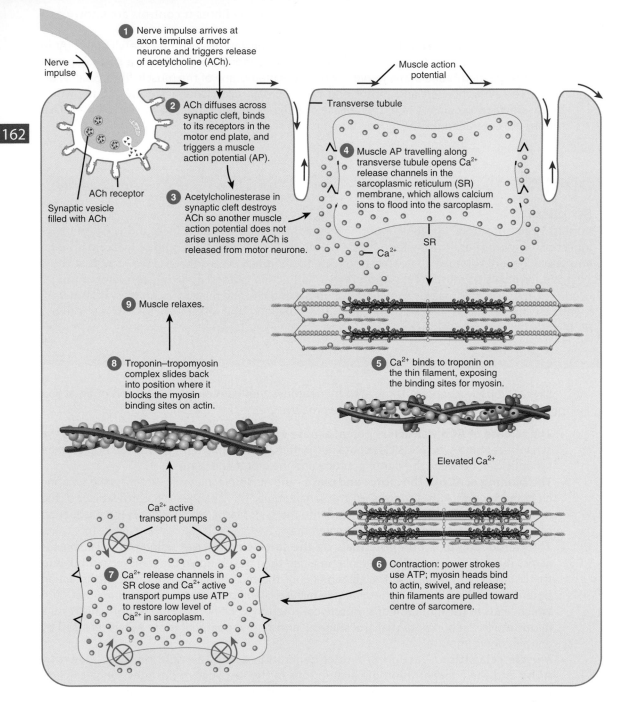

Figure 6.4 Summary of muscle contraction and relaxation. *Source*: Tortora and Derrickson (2009). Reproduced with permission of John Wiley & Sons.

Clinical considerations

Pyridostigmine is an anticholinesterase agent or AChE inhibitor and is used mainly to enhance neuromuscular transmission and improve muscle strength in voluntary and involuntary muscles of patients with myasthenia gravis. AChE inhibitors inhibit AChE, raising the concentration of ACh at the neuromuscular junction. In so doing they prolong the action of ACh by inhibiting the action of the enzyme AChE (BNF, 2014).

Cautions and contraindications

The drug should be used with caution in patients who have asthma, heart disease, epilepsy, Parkinsonism, thyroid disease or stomach ulcer. AChE inhibitors should not be given to patients with intestinal or urinary obstruction.

   Adverse effects of pyridostigmine include nausea, vomiting, abdominal cramps, diarrhoea, excessive salivation, sweating, bradycardia and bronchospasm. Adverse effects of the drug may be minimised by precise dosage adjustment.

Energy sources for muscle contraction

Muscle fibres require an energy source to enable them to contract as and when needed. This is provided initially in the form of ATP, which is stored in the muscle fibre. However, as only small amounts of ATP are stored in the muscle fibre, it is quickly depleted when the muscle is used and needs to be continuously available to power muscles. Therefore, working muscles require additional pathways to produce ATP, and these include:

- **Creatine phosphate:** This is broken down into creatine, phosphate and energy is the energy that is used to synthesise more ATP. Most of the creatine formed is used to resynthesise creatine phosphate and the creatine not used is converted to the waste product creatinine, which is excreted by the kidneys.
- **Anaerobic respiration:** Glycogen is the most abundant energy source found in muscle fibres and is broken down into glucose when it is needed to provide energy for muscle contraction. Glucose is initially broken down into pyruvic acid without the need for oxygen – a process known as glycolysis – and the small amounts of energy that are created by this process are captured by the bonds of ATP molecules.

During intensive muscle activity or when glucose and oxygen delivery are (temporarily) insufficient to meet the muscle requirements, the pyruvic acid generated during glycolysis converts to lactic acid. This pathway is much faster than that provided by aerobic respiration and can provide sufficient ATP for short spells of intensive exercise.

Aerobic respiration

Approximately 95% of the ATP used at rest and during moderate exercise comes from aerobic respiration involving a series of metabolic pathways that use oxygen – collectively known as oxidative phosphorylation (Marieb, 2013). In order to release energy from glucose, oxygen is necessary; muscles receive this either from the haemoglobin in red blood cells or from myoglobin, a protein that stores some oxygen within the muscle cells. During aerobic respiration,

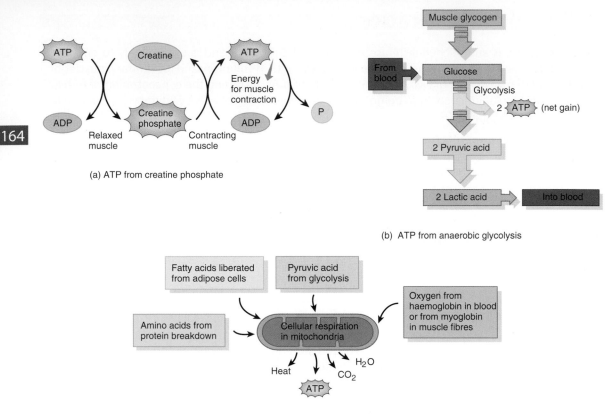

(a) ATP from creatine phosphate

(b) ATP from anaerobic glycolysis

(c) ATP from aerobic cellular respiration

Figure 6.5 (a–c) Sources of ATP for muscle energy. *Source*: Tortora and Derrickson (2009). Reproduced with permission of John Wiley & Sons.

glucose is broken down into carbon dioxide and water. The energy produced by the breakdown of these compounds is captured by the bonds of ATP molecules. While a rich source of ATP is obtained this way, it is a slow process that requires a continuous oxygen and fuel supply to the muscles.

Figure 6.5 provides an overview of the different ATP sources available for muscles.

Oxygen debt

When the body is moderately active or at rest, the cardiovascular and respiratory systems of the body can usually supply sufficient oxygen to skeletal muscles to support the aerobic reactions of cellular respiration (Shier *et al.*, 2012). However, when more strenuous activity is undertaken and a muscle relies on anaerobic respiration to supply its energy needs, it incurs an oxygen debt (Longenbaker, 2013), which requires the body to dispose of lactic acid and replenish creatinine phosphate in order to repay the debt.

Medicines management

Anabolic steroids

Anabolic steroids are synthetic substances related to testosterone and promote the growth of skeletal muscle (anabolic) by increasing protein within cells, particularly skeletal muscles and the development of male sexual characteristics (androgenic) – for example, the growth of the vocal cords, testicles (primary sexual characteristics) and body hair (secondary sexual characteristics). Anabolic steroids can be legally prescribed to treat conditions resulting from steroid hormone deficiency, such as delayed puberty, and, owing to their ability to stimulate muscle growth and appetite, diseases that result in loss of lean muscle mass, such as cancer and AIDS. But some athletes, bodybuilders and others abuse these drugs in an attempt to enhance performance and/ or improve their physical appearance. Doses taken by abusers may be 10 to 100 times higher than doses prescribed to treat medical conditions, and the abuse of anabolic steroids may lead to aggression and other psychiatric problems, including extreme mood changes, paranoid jealousy, manic-like symptoms and anger ('roid rage') that may lead to violence. Furthermore, steroid abuse may lead to serious, even irreversible, health problems, including kidney impairment or failure, damage to the liver and cardiovascular problems, including enlargement of the heart, high blood pressure and changes in blood cholesterol leading to an increased risk of stroke and heart attack (National Institute on Drug Abuse, 2012).

Muscle fatigue

Muscle fatigue occurs when a muscle fibre can no longer contract despite continued neural stimulation and occurs as a result of the oxygen debt that occurs during prolonged muscle activity.

Organisation of the skeletal muscular system

Every one of the body's skeletal muscles is attached at a minimum of two points to bone or other connective tissue. When one part of the skeleton is moved by muscle contraction, related parts have to be steadied by other muscles for the movement to be effective. The origin of a muscle is on the stationary bone where it begins, and the muscle ends at an insertion on the bone that moves (Longenbaker, 2013).

Muscles can be named according to size, shape, location and number of origins, associated bones and the action of the muscle. Table 6.3 provides examples of the criteria used to name muscles.

The body's skeletal muscles can be divided into four areas:

- head and neck muscles
- muscles of the upper limbs (shoulder, arm, forearm)
- trunk (thorax and abdomen)
- muscles of the lower limbs (hip, pelvis/thigh, leg).

The major muscles of the body are listed according to body area in Tables 6.4, 6.5, 6.6 and 6.7 and illustrated in Figures 6.6, 6.7, 6.8 and 6.9.

Figures 6.10 and 6.11 provide an overview of the major muscles of the body.

Table 6.3 Muscle names

Character/term	Definition	Example
Direction		
Transverse Oblique Rectus	Across Diagonal Straight	Transversus abdominis External oblique Rectus abdominis
Shape		
Trapezius Deltoid Obicularis Rhomboid Platys	Trapezoid Triangular Circular Diamond-shaped Flat	Trapezius Deltoid Obicularis oculi Rhomboideus Platysma
Size		
Major Minor Maximus Minimus Longus Latissimus	Larger Smaller Largest Smallest Longest Widest	Pectoralis major Pectoralis minor Gluteus maximus Gluteus minimus Adductor longus Latissimus dorsi
Number of origins		
Biceps Triceps Quadriceps	Two origins Three origins Four origins	Biceps brachii Triceps brachii Quadriceps femoris

Table 6.4 Muscles of the head and neck

Muscle	Origin	Insertion	Function
Frontalis	Skin and muscles around eye	Skin of eyebrow and bridge of nose	Wrinkles forehead Raises eyebrows
Occipitalis	Occipital bone	Galea aponeurotica (tendinous sheet)	Tenses and retracts scalp
Obicularis oculi	Maxillary and frontal bones	Skin around eye	Closes eye
Buccinator	Maxillary bone and mandible	Fibres of orbicularis oris	Compresses cheeks
Zygomaticus	Zygomatic bone	Obicularis oculi	Raises corner of mouth
Obicularis oris	Muscles near the mouth	Skin of central lip	Closes and protrudes lips
Masseter	Zygomatic arch/mandible	Lateral surface of mandible	Closes jaw
Temporalis	Temporal bone		Closes jaw
Pterygoids (medial and lateral)	Sphenoid and maxillary bones	Medial and anterior surface of mandible	Elevates and depresses mandible Moves mandible from side to side
Platysma	Fascia in upper chest	Lower mandible	Draws mouth downward
Stylohyoid	Temporal bone	Hyoid bone	Depresses hyoid bone and larynx
Mylohyoid	Mandible	Hyoid bone	Depresses mandible Elevates floor of mouth
Sternocleidomastoid	Margins of sternum of clavicle	Mastoid region of skull	Flexes the neck Rotates head

Table 6.5   Muscles of the upper limbs (shoulder, arm and hand)

Muscle	Origin	Insertion	Function
Levator scapulae	Transverse processes of cervical vertebrae	Scapula	Elevates scapula
Trapezius	Occipital bone and cervical and thoracic vertebrae	Clavicle, spine and scapula	Help to extend the head Adduct the scapulae when shoulders are shrugged or pulled back
Rotator cuff muscles: Supraspinatus Infraspinatus Subscapularis Teres minor Teres major	Posterior surface above and below scapula	Humerus	A group of muscles that are responsible for angular and rotational movements of the arm
Pectoralis major	Clavicle, sternum and upper ribs	Humerus	Flexes and adducts the arm
Muscles that move the forearm			
Biceps brachii	Between the scapula and forearm	Radius	Flexes and supinates the forearm
Triceps brachii	Between the scapula and forearm	Ulna	Extends the elbow/forearm
Brachialis	Between humerus and ulna	Ulna	Flexes forearm
Muscles that move the hand and fingers			
Flexor and extensor carpi	Base of second and third metacarpal bones	Base of second and third metacarpals	Flexion, extension abduction and adduction at wrist
Flexor and extensor digitorum	Posterior and distal phalanges	Base and surface of phalanges in fingers 2–5	Flexion and extension at finger joints and wrist
Palmaris longus	Distal end of humerus	Fascia of palm	Flexes the wrist

Table 6.6   Muscles of the trunk (thorax and abdomen)

Muscle	Origin	Insertion	Function
Internal intercostals	Superior border of each rib	Inferior border of preceding rib	Depress the rib cage and contract during forced expiration
External intercostals	Inferior border of each rib	Superior border of next rib	Elevate the ribs during inspiration
Diaphragm	Ribs 4–10, lumbar vertebrae	Tendon near to centre of diaphragm	Contracts to allow inhalation Relaxes to allow exhalation
Internal and external obliques	Between the lower ribs and pelvic girdle	Lower ribs, iliac crest and crest of pubis	Compress the abdominal cavity and protect and support the abdominal organs Rotation of the trunk
Transversus abdominis	Lower ribs, iliac crest and inguinal ligament	Extend horizontally across the abdomen from sternum to crest of pubis	Compress the abdominal cavity, protect and support the abdominal organs Rotation of the trunk
Rectus abdominis	Crest of pubic bone and symphysis pubis	Sternum and ribs	Compress the abdominal cavity, protect and support the abdominal organs Assists with flexing and rotating the lumbar spine

Table 6.7   Muscles of the lower limbs (hip, pelvis/thigh and leg)

Muscle	Origin	Insertion	Function
Psoas major	Lumbar vertebrae	Femur	Flexes thigh
Gluteus maximus	Sacrum, coccyx and surface of Ilium	Femur and fascia of thigh	Extends thigh at hip
Gluteus medius and minimus	Surface of Ilium	Femur	Abducts and rotates thigh
Adductor group	Pubic bone and Ischial tuberosity	Posterior surface of femur	Adducts, flexes, extends and rotates thigh
Quadriceps femoris group • Rectus femoris • Vastus lateralis • Vastus medialis • Vastus intermedius • Sartorius	Ilium, acetabulum and femur Ilium	Patella Tibia	Extends leg at knee Flexes, abducts and rotates thing to allow crossing of legs
Hamstring group • Biceps femoris • Semitendinosus • Semimembranosus	Femur, Ischial tuberosity, iliac spine	Tibia and head of fibula	Flexes and rotates leg, abducts, rotates and extends thigh
Posterior compartment • Gastrocnemius • Soleus • Tibialis posterior	Femur Fibula and tibia Tibia and fibula	Calcaneus (by means of the Achilles tendon) Second, third and fourth metatarsals	Flexes foot and leg at knee joint Flexes foot Flexes and inverts foot
Anterior compartment • Tibialis anterior • Extensor digitorum longus	Tibia Tibia and fibula	First metatarsal Middle and distal phalanges of each toe	Dorsiflexes and inverts foot Dorsiflexes and everts foot, extends toes
Lateral compartment • Fibularis longus	Fibula and tibia	First metatarsal	Flexes and everts foot

168

Skeletal muscle movement

Skeletal muscle movement occurs as a result of more than one muscle moving, and muscles invariably move in groups. As a general rule, when a muscle contracts at a joint, one bone remains fairly stationary and the other one moves. The origin of a muscle is on the stationary bone and the insertion of a muscle is on the bone that moves. The action of each muscle is dependent upon how the muscle is attached to either side of a joint and also the kind of joint it is associated with. When a muscle contracts it produces a specific action. However, muscles can only pull; they cannot push, as when a muscle contracts it becomes shorter. Usually, there are at least two opposing muscles (agonist and antagonist) acting on a joint that bring about movement in opposite directions. An agonist or prime mover is a muscle primarily responsible for producing an action, while an antagonist of a prime mover causes muscle movement in the opposite direction; for example, an agonist may cause an arm to bend, while the antagonist will cause it to straighten.

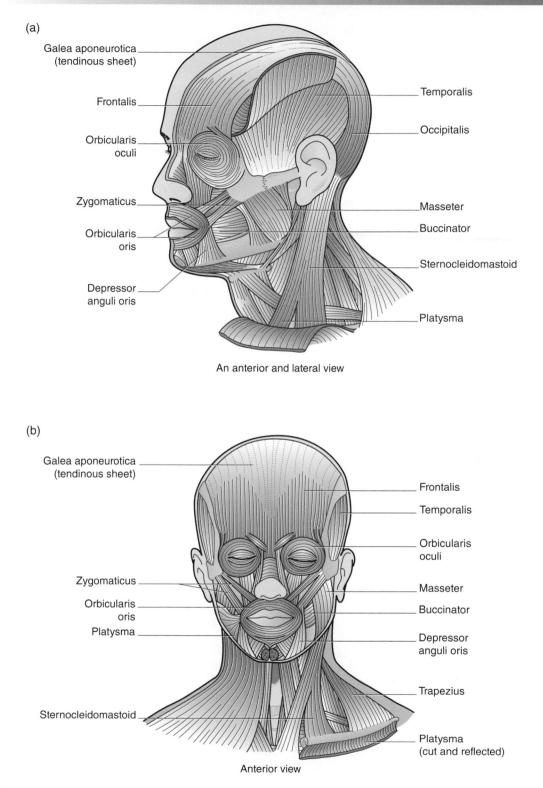

(a)

Galea aponeurotica (tendinous sheet)

Frontalis

Orbicularis oculi

Zygomaticus

Orbicularis oris

Depressor anguli oris

Temporalis

Occipitalis

Masseter

Buccinator

Sternocleidomastoid

Platysma

An anterior and lateral view

(b)

Galea aponeurotica (tendinous sheet)

Zygomaticus

Orbicularis oris

Platysma

Sternocleidomastoid

Frontalis

Temporalis

Orbicularis oculi

Masseter

Buccinator

Depressor anguli oris

Trapezius

Platysma (cut and reflected)

Anterior view

Figure 6.6 (a, b) Head and neck muscles.

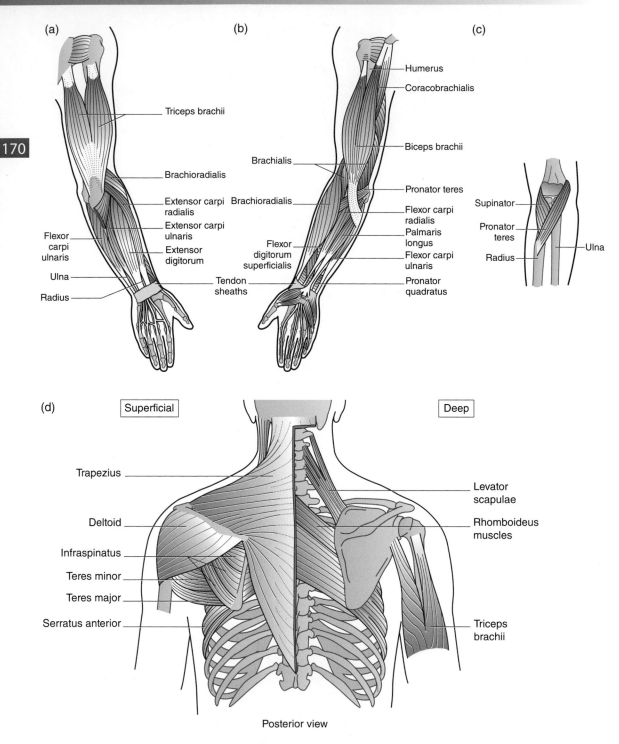

Figure 6.7   (a–g) Muscles of the upper limbs (shoulder, arm and hand).

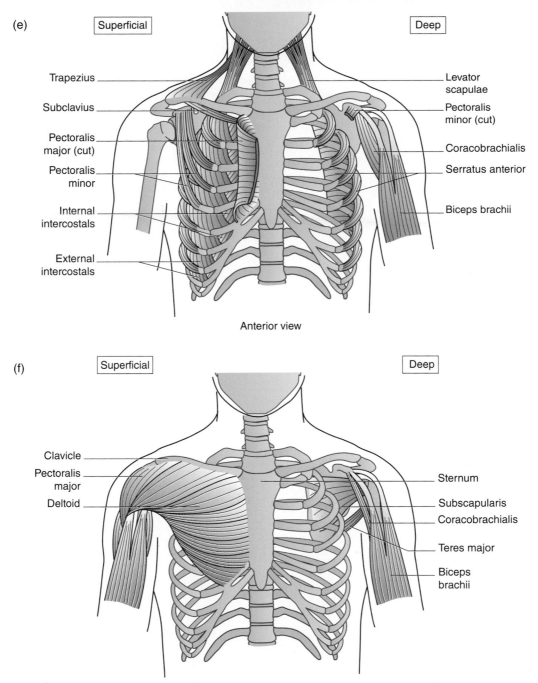

(e)

Superficial

Deep

Trapezius

Levator scapulae

Subclavius

Pectoralis minor (cut)

Pectoralis major (cut)

Coracobrachialis

Pectoralis minor

Serratus anterior

Internal intercostals

Biceps brachii

External intercostals

Anterior view

(f)

Superficial

Deep

Clavicle

Pectoralis major

Deltoid

Sternum

Subscapularis

Coracobrachialis

Teres major

Biceps brachii

Anterior view

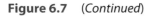

Figure 6.7 (*Continued*)

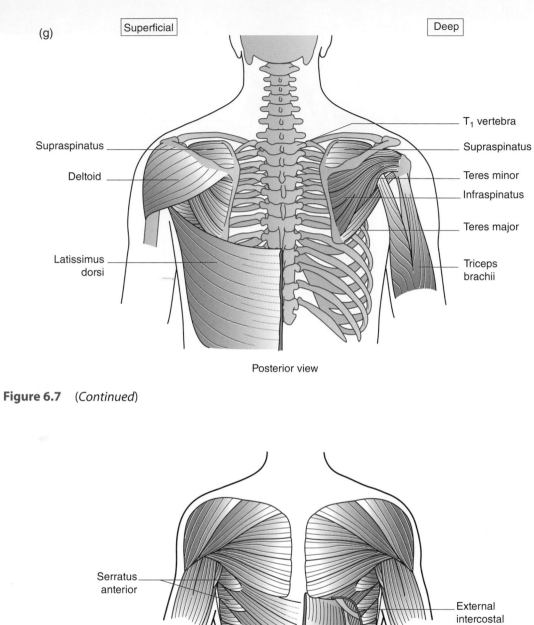

(g)

Superficial

Deep

T₁ vertebra

Supraspinatus

Supraspinatus

Deltoid

Teres minor

Infraspinatus

Teres major

Latissimus dorsi

Triceps brachii

Posterior view

Figure 6.7 (*Continued*)

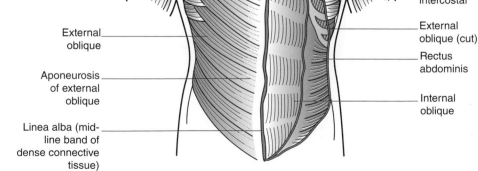

Serratus anterior

External intercostal

External oblique

External oblique (cut)

Aponeurosis of external oblique

Rectus abdominis

Internal oblique

Linea alba (mid-line band of dense connective tissue)

Figure 6.8 Trunk (thorax and abdomen).

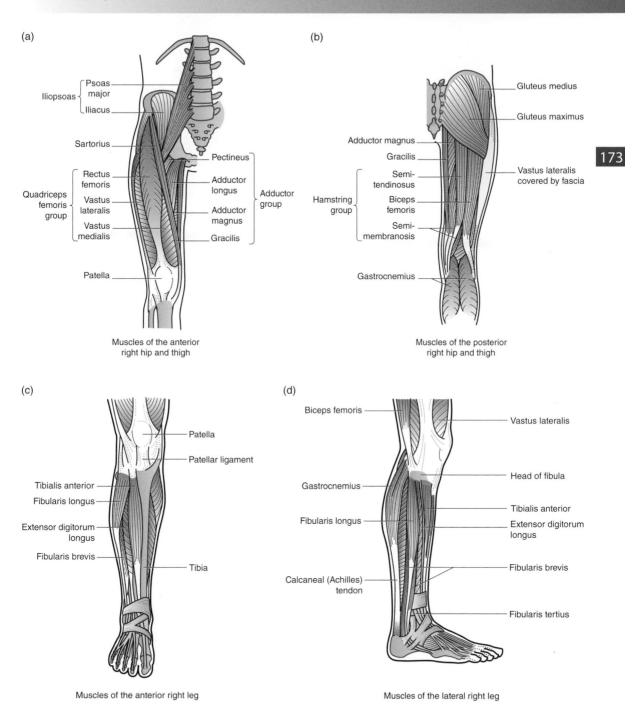

(a)

Iliopsoas { Psoas major, Iliacus

Sartorius

Quadriceps femoris group { Rectus femoris, Vastus lateralis, Vastus medialis

Patella

Pectineus

Adductor longus

Adductor magnus

Gracilis

Adductor group

Muscles of the anterior
right hip and thigh

(b)

Gluteus medius

Gluteus maximus

Adductor magnus

Gracilis

Hamstring group { Semi-tendinosus, Biceps femoris, Semi-membranosis

Vastus lateralis
covered by fascia

Gastrocnemius

Muscles of the posterior
right hip and thigh

(c)

Patella

Patellar ligament

Tibialis anterior

Fibularis longus

Extensor digitorum longus

Fibularis brevis

Tibia

Muscles of the anterior right leg

(d)

Biceps femoris

Gastrocnemius

Fibularis longus

Calcaneal (Achilles) tendon

Vastus lateralis

Head of fibula

Tibialis anterior

Extensor digitorum longus

Fibularis brevis

Fibularis tertius

Muscles of the lateral right leg

Figure 6.9   (a–f) Muscles of the lower limbs (hip, pelvis/thigh and leg).

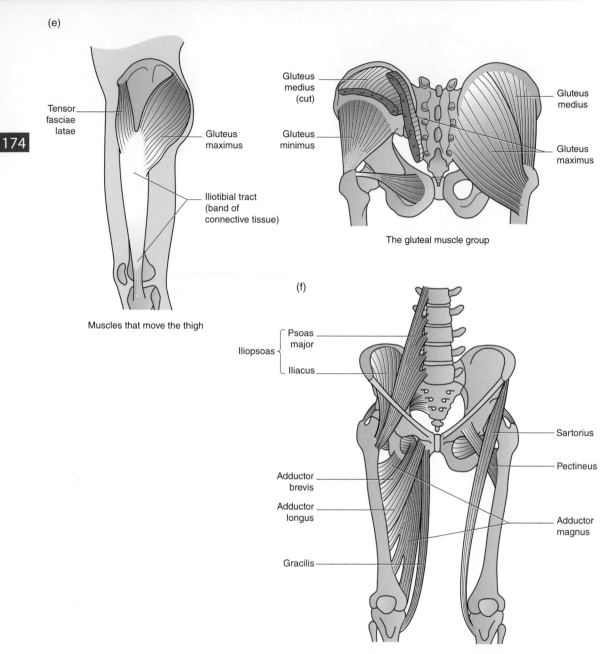

(e)

Tensor fasciae latae

Gluteus maximus

Iliotibial tract (band of connective tissue)

Muscles that move the thigh

Gluteus medius (cut)

Gluteus minimus

Gluteus medius

Gluteus maximus

The gluteal muscle group

(f)

Iliopsoas
Psoas major
Iliacus

Adductor brevis

Adductor longus

Gracilis

Sartorius

Pectineus

Adductor magnus

The iliopsoas muscle and the adductor group

Figure 6.9   (*Continued*)

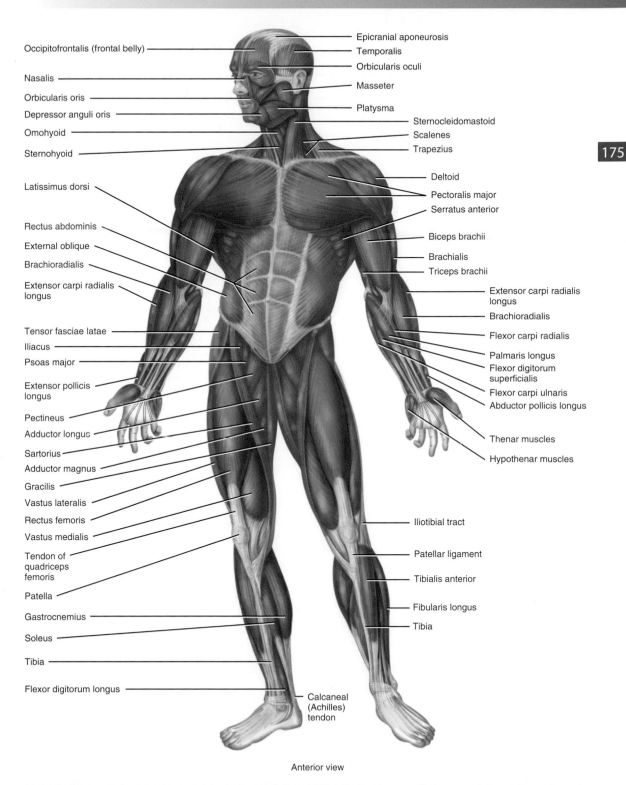

Occipitofrontalis (frontal belly)
Nasalis
Orbicularis oris
Depressor anguli oris
Omohyoid
Sternohyoid

Latissimus dorsi

Rectus abdominis
External oblique
Brachioradialis
Extensor carpi radialis longus

Tensor fasciae latae
Iliacus
Psoas major
Extensor pollicis longus
Pectineus
Adductor longus
Sartorius
Adductor magnus
Gracilis
Vastus lateralis
Rectus femoris
Vastus medialis
Tendon of quadriceps femoris
Patella
Gastrocnemius
Soleus
Tibia
Flexor digitorum longus

Epicranial aponeurosis
Temporalis
Orbicularis oculi
Masseter
Platysma
Sternocleidomastoid
Scalenes
Trapezius

Deltoid
Pectoralis major
Serratus anterior
Biceps brachii
Brachialis
Triceps brachii
Extensor carpi radialis longus
Brachioradialis
Flexor carpi radialis
Palmaris longus
Flexor digitorum superficialis
Flexor carpi ulnaris
Abductor pollicis longus
Thenar muscles
Hypothenar muscles

Iliotibial tract
Patellar ligament
Tibialis anterior
Fibularis longus
Tibia

Calcaneal (Achilles) tendon

Anterior view

Figure 6.10   Anterior view of the major muscles of the body. *Source*: Tortora and Derrickson (2009). Reproduced with permission of John Wiley & Sons.

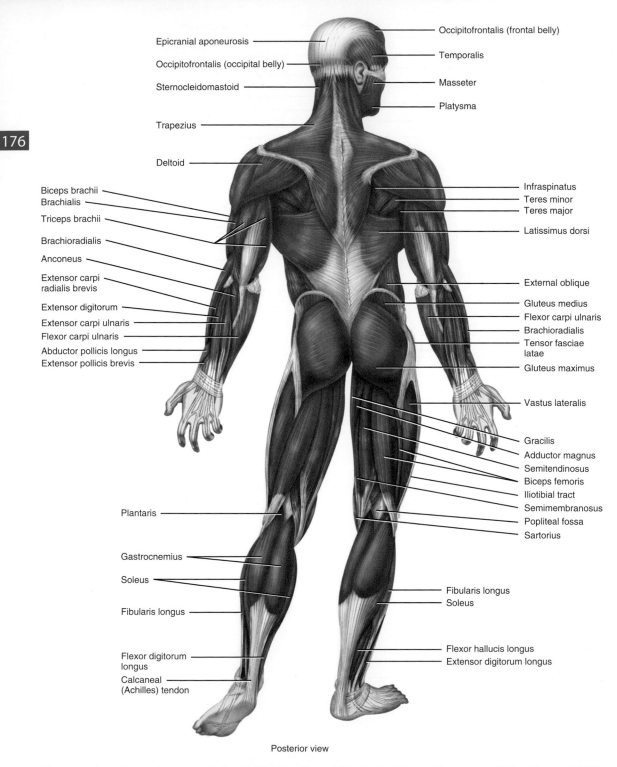

Epicranial aponeurosis

Occipitofrontalis (occipital belly)

Sternocleidomastoid

Trapezius

Deltoid

Biceps brachii
Brachialis

Triceps brachii

Brachioradialis

Anconeus

Extensor carpi
radialis brevis

Extensor digitorum

Extensor carpi ulnaris

Flexor carpi ulnaris

Abductor pollicis longus

Extensor pollicis brevis

Plantaris

Gastrocnemius

Soleus

Fibularis longus

Flexor digitorum
longus

Calcaneal
(Achilles) tendon

Occipitofrontalis (frontal belly)

Temporalis

Masseter

Platysma

Infraspinatus

Teres minor

Teres major

Latissimus dorsi

External oblique

Gluteus medius

Flexor carpi ulnaris

Brachioradialis

Tensor fasciae
latae

Gluteus maximus

Vastus lateralis

Gracilis

Adductor magnus

Semitendinosus

Biceps femoris

Iliotibial tract

Semimembranosus

Popliteal fossa

Sartorius

Fibularis longus

Soleus

Flexor hallucis longus

Extensor digitorum longus

Posterior view

Figure 6.11 Posterior view of the major muscles of the body. *Source*: Tortora and Derrickson (2009). Reproduced with permission of John Wiley & Sons.

Table 6.8   Types of muscle movement

Action	Definition
Extension	Increases the angle or distance between two bones or parts of the body
Flexion	Decreases the angle of a joint
Abduction	Moves away from the midline
Adduction	Moves closer to the midline
Circumduction	A combination of flexion, extension, abduction and adduction
Supination	Turns the palm up
Pronation	Turns the palm down
Plantar flexion	Lowers the foot (point the toes)
Dorsiflexion	Elevates the foot
Rotation	Moves a bone around its longitudinal axis

Common types of body movements include:

- extension – a movement that increases the angle or distance between two bones or parts of the body;
- hyperextension – an extension angle greater than 180°;
- flexion – the opposite of extension, in that it is a movement that decreases the angle or distance between two bones and brings the bones closer together and is a common movement of hinge joints – for example, bending the elbow or knee;
- abduction – moving a limb away from the midline of the body;
- adduction – (the opposite of abduction) the movement of a limb towards the midline of the body;
- rotation – a movement common to ball-and-socket joints and is the movement of a bone around its longitudinal axis;
- circumduction – a combination of abduction, adduction, extension and flexion.

Table 6.8 provides a summary of the different actions of muscle movement.

The effects of ageing

Generally, the size and power of all muscle tissues within the body decrease as the body ages. This can be attributed to:

- Loss of elasticity to skeletal muscle – as muscles age they lose their elasticity due to a process called fibrosis (Martini and Bartholomew, 2012). Fibrosis causes ageing muscles to develop increasing amounts of fibrous connective tissue, which results in a loss of flexibility, movement and circulation.
- Decrease in size of muscle fibres – as the muscle ages, the number of myofibrils decreases and results in a loss of muscle strength and an increased tendency for the muscle to fatigue more quickly. This tendency for rapid fatigue also means that, with age, there is a lower tolerance for exercise.
- Age-related reduction in cardiovascular performance – means that blood flow to muscles does not increase with exercise and the ability to recover from muscular injuries decreases and is likely to result in scar tissue formation.

Conclusion

Muscular tissue is either smooth, cardiac or skeletal and is a specialised tissue that is structured to contract. In so doing, it causes movement of bones at a joint or in soft tissues. Through its ability to sustain partial contraction of muscle, the muscular system also plays an important role in maintaining body posture for a long period of time. Skeletal muscle also plays an important role in heat production and is able to adjust heat production in extremes of environmental temperatures.

Glossary

Acetylcholine (ACh)   Neurotransmitter responsible for the transmission of a nerve impulse across a synaptic cleft.

Acetylcholinesterase (AChE)   Enzyme that breaks down acetylcholine.

Actin   One of the two major proteins of muscle that make up the myofibrils of muscle cells.

Adenosine triphosphate (ATP)   Molecule used by cells when energy is needed.

Aerobic   With oxygen.

Anaerobic   Without oxygen.

Antagonist   Muscle that acts in opposition to a prime mover.

Anterior   Pertaining to the front.

Aponeurosis   Membranous sheet connecting a muscle and the part it moves.

Glycogen   A polysaccharide that stores energy for muscle contraction.

Ligament   Strong connective tissue that connects bone.

Myofibril   A bundle of myofilaments that contracts.

Myasthenia gravis   Muscle weakness due to an inability to respond to the neurotransmitter ACh.

Myofibril   Portion of a muscle fibre that contracts.

Myoglobin   A red pigment that stores oxygen for muscle contraction.

Posterior   Pertaining to the back.

Sarcolemma   Plasma membrane of a muscle fibre that forms T tubules.

Sarcoplasm   Cytoplasm of a muscle fibre that contains organelles, including myofibrils.

Tendon   Tissue that connects muscle to bone.

T tubule   Extension of the sarcolemma that extends into the muscle fibre.

References

BNF (2014) https://www.medicinescomplete.com/mc/bnf/current/PHP6709-pyridostigmine-bromide.htm ?q=pyridostigmine&t=search&ss=text&p=1# (accessed 6 December 2015).

Harris, C. and Hobson, M. (2015) The management of soft tissue injuries and compartment syndrome. *Orthopaedics II: Spine and Pelvis* **33**(6): 251–256.

Longenbaker, S.N. (2013) *Mader's Understanding Human Anatomy and Physiology*, 6th edn. Maidenhead: McGraw-Hill.

Marieb, E.N. (2013) *Essentials of Human Anatomy and Physiology*, 9th edn. London: Pearson Benjamin Cummings.

Martini, F.H. and Bartholomew, E.F. (2012) *Essentials of Anatomy and Physiology*, 6th edn. Upper Saddle River, NJ: Pearson Education.

National Institute on Drug Abuse (2012) *DrugFacts; Anabolic Steroids*. http://www.drugabuse.gov/publications/drugfacts/anabolic-steroids (accessed 21 November 2015).

Public Health England (2014) *Botulism*. https://www.gov.uk/search?q=botulism (accessed 6 December 2015).

Shier, D., Butler, J. and Lewis, R. (2012) *Hole's Human Anatomy and Physiology*, 13th edn. Maidenhead: McGraw-Hill.

Tortora, G.J. and Derrickson, B.H. (2012) *Essentials of Anatomy and Physiology*, 9th edn. Chichester: John Wiley & Sons, Ltd.

Further reading

Myaware

http://www.myaware.org

Myaware is the name for the Myasthenia Gravis Association. This association offers support to people with myasthenia and their families; they aim to increase public and medical awareness of the condition and to raise funds for research and support staff.

Talk to Frank

http://www.talktofrank.com

Provides friendly confidential information about drugs.

Activities

Multiple choice questions

1. How much of the average adult human body is made up of skeletal muscle?
   (a) 40–50%
   (b) 10%
   (c) 30%
   (d) 70%
2. In an isotonic muscle contraction:
   (a) movement of bones does not occur
   (b) both muscle tension and length are changed
   (c) the length of the muscle remains constant
   (d) the muscle tension remains constant
3. The innermost layer of connective tissue surrounding a skeletal muscle is:
   (a) hypodermis
   (b) perimysium
   (c) endomysium
   (d) epimysium
4. Which of the following statement is *not* true of skeletal muscle?
   (a) is under voluntary control
   (b) is not striated
   (c) can have long muscle fibres
   (d) is usually attached to the skeleton

5. The energy for muscle contraction is most *directly* obtained from:
   (a) aerobic respiration
   (b) phosphocreatinine
   (c) anaerobic respiration
   (d) ATP
6. Extension of a muscle:
   (a) decreases the angle
   (b) increases the angle
   (c) is carried out by a flexor
   (d) (b) and (c)
7. The movable attachment of muscle to bone is referred to as:
   (a) the joint
   (b) the origin
   (c) the rotator
   (d) the insertion
8. Skeletal muscles move the body by:
   (a) means of neural stimulation
   (b) pulling on the bones of the skeleton
   (c) using the energy of ATP to form ADP
   (d) activation of enzyme pathways
9. If additional ATP is required, which of the following can be used as an alternative energy source?
   (a) myosin
   (b) troponin
   (c) creatine phosphate
   (d) myoglobin
10. Relaxing and contracting the masseter muscle would mean that you were:
   (a) blinking
   (b) running
   (c) chewing
   (d) bending downwards

True or false

1. There are two types of muscle tissue.
2. The majority of ATP used during moderate exercise comes from anaerobic respiration.
3. The body's skeletal muscles are divided into six sections.
4. When an oxygen debt occurs, the body is required to replenish creatine phosphate to repay the debt.
5. Adduction is the movement of a limb towards the midline of the body.
6. There are over 1000 muscles in your body.
7. Skeletal, or voluntary, muscles are the muscles you cannot control.
8. Tendons connect muscles to bones.
9. The liver is a muscle.
10. A muscle gets strained when it is stretched too much.

Label the diagram 1

Label the diagram using the following list of words:

Muscle glycogen, From blood, Glucose, Glycolysis, 2 ATP (net gain), 2 Pyruvic acid, 2 Lactic acid, Into blood

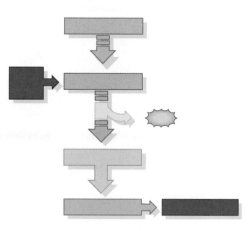

Label the diagram 2

Label the diagram using the following list of words:

Serratus anterior, External oblique, Aponeurosis of external oblique, Linea alba (midline band of dense connective tissue), External intercostal, External oblique (cut), Rectus abdominis, Internal oblique

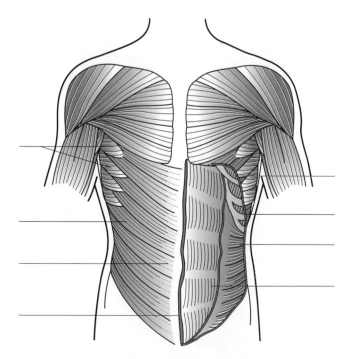

Crossword

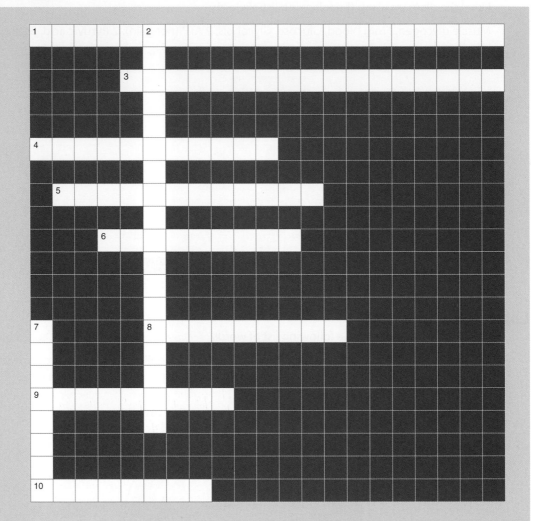

Across:

1. Produce the striations in skeletal muscle (5, 3, 4, 9).
3. Network of tubes that stores calcium (10, 7).
4. Glucose is converted to this during anaerobic respiration (7, 4).
5. One of the functions of the muscular system (8, 4).
6. The _____ of a muscle is on the bone that moves (9).
8. Movement away from the midline (9).
9. Reddish-brown pigment that stores oxygen (9).
10. Ageing results in this in muscle strength (8).

Down:

2. Provides 95% of the ATP required for moderate exercise (7, 11).
7. Diamond-shaped muscle (8).

Find out more

1. Name and describe the three forms of human muscle tissue and list where they are found in the body.
2. Outline how ATP is supplied to muscles.
3. Describe the processes that enable a muscle to contract.
4. Explain how ageing affects skeletal muscle.
5. Describe a neuromuscular junction.
6. Why does skeletal muscle appear striated when looked at under the microscope?
7. What role does calcium play in the muscle?
8. What do anabolic and catabolic mean?
9. What does myalgia mean?
10. What is the other name for the collarbone?

Conditions

The following is a list of conditions that are associated with the muscular system. Take some time and write notes about each of the conditions. You may make the notes taken from text books or other resources (e.g. people you work with in a clinical area), or you may make the notes as a result of people you have cared for. If you are making notes about people you have cared for you must ensure that you adhere to the rules of confidentiality.

Muscular dystrophy	
Myasthenia gravis	
Fibromyalgia	
Tetanus	
Rigor mortis	

Muscle cramps	
Poliomyelitis	
Rhabdomyolosis	
Sarcoma	
Fibrosis	
Botulism	

Chapter 7

Circulatory system

Muralitharan Nair

Test your prior knowledge

- Compare and contrast arteries and veins.
- List the formed elements of the blood.
- Functions of the blood cells.
- Discuss the life cycle of a red blood cell.
- List the functions of the lymphatic system.

Learning outcomes

After reading this chapter you will be able to:

- Discuss the normal composition of blood
- List the functions of the red blood cells, white blood cells and platelets
- Explain the life cycle of the red blood cells and the white blood cells
- List some of the differences between an artery and a vein
- Discuss the functions of the lymphatic circulation

Fundamentals of Anatomy and Physiology: For Nursing and Healthcare Students, Second Edition. Edited by Ian Peate and Muralitharan Nair.
© 2017 John Wiley & Sons, Ltd. Published 2017 by John Wiley & Sons, Ltd.
Student companion website: www.wileyfundamentalseries.com/anatomy
Instructor companion website: www.wiley.com/go/instructor/anatomy

Body map

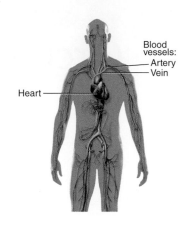

Introduction

The circulatory system is a complex system of distribution of nutrients, gases, electrolytes, removal of waste products of metabolism and other substances. The circulatory system includes the heart, the blood, the blood vessels and the lymphatic system. The blood vessels transport blood throughout the body. Blood consists of formed elements and a fluid portion called plasma. The blood vessels form a network that allows blood to flow from the heart to all living cells and back to the heart. Blood has numerous functions, including transportation of nutrients, respiratory gases such as oxygen and carbon dioxide, nutrients, metabolic wastes such as urea and uric acid, hormones, electrolytes and antibodies. As the blood is circulating throughout the body, cells are constantly extracting nutrients, hormones, electrolytes, oxygen and other substances and excreting unwanted wastes into the blood. Blood is transported throughout the body by a network of blood vessels leading away and returning to the heart. The main types of blood vessels include arteries, arterioles, capillaries, venules and veins. Another important part of the circulatory system is the lymphatic system, which drains the fluid called lymph. The lymphatic system consists of the lymph vessels, lymph nodes and lymph glands such as the spleen and the thymus gland. This chapter will focus on the composition, structure and functions of various blood cells, discuss the structure and functions of the blood vessels, factors affecting blood pressure and the structure and functions of the lymphatic system.

Components of blood

Blood consists of formed elements such as red blood cells (erythrocytes), leucocytes (white blood cells) and platelets. The fluid portion of blood is called plasma, which contains different types of proteins and other soluble molecules. When a blood sample is centrifuged, the formed elements account for 45% of the blood and plasma makes up 55% of the total blood volume. Normally, more than 99% of the formed elements are cells named for their red colour (red blood cells). White blood cells (pale in appearance) and platelets comprise less than 1% of the formed elements. Between the plasma and erythrocytes lies the buffy coat, which consists of white blood cells and platelets (see Figure 7.1). The percentage of the formed elements constitutes the haematocrit or packed cell volume. Haematocrit is a blood test that measures the percentage of red blood cells in whole blood. The volume of blood is constant unless a person has physiological problems, such as haemorrhage.

Thus, blood is composed of plasma, a yellowish liquid containing nutrients, hormones, minerals and various cells, mainly red blood cells, white blood cells and platelets (see Figure 7.2). Both the formed elements and the plasma play an important role in homeostasis.

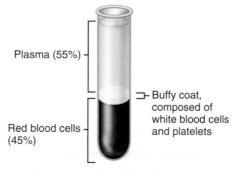

Plasma (55%)

Buffy coat, composed of white blood cells and platelets

Red blood cells (45%)

Appearance of centrifuged blood

Figure 7.1 Components of blood. *Source*: Tortora and Derrickson (2009). Reproduced with permission of John Wiley & Sons.

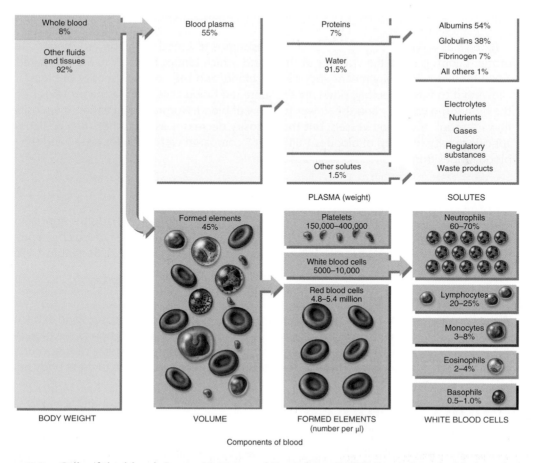

Components of blood

Figure 7.2 Cells of the blood. *Source*: Tortora and Derrickson (2009). Reproduced with permission of John Wiley & Sons.

Properties of blood

The average adult has a blood volume of approximately 5 L, which comprises about 7–9% of the body's weight. Men have 5–6 L and women 4–5 L. Blood is thicker, denser and flows much slower than water due to the red blood cells and plasma proteins such as albumin and fibrinogen. Plasma proteins, including albumin, fibrinogen, prothrombin and the gamma globulins, constitute about 8% of the blood plasma in the body. These proteins help maintain water balance, and they affect osmotic pressure, increase blood viscosity and help maintain blood pressure. All the plasma proteins except the gamma globulins are synthesised in the liver.

The normal osmolality of extracellular fluid is 285–295 mosmol/kg. The osmolality of the blood is important for the cells to survive. If the osmolality is approximately 600 mosmol, the red blood cells could crenate (shrivel up) and die, and if the osmolality is below 150 mosmol, haemolysis (rupture) of the red blood cells could occur. Massive haemolysis can be fatal. Plasma osmolality is tightly controlled by homeostatic mechanisms. Changes in plasma osmolality are detected by osmoreceptors in the circulatory system. If the osmolality is too low (i.e. the blood is too dilute) the secretion of antidiuretic hormone (ADH) is switched off, and the blood slowly concentrates as water is excreted into the urine. Dehydration causes ADH to be switched on and water conserved. In order to avoid crenation or haemolysis, intravenous infusion fluids should have an osmolality as close to plasma as possible. A solution that has the same osmotic pressure as another is called isotonic. An isotonic solution generally assumes that a solution will have the same osmolality as blood.

Blood has a high viscosity, which offers resistance to blood flow. The red blood cells and proteins contribute to the viscosity of the blood, which ranges from 3.5 to 5.5 compared with 1.000 for water. Viscosity means stickiness of blood, and the normal viscosity of blood is low, allowing it to flow smoothly. However, the more red blood cells and plasma proteins in blood, the higher the viscosity and the slower the flow of blood. Normal blood varies in viscosity as it flows through the blood vessels, but the viscosity decreases as it reaches the capillaries. The specific gravity (density) of blood is 1.045–1.065 compared with 1.000 for water, and the pH of blood ranges from 7.35 to 7.45 (Nair, 2013).

Plasma

Blood plasma is a pale yellow-coloured fluid and its total volume in an adult is approximately 2.5–3 L. Blood plasma is approximately 91% water and 10% solutes, most of which are proteins. Plasma constitutes approximately 55% of blood's volume (see Figure 7.2). See Table 7.1 for the composition of plasma.

Water in plasma

Water constitutes approximately 91% of plasma and is available to cells, tissues and extracellular fluid of the body to maintain homeostasis. It is considered the liquid portion of the blood. It is a solvent where chemical reactions between intracellular and extracellular reactions occur. Water contains solutes, for example, electrolytes whose concentrations change to meet body needs.

Functions of blood

The functions of the blood are

- **Transportation:** The blood is the means whereby all nourishment and respiratory gases are transported into and out of the cells.

188

Table 7.1 Compositions of plasma and their functions

Substances	Functions
Water 91%	Lubricates, transports, heat distribution and a solvent
Plasma protein • Albumin • Globulin • Prothrombin • Fibrinogen	Responsible for colloid osmosis, provides blood viscosity, transports hormones, fatty acids and calcium. Protection from infections. Transport of insoluble substances by allowing them to bind to protein molecules. Regulates pH of blood. An imbalance of plasma proteins can lead a patient to experience symptoms ranging from abnormally dilated blood vessels to a weakened immune system.
Electrolytes • Sodium • Potassium • Calcium • Bicarbonate • Phosphate • Chloride	Help maintain osmotic pressure and cell functions
Nutrients • Amino acids • Fatty acids • Glucose • Glycerol • Vitamins • Minerals	Cell function growth and development
Gases	Cellular function and regulation of blood pH
Enzymes, hormones and vitamins	Chemical reactions, regulate growth and development and cofactors for enzymatic reaction
Waste products • Urea • Uric acid • Creatinine • Bilirubin • Ammonia	Broken down and transported by blood to organs of excretion

Source: Adapted from Jenkins and Tortora (2013).

- **Maintaining body temperature:** Blood helps to maintain the body temperature by distributing the heat produced by the chemical activity of the cells evenly, throughout the body.
- **Maintaining the acid–base balance:** Blood pH is maintained by the excretion or reabsorption of hydrogen ions and bicarbonate ions.
- **Regulation of fluid balance:** When the blood reaches the kidneys, excess fluid is excreted or reabsorbed to maintain fluid balance.
- **Removal of waste products:** The blood removes all waste products from the tissues and cells. These waste products are transported to the appropriate organs for excretion – lungs, kidneys, intestine, skin and so on.
- **Blood clotting:** By the mechanism of clotting, loss of blood cells and body fluids is prevented.
- **Defence action:** The blood aids in the defence of the body against the invasion of microorganisms and their toxins due to
  - the phagocyte action of neutrophils and monocytes;
  - the presence of antibodies and antitoxins.

Clinical considerations

Blood transfusion

The main reason for a red blood cell transfusion is to treat anaemia. Anaemia occurs when the body does not have enough red, oxygen-carrying blood cells, which means the body's tissues and cells are not getting enough oxygen. Blood is usually administered through a plastic tube inserted into a vein in the arm. It can take between 30 min and 4 h, depending on how much blood is needed.

In the UK and other Western countries, there are rigorous regulations regarding blood donations and blood transfusions. The aim of the regulations is to minimise the risk of a person being given blood contaminated with a virus, such as hepatitis C, or receiving blood from a blood group that is unsuitable for them.

Nurses need to adhere to local and professional policies when setting up a blood transfusion. Some of the checks carried out include:

- that the patient is wearing an identification bracelet with their last name, first name, date of birth and NHS number;
- date and time the transfusion is required;
- patient's blood group;
- presence of known antibodies/allergies;
- gender;
- diagnosis;
- informed consent.

See Dougherty and Lister (2011).

Formation of blood cells

Red blood cells and most white blood cells and platelets are produced in the bone marrow. The red blood and white blood cells and the platelets are the formed elements of blood (see Figure 7.3). The bone marrow is the soft fatty substance found in bone cavities. Within the bone marrow, all blood cells originate from a single type of unspecialised cell called a stem cell. When a stem cell divides, it first becomes an immature red blood cell, white blood cell or platelet-producing cell. The immature cell then divides, matures further and ultimately becomes a mature red blood cell, white blood cell or platelet (see Figure 16.1).

In order to produce blood cells, multipotent (also called pluripotent) stem cells divide into myeloid and lymphoid stem cells in the bone marrow. The myeloid stem cells further subdivide in the bone marrow to produce red blood cells, platelets (thrombocytes), basophils, eosinophils, neutrophils and monocytes. The lymphoid stem cells begin the development in the bone marrow as B- and T-lymphocytes. B-lymphocytes continue development in bone marrow, before migrating to other lymph organs such as lymph nodes, spleen or tonsils. T-lymphocytes continue their development in the thymus, and may then migrate to other lymph tissues.

Red blood cells

Red blood cells (also known as erythrocytes) are the most abundant blood cells. They are biconcave discs (see Figure 7.4) and contain oxygen-carrying protein called haemoglobin. The biconcave shape is maintained by a network of proteins called spectrin. This network of

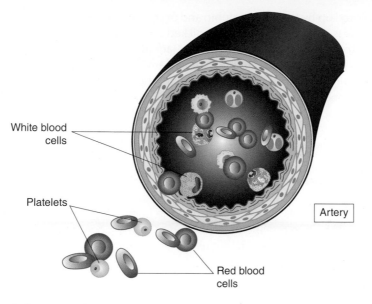

White blood cells

Platelets

Red blood cells

Artery

Figure 7.3 Formed elements of blood.

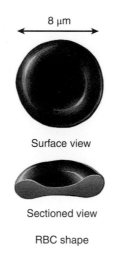

8 μm

Surface view

Sectioned view

RBC shape

Figure 7.4 Red blood cells. *Source*: Tortora and Derrickson (2009). Reproduced with permission of John Wiley & Sons.

protein allows the red blood cells to change shape as they are transported through the blood vessel. The plasma membrane of a red blood cell is strong and flexible. There are approximately 4 million to 5.5 million red blood cells in each cubic millimetre of blood. They are a pale buff colour that appears lighter in the centre. Young red blood cells contain a nucleus; however, the nucleus is absent in a mature red blood cell and without any organelles such as mitochondria, thus increasing the oxygen-carrying capacity of the red blood cell.

The main function of haemoglobin in the red blood cell is to transport oxygen and carbon dioxide (approximately 20%). As the blood flows through the capillaries in the tissues, carbon dioxide is picked up by the haemoglobin and oxygen is released. As the blood reaches the lungs, carbon dioxide is released and oxygen is picked up by the haemoglobin molecules. As red blood cells lack mitochondria to produce energy (adenosine triphosphate), they utilise anaerobic respiration to produce energy and do not use any of the oxygen they are transporting. Apart from transporting oxygen and carbon dioxide, the haemoglobin plays an important role in maintaining blood pressure and blood flow.

Medicines management

Iron deficiency anaemia

Treatment for iron deficiency anaemia usually involves taking iron supplements and changing the diet to increase the iron levels, as well as treating the underlying cause. Iron supplement may be prescribed to restore the iron missing from the body. The most commonly prescribed supplement is ferrous sulphate which is taken as a tablet two or three times a day. Nurses need to be aware that patients on iron tablets may experience:

- abdominal pain
- constipation or diarrhoea
- heartburn
- feeling sick
- black stools (faeces).

Black stools may also result from an upper gastrointestinal bleed. If these symptoms persist, advise the patient to see their GP so that prompt action can be taken to alleviate the side effects.

See NHS Choices (2014).

Haemoglobin

Haemoglobin is composed of a protein called globin bound to the iron-containing pigments called haem. Each globin molecule has four polypeptide chains consisting of two alpha and two beta chains (see Figure 7.5). Each haemoglobin molecule has four atoms of iron, and each atom of iron transports one molecule of oxygen; therefore, one molecule of haemoglobin transports four molecules of oxygen. There are approximately 250 million haemoglobin molecules in one red blood cell; therefore, one red blood cell transports 1 billion molecules of oxygen. At the capillary end the haemoglobin releases the oxygen molecule into the interstitial fluid, which is then transported into the cells.

Formation of red blood cells

Erythroblasts undergo development in the red bone marrow to form red blood cells (see Figure 16.1). During maturation, red blood cells lose their nucleus and organelles and gain more haemoglobin molecules, thus increasing the amount of oxygen they transport. Mature red blood cells do not have a nucleus; their life span is approximately 120 days. It is estimated that approximately 2 million red blood cells are destroyed per second; however, an equal number are replaced each time to maintain the balance. The production of red blood

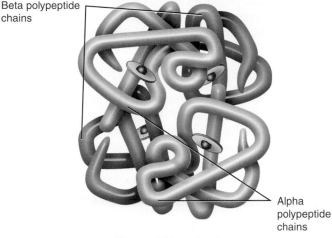

Beta polypeptide chains

Alpha polypeptide chains

Haemoglobin molecule

Figure 7.5   Haemoglobin molecule. *Source*: Tortora and Derrickson (2009). Reproduced with permission of John Wiley & Sons.

Snapshot

A patient with folic acid deficiency anaemia

Boon Sew is an 84-year-old man who lives alone. His wife passed away 3 years ago and he still misses her company. He has two grown-up children and they visit him regularly. He tells his son, when he visited him on Father's Day, that lately he is feeling very tired and does not feel like cooking a meal for himself. All he wants to do is rest and go to sleep. Concerned, his son informs him to see his GP for a check-up.

Boon made an appointment and saw his GP. At the surgery, he informs the doctor that preparing a meal for one person seems senseless and at times he just has light breakfast and couple of slices of bread at lunch time and soup with bread at 7 p.m. and that has been his meal for a couple of weeks.

Boon's physical assessment and vital signs recording are as follows: weight 65 kg; temperature 36 °C; pulse 110 beats per minute; respiration 23 breaths per minute; blood pressure 90/52 mmHg.

His GP carried out some blood tests and sees Boon when the results of his blood tests are ready. The test revealed that Boon has folic acid deficiency anaemia. He is commenced on oral folic acid supplement and referred to the practice nurse for dietary advice.

Boon is seen by his GP after a couple of weeks. He has gained weight (0.55 kg) and informs the doctor that he feels that he has more energy in him and he is able to do his housework and shopping without feeling too tired.

cells is controlled by the hormone erythropoietin. Other essential components for the synthesis of red blood cells include:

- iron
- folic acid
- vitamin B$_{12}$.

Erythropoietin is a hormone produced by the kidneys, which is then transported by the blood to the bone marrow. In the bone marrow erythropoietin stimulates the production of red blood cells, which then enter the bloodstream. The production and release of erythropoietin is through a negative feedback system (see Figure 7.6).

Life cycle of the red blood cell

Without a nucleus and other organelles the red blood cell cannot synthesise new structures to replace the ones that are damaged. The breakdown (haemolysis) of the red blood cell is carried out by macrophages in the spleen, liver and the bone marrow (see Figure 7.7). The globin is broken down into amino acids and reused for protein synthesis. Iron is separated from haem and is stored in the muscles and the liver and reused in the bone marrow to manufacture new red blood cells. Haem is the portion of the haemoglobin that is converted to bilirubin and is transported by plasma albumin to the liver and eventually secreted in bile. In the large intestine, bacteria convert bilirubin into urobilinogen, some of which is reabsorbed into the bloodstream where it is converted into a yellow pigment called urobilin, which is excreted in urine, giving the urine a yellowish colour. The remainder of the urobilinogen is eliminated in faeces as a brown pigment called stercobilin.

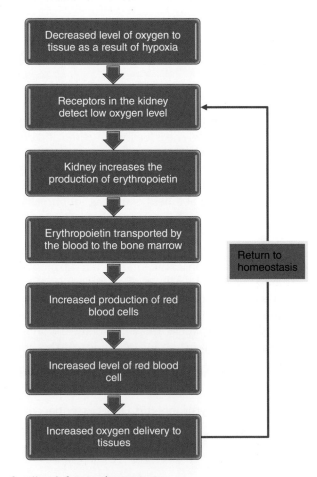

Figure 7.6   Negative feedback for erythropoiesis.

194

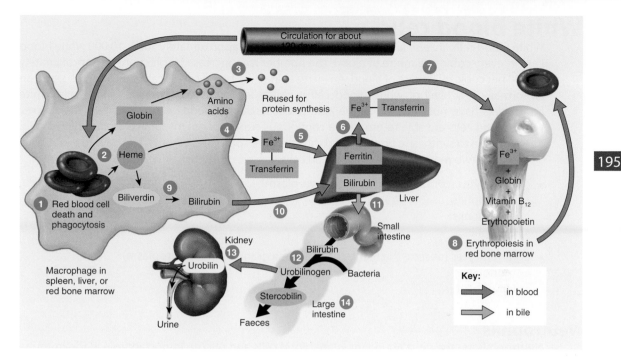

Figure 7.7 Destruction of the red blood cell. *Source*: Tortora and Derrickson (2009). Reproduced with permission of John Wiley & Sons.

Transport of respiratory gases

The major role of red blood cells is to transport oxygen from the lungs to the tissues. The oxygen in the alveoli (air sac) of the lungs combines with iron molecules in the haemoglobin to form oxyhaemoglobin. This is then transported by the blood to the tissues. As the oxygen level in the red blood cell increases it becomes bright red, and when the level of oxygen content drops the colour changes to dark bluish-red.

In addition to transporting oxygen from the lungs to the body tissues, red blood cells transport carbon dioxide from the tissues to the lungs. Carbon dioxide is transported in three ways:

- 10% of the carbon dioxide is dissolved in the plasma;
- 20% of the carbon dioxide combines with haemoglobin of the red blood cell to form carbaminohaemoglobin;
- 70% of the carbon dioxide reacts with water to form carbonic acid, which is converted to bicarbonate and hydrogen ions:

$$\text{CO}_2 + \text{H}_2\text{O} \xleftrightarrow[\text{anhydrase}]{\text{carbonic}} \text{H}_2\text{CO}_3 \longleftrightarrow \text{HCO}_3^- + \text{H}^+$$

carbonic   bicarbonate   hydrogen
acid   ion   ion

The reaction occurs primarily in red blood cells, which contain large amounts of carbonic anhydrase (an enzyme that facilitates the reaction). Once the bicarbonate ions are formed, they move out of the red blood cells into the plasma.

White blood cells

White blood cells are also known as leucocytes. There are approximately 5000–10,000 white blood cells in every cubic millimetre of blood. The number may increase in infections to approximately 25,000 per cubic millimetre of blood. An increase in white blood cells is called leukocytosis, and an abnormally low level of white blood cell is called leukopenia. Unlike red blood cells, white blood cells have nuclei and they are able to move out of blood vessel walls into the tissues. White blood cells are able to produce a continuous supply of energy, unlike the red blood cells. They are able to synthesise proteins, and thus their life span can be from a few days to years.

There are two main types of white blood cells:

- granulocytes (contain granules in the cytoplasm)
  - neutrophils
  - eosinophils
  - basophils;

- agranulocytes (despite the name contain a few granules in the cytoplasm)
  - monocytes
  - lymphocytes.

Neutrophils

Neutrophils are the most abundant white blood cells and play an important role in the immune system. They form approximately 60–65% of granulocytes and are phagocytes. They are approximately 10–12 µm in diameter and capable of ingesting microorganisms. They contain lysozymes; therefore, their main function is to protect the body from any foreign material. They are capable of moving out of blood vessel walls by a process called diapedesis and are actively phagocytic. A non-active neutrophil lasts approximately 12 h, while an active neutrophil may last 1–2 days. Neutrophils are the first immune cells to arrive at a site of infection, through a process known as **chemotaxis**. A deficiency of neutrophils is called **neutropenia**, which may be congenital or acquired; for example, in certain kinds of anaemia and leukaemia, or as a side effect of chemotherapy. Since neutrophils are such an important part of the immune response, a lowered neutrophil count results in a compromised immune system.

The nuclei of the neutrophils are multi-lobed (see Figure 7.8). The number of neutrophils increases in

- pregnancy
- infection

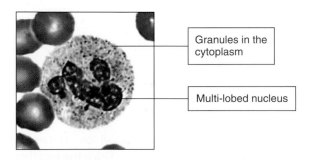

Figure 7.8   Neutrophil. *Source*: Tortora and Derrickson (2009). Reproduced with permission of John Wiley & Sons.

- leukaemia
- metabolic disorders such as acute gout
- inflammation
- myocardial infarction.

Eosinophils

These form approximately 2–4% of granulocytes and have B-shaped nuclei (see Figure 7.9). Like neutrophils, they too migrate from blood vessels and they are 10–12 μm in diameter. They are phagocytes; however, they are not as active as neutrophils. They contain lysosomal enzymes and peroxidase in their granules, which are toxic to parasites, resulting in the destruction of the organism. Numbers increase in allergy (e.g. hay fever and asthma) and parasitic infection (e.g. tapeworm infection).

Basophils

Basophils are least abundant, accounting for approximately 1% of granulocytes, and contain elongated lobed nuclei (see Figure 7.10). Basophils are 8–10 μm in diameter. In inflamed tissue they become mast cells and secrete granules containing heparin, histamine and other proteins that promote inflammation. They also secrete lipid mediators like leukotrienes and several cytokines. Basophils play an important role in providing immunity against parasites and also in the allergic response, as they have immunoglobulin E (IgE) on their surface and release chemical mediators that cause allergic symptoms when the IgE binds to its specific allergen.

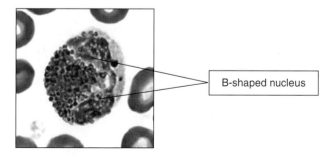

Figure 7.9   Eosinophil. *Source*: Tortora and Derrickson (2009). Reproduced with permission of John Wiley & Sons.

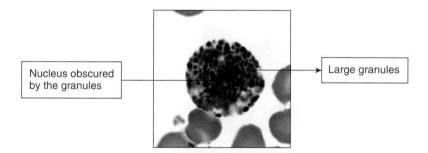

Figure 7.10   Basophil. *Source*: Tortora and Derrickson (2009). Reproduced with permission of John Wiley & Sons.

Monocytes

Monocytes account for 5% of the agranulocytes and are circulating leucocytes (see Figure 7.11). Monocytes develop in the bone marrow and spread through the body in 1–3 days. They are approximately 12–20 µm in diameter. The nucleus of the monocyte is kidney- or horseshoe-shaped. Some of the monocytes migrate into the tissue, where they develop into macrophages and engulf pathogens or foreign proteins. Macrophages play a vital role in immunity and inflammation by destroying specific antigens.

198 Lymphocytes

Lymphocytes account for 25% of the leucocytes, and most are found in the lymphatic tissue such as the lymph nodes and the spleen (see Figure 7.12). Small lymphocytes are approximately 6–9 µm in diameter, while the larger ones are 10–14 µm in diameter. They get their name from the lymph, the fluid that transports them. They can leave and re-enter the circulatory system, and their life span ranges from a few hours to years. The main difference between lymphocytes and other white blood cells is that lymphocytes are not phagocytes. Two types of lymphocytes are identified, and they are T- and B-lymphocytes. T-lymphocytes originate from the thymus gland (hence the name), while B-lymphocytes originate in the bone marrow. T-lymphocytes mediate cellular immune response, which is part of the body's own defence. The B-lymphocytes, on the other hand, become large plasma cells and produce antibodies that attach to antigen.

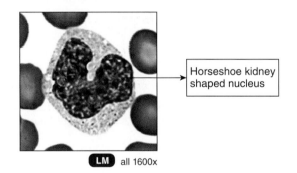

Horseshoe kidney shaped nucleus

LM   all 1600x

Figure 7.11   Monocytes. *Source*: Tortora and Derrickson (2009). Reproduced with permission of John Wiley & Sons.

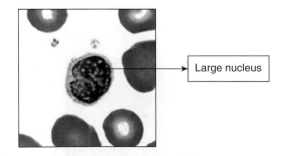

Large nucleus

Figure 7.12   Lymphocyte. *Source*: Tortora and Derrickson (2009). Reproduced with permission of John Wiley & Sons.

Platelets

Platelets are small blood cells consisting of some cytoplasm surrounded by a plasma membrane. They are produced in the bone marrow from megakaryocytes and fragments of megakaryocytes break off to form platelets. They are approximately 2–4 µm in diameter but have no nucleus and the life span is approximately 5–9 days. Old and dead platelets are removed by macrophages in the spleen and the Kupffer cells in the liver. The surface of platelets contains proteins and glycoproteins that allow them to adhere to other proteins such as collagen in the connective tissues. Platelets play a vital role in blood loss by the formation of platelet plugs, which seal the holes in the blood vessels and release chemicals that aid blood clotting. If the platelet number is low, excessive bleeding can occur; however, if the number increases, blood clots (thrombosis) can form, leading to cerebrovascular accident, deep vein thrombosis, heart attack or pulmonary embolism.

Haemostasis

Haemostasis is a sequence of responses that stops bleeding and can prevent haemorrhage from smaller blood vessels. Haemostasis plays an important part in maintaining homeostasis, and it consists of three main components:

- vasoconstriction
- platelet aggregation
- coagulation.

Vasoconstriction

- Results from contraction of the smooth muscle of the vessel wall, a reaction called vascular spasm.
- Constriction blocks small blood vessels, thus preventing blood flow through them.
- The action of the sympathetic nervous system is to cause vasoconstriction, which restricts blood flow for several minutes or several hours.
- Platelets release thromboxanes, which belong to the lipid group eicosanoids. Thromboxanes are vasoconstrictors and potent hypertensive agents; they facilitate platelet aggregation.

Platelet aggregation

- Platelets adhere to the exposed collagen fibres of the connective tissue of the damaged blood vessels.
- Platelets release adenosine diphosphate, thromboxane and other chemicals that make other platelets in the area stick, and they all clump together to form a platelet plug. Platelet plugs are very effective in preventing blood loss in small blood vessels, and with fibrin threads form tight plugs.

Coagulation

Blood coagulation is an important process to maintain homeostasis. If blood vessel damage is so extensive that platelet aggregation and vasoconstriction cannot stop the bleeding, the complicated process of coagulation (blood clotting) will begin to take place with the aid of clotting factors (see Table 7.2). Coagulation factors are a group of proteins essential for clotting, and most of the clotting factors are synthesised in the liver and some are obtained from our diet.

Table 7.2 Blood clotting factors

Factor	Common name
I	Fibrinogen
II	Prothrombin
V	Proaccelerin, labile factor
VII	Proconvertin
VIII	Antihaemophilic factor A
IX	Antihaemophilic factor B
X	Thrombokinase, Stuart–Prower factor
XI	Antihaemophilic factor C
XII	Hageman factor
XIII	Fibrin stabilising factor

The simplified clotting stages involve the following:

1. Thromboplastinogenase is an enzyme released by the blood platelets and combines with antihaemophilic factor to convert the plasma protein thromboplastinogen into thromboplastin.
2. Thromboplastin combines with calcium ions to convert the inactive plasma protein prothrombin into thrombin.
3. Thrombin acts as a catalyst to convert the soluble plasma protein fibrinogen into insoluble plasma protein fibrin.
4. The fibrin threads trap blood cells to form a clot.
5. Once the clot is formed, the healing of the damaged blood vessel takes place, which restores the integrity of the blood vessel.

Two pathways were identified in triggering a blood clot: intrinsic and extrinsic pathways. The extrinsic pathway is a rapid clotting system activated when the blood vessels are ruptured and tissue damage takes place. The intrinsic pathway is slower than the extrinsic pathway and is activated when the inner walls of the blood vessels are damaged.

Clinical considerations

Clotting disorders
Sometimes a blood clot forms within a blood vessel that has not been injured or cut. For example:

- A blood clot that forms within an artery supplying blood to the heart or brain is the common cause of heart attack and stroke. The platelets become sticky and clump next to patches of atheroma (fatty material) in blood vessels and activate the clotting mechanism.

(Continued)

- Sluggish blood flow can make the blood clot more readily than usual. This is a factor in deep vein thrombosis, which is a blood clot that sometimes forms in a leg vein.
- Certain genetic conditions can make the blood clot more easily than usual.
- Certain medicines can affect the blood clotting mechanism, or increase the amount of some clotting factors, which may result in the blood clotting more readily.
- Liver disorders can sometimes cause clotting problems, as your liver makes some of the chemicals involved in preventing and dissolving clots.

There are a number of different tests. The ones chosen depend on the circumstances and the suspected problem. Some of them include:

- Blood count – full blood count is a routine blood test that can count the number of red cells, white cells and platelets per millilitre of blood. It will detect a low level of platelets.
- Bleeding time – in this test, a tiny cut is made in your earlobe or forearm and the time taken for the bleeding to stop is measured. It is normally 3–8 min.
- Blood clotting tests – there are a number of tests that may be done. For example, the 'prothrombin time' and the 'activated partial thromboplastin time' are commonly done. These tests measure the time it takes for a blood clot to form after certain activating chemicals are added to the blood sample.
- Platelet aggregation test – this measures the rate at which, and the extent to which, platelets form clumps (aggregate) after a chemical is added that stimulates aggregation. It tests the function of the platelets.

See Knott (2012).

Medicines management

Anticoagulants

Anticoagulant medicines reduce the ability of the blood to clot. This is necessary if the blood clots too much, as blood clots can block blood vessels and lead to conditions such as a stroke or a heart attack. The two most common anticoagulant medicines are:

- heparin
- warfarin.

Rixaroxaban, dabigatran and apixaban are newer anticoagulants that may be used as an alternative to warfarin for certain conditions. Some of the side-effects include:

- passing blood in the urine or stool
- severe bruising
- excessive bleeding (haemorrhages)
- bleeding gums
- prolonged nose bleeds

(Continued)

- passing black faeces
- difficulty in breathing/chest pain
- in women, heavy or increased bleeding during your period, or any other bleeding from your vagina.

Patients taking anticoagulant medicines should be monitored closely to check that they are on the correct dose and not at risk of excessive bleeding (haemorrhages). The most common test for this is the international normalisation ratio.

See NHS Choices (2015).

Snapshot

Haemophilia

Jonathan Gray is a 25-year-old student nurse in his third year of nursing education. He loves playing rugby during the weekend. One Saturday, when playing rugby, Jonathan received a blow to his face during a rugby tackle. His nose started to bleed heavily and did not stop. He was rushed to the local A&E department with a severe nose bleed.

He was seen by the triage nurse and during the assessment Jonathan informed the nurse that he has haemophilia. The nurse recorded his vital signs as temperature 37 °C, pulse 68 beats per minute, respiration 16 breaths per minute and blood pressure 116/60 mmHg. He also informed the nurse that he was told to avoid contact sports but said that 'playing rugby is in my blood'.

He was also seen by the duty doctor, who carried out some blood tests. The result of the test indicated that his prothrombin and bleeding times were normal.

Jonathan was treated with desmopressin, a synthetic hormone. Hormones are powerful chemicals that can have a wide range of effects on the body. Desmopressin works by stimulating the production of clotting factor VIII (8) and is usually given by injection.

He was admitted for overnight observations and to assess the effect of the treatment.

Blood groups

It is the red blood cells that define which blood group an individual belongs to. On the surface of the red cells there are markers called antigens, which are so small they cannot even be seen under a microscope. Apart from identical twins, each person has different antigens, and these antigens are the key to identifying blood types and must be matched in transfusions to avoid serious complications. The structure for defining blood groups is known as the ABO system. If an individual has blood group A, then they have A antigens covering their red cells. Group B has B antigens on their red blood cell, while group O has neither antigens and group AB has both antigens (Tortora and Derrickson, 2011).

The ABO system also covers antibodies in the plasma that are the body's natural defence against foreign antigens. So, for example, blood group A has anti-B in their plasma, B has anti-A, and so on. However, group AB has no antibodies and group O has both (see Figure 7.13). If these antibodies find the wrong red blood cells, they will attack them and destroy them. That is why transfusing the wrong blood to a patient can be fatal.

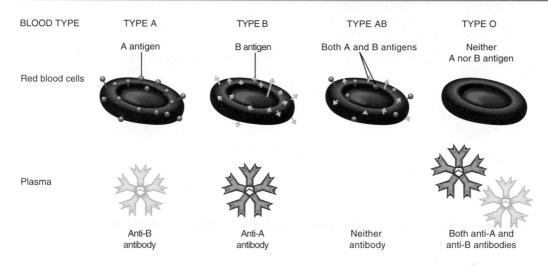

Figure 7.13 ABO blood groups. *Source*: Tortora and Derrickson (2009). Reproduced with permission of John Wiley & Sons.

Table 7.3 Blood groups

Blood type	Antigens	Antibodies	Can donate blood to	Can receive blood from
A	Antigen A	Anti-B	A, AB	A, O
B	Antigen B	Anti-A	B, AB	B, O
AB	Antigen A	None	AB	A, B, AB, O
	Antigen B			
O	None	Anti-A	A, B, AB, O	O
		Anti-B		

There is also another factor (factor D) to be considered – the rhesus factor (Rh) system. Rh antigens can be present in each of the blood groups. Not everyone has the Rh antigen on the red blood cell; however, if a person has Rh antigen on their red blood cells then they are Rh positive and if they do not have the Rh antigen then they are Rh negative. A person with blood group A and Rh positive is known as A+, while if the Rh is negative they are A−. The same applies for B, AB and O. In the UK, approximately 85% of the population are rhesus positive; that is, they possess factor D on their red blood cells. The remaining 15% of the population are rhesus negative as their red blood cells do not have factor D. It is important to consider the rhesus factor when cross-matching and transfusing blood to patients to avoid unnecessary complications such as agglutination (see Table 7.3).

Blood vessels

Blood vessels are part of the circulatory system that transports blood throughout the body. There are three major types of blood vessels: the arteries, which carry the blood away from the heart, the capillaries, which enable the actual exchange of water, nutrients and chemicals between the blood and the tissues; and the veins, which carry blood from the capillaries back

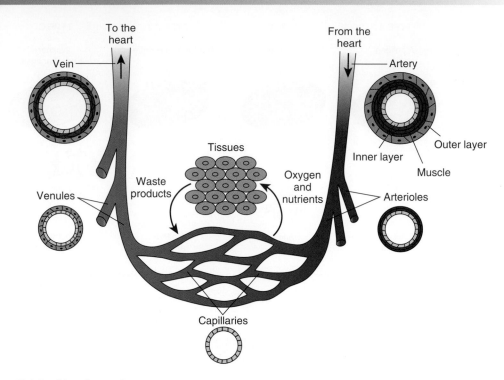

Figure 7.14   Blood vessels.

towards the heart (see Figure 7.14). All arteries, with the exception of the pulmonary and umbilical arteries, carry oxygenated blood, while most veins carry deoxygenated blood from the tissues back to the heart; exceptions are the pulmonary and umbilical veins, both of which carry oxygenated blood. The capillaries form the microcirculatory system, and it is at this point that nutrients, gases, water and electrolytes are exchanged between the blood and the tissue fluid. Capillaries are tiny, extremely thin-walled vessels and act as a bridge between arteries and veins. The thin walls of the capillaries allow oxygen and nutrients to pass from the blood into tissue fluid and allow waste products to pass from tissue fluid into the blood.

Structure and function of arteries and veins

For most of the blood vessels, the walls consist of three layers:

- the tunica interna
- the tunica media
- the tunica externa (adventia).

See Figure 7.15.

The **tunica interna** is a thin layer (only a few cells thick) of a vein and artery. It is sometimes referred to as the intima membrane. It is this layer that gives smoothness to the lining of the vessel, enhancing blood flow. It is lined by endothelial cells and elastic tissues; however, it varies in thickness between the blood vessels:

- arteries – most elastic tissue;
- veins – very little tissue;
- capillaries – no elastic layer.

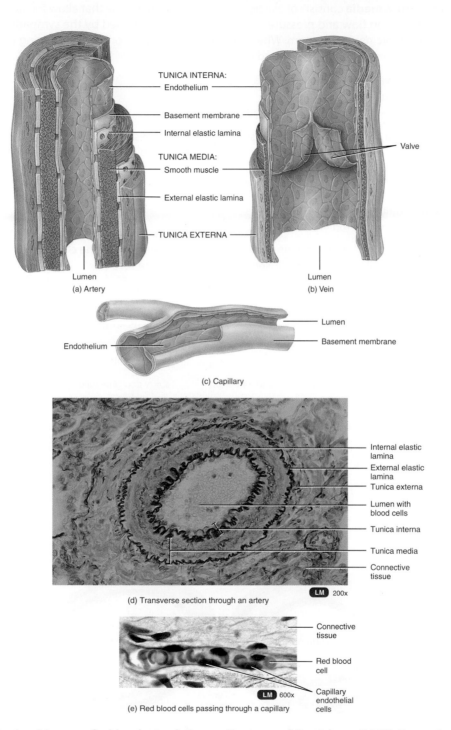

TUNICA INTERNA:
Endothelium

Basement membrane

Internal elastic lamina

TUNICA MEDIA:
Smooth muscle

External elastic lamina

TUNICA EXTERNA

Valve

Lumen
(a) Artery

Lumen
(b) Vein

Lumen

Basement membrane

Endothelium

(c) Capillary

Internal elastic lamina

External elastic lamina

Tunica externa

Lumen with blood cells

Tunica interna

Tunica media

Connective tissue

LM 200x

(d) Transverse section through an artery

Connective tissue

Red blood cell

Capillary endothelial cells

LM 600x

(e) Red blood cells passing through a capillary

Figure 7.15 (a–e) Layers of a blood vessel. *Source*: Tortora and Derrickson (2009). Reproduced with permission of John Wiley & Sons.

The **tunica media** consists of elastic fibres and smooth muscle that allow for vasoconstriction, changing blood flow and pressure. The tunica media is supplied by the sympathetic branch of the autonomic nervous system. When stimulated, the walls contract, narrowing the lumen and increasing pressure within the blood vessel:

- arteries – varies by the size of the artery;
- veins – thin layer;
- capillaries – do not have tunica media.

The **tunica externa** (adventia) consists of collagen fibres and varies in thickness between the vessels. The collagen serves to anchor the blood vessel to nearby organs, giving it support and stability:

- arteries – relatively thick;
- veins – relatively thick;
- capillaries – very delicate.

Although the arteries and veins have similar layers, there are some clear differences between these two vessels. For a summary, see Table 7.4 and Figure 7.16.

Table 7.4   Differences between arteries and veins

Arteries	Veins
Transport blood away from the heart	Transport blood to the heart
Carry oxygenated blood, except the pulmonary and umbilical arteries	Carry deoxygenated blood, except the pulmonary and umbilical veins
Have a narrow lumen	Have a wider lumen
Have more elastic tissue	Have less elastic tissue
Do not have valves	Do have valves
Transport blood under pressure	Transport blood under low pressure

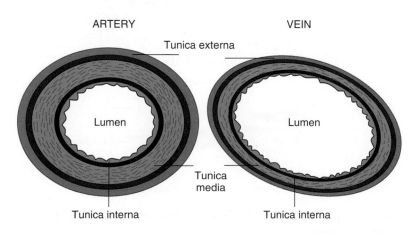

Figure 7.16   Artery and vein.

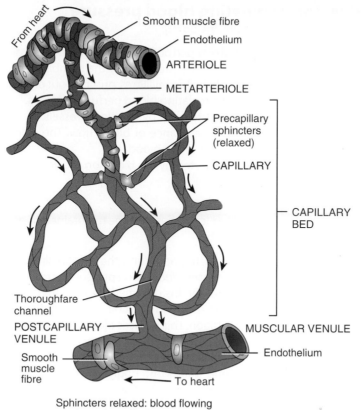

Figure 7.17 Capillary. *Source*: Tortora and Derrickson (2009). Reproduced with permission of John Wiley & Sons.

Capillaries

Capillaries are tiny blood vessels, approximately 5–20 μm in diameter. There are networks of capillaries (see Figure 7.17) in most of the organs and tissues of the body. Capillary walls are only one cell thick, which allows exchange of material between the contents of the capillary and the surrounding tissue fluid. The walls of capillaries are composed of a single layer of cells, the endothelium. This layer is so thin that molecules such as oxygen, water and lipids can pass through them by diffusion and enter the tissues. Waste products such as carbon dioxide and urea can diffuse back into the blood to be carried away for removal. Capillaries are so small that the red blood cells need to change shape in order to pass through them in single file.

Blood pressure

Blood pressure is the pressure exerted by blood within the blood vessel. The pressure is at its greatest near the heart and decreases as the blood moves further from the heart. Three factors regulate blood pressure. They are:

- Neuronal regulation – through the autonomic nervous system
- Hormonal regulation – adrenaline, noradrenaline, renin and others
- Autoregulation – through the renin-angiotensin system.

Physiological factors regulating blood pressure

Several factors affect blood pressure, including:

- Cardiac output, the volume of blood pumped out by the heart in 1 min. Cardiac output is a function of heart rate and stroke volume. The heart rate is simply the number of heart beats per minute. The stroke volume is the volume of blood, in millilitres, pumped out of the heart with each beat.
- Circulating volume, the volume of circulating blood perfusing tissues.
- Peripheral resistance, the resistance provided by the blood vessels.
- Blood viscosity, the measure of the resistance of blood flow. The resistance is provided by plasma proteins and other substances in the blood.
- Hydrostatic pressure, the pressure exerted by the blood on the vessel wall.

Control of arterial blood pressure

Blood pressure within the large systemic arteries must be maintained to ensure adequate blood flow to the tissues. This is maintained by:

- Baroreceptors situated in the arch of the aorta and the carotid sinus, which are sensitive to pressure changes within the blood vessel. When blood pressure increases, signals are sent to the cardio-regulatory centre (CRC) in the brainstem (medulla oblongata). The CRC increases the parasympathetic activity to the heart, reducing heart rate and inhibiting sympathetic activity to the blood vessels, causing vasodilatation. This reduces blood pressure. On the other hand, if the blood pressure falls, the CRC increases the sympathetic activity to the heart and the blood vessels, thus increasing heart rate and vasoconstriction, resulting in increased blood pressure.
- Chemoreceptors situated in carotid and aortic bodies help to regulate blood pressure by detecting changes in the levels of oxygen, carbon dioxide and hydrogen ions. Changes in the levels of carbon dioxide, oxygen and hydrogen ions can affect heart and respiration rates.
- Circulating hormones, such as antidiuretic and atrial natriuretic peptide hormones, help to regulate circulating blood volume, thus affecting blood pressure.
- The renin–angiotensin system helps to maintain blood pressure though its action on vasoconstriction.
- The hypothalamus responds to stimuli such as emotion, pain and anger and stimulates sympathetic nervous activity, affecting blood pressure.

Lymphatic system

The lymphatic system (see Figure 7.18) is part of the circulatory system and it transports a clear fluid called lymph. The lymphatic system begins with very small, closed-end vessels called lymphatic capillaries (see Figure 7.19), which are in contact with the surrounding tissues and the interstitial fluid. The lymphatic system consists of:

- lymph
- lymph vessels
- lymph nodes
- lymphatic organs such as spleen and the thymus.

Lymph

Lymph is a clear fluid found inside the lymphatic capillaries and has a similar composition to plasma. Lymph is the ultrafiltrate of the blood, which occurs at the capillary ends of the blood vessels. Blood pressure in the blood vessel forces fluid and other substances such as small

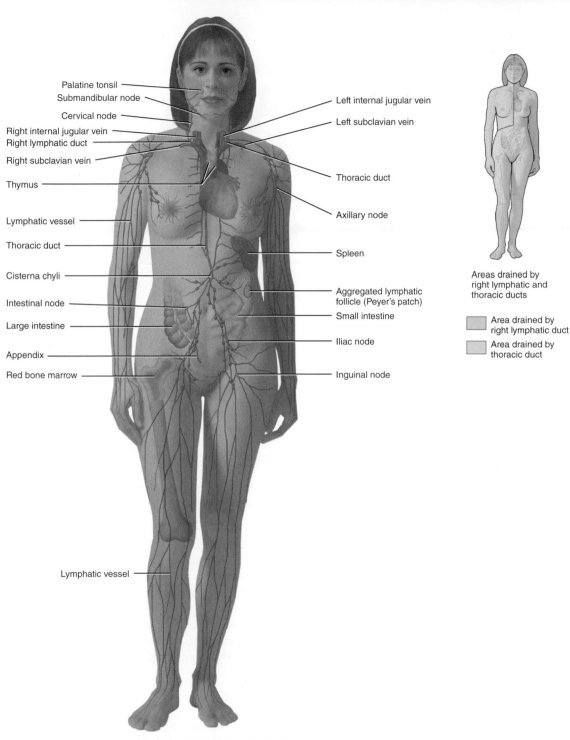

Anterior view of principal components of lymphatic system

Figure 7.18 Lymphatic system. *Source*: Tortora and Derrickson (2009). Reproduced with permission of John Wiley & Sons.

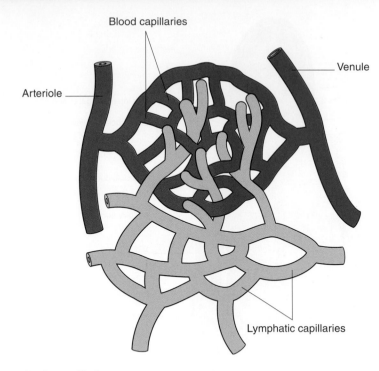

Figure 7.19 Lymphatic capillaries.

protein (albumin) from the capillaries into the tissue space as interstitial fluid, which then enters the lymphatic capillaries as lymph. The body contains approximately 1–2 L of lymph, which forms about 1–3% of body weight. Lymph transports plasma proteins, bacteria, fat from the small intestine and damaged tissues to the lymph nodes for destruction. The lymph contains lymphocytes and macrophages, which play an important role in the immune system.

Lymph capillaries and large lymph vessels

Both the blood and the lymphatic capillaries have a similar structure, in that they both consist of a single-layered endothelial cell that allows movement of substances from the interstitial space into the lymphatic capillaries (see Figure 7.19). However, lymphatic capillaries are one-way vessels with a blind end (see Figure 7.20) in the interstitial space. Lymphatic vessels resemble veins in structure; however, the lymphatic vessels have thinner walls and more valves in them. The larger lymphatic vessels have numerous valves to prevent backflow of lymph. The lymphatic vessels combine to form two large ducts, the right lymphatic and thoracic ducts, which then empty into the subclavian veins.

Lymph nodes

Lymph nodes are bean-shaped organs located along the lymphatic vessels. These nodes are found in the largest concentrations in the neck, armpit, thorax, abdomen and the groin; lesser concentrations are found behind the elbows and knees. The lymphocytes in the lymph nodes filter out harmful substances from the lymph and are sites for specific defences of the immune

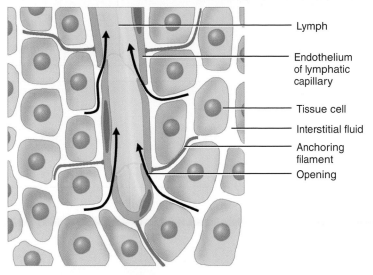

Details of a lymphatic capillary

Figure 7.20   Lymphatic circulation. *Source*: Tortora and Derrickson (2009). Reproduced with permission of John Wiley & Sons.

Clinical considerations

Oedema

Oedema, also known as dropsy, is the medical term for fluid retention in the body. The build-up of fluid causes affected tissue to become swollen. The swelling can occur in one particular part of the body – for example, as the result of an injury – or it can be more general.

The latter is usually the case with oedema that occurs as a result of certain health conditions, such as heart failure or kidney failure. Some of the possible symptoms include:

- skin discolouration
- areas of skin that temporarily hold the imprint of the finger when pressed (known as pitting oedema)
- aching, tender limbs
- stiff joints
- weight gain or weight loss
- raised blood pressure and pulse rate.

The treatment includes treating the underlying cause, including losing weight, exercise and diuretics to get rid of excess body water.

See Robinson (2012).

system. The lymph node is made up of an outer fibrous capsule that dips down into the node to form partitions (trabeculae), thus dividing the node into compartments (see Figure 7.21). Approximately four or five afferent vessels may enter a lymph node; however, only one efferent vessel will transport the lymph out of the node.

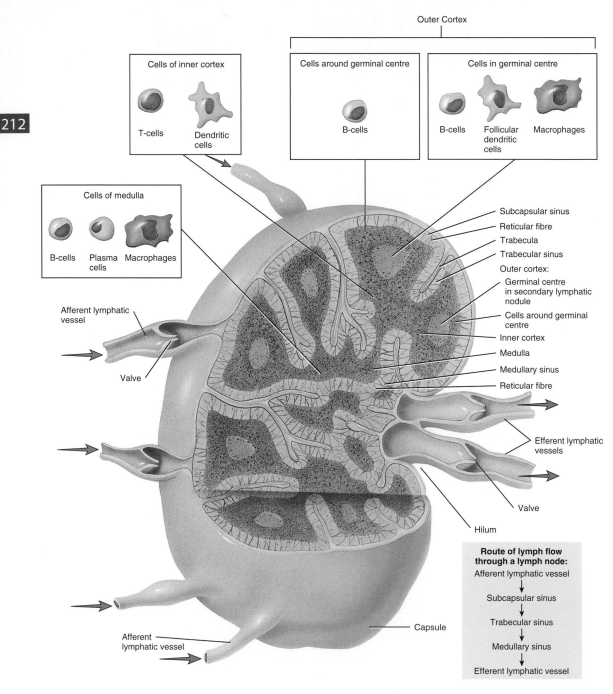

Figure 7.21 A lymph node. *Source*: Tortora and Derrickson (2009). Reproduced with permission of John Wiley & Sons.

Medicines management

ABVD and chemotherapy treatments for Hodgkin lymphoma

Hodgkin lymphoma is a blood cancer. Hodgkin lymphoma is a cancer that develops in the lymph nodes of the lymphatic system. It is the most common form of blood cancer in teenagers and young adults. It appears as a solid tumour in the glands in the neck, chest, armpit or groin.

Chemotherapy for Hodgkin lymphoma uses combinations of different anti-cancer drugs rather than just one drug. This reduces the chances of the patient developing resistance to any one of the drugs. It also reduces the side effects, because lower doses of individual drugs are used. The drug combination most widely used for Hodgkin lymphoma is called ABVD (adriamycin, bleomycin, vinblastine and dacarbazine). This regime is usually given in 4-week cycles by administering the drugs into the vein on days 1 and 15 of each cycle. Patients with late-stage Hodgkin lymphoma are given more cycles of treatment.

Side effects of chemotherapy:

- nausea, which can be relieved using other medication;
- hair loss;
- low white blood cell count.

Side effects of ABVD:

- heart problems caused by adriamycin;
- fever or rash caused by bleomycin;
- lung condition called fibrosis caused by bleomycin;
- ulcers or blisters caused by vinblastine;
- headaches, fatigue or diarrhoea caused by dacarbazine.

See Bloodwise home page at https://bloodwise.org.uk/hodgkin-lymphoma-hl.

Lymphatic organs

Spleen

The two main organs of the lymphatic system are the spleen and the thymus gland. The spleen is the largest lymphoid organ and is approximately 12 cm in length, 7 cm wide and 2.5 cm thick. It weighs about 200 g and is purplish in colour. The main functions of the spleen are:

- filtering the blood – the destruction of old red blood cells and the remnants of manufacturing phagocytic lymphocytes and monocytes;
- storage of blood – approximately 350 mL.

The structure of the spleen is similar to the lymph node. The spleen is surrounded by a capsule of connective tissue and, like the lymph nodes, it is divided into compartments by trabeculae. The two main functional sections of the spleen are the red and the white pulp. It is in contact with the stomach, the left kidney and the diaphragm. The blood supply to the spleen derives from the splenic artery, and the splenic vein transports the blood out of the spleen.

The thymus gland

The thymus gland is a ductless, pinkish-grey mass of lymphoid tissue located in the thorax. At birth it is about 5 cm in length, 4 cm in breadth and about 6 mm in thickness. The organ enlarges during childhood and atrophies at puberty. The thymus gland consists of two lobes joined by connective tissue, and each lobe is covered by an outer cortex and an inner portion called the medulla. Each lobe is divided into lobules by trabeculae, and each lobule has an outer cortex and inner medulla. The cortex contains many immature lymphocytes, which migrate from the bone marrow to the thymus gland to become specialised T-lymphocytes (T-cells). Mature T-cells then migrate to the medulla and it is from the medulla the mature T-cells enter the general circulation, where they are transported by the blood to the spleen and the lymph nodes.

Functions of the lymphatic system

- The lymphatic system aids the immune system in destroying pathogens and filtering waste so that the lymph can be safely returned to the circulatory system.
- The lymphatic system removes excess fluid, waste, debris, dead blood cells, pathogens, cancer cells and toxins from these cells and the tissue spaces between them.
- The lymphatic system also works with the circulatory system to deliver nutrients, oxygen and hormones from the blood to the cells that make up the tissues of the body.
- Important protein molecules are created by cells in the tissues. These molecules are too large to enter the capillaries of the circulatory system; thus, these protein molecules are transported by the lymph to the bloodstream.

Snapshot

Hodgkin's disease

Dorothy Perkins, a 25-year-old, is a qualified nurse on a busy surgical ward. She is married to Peter and they have a child aged 2 years. Lately, she has been feeling more tired than usual, waking up at night covered with sweats and unwell. She put this down to stress at work.

One evening, while having a shower, she felt a large swollen lump on the left side of her neck. Encouraged by her husband, Dorothy made an appointment to see her GP. During the conversation Dorothy informs her GP that she has lost 2 kg over a 2-month period. Concerned, her GP referred Dorothy to hospital for tests.

Dorothy was seen in the haematology clinic. After taking a medical history, the haematologist carried out some blood tests and a biopsy of the lump in the neck. Dorothy returned to the hospital after a couple of weeks for the results with her husband. Dorothy was informed that blood tests revealed mild anaemia and an increased neutrophil count. The lymph node biopsy showed Reed–Sternberg cells, but the prognosis is good.

The haematologist recommended a short course of chemotherapy followed by radiotherapy to the affected site. After these treatments, Dorothy was returned to the community under the care of her GP.

Conclusion

The circulatory system is a very efficient and complex system. It ensures that all the cells and tissues of the body receive all they need, including oxygen, nutrients and electrolytes to ensure that all systems are functioning efficiently. The blood transports many substances, such as red blood cells, white blood cells, hormones and electrolytes essential for cellular function. It also plays a major role in the body's defence against bacteria and other organisms through the action of the white blood cells. The blood also transports waste products of metabolism; for example, urea, carbon dioxide and uric acid.

Blood that is pumped out of the left ventricle of the heart is transported by a network of vessels called arteries and the blood is returned to the heart by the veins. There are three types of blood vessels: arteries, veins and capillaries. Arteries carry blood away from the heart, while the veins transport blood to the heart. The blood vessels of the circulatory system are a closed system, in that blood does not leave or leak out of the blood vessels unless they are damaged. It is at the capillary end that nutrients and other products essential for cellular function leave the blood vessels. White blood cells may also leave the blood vessels at the capillary end; however, red blood cells are contained within the circulatory system.

The lymphatic system is also known as the secondary circulation. It transports fluid called lymph, which is an ultrafiltrate of the blood. It plays an important part in the immune system. The fluid lymph is transported by the lymphatic system from all parts of the body and returned to the circulatory system via the right lymphatic and thoracic ducts, which then empty into the subclavian veins.

Glossary

Active transport   The process by which substances move against a concentration gradient by utilising cellular energy.

Adenosine diphosphate   The end product that results when adenosine triphosphate loses one of its phosphate groups located at the end of the molecule.

Adenosine triphosphate   Compound that is necessary for cellular energy.

Chemical reactions   Reactions that involve molecules, in which they are formed, changed or broken down.

Compartments   Spaces.

Cytoplasm   Fluid found inside the cell.

Diffusion   The most common form of passive transport of materials; it is the means by which gases, liquids and solutes disperse randomly and occupy any space available so that there is an equal distribution.

Electrolytes   Substances that dissociate in water to form ions.

Endocytosis   Processes by which cells ingest foodstuffs and infectious microorganisms.

Extracellular   Space found outside the cell.

Exocytosis   The system of transporting material out of cells.

Facilitated diffusion   Diffusion with the aid of a transport protein.

Hydrophilic   Water loving.

Hydrophobic   Water hating.

Hypertonic   Solution that has a large amount of solutes dissolved in it.

Hypotonic   Solution that has a low concentration of solutes.

Interstitial   Space between cells.

Intracellular   Space inside the cell.

Organelles   Structural and functional parts of a cell.

Osmosis   Movement of water through a selectively permeable membrane so that concentrations of substances in water are the same on either side of the membrane.

Osmotic pressure   The pressure that must be exerted on a solution.

Passive transport   The process by which substances move on their own down a concentration gradient without utilising cellular energy.

Plasma membrane   Outer layer of the cell.

Transport protein   Small molecules that help in the movement of ions across a cell membrane.

References

Dougherty, L. and Lister, S. (2011) *The Royal Marsden Hospital Manual for Clinical Nursing Procedures*, 8th edn. Chichester: John Wiley & Sons, Ltd.

Jenkins, G. and Tortora, G.J. (2013) *Anatomy and Physiology: From Science to Life*, vol. 2, 3rd edn. Hoboken, NJ: John Wiley & Sons, Inc.

Knott, L. (2012) *Blood Clotting Tests*. http://www.patient.co.uk/health/blood-clotting-tests (accessed 22 November 2015).

Nair, M. (2013) The blood and associated disorders. In Nair, M. and Peate, I. (eds), *Fundamentals of Applied Pathophysiology – An Essential Guide for Nursing and Healthcare Students*, 2nd edn. Chichester: John Wiley & Sons, Ltd.

NHS Choices (2014) *Iron Deficiency Anaemia – Treatment*. http://www.nhs.uk/Conditions/Anaemia-iron-deficiency-/Pages/Treatment.aspx (accessed 22 November 2015).

NHS Choices (2015) *Anticoagulant Medicines*. http://www.nhs.uk/conditions/anticoagulant-medicines/Pages/Introduction.aspx (accessed 22 November 2015).

Robinson, A. (2012) *Oedema (Swelling)*. http://www.patient.co.uk/health/oedema-swelling (accessed 22 November 2015).

Tortora, G.J. and Derrickson, B.H. (2009) *Principles of Anatomy and Physiology*, 12th edn. Hoboken, NJ: John Wiley & Sons, Inc.

Tortora, G.J. and Derrickson, B.H. (2012) *Principles of Anatomy and Physiology*, 13th edn. Hoboken, NJ: John Wiley & Sons, Inc.

Further reading

Non-Hodgkin's lymphoma – rituximab

http://guidance.nice.org.uk/TA65

Use this to find out National Institute for Health and Care Excellence (NICE) guidance on the use of rituximab (Mab Thera) to treat aggressive non-Hodgkin's lymphoma.

Anaemia – iron deficiency

http://cks.nice.org.uk/anaemia-iron-deficiency#!scenariorecommendation:6

In this link you will find National Institute for Health and Care Excellence recommendation in the treatment and management of iron deficiency anaemia.

Blood clotting disorders

http://www.patient.co.uk/doctor/bleeding-disorders

Use this link to find out more about clotting disorders. It provides information on investigation and diagnosis, treatment and management.

Activities
Multiple choice questions

1. What is the normal pH of blood?
    (a) 7.45
    (b) 7.35
    (c) 7.00
    (d) 8.02
2. The most abundant plasma protein in the blood is:
    (a) albumin
    (b) globulin
    (c) amino acid
    (d) clotting factors
3. Blood flow to the skin:
    (a) increases in stress
    (b) is controlled when pH of the blood drops
    (c) increases when environmental temperature increases
    (d) increases when there is a lack of ADH in the bloodstream
4. Which of the following is *not* true about veins?
    (a) venous valves are formed from tunica media
    (b) the volume of blood in the veins is greater than in the arteries at any given time
    (c) veins have thinner muscular layers than arteries
    (d) veins take blood away from the heart
5. Nutrient and gas exchange take place in:
    (a) the arteries
    (b) the capillaries
    (c) the veins
    (d) the arterioles
6. Arteries transport oxygenated blood except:
    (a) the pulmonary artery
    (b) the brachial artery
    (c) the cephalic artery
    (d) the cerebral artery
7. The life span of a red blood cell is approximately:
    (a) 120 days
    (b) 90 days
    (c) 30 days
    (d) 1 year
8. Lymphatic capillaries are:
    (a) non-permeable
    (b) more permeable than blood capillaries
    (c) less permeable than blood capillaries
    (d) equally permeable
9. Lymph exits the lymph node via:
    (a) the afferent lymphatic vessel
    (b) the efferent lymphatic vessel
    (c) the inferior vena cava
    (d) the superior vena cava

10. The red pulp of the lymph node primarily consists of:
    (a) monocytes
    (b) platelets
    (c) erythrocytes
    (d) lymphocytes

True or false

1. Most of the iron store of the body is found in the heart.
2. Haemoglobin is found in the white blood cells.
3. Clumping of red blood cells occurs as a result of mismatched blood.
4. Lymphocytes are leucocytes but not all leucocytes are lymphocytes.
5. Arteries have a thicker middle layer compared with veins.
6. Osmotic pressure occurs as a result of fluid pressing against the blood vessel wall.
7. The inner most layer of a blood vessel is called tunica adventitia.
8. Lymph flows away from the heart.
9. Lymphocytes reside in the lymphoid tissue.
10. All the lymphatic tissues are fully formed at birth.

Label the diagram 1

Label the diagram using the following list of words:

Decreased level of oxygen to tissue as a result of hypoxia, Receptors in the kidney detect low oxygen level, Kidney increases the production of erythropoietin, Erythropoietin transported by the blood to the bone marrow, Increased production of red blood cells, Increased level of red blood cell, Increased oxygen delivery to tissues, Return to homeostasis

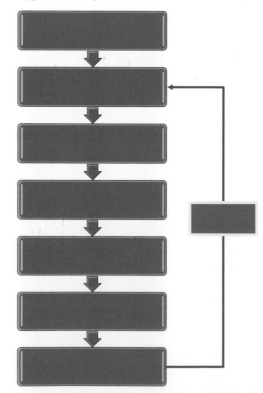

Label the diagram 2

Label the diagram using the following list of words:

TUNICA INTERNA, Endothelium, Basement membrane, Valve, Internal elastic lamina, TUNICA MEDIA, Smooth muscle, External elastic lamina, TUNICA EXTERNA, Lumen, Lumen, Lumen, Basement membrane, Endothelium, Internal elastic lamina, External elastic lamina, Tunica externa, Lumen with blood cells, Tunica interna, Tunica media, Connective tissue, Connective tissue, Red blood cell, Capillary endothelial cells

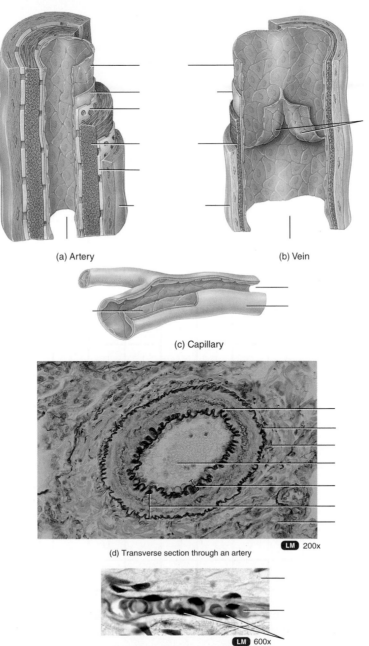

(a) Artery

(b) Vein

(c) Capillary

(d) Transverse section through an artery   LM 200x

(e) Red blood cells passing through a capillary   LM 600x

Blood groups

Complete the following table for the ABO blood groups:

Blood type	Antigens	Agglutinins	Can donate to	Can receive from
Type A	Antigen A			
Type B		Anti-A		
Type AB			AB	
Type O	None			

220

Word search

P	X	D	M	H	S	Q	S	S	L	O	H	T	K	E
N	G	A	I	A	E	D	S	E	Y	S	A	P	M	Y
O	H	V	O	R	T	L	N	I	M	T	E	S	P	L
I	L	K	A	R	Y	I	I	R	P	E	M	L	L	M
S	M	S	V	R	C	H	E	A	H	L	O	F	A	N
U	N	O	S	E	O	P	V	L	O	E	G	L	S	J
F	S	G	I	T	N	O	V	L	I	T	L	E	M	U
F	E	N	S	Y	O	S	I	I	D	A	O	U	A	N
I	V	I	O	C	M	A	S	P	N	L	B	C	Y	W
D	L	T	M	O	Q	B	C	A	L	P	I	O	N	O
D	A	T	S	H	U	B	O	C	B	S	N	C	R	Y
O	V	O	O	P	S	T	S	O	C	R	B	Y	J	X
O	N	L	Y	M	E	F	I	D	R	A	M	T	C	U
L	H	C	H	Y	V	F	T	V	D	Q	C	E	A	O
B	R	M	L	L	V	O	Y	X	Z	S	F	S	R	F

Plasma, Lymphocyte, Lymphoid, Veins, Capillaries, Valves, Osmosis, Diffusion, Viscosity, Basophil, Leucocytes, Platelets, Haemoglobin, Blood, Clotting, Monocytes

Fill in the blanks

Blood

In adults, the most active bone marrow is found in the _____, _____, _____, ribs, breastbone and skull. _____ cells found within the bone marrow are called <u>stem cells</u>. Stem cells can also be found in smaller amounts in the _____. These are called peripheral _____.

The process of blood cell development is called haematopoiesis. In the earliest stage of blood cell development, _____ begin to develop either along the _____ line or the myeloid cell line. In both cell lines the stem cells become _____, which are still _____. During the last stage of cell development the blasts mature into three types of blood cells, called _____, _____ and _____.

blasts, blood stem cells, bloodstream, Immature blood, immature cells, lymphoid cell, pelvic, platelets, red bloods cells, shoulder bones, stem cells, stem cells, vertebrae, white blood cells

Blood vessels

_____ carry blood away from the heart to other organs. They can vary in size. The _____ have special _____ in their walls. This helps to complement the work of the heart, by _____ along when heart muscle relaxes. Arteries also respond to signals from our _____, either constricting or _____.

_____ are the smallest arteries in the _____. They deliver _____ to _____. Arterioles are also capable of constricting or dilating and, by doing this, they _____ how much blood enters the capillaries.

_____ are tiny vessels that connect _____ to _____. They have very thin walls that allow _____ from the blood to pass into the _____. _____ products from body tissues can also pass into the capillaries. For this reason, capillaries are known as _____.

arteries, arterioles, arterioles, blood, body, body tissues, capillaries, capillaries, control, dilating, elastic fibres, exchange vessels, largest arteries, nervous system, nutrients, squeezing blood, venules, waste

Lymphatic

The lymphatic system is like the blood circulation – the vessels branch through all parts of the body like the _____ and _____ that carry blood. But the lymphatic system vessels are much _____ and carry a colourless liquid called _____. Lymph contains a high number of lymphocytes. Plasma leaks out of the capillaries to surround and _____ the _____. This then drains into the _____.

arteries, bathe, body tissues, lymph, lymph vessels, thinner, veins

Find out more

1. Explain why blood is called connective tissue.
2. In the white blood cells there are some grouped under the term granulocytes. List these white blood cells and their functions.
3. What is acute myeloid leukaemia?
4. List the checks you would make to ensure that the patient is receiving the correct blood transfusion.

5. Describe the forces that move fluid across capillary walls.
6. Describe the physiological factors affecting blood pressure.
7. Explain the term 'essential hypertension'.
8. Describe the flow of lymphatic fluid through the lymphatic.
9. In our body there are MALT tissues. Explain the term MALT and its function.
10. How does the structure of a lymph node aid lymphocytes and macrophages in their protective function?

Conditions

Below is a list of conditions that are associated with the circulatory system. Take some time and write notes about each of the conditions. You may make the notes taken from text books or other resources (e.g. people you work with in a clinical area) or you may make the notes as a result of people you have cared for. If you are making notes about people you have cared for you must ensure that you adhere to the rules of confidentiality.

Thrombocyte disorders	
Aplastic anaemia	
Deep vein thrombosis	
Peripheral vascular disease	
Non-Hodgkin's lymphoma	

Chapter 8

The cardiac system

Carl Clare

Test your prior knowledge

- Name the chambers of the heart.
- Describe blood flow through the heart.
- Name one of the valves in the heart.
- Describe the position of the heart in the body.
- Describe the factors that affect heart rate.

Learning outcomes

After reading this chapter you will be able to:

- Describe the structure of the heart
- List the arteries that supply blood to the heart muscle
- Describe the electrical excitation of the heart
- Describe the cardiac action potential
- Discuss the cardiac cycle

Fundamentals of Anatomy and Physiology: For Nursing and Healthcare Students, Second Edition. Edited by Ian Peate and Muralitharan Nair.
© 2017 John Wiley & Sons, Ltd. Published 2017 by John Wiley & Sons, Ltd.
Student companion website: www.wileyfundamentalseries.com/anatomy
Instructor companion website: www.wiley.com/go/instructor/anatomy

Body map

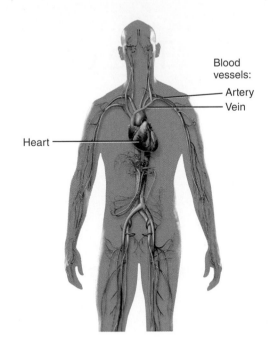

Blood
vessels:

Artery

Vein

Heart

Introduction

The heart is a muscular organ containing four chambers. Its main function is to pump blood around the circulatory system of the lungs and the systemic circulation of the rest of the body. In the average day the heart beats about 100,000 times and never rests. It must continue its cycle of contraction and relaxation in order to provide a continuous blood supply to the tissues and ensure the delivery of nutrients and oxygen and the removal of waste products. The purpose of this chapter is to review the structure and function of the heart, including:

- the size and location of the heart;
- the overall structure of the heart;
- the heart muscle and the cells of the heart;
- the blood supply to the heart muscle;
- the flow of blood through the heart;
- the electrical pathways of the heart;
- the cardiac cycle;
- factors affecting cardiac output.

Size and location of the heart

The heart weighs 250–390 g in men and 200–275 g in women and is a little larger than the owner's closed fist, being approximately 12 cm long and 9 cm wide (Jenkins and Tortora, 2013). It is located in the thoracic cavity (chest) in the mediastinum (between the lungs), behind and to the left of the sternum (breastbone) (see Figure 8.1).

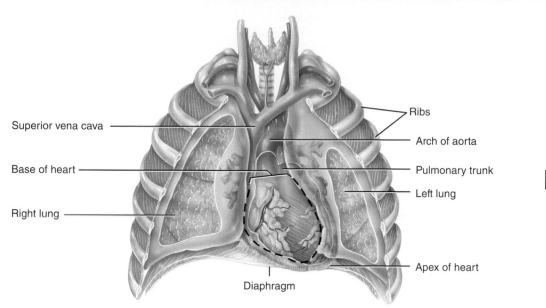

Figure 8.1   Location of the heart. *Source*: Tortora and Derrickson (2009). Reproduced with permission of John Wiley & Sons.

As can be seen, the apex of the heart (the pointed end) is below the base of the heart and lies on the diaphragm. The base of the heart is itself made up of two of the chambers of the heart known as the atria (atrium is the singular of atria).

The structures of the heart
Heart wall
Pericardium

The heart is surrounded by a membrane called the pericardium (peri = around). This is often referred to as a single sac surrounding the heart but is in fact made up of two sacs (the fibrous pericardium and the serous pericardium) that are closely connected to each other (see Figure 8.2). These two sacs have very different structures (Jenkins and Tortora, 2013):

- The fibrous pericardium, a tough, inelastic layer made up of dense, irregular, connective tissue. The role of this layer is to prevent the overstretching of the heart. It also provides protection to the heart and anchors it in place.
- The serous pericardium, a thinner, more delicate, layer that forms a double layer around the heart:
  - the parietal pericardium, the outer layer fused to the fibrous pericardium;
  - the visceral pericardium (otherwise known as the epicardium) adheres tightly to the surface of the heart.

Between the parietal and visceral pericardium is a thin film of fluid (pericardial fluid) that reduces the friction between the membranes as the heart moves during its cycle of contraction and relaxation. The space containing the pericardial fluid is known as the pericardial cavity; however, it must be noted that this 'space' is so small it is normally considered to be a 'virtual' space.

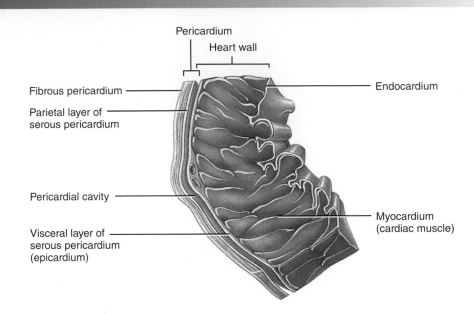

Pericardium

Heart wall

Fibrous pericardium

Parietal layer of
serous pericardium

Endocardium

Pericardial cavity

Myocardium
(cardiac muscle)

Visceral layer of
serous pericardium
(epicardium)

Figure 8.2   Heart wall. *Source*: Tortora and Derrickson (2009). Reproduced with permission of John Wiley & Sons.

Myocardium

Underlying the pericardium is the heart muscle known as the myocardium (myo = muscle). The myocardium makes up the majority of the bulk of the heart. It is a type of muscle only found within the heart and is specialised in its structure and function. The myocardium can be divided into two categories: the majority is specialised to perform mechanical work (contraction); the remainder is specialised to the task of initiating and conducting electrical impulses (this second type of cardiac muscle cell will be reviewed later in the chapter). The cardiac muscle cells (myocytes) are held together in interlacing bundles of fibres that are arranged in a spiral or circular bundles. Compared with skeletal muscle fibres, cardiac muscle fibres are shorter in length and have branches (see Figure 8.3). The ends of the cardiac myocytes are attached to the adjacent cells in an end-to-end fashion. At this point there is a thickening of the sarcolemma (plasma membrane) known as intercalated discs. These discs contain two types of junction:

- desmosomes hold the cells together so that the fibres do not pull apart;
- gap junctions allow the rapid passage of action potentials (electrical current) between cells.

Compared with skeletal muscle cells, the cardiac myocyte contains one nucleus (or occasionally two nuclei) and the mitochondria are larger and more numerous, making cardiac muscle cells less prone to fatigue. However, cardiac muscle requires a large supply of oxygen and is less able to cope with reductions in the amount of available oxygen.

The cardiac muscle cells are divided into two discrete networks separated by a fibrous layer, the atria and the ventricles, and these two networks contract as separate units. Thus, the atria contract separately from the ventricles (see later). Within each myocyte are long contractile bundles of myofibrils. Myofibrils are in turn made up of smaller units known as sarcomeres. Contraction of the cardiac muscle is by the shortening of its sarcomeres.

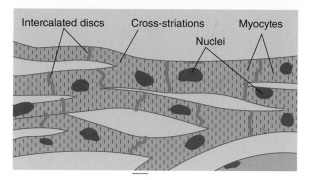

Figure 8.3   Cardiac muscle cells (cardiac myocytes).

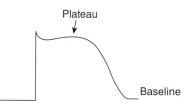

Figure 8.4   Cardiac action potential.

The cardiac action potential

Unlike the normal skeletal muscle, in response to a single action potential a cardiac muscle fibre develops a prolonged contraction that is approximately 10–15 times longer in duration than a skeletal muscle contraction due to a plateau phase. Cardiac muscle fibres also have a longer refractory period, and thus a new contraction cannot be initiated until muscle relaxation is well advanced. Thus, a maintained contraction (tetany) cannot occur in cardiac muscle (Figure 8.4).

Endocardium

The endocardium (endo = within) is a layer of smooth simple epithelium lining the inside of the heart muscle (see Figure 8.2) and the heart valves. It is connected seamlessly with the lining of the large blood vessels that are connected to the heart.

The heart chambers

The heart is divided into four chambers (see Figure 8.5): the atria (entry halls or chambers) and the ventricles (little bellies). Even though the heart is referred to as a pump, it is better to think of it as two pumps:

- The right heart pump receives deoxygenated blood (blood that has given up some of its oxygen to the cells) from the tissues and pumps it out into the pulmonary circulation (the lungs).
- The left heart pump receives oxygenated blood from the pulmonary circulation and pumps it out to the rest of the body (the systemic circulation).

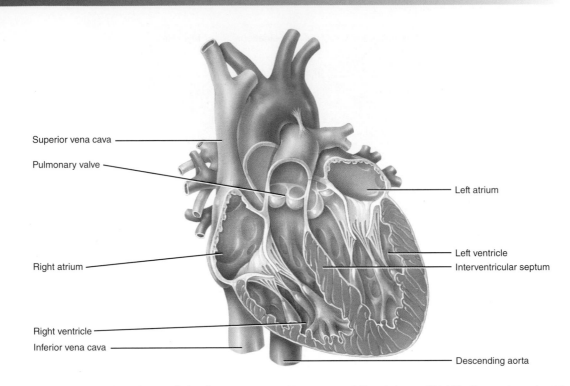

Superior vena cava

Pulmonary valve

Left atrium

Left ventricle
Interventricular septum

Right atrium

Right ventricle
Inferior vena cava

Descending aorta

Figure 8.5 The chambers of the heart. *Source*: Tortora and Derrickson (2009). Reproduced with permission of John Wiley & Sons.

Atria

The atria are the smaller chambers of the heart and lie superior to (above) the ventricles. There are two atria:

- The right atrium receives blood from three veins – the superior vena cava, the inferior vena cava and the coronary sinus. The superior vena cava drains blood from the upper parts of the body, the inferior vena cava drains blood from the lower parts of the body and the coronary sinus drains blood from the circulation of the heart itself.
- The left atrium forms most of the base of the heart and receives blood from the lungs through four pulmonary veins.

Between the atria is a thin dividing wall, the interatrial septum (inter = between, septum = dividing wall).

The thickness of a chamber's wall varies according to the work the chamber has to perform. As the atria are only pumping blood into the ventricles they have much thinner walls than the ventricles, which have to pump blood around the pulmonary and systemic circulation.

Between the atria and the ventricles are two valves (the atrioventricular (AV) valves):

- the tricuspid valve is made up of three cusps (leaflets) and lies between the right atrium and the right ventricle;
- the bicuspid (mitral) valve is made up of two cusps and lies between the left atrium and the left ventricle.

The purpose of the AV valves is to prevent the backward flow of blood from the ventricles into the atria.

Ventricles

There are two ventricles: the right ventricle and the left ventricle. Each ventricle pumps the same amount of blood per beat but they have very different pressures.

- The right ventricle receives blood from the right atrium and pumps this blood out into the pulmonary circulation (the lungs). As the pressure in the pulmonary circulation is quite low the right ventricle has a thinner wall than the left ventricle.
- The left ventricle receives blood from the left atrium and pumps this blood out into the systemic circulation (the rest of the body) via the aorta. As the left ventricle has to pump against a higher pressure and over a greater distance it has a much thicker (more muscular) wall.

Between the ventricles is a dividing wall, the interventicular septum. Thus, with the septum between the atria and the septum between the ventricles there is no mixing of blood between the two sides.

At the outlet of each ventricle is a valve. Both of these valves are made up of three semilunar (half-moon-shaped) cusps (leaflets):

- the pulmonary valve lies between the right ventricle and the pulmonary arteries and prevents the backward flow of blood into the right ventricle from the pulmonary arteries;
- the aortic valve lies between the left ventricle and the aorta (the main artery leading to the systemic circulation) and prevents the backward flow of blood into the left ventricle from the systemic circulation.

Snapshot

Betty is an 80-year-old lady who has been reporting increasing shortness of breath on exertion and regular chest pain. Betty was diagnosed with aortic valve stenosis several years ago after her GP noted a cardiac murmur on auscultation. She has yearly cardiology outpatient appointments at the local hospital, but owing to her worsening symptoms the GP has asked for an urgent review.

The cardiologist refers Betty for an echocardiogram, which shows worsening stenosis of the aortic valve. As Betty is unsuitable for surgery he referred her to a specialist unit for balloon valvuloplasty, which is the dilatation of the aortic valve using a balloon during cardiac catheterisation and is considerably safer than open heart surgery (National Institute for Health and Care Excellence, 2004).

Any of the four valves of the heart can become disordered in their functioning. There are two main processes that can affect the valves (Clare, 2007):

- **Valvular incompetence (regurgitation).** The valve becomes unable to close properly and thus there is backward flow of blood into the heart chamber behind the valve. Incompetence is most common in the mitral and aortic valves; it is very rare in both the tricuspid and pulmonary valves. Common causes of incompetence include age-related degeneration of the valve, infection of the valve and coronary heart disease.
- **Valve stenosis.** The valve becomes stiff and the leaflets of the valve may fuse together, thus narrowing the opening that blood can pass through. Stenosis is rare in the pulmonary valve and is usually only found in the tricuspid valve in conjunction with aortic and/or mitral valve stenosis. Common causes of stenosis are rheumatic fever, and age-related changes in the case of aortic valve stenosis.

The blood supply to the heart

Although small, the heart receives about 5% of the body's blood supply. Ensuring that the heart receives a plentiful supply of blood is essential to ensure the constant supply of oxygen and nutrients and the efficient removal of waste products required by the myocardium.

Only the inner part of the endocardium (about 2 mm in thickness) is supplied with blood directly from the inside of the heart chambers. The rest of the heart is supplied by the coronary arteries. The coronary arteries come directly off the aorta just after the aortic valve. They continuously divide into smaller branches, forming a web of blood vessels to supply the heart muscle. Figure 8.6 shows the main coronary arteries.

Each artery (and its branches) supplies different areas of the heart muscle; Table 8.1 gives a summary of the main arteries, their branches and the areas of the heart they supply. It is important to note that Table 8.1 gives the anatomy as it pertains to most people, but there are normal variations in this pattern of blood supply in as much as 30% of the population. These variations have no significance in the normal, healthy person but can be important in the treatment of cardiac patients.

As the coronary arteries are compressed during each heart beat, blood does not flow through the coronary arteries at this time. Thus, blood flow to the myocardium occurs during the relaxation phase; this is the opposite of every other part of the body.

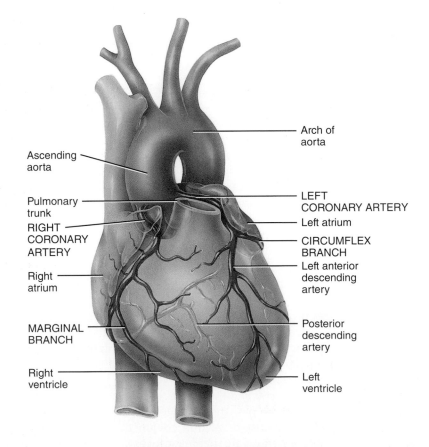

Figure 8.6   Coronary arteries. *Source*: Tortora and Derrickson (2009). Reproduced with permission of John Wiley & Sons.

Table 8.1 Names of the coronary arteries, their major branches and the areas of the heart they supply

Artery	Area of the heart supplied	Major branches
Left anterior descending (LAD)	Front and side of the left ventricle, apex of the heart	Diagonals Septals
Circumflex artery	Back and side of the left ventricle	Oblique marginal
Right coronary artery (RCA)	Right ventricle, base of the heart and interventricular septum	Posterior descending artery

Snapshot

George is a 50-year-old gentleman who has been complaining of recurrent chest pain for the last few weeks. His GP has referred him to the local hospital for investigation and the cardiologist has decided that, given George's test results and his risk factors for coronary heart disease, George should undergo an angiogram (cardiac catheter).

Cardiac catheterisation is the insertion of a catheter through a large artery (normally in the groin or the arm) to the heart where X-ray dye can be injected into the coronary arteries in order to gain an image of any narrowing of the lumen that may be reducing blood flow to the cardiac muscle (Figure 8.7).

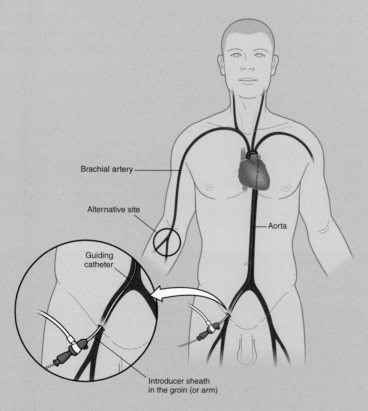

Brachial artery

Alternative site

Guiding catheter

Aorta

Introducer sheath in the groin (or arm)

Figure 8.7 Cardiac catheterisation.

(Continued)

The procedure is safe and is usually carried out as a day-case procedure under local anaesthetic. As with all procedures there is some risk, but the patient should be reassured that complications are rare and usually minor.

George undergoes cardiac catheterisation through the femoral artery. After the procedure George will be required to remain on flat bed rest and then bed rest sat up at a 30° angle before he can be allowed to mobilise. The insertion site should be monitored for active bleeding or the development of a haematoma, and regular blood pressure, pulse and pedal pulse monitoring should take place according to local practice.

The patient should be encouraged to drink to help the kidneys excrete the radio-opaque dye that has been injected into the blood.

See O'Grady (2007).

232

Medicines management

Cardiac medication

Following his angiogram George is informed that he has narrowing in some of his coronary arteries and the pain he is experiencing is angina due to an imbalance between the heart muscles' need for oxygen and the ability of blood to flow through the narrowed arteries. The cardiologist prescribed George a drug called diltiazem to help stop the pain from affecting his day-to-day life.

Diltiazem is one of a class of drugs known as calcium channel blockers. In angina they work by reducing the force of contraction of the heart by reducing the influx of calcium into the myocytes. This reduction in the force of contraction reduces the work of the heart, and therefore the need for oxygen.

Calcium channel blockers are also commonly used in the treatment of hypertension.

The side effects of calcium channel blockers include swollen ankles, ankle or foot pain, constipation, skin rashes, a flushed face, headaches, dizziness or tiredness (National Institute for Health and Care Excellence, 2013).

While diltiazem is not known to be affected, many of the calcium channel blockers are affected by grapefruit, and thus patients are generally advised not to drink grapefruit juice or eat grapefruit when taking calcium channel blockers. Other citrus fruits do not seem to have the same effect and can be eaten as normal.

A list of medications that can interact with grapefruit can be found at http://www.evidence.nhs.uk/formulary/bnf/current/a1-interactions/list-of-drug-interactions/grapefruit-juice.

Clinical considerations

Myocardial infarction

When one of the arteries supplying the heart muscle with blood becomes blocked by a thrombus (blood clot) the patient needs rapid treatment in order to try to limit the damage to the heart muscle. There are two main treatment options available:

- **Thrombolysis** – the administration of a thrombolytic drug in order to try to break up the clot and return blood flow through the artery. This form of treatment is very common and requires no specialist equipment to administer. However, patients are closely monitored for side effects, including bleeding, hypotension and disturbances in the heart rhythm.

(Continued)

- **Percutaneous coronary intervention (PCI)** – this is a specialist procedure requiring a dedicated cardiac catheterisation suite (a form of operating theatre with special imaging equipment), trained staff and various cardiac catheters, balloons and stents (Figure 8.8). The patient has a catheter inserted through a hole made in the femoral artery and the catheter is manoeuvred to the artery where the blockage is situated. A balloon is then passed through and inflated to push the thrombus into the walls of the artery and if necessary a metal cage (a stent) is inserted into the artery to keep the artery open. Though a specialist procedure, PCI is becoming more common in the UK.

See University of Michigan Health System (2014) for diagrams on coronary stent placement.

233

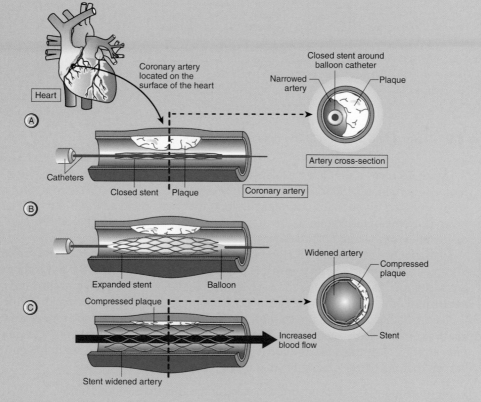

Figure 8.8 Percutaneous coronary intervention. *Source*: National Heart, Lung, and Blood Institute, National Institutes of Health.

Blood flow through the heart

As noted earlier in the chapter, though the heart is a single organ it is best to think of it as two pumps, the right and the left heart pumps. Each pump is made up of two chambers (atrium and ventricle) and their associated valves.

- The right heart pump receives blood from the systemic circulation (the body) and pumps it through the pulmonary circulation (the lungs).
- The left heart pump receives blood from the pulmonary circulation and pumps it out around the systemic circulation.

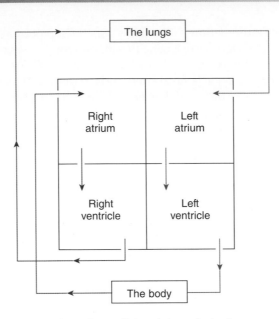

Figure 8.9   A simplified diagram of the flow of blood though the heart.

Figure 8.9 gives a simplified explanation of the flow of blood through the heart. In this diagram, deoxygenated blood is in blue and oxygenated blood is in red. It is important to note that 'deoxygenated blood' does not refer to blood that has no oxygen in it but to blood that has given up some of its oxygen to the tissues. Typically, deoxygenated blood contains 75% of the oxygen that oxygenated blood carries.

So as can be seen, deoxygenated blood returns from the body to the right atrium and then into the right ventricle, from where it is pumped out to the lungs. In the lungs the waste gases are exchanged for oxygen and the oxygenated blood flows into the left atrium and into the left ventricle. From the left ventricle the blood is then pumped into the circulation of the body.

A more detailed and anatomical view can be seen in Figure 8.10. Blood enters the right atrium via the superior vena cava and inferior vena cava and leaves the right ventricle via the pulmonary arteries. Note that even though it is deoxygenated blood leaving the right ventricle it is the vessels that the blood is carried in that make it arterial or venous. Thus:

- blood entering the atria is carried in veins and is therefore venous blood;
- blood leaving the ventricles is carried in arteries and is arterial blood.

Blood is transported through the pulmonary circulation and returned to the left atrium through the pulmonary veins; it is then pumped out by the left ventricle into the aorta.

The electrical pathways of the heart

Within the heart there is a specialised network of electrical pathways dedicated to ensuring the rapid transmission of electrical impulses. This ensures that the myocardium is excited rapidly in response to an initiating impulse so that the chambers contract and relax in the right order and the different pairs of chambers (atria and ventricles) contract at the same time. So, for instance, the left and right ventricles will contract simultaneously in response to an impulse (but after the atria). Also, the way in which the conduction system is organised means that the ventricles contract in a

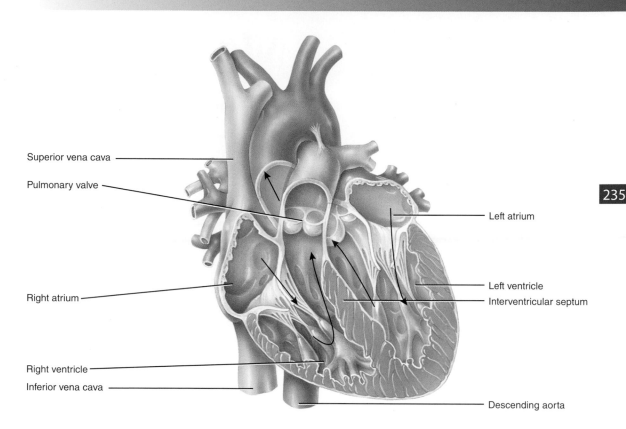

Superior vena cava

Pulmonary valve

Left atrium

Right atrium

Left ventricle
Interventricular septum

Right ventricle

Inferior vena cava

Descending aorta

Figure 8.10 Anatomical view of the blood flow through the heart. *Source*: Tortora and Derrickson (2009). Reproduced with permission of John Wiley & Sons.

certain way to ensure they eject blood effectively. For example, if you wanted to empty out a tube of toothpaste you would squeeze from the base to ensure maximum effect. Likewise, the ventricles contract in such a way as to push blood towards and through the semilunar valves.

The cardiac muscles have a specialised property not seen in any other part of the body. All cells within the myocardium have the ability to create their own action potential without external excitation from another cell or a hormone. This is known as automaticity (or auto-rhythmicity). The problem with this is that, uncontrolled, the cells would all act independently and the heart would not beat effectively as there would be no coordination of the electrical activity and the subsequent muscle contractions. This is overcome by the use of the specialised cells in the conduction system. These cells create and distribute an electrical current that leads to a controlled and effective heart contraction. An overview of the anatomy of the conduction system can be seen in Figure 8.11.

Normal electrical excitation/distribution begins in the sinoatrial (SA) node, which is located in the right atrium, and is rapidly transmitted across the atria by fast pathways. This ensures that the right and left atria are excited together and beat as one unit. The impulse is transmitted to the AV node, where further transmission is delayed for approximately 0.1 s (Martini *et al.*, 2014). This ensures that the atria have completely contracted before ventricular contraction is initiated. It should be noted that the atria and the ventricles are electrically isolated from each other by a band of non-conducting fibrous tissue, and thus the only electrical connection between the two is the bundle of His (AV bundle) (Figure 8.12).

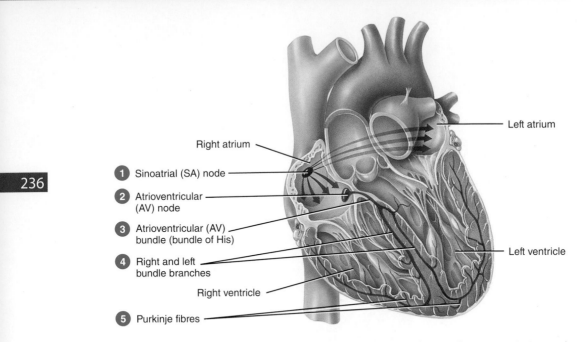

Figure 8.11 Conduction system of the heart. *Source*: Tortora and Derrickson (2009). Reproduced with permission of John Wiley & Sons.

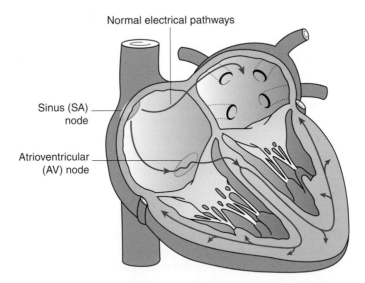

Figure 8.12 Normal electrical conduction. *Source*: Tortora and Derrickson (2009). Reproduced with permission of John Wiley & Sons.

Once the impulse has been 'held' in the AV node it is then transmitted down the bundle of His (AV bundle) to the fast pathways of the two bundle branches (one bundle branch per ventricle). The bundles then divide into the smaller and smaller branches of the Purkinje system, which transmits the impulses to the muscles of the ventricles.

Medicines management

Digoxin

Pauline is a 72-year-old lady admitted to the coronary care unit with a heart rate of 35 and a blood pressure of 90/40 mmHg. She is feeling very unwell and is restless, confused and agitated. The electrocardiogram (ECG) recording of her heart shows signs of digoxin toxicity, and on questioning Pauline's daughter it appears Pauline had been prescribed digoxin a few months ago.

Digoxin is a cardiac glycoside used in the treatment of heart failure and arrhythmias of the atria. Once a very popular drug its use has reduced, but it is still commonly prescribed. Digoxin slows and strengthens the heart beat (decreasing heart rate and increasing force of contraction). Owing to these effects, an excess of digoxin in the blood can lead to slow heart rates, leading to dizziness. In the elderly, excretion of digoxin is reduced, and thus digoxin levels can rise above the therapeutic threshold even on normal doses.

The signs of digoxin toxicity include nausea, vomiting, confusion, delirium and headache. It can also lead to very high levels of blood potassium. In life-threatening cases the digoxin can be counteracted by the use of digoxin-specific antibodies (digibind) infused into the blood. Otherwise supportive treatment and monitoring may be instituted and the digoxin withheld.

When administering digoxin, the nurse is expected to take the pulse of the patient and if it is below 60 beats per minute the drug should be withheld and medical advice sought.

See British National Formulary (2015).

237

Clinical considerations

Nodal cells

Otherwise known as pacemaker cells, these are specialised cells that not only create electrical impulses but also create them at regular intervals.

Nodal cells are divided into two groups:

1. The SA node located in the right atrium, which generates electrical impulses at approximately 70–80 impulses per minute.
2. The AV node, located just above the point where the atria and ventricles meet. This node generates impulses at 40–60 impulses per minute.

The difference in the rate of impulse creation is important in the normal functioning of the heart as every time an impulse is transmitted down the electrical system it 'resets' the cells 'lower down'. Hence, the SA node is the normal pacemaker of the heart as it creates impulses faster than the AV node.

Thus, like a military command structure, the SA node could be seen to be a general who commands the captain (AV node), but if the general no longer issues commands then the captain will take over command.

Even with the 'command structure' created by the nodal cells the conduction system of the heart can slow considerably and the patient can become very unwell. For instance, if the AV node no longer transmits impulses into the bundle of His (bundle of His), the cells in the lower parts of the conduction system can produce action potentials of their own, but this will be at a very slow rate (between 20 and 35 impulses per minute). In order to deal with this problem the patient would need to have a permanent pacemaker fitted (Figure 8.13).

(Continued)

The 'generator' (battery and circuitry) is contained in a small box that is buried beneath the skin of the chest wall. Wires lead from the generator through a vein into the patient's heart. Depending on the type of pacemaker fitted, there may be one or two wires. So, for instance, in the case of a failed AV node the pacemaker would have two wires: one in the right atrium and one in the right ventricle. The pacemaker would sense the atrial action potential and then (after a short delay to mimic the action of the AV node) the ventricle would receive an electrical impulse, causing it to contract. Thus, the pacemaker acts as a replacement AV node (O'Grady, 2007).

238

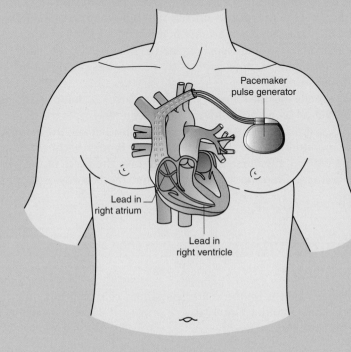

Figure 8.13   Pacemaker.

Snapshot

On admission to the coronary care unit Pauline required a 12-lead ECG and cardiac monitoring. While they both record the electrical activity of the heart, 3-lead monitoring and a 12-lead ECG have different purposes.

Three-lead cardiac monitoring is used for the continuous monitoring of the heart rhythm in patients thought to be at risk of a heart rhythm disturbance. The lead placement is as follows:

Red lead	Right arm
Yellow lead	Left arm
Green lead	Left leg
or	
Black lead	Right leg

(Continued)

It should be noted that the leads of a monitoring system are normally attached to the relevant shoulder for the arm leads and the lower chest for the leg leads, thus leaving the patient freedom of movement and leaving the chest clear for resuscitation (if required).

For a 12-lead ECG the limb leads are placed as noted above but at the wrists and ankles; the chest leads are then attached. Many nurses use mnemonics to remember limb lead placement such as: '**R**ide **Y**our **G**reen **B**ike'; others will think of *red for right* and *lemon for left*.

Twelve-lead ECGs are used for diagnostic purposes, and correct lead placement is essential.

Chest lead placement for a 12-lead ECG is a skill that should be practised under supervision until competent. Figure 8.14 shows the lead placement.

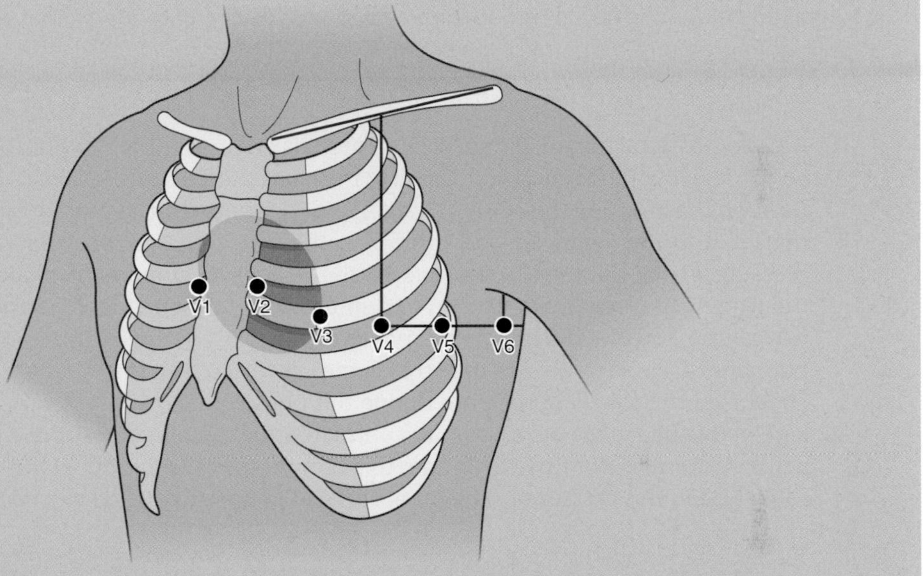

Figure 8.14   Chest lead placement for a 12-lead ECG.

- V1: fourth intercostal space, right sternal border.
- V2: fourth intercostal space, left sternal border.
- V3: midway between V2 and V4.
- V4: fifth intercostal space, left midclavicular line.
- V5: level with V4, left anterior axillary line.
- V6: level with V4, left mid axillary line.

In female patients electrodes are *never* placed on top of the breast unless you cannot gain access to the normal position. If you do have to move onto the breast, write it on the recording.

The cardiac cycle

The cardiac cycle is the name given to the mechanical activity of the heart and is best understood by looking at the pressure changes in the heart chambers and the aorta and relating these to the mechanical activity of the heart and its chambers.

Systole and diastole

These are two terms that require definition as they are unique in anatomy and physiology to the functioning of the heart.

Systole: the contraction of a heart chamber (atrium or ventricle).

Diastole: the relaxation of a heart chamber (atrium or ventricle).

The cardiac cycle can be seen in Figure 8.15. Note, the diagram refers to the pressures in the left side of the heart (atrium and ventricle); the cardiac cycle is the same on the right side but the pressures are lower. The cardiac cycle can be broken down into a series of steps that are detailed below. The flow of blood in the heart and the circulatory system is always from a point of higher pressure to a point of lower pressure.

The cardiac cycle is usually divided into five phases:

1. A period of ventricular filling in mid to late relaxation (ventricular diastole). Pressure in the ventricle is low. Blood that is returning to the heart through the vena cava is flowing passively through the atria and the open AV valves into the ventricle. The pressure in the atria is higher than that in the ventricles and this forces the bicuspid and tricuspid valves open. As the pressure in the ventricles rises due to the increased amount of blood in the ventricles the leaflets of the AV valves begin to drift upwards to their closed positions. The semilunar valves (the aortic and the pulmonary valves) are closed; the pressure in the aorta and the pulmonary arteries is greater than that in the ventricles, thus forcing these valves shut. About 70% of ventricular filling happens during this phase.

2. Late in this phase the atria begin to contract (atrial systole) in response to excitation by an action potential from the SA node; this compresses the blood in the atria, leading to a slight rise in the pressure in the atria. This rise in pressure leads to a greater flow of blood

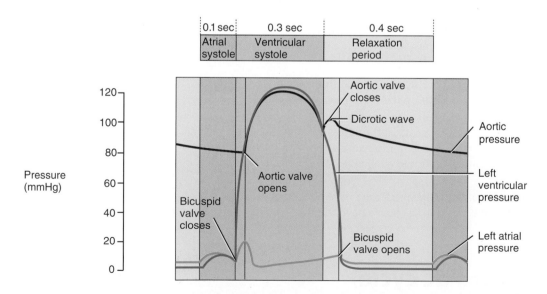

Figure 8.15 The cardiac cycle. *Source*: Tortora and Derrickson (2009). Reproduced with permission of John Wiley & Sons.

into the ventricles from the atria. The ventricles remain in diastole as the electrical excitation that led to atrial contraction is delayed in the AV node. By the end of this point in time the ventricles are in the last part of their relaxation phase and contain the largest amount of blood they will contain during the cardiac cycle. This is known as the end diastolic volume (EDV) and is about 130 mL of blood (Jenkins and Tortora, 2013); that is, the volume of blood contained in the ventricles at the end of their relaxation phase (diastole). The EDV is the main factor in the creation of the end diastolic pressure, as the pressure is directly related to the amount of blood within the ventricle when the ventricle is relaxed.

3. Ventricular contraction (systole). The atria relax, leading to a drop in atrial pressure. The ventricles begin to contract as the electrical excitation is transmitted from the AV node to the ventricles through the bundle of His, then the bundle branches and finally the Purkinje fibres; this leads to a sharp rise in ventricular pressure without any change in ventricular volume (i.e. the amount of blood in the ventricles does not change). Once this pressure rises above the pressure in the atria the AV valves are forced closed. As the semilunar valves remain closed at this point (the ventricular pressure is still lower than the pressure in the aorta and the pulmonary arteries), the ventricles are completely closed off and blood volume in the ventricles remains the same while pressure rises. This is known as the isovolumetric contraction phase ('iso' means remaining the same). Eventually, the pressure in the ventricles becomes greater than the pressure in the aorta and the pulmonary arteries. At this point the semilunar valves are forced open and blood is ejected from the ventricles.

4. Early ventricular diastole (relaxation). The ventricles begin to relax. The blood in the ventricles is no longer compressed by the action of the heart muscle, and the pressure within the ventricles drops rapidly. As the blood volume in the ventricles remains constant (the AV valves are closed) the pressure in the aorta and the pulmonary arteries becomes greater than the pressure in the ventricles, and the semilunar valves are forced closed. This is the ventricular isovolumetric relaxation phase. Closure of the semilunar valves causes a brief rise in the pressure in the aorta as backflowing blood rebounds off the closed aortic valve; this can be seen as a slight 'bump' in the pressure tracing known as the 'dicrotic notch'.

5. During the period of ventricular systole the atria have been in diastole and filling with blood from the veins. When the pressure in the atria is greater than the pressure in the ventricles the AV valves are forced open and blood begins to flow into the ventricles again.

Clinical considerations

Electrocardiogram and the cardiac cycle

Though the cardiac cycle refers to the mechanical action of the heart, the electrical activity that stimulates this mechanical action can be seen by the use of an ECG, an electrical tracing produced by attaching electrodes to the patient's skin and generated by an ECG machine. However, it is possible for the electrical tracing to be present without mechanical activity in certain types of cardiac arrest.

The normal ECG of one cycle of the heart is shown in Figure 8.16 (adapted from Jenkins and Tortora, 2013):

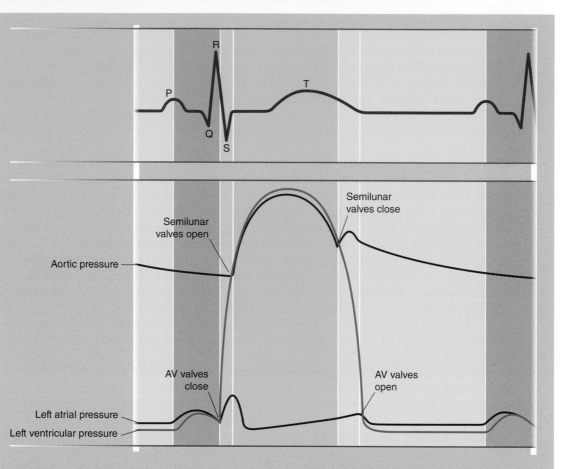

Figure 8.16 Normal ECG of one cycle of the heart. *Source*: Adapted from Jenkins and Tortora (2013). Reproduced with permission of John Wiley & Sons.

The changes from the baseline on the ECG are labelled by letters of the alphabet:
P – atrial depolarisation; corresponds to atrial contraction
QRS – ventricular depolarisation; corresponds approximately to ventricular contraction (though this happens just after the peak of the R wave)
T – ventricular repolarisation; corresponds to the relaxation phase of the ventricle; atrial repolarisation cannot be seen as it is hidden by the greater electrical activity of ventricular depolarisation.

Despite this appearing to be a long process, if we assume a heart rate of 75 beats per minute then the average cardiac cycle would take approximately 0.8 s. The atria are in systole for 0.1 s and then in diastole for 0.7 s, while the ventricles are in systole for 0.3 s and diastole for 0.5 s. As heart rate increases, the cardiac cycle becomes shorter due to the shortening of the diastolic phase; the systolic phase remains the same. As already noted, the heart muscle is supplied with blood during the diastolic (relaxation) phase, as blood cannot flow in the coronary arteries when the heart is contracting; thus, as heart rate increases, blood flow in the coronary arteries (and blood supply to the heart muscle) is reduced.

Factors affecting cardiac output

This section gives an overview of the factors affecting the cardiac output. 'Cardiac output' is a term relating to the amount of blood the heart pumps out in 1 min and is defined by

$$\text{Cardiac Output}\,(CO) = \text{Stroke Volume}\,(SV) \times \text{Heart Rate}\,(HR)$$

Thus, the amount of blood the heart pumps out in a minute is made up of the amount of blood ejected from the ventricle in one beat (SV) times the heart rate (HR) in beats per minute. This gives a total volume. Thus, if we said that SV is 70 mL and the heart rate is 75, then cardiac output is $70 \times 75 = 5250$ mL (or 5.25 L) per minute.

To review the factors affecting cardiac output, the following sections will look at the factors regulating stroke volume and the factors regulating heart rate separately.

Regulation of stroke volume

Stroke volume is effectively the difference between the EDV (i.e. the amount of blood in the ventricle at the end of relaxation) and the end systolic volume (ESV – i.e. the amount of blood in the ventricle at the end of systole). The factors that affect stroke volume are preload, force of contraction and afterload.

Preload

The force the cardiac muscle fibres contract with during systole is affected by the amount of stretch they are subjected to (the greater the stretch, the greater the force). This is known as the Frank–Starling law.

The stretch of the cardiac muscle is directly related to the amount of blood in the ventricle at the end of diastole (EDV), which is, in turn, dependent on the volume of blood returned to the heart via the veins (venous return). Thus, venous return is related to the force of contraction of the ventricles. Anything that affects the speed or volume of venous return affects EDV, and therefore force of contraction. So, for instance:

- A slower heart rate allows for more time for blood to fill the ventricle, increasing the volume of blood in the ventricle at the end of diastole.
- Exercise increases venous return, as the increase in heart rate increases the pressure in the veins and the speed of venous return and the effect of skeletal muscle activity squeezes the veins 'pushing' blood back to the heart (skeletal muscle pumps). Conversely, standing still means that venous return is reduced. Thus, the guardsmen who have to stand still outside Buckingham Palace are taught to discretely contract and relax their feet to aid venous return and prevent fainting.
- Hormonal and nervous influences. The release of adrenaline or the excitation of the sympathetic nervous system leads to the contraction of the veins and the 'squeezing' of blood back to the heart.
- Very fast heart rates reduce the diastolic filling time, and thus there is less time for the ventricle to receive blood before systole starts.
- Certain heart arrhythmias stop the atria contracting effectively, and thus atrial systole is no longer effective at 'pushing' the last bit of blood into the ventricles.
- A reduced blood volume (for instance, due to a haemorrhage) reduces venous return.

Force of contraction

Though EDV is a major component of the force of contraction (because of the Frank–Starling law), force of contraction can also be affected by other factors. The contractility of the heart can be affected by several factors:

- Hormones, such as adrenaline, glucagon and thyroxine, all increase the force of contraction.
- Sympathetic nervous system activity increases the force of contraction through the action of noradrenaline.
- Contractility can be reduced by acidaemia (excess hydrogen ions in the blood) and high potassium levels in the blood.

Afterload

Afterload refers to the pressure in the arteries leading from the ventricles (aorta or pulmonary arteries) that the ventricle must overcome in order to eject blood. In the normal adult the pressure is 80 mmHg in the aorta and 8 mmHg in the pulmonary arteries. This difference in the pressure to be overcome is reflected in the relative thickness of the ventricular walls, with the left ventricular wall being thicker (more muscular) than the right (see previous discussion on the structure of the heart).

In the average adult, aortic and pulmonary pressure is not an important factor in determining afterload as it is constant, but changes in anatomy and/or physiology, such as hypertension or aortic valve disease, can increase afterload. Increased afterload increases the amount of blood left in the ventricle after each systole, and thus also has an effect in increasing the preload (by increasing ventricular ESV and therefore pressure).

Medicines management

Myocardial infarction

Dave is a 45-year-old office worker who has recently returned to work after a myocardial infarction (MI). The rehabilitation nurse has given Dave a lot of information on healthy eating and exercise but she notes his blood cholesterol test result is significantly higher than is advisable for someone who has had an MI. The nurse consults with the medical team and Dave is prescribed 80 mg atorvastatin once a day.

Atorvastatin is a cholesterol-lowering medication that lowers the amount of cholesterol produced in the body. It is commonly used in patients who have had an MI and have high cholesterol as it has been shown to reduce the chance of another MI. The patient is still required to maintain a healthy diet as atorvastatin will not treat the dietary intake of cholesterol and fat by the patient.

The nurse advises Dave to take the atorvastatin at night as one of the more common side effects is muscle pain and the patient is less likely to notice this when asleep. Dave is also advised not to eat grapefruit or drink grapefruit juice while taking atorvastatin as it can interact.

See National Institute for Health and Care Excellence (2014).

Regulation of heart rate

Heart rate is controlled by two main mechanisms:

- autononomic nervous system activity;
- hormone activity.

Resting heart rate is also affected by factors such as age, gender, temperature and physical fitness (Jenkins and Tortora, 2013).

Autonomic nervous system activity

When activated by a stimulus, such as exercise or stress, the sympathetic nerve fibres release the neurotransmitter noradrenaline at their cardiac endings. This leads to the excitation of the SA node and an increase in its production of action potentials and thus an increase in heart rate.

Alternatively, when the parasympathetic nervous system is stimulated this results in the release of acetylcholine at the parasympathetic cardiac nerve endings, which has the effect of reducing the rate of action potential generation in the SA node and thus reducing heart rate.

Both the sympathetic and parasympathetic nervous systems are active at all times, but the parasympathetic nervous system is normally the dominant influence. This can be seen if the vagus nerve (cranial nerve X) is cut, for instance in heart transplant patients. In these situations the SA node will normally produce action potentials at a rate of 100 a minute and therefore the heart rate increases to 100 beats per minute. The removal of the influence of the parasympathetic nervous system (by the disconnection of the vagus nerve) removes the heart rate reducing effect of this system.

Baroreceptors and the cardiovascular centre

Baroreceptors are specialised mechanical receptors located in the carotid sinus and the aortic arch. They are sensitive to the amount of stretch in these blood vessels and have direct outflow via the autonomic nervous system to the cardiovascular centre in the medulla oblongata.

The cardiovascular centre of the medulla oblongata is the main centre for the control of autonomic nervous activity that affects the heart. As can be seen in Figure 8.17, the cardiovascular centre is made up of two sub-centres:

- The cardioinhibitory centre directly controls parasympathetic outflow to the heart (especially the SA node); thus, increased outflow from this centre has the effect of reducing heart rate.
- The vasomotor centre is further divided into the pressor area and the depressor area. The pressor area has a relatively constant outflow of action potentials to the heart via the sympathetic nervous system. This has a direct effect on both heart rate and the force of ventricular contraction (and therefore stroke volume) as well as effects on the vasculature, which subsequently will affect heart function by changing preload and afterload. Outflow from the pressor area is moderated by nerves transmitting impulses from the depressor area that have a directly inhibiting effect on the transmission of impulses from the pressor area. Thus, it can be thought that the nerve impulses of the depressor area act like a 'collar' or tap: the greater the number of impulses from the depressor area the tighter the collar or tap is made, reducing the number of impulses from the pressor area to the heart, and thus the effect on heart rate and force of contraction.

Hormone activity

Two hormones are normally associated with the control of heart rate:

- Adrenaline – from the adrenal medulla. Adrenaline has the same effect as noradrenaline released by the sympathetic nervous system.
- Thyroxine – from the thyroid gland. Released in large quantities, thyroxine has the effect of increasing the heart rate.

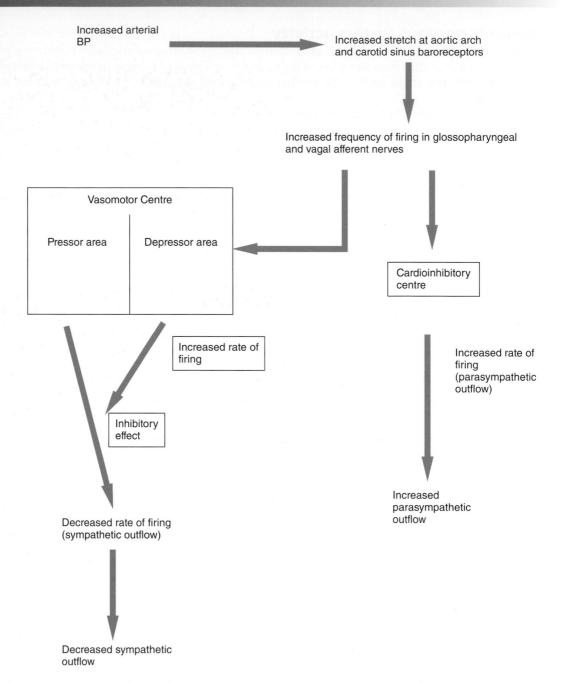

Figure 8.17 Baroreceptor reflex.

Conclusion

The heart is a single organ situated in the thoracic cavity between the lungs. Though a single organ, the heart is effectively two separate pumps made up of four chambers:

- The right heart pump, comprised of the right atrium and right ventricle, pumps blood through the pulmonary circulation.
- The left heart pump, comprised of the left atrium and the left ventricle, pumps blood through the systemic circulation.

Surrounding the heart is a double protective sac called the pericardium. Underlying the pericardium is the heart muscle (myocardium), which is a specialised type of muscle that is branched in its structure and is laid down in spiral bundles to make up the walls of the various heart chambers.

Control of the heart muscle is achieved by the use of a specialised series of nerve cells that make up the conduction system of the heart, including:

- the SA node, the pacemaker of the heart;
- the AV node, an area of the heart's conduction system that controls the delivery of the action potential to the ventricles;
- Purkinje fibres, conductive fibres that aid rapid distribution of the action potential throughout the ventricles.

Blood flow through the heart is based on changes of pressure in the cardiac cycle. These pressure changes also lead to the opening and closing of the cardiac valves, thus further controlling blood flow.

Regulation of the heart's activity is based on the actions of:

- hormones, especially adrenaline;
- autonomic nervous system activity, for instance via the cardiovascular centres.

Glossary

Action potential   Momentary change in the electrical status of a cell wall.

Afterload   The 'load' that the heart has to pump against, mostly created by the blood pressure in the arteries.

Aorta   Main artery leading from the left ventricle.

Aortic valve   Semilunar valve that lies between the left ventricle and the aorta.

Arterial   Pertaining to the arteries.

Arterial blood   Blood carried in the arteries.

Atria   Upper chambers of the heart (singular = atrium).

Atrioventricular bundle   Bundle of conductive nerve fibres that transmit action potentials from the AV node to the ventricular conduction system. Otherwise known as the bundle of His.

Atrioventricular node   Otherwise known as the AV node. Specialised area of cardiac cells located just above the point where the right atrium and right ventricle meet.

Atrioventricular valve Collective name for the two valves that lie between the atria and the ventricles (bicuspid and tricuspid).

Automaticity The ability of certain cells to generate their own action potential without an external stimulus.

Baroreceptors Specialised mechanical receptors located in the aortic arch and the carotid sinus.

Bicuspid valve The AV valve that lies between the left atrium and the left ventricle. Also known as the mitral valve.

Bundle of His See **atrioventricular bundle**.

Cardiac action potential Specialised action potential of the heart muscle cells, it is of longer duration than normal cellular action potentials.

Cardiac cycle The sequence of events that occurs when the heart beats.

Cardiac output The amount of blood pumped out by a ventricle in millilitres per minute.

Cardioinhibitory centre Part of the cardiovascular centre; when stimulated, the major effect is to slow down the heart rate.

Cardiovascular centre Located in the medulla oblongata, this centre controls most of the nervous activity that affects the heart.

Coronary arteries Arteries that supply the myocardium with oxygenated blood.

Coronary sinus Collection of veins that come together to form a single large vessel that returns blood from the myocardium to the right atrium.

Depolarisation Change in the electrical potential of a cell membrane to a more positive charge.

Desmosomes A specialised cell structure whose function is to hold cells together.

Diastole The relaxation of a heart chamber (atrium or ventricle).

Dicrotic notch A small bump in the pressure tracing of the arteries created by a backflow of blood after the closure of the aortic valve.

End diastolic pressure The pressure created by the blood in a named chamber (usually the left ventricle) at the end of diastole.

End diastolic volume The volume of blood in a named chamber (usually the left ventricle) at the end of diastole.

Endocardium Innermost layer that lines the chambers of the heart and also lines the cardiac valves.

Epithelium Layer of body tissue that lines the inside of cavities and the surface of many structures.

Fibrous pericardium The outer, tough layer of the pericardium that provides protection to the heart, prevents overstretching of the heart and helps to anchor the heart in place.

Gap junction A specialised connection between cell membranes that allows the passage of ions and molecules.

Hormone Chemical substance that is released into the blood by the endocrine system and has a physiological control over the function of cells or organs other than those that created it.

Inferior vena cava Large vein that returns blood to the right atrium from the lower parts of the body.

Interatrial septum   Dividing wall between the atria.

Interventricular septum   Dividing wall between the ventricles.

Ion   An electrically charged atom or molecule.

Isovolumetric   No change in volume (amount).

Medulla oblongata   The lower half of the brainstem.

Mitral valve   See **bicuspid valve**.

Myocardium   Muscle layer of the heart.

Myocyte   Cardiac muscle cell.

Nodal cells   Otherwise known as pacemaker cells, these are specialised cells that not only create electrical impulses but create them at regular intervals. The two main groupings of these cells are located in the SA node and the AV node.

Parietal pericardium   The outer layer of the serous pericardium, it is fused to the fibrous pericardium.

Pericardial fluid   A thin film of fluid that reduces the friction between the pericardial membranes as the heart moves during its cycle of contraction and relaxation.

Pericardium   Double-layered sac that surrounds the heart.

Pulmonary circulation   Circulatory system of the lungs.

Pulmonary valve   Semilunar valve that lies between the right ventricle and the pulmonary circulation.

Pulmonary veins   Veins of the pulmonary circulation that return blood from the lungs to the left atrium.

Purkinje fibres (system)   Specialised conductive fibres that rapidly transport action potentials through the ventricle walls.

Repolarisation   Return of the electrical potential of a cell membrane to a negative resting state.

Sarcolemma   Cell membrane of a muscle cell.

Semilunar valves   The valves that lie between the ventricles and the pulmonary or systemic circulation (aortic valve and pulmonary valve).

Septum   A dividing wall.

Serous pericardium   Inner (double) layer of the pericardium comprised of the parietal and visceral pericardial layers.

Sinoatrial node   Otherwise known as the SA node. Specialised area of cardiac cells located in the upper part of the right atrium. Usually referred to as the pacemaker of the heart.

Stroke volume   The amount of blood ejected by a ventricle in one beat.

Superior vena cava   The large vein that returns blood to the right atrium from the upper part of the body.

Systemic circulation   The circulatory system of the body (excluding the lungs).

Systole   The contraction of a heart chamber (atrium or ventricle).

Tetany   Sustained involuntary contraction of a muscle.

Tricuspid valve   The AV valve that lies between the right atrium and ventricle.

Vasomotor centre   Part of the cardiovascular centre; has effects on heart rate and the force of contraction of the heart.

Venous   Pertaining to the veins.

Venous blood   Blood carried in the veins.

Ventricles   The large lower chambers of the heart.

Visceral pericardium   The inner layer of the serous pericardium (otherwise known as the epicardium); adheres tightly to the surface of the heart.

References

British National Formulary (2015) *Cardiac Glycosides*. http://www.evidence.nhs.uk/formulary/bnf/current/2-cardiovascular-system/21-positive-inotropic-drugs/211-cardiac-glycosides (accessed 24 November 2015).

Clare, C. (2007) Valve disorders. In Hatchett, R. and Thompson, D.R. (eds), *Cardiac Nursing: A Comprehensive Guide*. London: Churchill Livingstone Elsevier; pp. 357–382.

Jenkins, G.W. and Tortora, G.J. (2013) *Anatomy and Physiology: From Science to Life*, 3rd edn. Hoboken, NJ: John Wiley & Sons, Inc.

Martini, F.H., Nath, J.L. and Bartholemew, E.F. (2014) *Fundamentals of Anatomy and Physiology*, 10th edn. San Francisco, CA: Pearson Benjamin Cummings.

National Institute for Health and Care Excellence (2004) *Balloon Valvuloplasty for Aortic Valve Stenosis in Adults and Children*. NICE interventional procedures guidance [IPG78]. http://www.nice.org.uk/Guidance/IPG78# (accessed 24 November 2015).

National Institute for Health and Care Excellence (2013) *Myocardial Infarction: Cardiac Rehabilitation and Prevention of Further MI*. NICE guidelines [CG172]. https://www.nice.org.uk/guidance/cg172 (accessed 24 November 2015).

National Institute for Health and Care Excellence (2014) *Lipid Modification Therapy for Preventing Cardiovascular Disease: Secondary Prevention*. NICE Pathways. http://pathways.nice.org.uk/pathways/cardiovascular-disease-prevention#path=view%3A/pathways/cardiovascular-disease-prevention/lipid-modification-therapy-for-preventing-cardiovascular-disease.xml&content=view-node%3Anodes-secondary-prevention (accessed 24 November 2015).

O'Grady, E (2007) *A Nurse's Guide to Caring for Cardiac Intervention Patients*. Chichester: John Wiley & Sons, Ltd.

Tortora, G.J. and Derrickson, B.H. (2009) *Principles of Anatomy and Physiology*, 12th edn. Hoboken, NJ: John Wiley & Sons, Inc.

University of Michigan Health System (2014) *Coronary Angioplasty and Stenting*. http://www.med.umich.edu/cardiac-surgery/patient/adult/adultcandt/coronary_angioplasty.shtml (accessed 5 December 2015).

Further reading

British Heart Foundation

https://www.bhf.org.uk/

The British Heart Foundation is the UK's largest charity for heart disease. The website has many useful resources for patients and professionals.

Arrhythmia Alliance

http://www.heartrhythmcharity.org.uk/www/436/0/About/
The Arrhythmia Alliance is an alliance of several independent charities devoted to raising awareness of heart arrhythmias, improving diagnosis and improving the life of people with arrhythmias.

Resuscitation Council (UK)

https://www.resus.org.uk/index.html
The Resuscitation Council (UK) is an organisation devoted to promoting evidence-based resuscitation guidelines and contributing to saving lives through training and education.

Activities
Multiple choice questions

1. The double sac surrounding the heart is:
   (a) the myocardium
   (b) the pericardium
   (c) the endocardium
   (d) the epicardium
2. Which heart chamber has the thickest muscle wall?
   (a) right ventricle
   (b) right atrium
   (c) left ventricle
   (d) left atrium
3. Blood flowing into the right atrium comes from:
   (a) the lungs
   (b) the body (systemic circulation)
   (c) the left heart
   (d) the right heart
4. Blood pumped out from the left heart is carried by:
   (a) the vena cava
   (b) the pulmonary arteries
   (c) the aorta
   (d) the coronary arteries
5. The contraction of a heart chamber is known as:
   (a) automaticity
   (b) diastole
   (c) isovulmetric
   (d) systole
6. The blood flow through the heart is caused by changes in:
   (a) pressure
   (b) electricity
   (c) transport molecules
   (d) oxygen

7. The artery supplying blood to the front of the left ventricle is:
   (a) the posterior descending artery
   (b) the circumflex artery
   (c) the right coronary artery
   (d) the left anterior descending artery
8. Normal electrical excitation of the heart begins in:
   (a) the bundle of His
   (b) the Purkinje fibres
   (c) the AV node
   (d) the SA node

9. The effect of increased parasympathetic nervous system activity is to:
   (a) increase heart rate
   (b) decrease heart rate
   (c) increase force of contraction
   (d) decrease force of contraction
10. Preload is mostly a factor of:
    (a) ESV
    (b) EDV
    (c) the Frank–Starling law
    (d) adrenaline release

True or false

1. Cardiac muscle contractions last 10–15 times longer than skeletal muscle contractions.
2. The right ventricle has a thinner wall than the left ventricle.
3. Age is a risk factor for heart valve incompetence.
4. The volume of blood remaining in the ventricle at the end of a ventricular contraction is the EDV.
5. Thyroxine hormone release only affects heart rate.
6. The cardioinhibitory centre controls the sympathetic nervous outflow to the heart.
7. Cardiac catheterisation can be performed through the femoral artery.
8. It is possible for there to be electrical activity in the heart in cardiac arrest.
9. Endothelium covers the heart valves as well as the inner layer of the heart.
10. The AV node is the pacemaker of the heart.

Label the diagram 1

Label the diagram using the following list of words:

Superior vena cava, Pulmonary valve, Right atrium, Right ventricle, Inferior vena cava, Left atrium, Left ventricle, Interventricular septum, Descending aorta

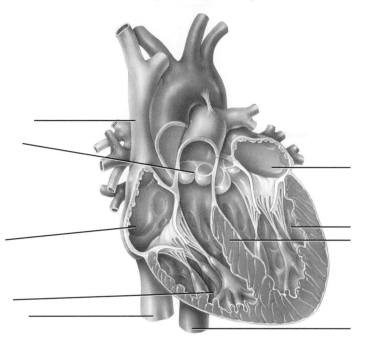

Label the diagram 2

Draw arrows on the diagram below to show blood flow through the heart.

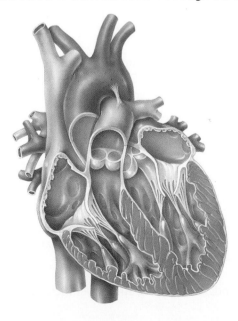

Word search

S	Z	Q	P	U	L	L	E	A	V	K	M	W	V	J	I	F	J	O	Q
I	H	R	E	F	R	A	C	T	O	R	Y	H	H	G	P	J	P	K	F
N	S	P	R	O	N	K	I	J	P	M	O	T	B	T	X	I	U	Y	L
O	R	T	I	O	M	R	H	I	L	U	F	J	D	R	F	G	L	K	A
A	W	R	C	N	O	V	D	C	A	O	I	U	H	I	K	Z	M	F	C
T	N	V	A	L	V	E	V	Y	A	D	B	I	M	C	N	D	O	M	L
R	G	F	R	G	E	N	D	O	C	A	R	D	I	U	M	G	N	M	D
I	Q	M	D	E	R	O	N	F	C	S	I	J	T	S	F	F	A	H	F
A	C	P	I	B	E	U	E	H	B	T	L	C	R	P	W	O	R	A	P
L	I	M	U	F	M	S	R	J	E	U	D	E	A	I	S	B	Y	I	S
X	S	P	M	G	O	D	P	R	N	K	M	J	L	D	M	F	T	R	A
A	Q	J	U	E	C	J	I	A	P	I	T	E	R	U	Y	U	X	U	R
C	L	T	C	F	R	S	S	N	A	Z	K	N	I	A	O	R	T	I	C
Y	T	D	E	Q	A	I	S	U	V	Y	T	R	W	G	C	N	H	K	O
A	S	I	N	U	S	Q	I	L	U	V	T	M	U	P	Y	X	O	K	L
B	C	B	K	O	S	R	C	I	R	A	C	U	S	P	T	B	R	T	E
Z	R	X	N	K	R	T	W	M	P	J	O	T	J	B	E	S	A	L	M
G	L	E	H	O	L	E	D	E	T	J	L	P	S	P	S	Q	C	B	M
B	T	P	O	R	D	I	A	S	T	O	L	E	Y	P	R	S	I	D	A
S	T	A	R	U	V	E	S	G	Z	Y	C	S	A	I	T	L	C	C	A

Aortic, Endocardium, Pericardium, Sarcomere, Stenosis, Apex, Mitral, Pulmonary, Semilunar, Thoracic, Atrium, Myocyte, Purkinje, Septum, Tricuspid, Cusp, Myofibril, Refractory, Sinoatrial, Valve, Diastole, Node, Sarcolemma, Sinus, Venous

Fill in the blanks

Normal electrical excitation/distribution begins in the _____ node, which is located in the right _____, and is rapidly transmitted across the atria by fast pathways. The impulse is transmitted to the _____ (AV) node where further transmission is delayed for approximately 0.1 _____. This ensures that the atria have completely contracted before ventricular _____ is initiated. Once the impulse has been 'held' in the AV node it is then transmitted down the bundle of His (AV bundle) to the fast pathways of the two _____ branches. The bundles then divide into the smaller and smaller branches of the _____ system which transmits the impulses to the muscles of the _____.

atrioventricular, seconds, contraction, atrium, ventricles, sinoatrial, Purkinje, bundle

Find out more

1. What preparation does a patient require prior to a cardiac catheter (angiogram)?
2. What is cardiac rehabilitation?
3. What are the risk factors for coronary artery disease?
4. What advice should be given to a patient after they have had a pacemaker implanted?
5. A patient you are caring for requires coronary artery bypass graft surgery. Find out what you can do to help the patient understand the operation they are going to have?
6. What would you advise a patient who wants to know how to start exercise after a myocardial infarction?
7. What blood tests are carried out to detect a myocardial infarction?
8. Why is aspirin prescribed to patients with coronary heart disease?
9. Different leads on a 12-lead ECG reading correspond to different parts of the heart. Find out which lead represents which territory of the heart.
10. Why does a person's resting heart rate decrease the fitter they are?

Conditions

The following is a list of conditions that are associated with the cardiac system. Take some time and write notes about each of the conditions. You may make the notes taken from text books or other resources (e.g. people you work with in a clinical area), or you may make the notes as a result of people you have cared for. If you are making notes about people you have cared for you must ensure that you adhere to the rules of confidentiality.

Heart failure	
Myocardial infarction	
Aortic stenosis	

Mitral regurgitation	
Pericarditis	

Chapter 9

The digestive system

Louise McErlean

Test your prior knowledge

- What is the main function of the digestive system?
- List the structures that form the digestive system.
- List the hormones and enzymes involved in the digestive system.
- Name the main food groups.
- Differentiate between macronutrients and micronutrients.

Learning outcomes

After reading this chapter you will be able to:

- Identify the organs of the digestive system, including the accessory organs of the digestive system
- Describe the functions of each of these organs, as well as the overall function of the digestive system
- Explain the action of the enzymes and hormones associated with the digestion of proteins, carbohydrates and fats
- Describe what proteins, carbohydrates and fats are broken down into and how the body uses these constituent parts
- Describe the structure and function of the accessory organs of the digestive system
- List the common vitamins and minerals and the problems associated with a deficit or excess

Fundamentals of Anatomy and Physiology: For Nursing and Healthcare Students, Second Edition. Edited by Ian Peate and Muralitharan Nair.
© 2017 John Wiley & Sons, Ltd. Published 2017 by John Wiley & Sons, Ltd.
Student companion website: www.wileyfundamentalseries.com/anatomy
Instructor companion website: www.wiley.com/go/instructor/anatomy

Body map

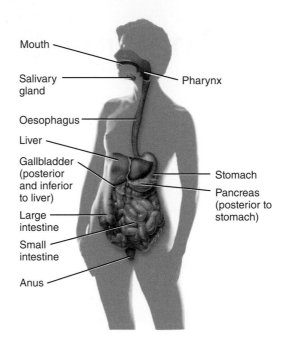

Mouth

Salivary
gland

Pharynx

Oesophagus

Liver

Gallbladder
(posterior
and inferior
to liver)

Stomach

Pancreas
(posterior to
stomach)

Large
intestine

Small
intestine

Anus

258

Introduction

The digestive system is also known as the gastrointestinal system or the alimentary canal. This vast system is approximately 10 m long. It travels the length of the body from the mouth through the thoracic, abdominal and pelvic cavities, where it ends at the anus (see Figure 9.1). The digestive system has one major function: to convert food from the diet into a form that can be utilised by the cells of the body in order to carry out their specific functions. This chapter discusses the structure and function of the digestive system and explains how dietary nutrients are broken down and used by the body for cell metabolism and for growth and repair.

The activity of the digestive system

The activity of the digestive system can be categorised into five processes:

- **Ingestion:** taking food into the digestive system.
- **Propulsion:** moving the food along the length of the digestive system.
- **Digestion:** breaking down food. This can be achieved *mechanically* as food is chewed or moved through the digestive system, or *chemically* by the action of *enzymes* mixed with the food as it moves through the digestive system.
- **Absorption:** the products of digestion exit the digestive system and enter the blood or lymph capillaries for distribution to where they are required.
- **Elimination:** the waste products of digestion are excreted from the body as faeces.

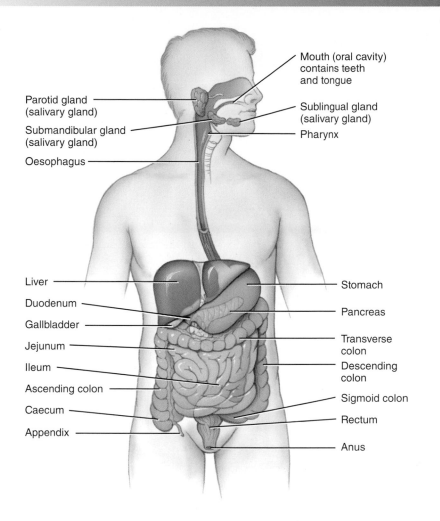

Mouth (oral cavity)
contains teeth
and tongue

Parotid gland
(salivary gland)

Sublingual gland
(salivary gland)

Submandibular gland
(salivary gland)

Pharynx

Oesophagus

Liver

Stomach

Duodenum

Pancreas

Gallbladder

Jejunum

Transverse
colon

Ileum

Descending
colon

Ascending colon

Sigmoid colon

Caecum

Rectum

Appendix

Anus

Figure 9.1   The digestive system. *Source*: Tortora and Derrickson (2009). Reproduced with permission of John Wiley & Sons.

The organisation of the digestive system

The digestive system consists of the main digestive system structures and the accessory organs. The main digestive system structures include the mouth, pharynx, oesophagus, stomach, small intestine and large intestine. Accessory organs also contribute to the function of the digestive system. The accessory organs are the salivary glands, the liver, the gallbladder and the pancreas.

The digestive system organs

The mouth (oral cavity)

Food enters the mouth or oral cavity, and this is where the process of digestion begins. The oral cavity consists of several structures (see Figure 9.2). Food enters the oral cavity in a process called **ingestion**. The food mixes with saliva.

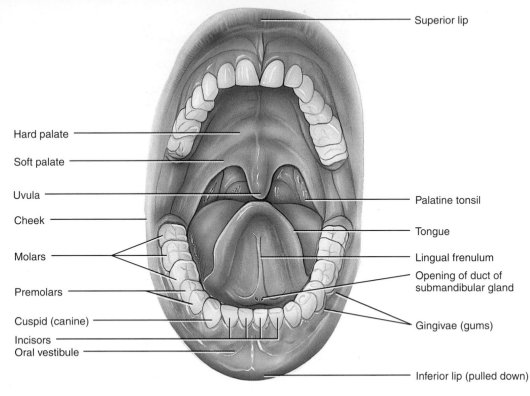

Anterior view

Figure 9.2   The oral cavity. *Source*: Tortora and Derrickson (2009). Reproduced with permission of John Wiley & Sons.

The **lips** and **cheeks** are formed of muscle and connective tissue. This allows the lips and cheeks to move food mixed with saliva around the mouth and begin **mechanical digestion**. The teeth contribute to mechanical digestion by grinding and tearing food. This process of chewing and mixing food with saliva is called **mastication**. The oral cavity can be exposed to very hot and very cold food as well as rough food particles. It is lined with mucus-secreting, stratified squamous epithelial cells. This layer provides some protection against abrasion, the effects of heat and continuous wear and tear.

The lips and cheeks are also involved in speech and facial expression.

Tongue

The tongue is a large, voluntary muscular structure that occupies much of the oral cavity. It is attached posteriorly to the **hyoid** bone and inferiorly by the **frenulum** (see Figure 9.2).

The superior surface of the tongue is covered in stratified squamous epithelium for protection against wear and tear. This surface also contains many little projections called papillae. The papillae (or taste buds) contain the nerve endings responsible for the sense of taste (Tortora and Derrickson, 2012). The taste buds contribute to our enjoyment of food. As well as taste, other functions of the tongue include swallowing (deglutition), holding and moving food around the oral cavity and speech.

Palate

The palate forms the roof of the mouth and consists of two parts: the hard palate and the soft palate. The hard palate is located anteriorly and is bony. The soft palate lies posteriorly and consists of skeletal muscle and connective tissue (see Figure 9.2). The palate plays a part in swallowing. The **palatine tonsils** lie laterally and are lymphoid tissue. The **uvula** is a fold of tissue that hangs down from the centre of the soft palate.

Teeth

Temporary teeth are also known as deciduous teeth or milk teeth. Temporary teeth begin to appear at about 6 months old. There are 20 temporary teeth, and these are replaced by permanent teeth from about the age of 6 years (Nair and Peate, 2013). There are 32 permanent teeth. Sixteen are located in the maxilla arch (upper) and 16 are located in the mandible (lower) (see Figure 9.3).

Canines and incisors are cutting and tearing teeth. Premolars and molars are used for the grinding and chewing of food. Despite their different functions and shape, the structure of each tooth is the same. The visible part of the tooth is called the **crown**. The crown sits above the gum

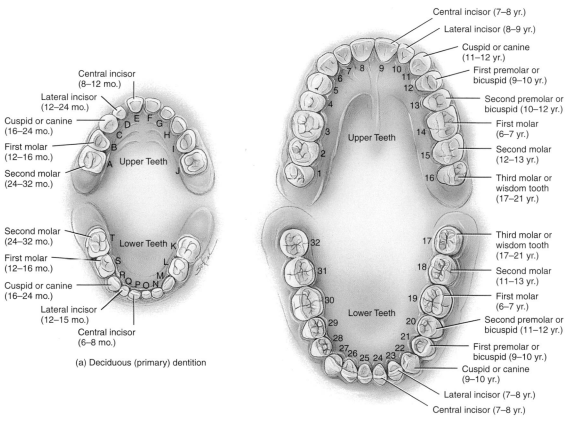

(a) Deciduous (primary) dentition

(b) Permanent (secondary) dentition

Figure 9.3 (a, b) Teeth. *Source*: Tortora and Derrickson (2009). Reproduced with permission of John Wiley & Sons.

or **gingiva**. The centre of the tooth is called the **pulp cavity**. Blood and lymph vessels as well as nerves enter and leave the tooth here. The tooth receives nutrients and sensations via the pulp. Surrounding this is a calcified matrix, not unlike bone, called the **dentine**. Surrounding the dentine is a very hard, protective material called **enamel**. The neck of the tooth is where the crown meets the root. The teeth are anchored in a socket with a bone-like material called **cementum**, and the function of the teeth is to chew (masticate) food.

Salivary glands

There are three pairs of salivary glands (see Figure 9.4). The **parotid glands** are the largest and they are located anterior to the ears. Saliva from the parotid glands enters the oral cavity close to the level of the second upper molar tooth. The submandibular glands are located below the jaw on each side of the face. Saliva from these glands enters the oral cavity from beside the frenulum of the tongue. The sublingual glands are the smallest. They are located in the floor of the mouth.

Although saliva is continuously secreted in order to keep the oral cavity moist, the activity of the parasympathetic fibres that innervate the salivary glands will lead to an increased production of saliva in response to the sight, smell or taste of food. The action of sympathetic fibres leads to a decreased secretion of saliva.

In health, approximately 1–1.5 L of saliva are secreted daily. Saliva consists of:

- water
- salivary amylase
- mucus

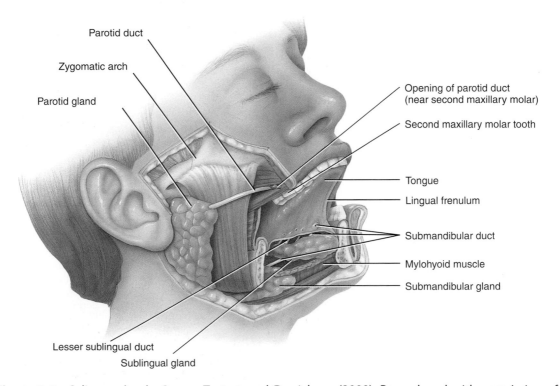

Figure 9.4   Salivary glands. *Source*: Tortora and Derrickson (2009). Reproduced with permission of John Wiley & Sons.

- mineral salts
- lysozyme
- immunoglobulins
- blood clotting factors.

  Saliva has several important functions:

- Salivary amylase is a digestive enzyme responsible for beginning the breakdown of carbohydrate molecules from complex polysaccharides to the disaccharide maltase.
- The fluid nature of saliva helps to moisten and lubricate food that enters the mouth. This makes it easier to hold the food in the mouth and also assists in forming the food into a bolus in preparation for swallowing.
- The continuous secretion of saliva is cleansing and helps to maintain moisture in the oral cavity. A lack of moisture can lead to oral mucosal infections and formation of mouth ulcers.
- The oral cavity is an entry route for pathogens from the external environment. Lysozyme, a constituent of saliva, has an antibacterial action. Immunoglobulin and clotting factors also contribute to the prevention of infection.
- Taste is only possible when food substances are moist. Saliva is required to moisten food.

263

Clinical considerations

Mouth care

Patients who are ill are often dehydrated and therefore the production of saliva is reduced. This can lead to an increased risk of oral infections, as wear and tear within the oral cavity increases. Reduced amounts of saliva lead to less washing away of pathogens to the acid environment of the stomach where they may be destroyed. The oral cavity provides a route for pathogens to enter the respiratory tract, and therefore good oral hygiene practices may help prevent respiratory infections, particularly in patients who are vulnerable because of acute illness, cancer treatments or immobility.

When patients are ill, diet is essential for tissue repair and healing; however, a lack of saliva will lead to the food not tasting as it should. The food will not easily form into the required bolus size for ease of swallowing. This may put the patient off eating and drinking and may lead to the patient losing their appetite and potentially delayed healing.

Ill health can lead to neglect of hygiene standards for individuals. Mouth care is easy for patients to ignore when they are feeling poorly. However, it is an essential consideration for nursing.

Pharynx

The pharynx consists of three parts: the **oropharynx**, the **nasopharynx** and the **laryngopharynx**. The nasopharynx is considered a structure of the respiratory system. The oropharynx and the laryngopharynx are passages for both food and respiratory gases (see Figure 9.5). The **epiglottis** is responsible for closing the entrance to the larynx during swallowing, and this essential action prevents food from entering the larynx and obstructing the respiratory passages.

Swallowing (deglutition)

Once ingested food has been adequately chewed and formed into a bolus it is ready to be swallowed. Swallowing (deglutition) occurs in three phases.

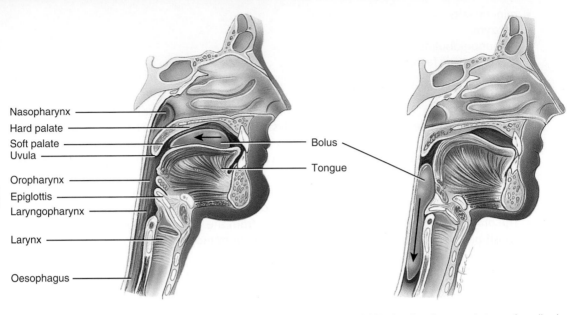

Nasopharynx
Hard palate
Soft palate
Uvula
Oropharynx
Epiglottis
Laryngopharynx
Larynx
Oesophagus

Bolus
Tongue

(a) Position of structures before swallowing

(b) During the pharyngeal stage of swallowing

Figure 9.5   (a, b) Swallowing. *Source*: Tortora and Derrickson (2009). Reproduced with permission of John Wiley & Sons.

1. **The voluntary phase:** During this phase the action of the voluntary muscles serving the oral cavity manipulates the food bolus into the oropharynx. The tongue is pressed against the palate and this prevents the food from moving forward again.
2. **The pharyngeal phase:** During this phase a reflex action is initiated in response to the sensation of the food bolus in the oropharynx. This reflex is coordinated by the swallowing centre in the medulla oblongata, and the motor response is contraction of the muscles of the pharynx. The soft palate elevates, closing off the nasopharynx and preventing the food bolus from using this route. The larynx moves up and moves forward, allowing the epiglottis to cover the entrance to the larynx so the food bolus cannot move into the respiratory passages.
3. **The oesophageal phase:** The food bolus moves from the pharynx into the oesophagus. Waves of oesophageal muscle contractions move the food bolus down the length of the oesophagus and into the stomach. This wave of muscle contraction is known as **peristalsis** (see Figure 9.6).

Oesophagus

The food bolus leaves the oropharynx and enters the oesophagus. The oesophagus extends from the laryngopharynx to the stomach. It is a thick-walled structure, measuring about 25 cm in length and lies in the thoracic cavity, posterior to the trachea. The function of the oesophagus is to transport substances (the food bolus) from the mouth to the stomach. Thick mucus is secreted by the mucosa of the oesophagus, and this aids the passage of the food bolus and also protects the oesophagus from abrasion.

The upper oesophageal sphincter regulates the movement of substances into the oesophagus, and the lower oesophageal sphincter (also known as the cardiac sphincter) regulates the

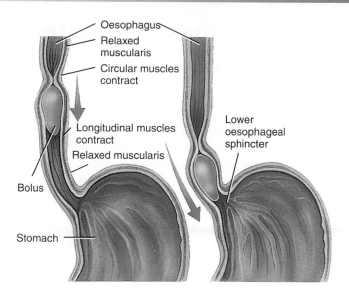

Anterior view of frontal sections of peristalsis in oesophagus

Figure 9.6 Peristalsis in the oesophagus. *Source*: Tortora and Derrickson (2009). Reproduced with permission of John Wiley & Sons.

movement of substances from the oesophagus to the stomach. The muscle layer of the oesophagus differs from the rest of the digestive tract, as the superior portion consists of skeletal (voluntary) muscle and the inferior portion consists of smooth (involuntary) muscle. Breathing and swallowing cannot occur at the same time (Nair and Peate, 2013).

Medicines management

Omeprazole

Omeprazole is a medicine used to treat a number of digestive system conditions, including dyspepsia, acid reflux, oesophagitis and peptic ulcer disease. It belongs to a group of medicines known as proton pump inhibitors (Galbraith *et al.*, 2007). Hydrochloric acid produced in the stomach can escape into the oesophagus or the duodenum of the small intestine and irritate the delicate epithelium in these areas. Omeprazole works on the parietal cells in the stomach, inhibiting the production of hydrochloric acid.

Omeprazole is usually prescribed as 20–40 mg once daily.

The common side effects for patients taking omeprazole are:

- vomiting
- diarrhoea
- constipation
- pain (stomach)
- headaches
- increased flatulence
- nausea.

NICE (2014a) produces guidance on the investigation and management of dyspepsia.

The structure of the digestive system

There are four layers of tissue or tunicas that exist throughout the length of the digestive tract from oesophagus to anus (see Figure 9.7).

The **mucosa** is the innermost layer. The products of digestion are in contact with this layer as they pass through the digestive tract. The mucosa consists of three layers: the mucous epithelium (mucous membrane), which is involved in the **secretion** of mucus and other digestive system secretions such as saliva or gastric juice. This layer helps to **protect** the digestive system from the continuous wear and tear it endures. In the small intestine this layer is involved in **absorption** of the products of digestion. The next layer is the **lamina propria**, which consists of loose connective tissue that has a role in supporting the blood vessels and lymphatic tissue of the mucosa. The outermost layer is called the **muscularis mucosa** and consists of a thin smooth muscle layer that helps to form the gastric pits or the microvilli of the digestive system.

The **submucosa** is a thick layer of connective tissue. It contains blood and lymphatic vessels and some small glands. It also contains **Meissner's plexus** – nerves that stimulate the intestinal glands to secrete their products.

The **muscularis** consists of an inner layer of circular smooth muscle and an outer layer of longitudinal smooth muscle. The stomach has three layers of smooth muscle, and the upper oesophagus has skeletal muscle. Blood and lymph vessels and the **myenteric plexus** (a network

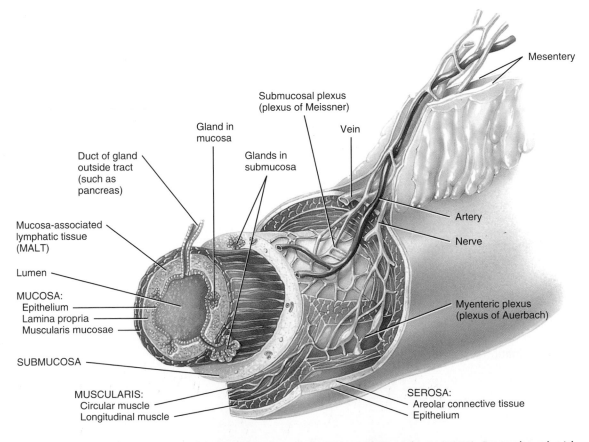

Figure 9.7   Structure of the digestive tract. *Source*: Tortora and Derrickson (2009). Reproduced with permission of John Wiley & Sons.

of sympathetic and parasympathetic nerves) are located between the two layers of smooth muscle. The wave-like contraction and relaxation of this muscle layer are responsible for moving food along the digestive tract – a process known as **peristalsis** (see Figure 9.7). Peristalsis helps to churn and mechanically digest food.

The outer layer of the digestive tract is the **serosa (adventitia)**. The largest area of serosa is found in the abdominal and pelvic cavities and is known as the **peritoneum**. The peritoneum is a closed sac. The visceral peritoneum covers the organs of the abdominal and pelvic cavity, and the parietal peritoneum lines the abdominal wall. A small amount of serous fluid lies between the two layers. The peritoneum has a good blood supply and contains many lymph nodes and lymphatic vessels. It acts as a barrier, protecting the structures it encloses, and can act to isolate areas of infection to prevent damage to neighbouring structures.

Stomach

The stomach lies in the abdominal cavity. It lies between the oesophagus superiorly and the duodenum of the small intestine inferiorly. It is divided into regions (see Figure 9.8).

The entrance to the stomach from the oesophagus is via the lower oesophageal sphincter or cardiac sphincter. This leads to a small area within the stomach called the **cardiac region** or **cardia**. The **fundus** is the dome-shaped region in the superior part of the stomach. The **body region** occupies the space between the lesser and greater curvature of the stomach, and the **pyloric region** narrows into the **pyloric canal**. The **pyloric sphincter** controls the exit of **chyme** from the stomach into the small intestine. Chyme is the name given to the food bolus as it leaves the stomach.

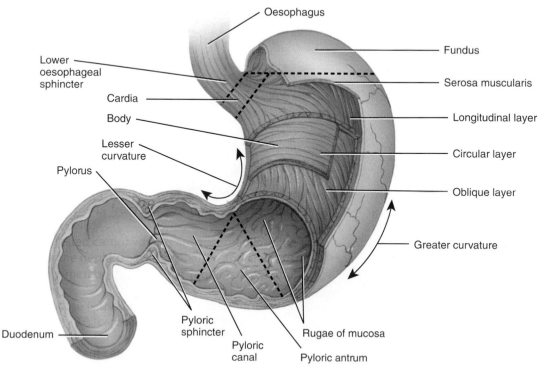

Anterior view of regions of stomach

Figure 9.8 The stomach. *Source*: Tortora and Derrickson (2009). Reproduced with permission of John Wiley & Sons.

The stomach is supplied with arterial blood from a branch of the celiac artery, and venous blood leaves the stomach via the hepatic vein. The vagus nerve innervates the stomach with parasympathetic fibres that stimulate gastric motility and the secretion of gastric juice. Sympathetic fibres from the celiac plexus reduce gastric activity.

The stomach has the same four layers of tissue as the digestive tract, but with some differences. The muscularis contains three layers of smooth muscle instead of two. It has longitudinal, circular and oblique muscle fibres. The extra muscle layer facilitates the churning, mixing and mechanical digestion of food that occurs within the stomach, as well as supporting the onward journey of the food by peristalsis.

The mucosa within the stomach is also different from the rest of the digestive tract. When the stomach is empty, the mucosal epithelia falls into long folds known as **rugae**. The rugae fill out when the stomach is full. A very full stomach can contain approximately 4 L, while an empty stomach contains only about 50 mL (Marieb and Hoehn, 2010). The shape and size of the stomach vary from person to person and depending on the quantity of food stored within it.

The mucosa also contains many gastric glands that secrete many different substances (see Figure 9.9).

- **Surface mucous cells** produce thick bicarbonate-coated mucus. This thick layer of mucus protects the stomach mucosal epithelia from corrosion by acidic gastric juice. When these cells become damaged they are quickly shed and replaced.

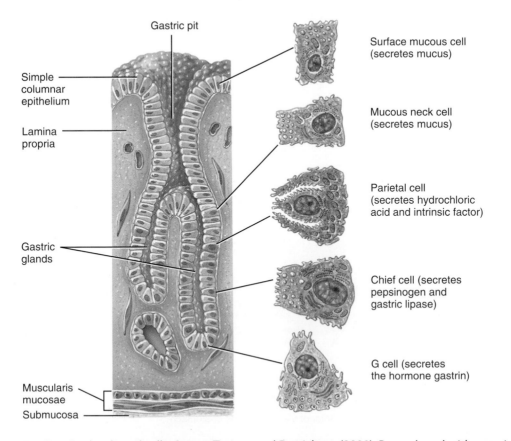

Figure 9.9   Gastric glands and cells. *Source*: Tortora and Derrickson (2009). Reproduced with permission of John Wiley & Sons.

- **Mucous neck cells** also secrete mucus – this mucus is different from surface cell mucus.
- **Parietal cells** produce **hydrochloric acid** and **intrinsic factor**. Intrinsic factor is necessary for the absorption of vitamin B_{12}. This vitamin is essential for the production of mature erythrocytes. Hydrochloric acid creates the acidic environment of the stomach (pH 1–3) and begins denaturing dietary protein in preparation for the action of pepsin.
- **Chief cells** produce pepsinogen, which is converted to **pepsin** in the presence of hydrochloric acid. Pepsin is necessary for the breakdown of protein into smaller peptide chains.
- **Enteroendocrine cells**, such as g cells, produce a variety of hormones, including **gastrin**. These hormones help regulate gastric motility.

This concoction of secretions plus water and mineral salts is more commonly called gastric juice. About 2 L of gastric juice is produced daily.

Snapshot

Hydrogen breath test

This is a test that uses the measurement of hydrogen in the breath to diagnose a number of conditions that cause gastrointestinal symptoms. Limited hydrogen is produced from the small amounts of unabsorbed food that reach the colon; large amounts of hydrogen may be produced when there is a problem with the digestion or absorption of food in the small intestine, which allows more unabsorbed food to reach the colon.

The hydrogen-containing blood travels to the lungs where the hydrogen is released and exhaled in the breath, where it can be measured. Hydrogen breath testing is used in the diagnosis of three conditions. The first is a condition in which dietary sugars are not digested normally. The most common sugar that is poorly digested is lactose. The second condition is to diagnose bacterial overgrowth of the small bowel. The final condition is to diagnose rapid passage of food through the small intestine. All of these conditions may cause abdominal pain, abdominal bloating and distension, flatulence and diarrhoea.

Before the test, the patient fasts for at least 12 h. At the start of the test, the patient blows into and fills a balloon with a breath of air. The concentration of hydrogen is measured in a sample of breath removed from the balloon. The patient then ingests a small amount of the test sugar (lactose, sucrose, sorbitol, fructose, lactulose, depending on the purpose of the test). Additional samples of breath are collected and analysed for hydrogen every 15 min for 3 h and up to 5 h.

The interpretation of the results of hydrogen breath testing depends on the sugar that is used for testing, and the pattern of hydrogen production after the sugar is ingested.

After ingestion of test doses of the dietary sugars, any production of hydrogen means that there has been a problem with digestion or absorption of the test sugar and that some of the sugar has reached the colon.

Regulation of gastric juice secretion is divided into three phases (see Figure 9.10).

1. **The cephalic phase:** The sight, taste or smell of food stimulates the secretion of gastric juice.
2. **The gastric phase:** When food enters the stomach, the hormone gastrin is secreted into the bloodstream, and this stimulates the secretion of gastric juice. The secretion of hydrochloric acid reduces the pH of the stomach contents, and when the pH drops below 2 the secretion of gastrin is inhibited.

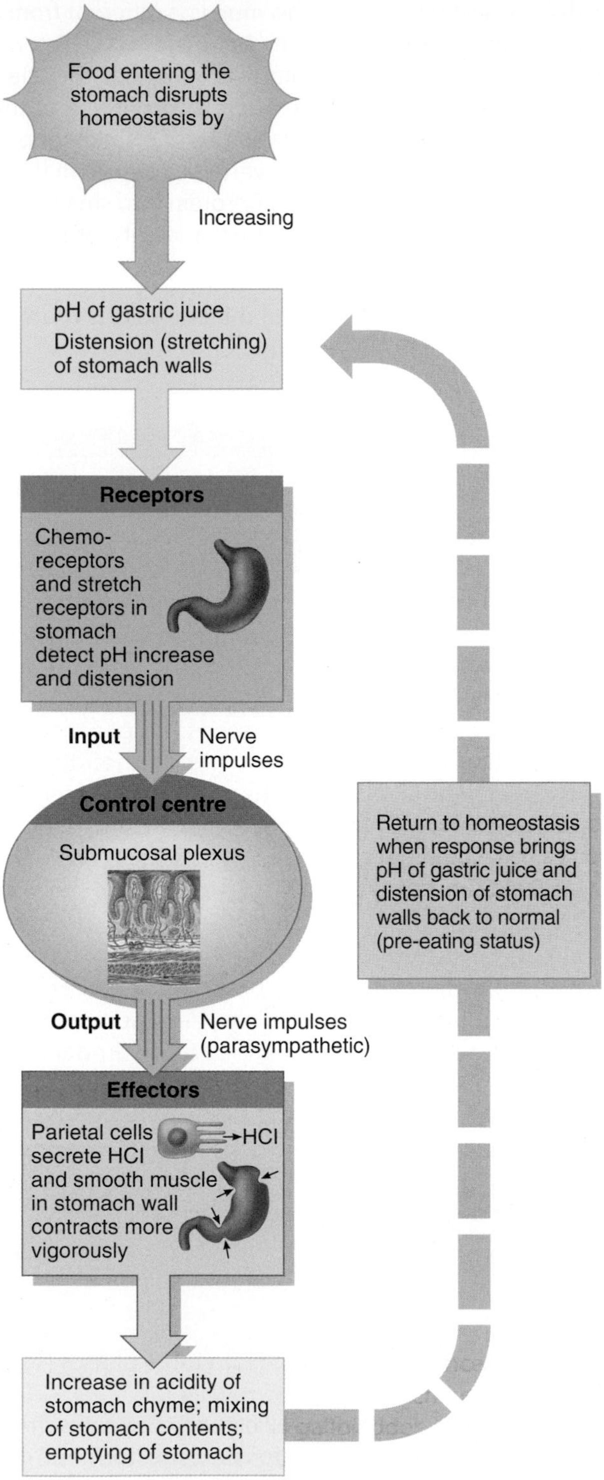

Figure 9.10 Phases of gastric juice secretion. *Source*: Tortora and Derrickson (2009). Reproduced with permission of John Wiley & Sons.

3. **The intestinal phase:** As the acidic contents of the stomach enter the duodenum of the small intestine the hormones secretin and cholecystokinin (CKK) are secreted. These hormones also act to reduce the secretion of gastric juice and gastric motility.

The rate of gastric emptying depends on the size and content of the meal. A large meal takes longer than a small meal. Liquids quickly pass through the stomach, while solids require longer to be thoroughly mixed with gastric juice. Most meals will have left the stomach 4 h after ingestion.

The functions of the stomach are:

- to act as a store for food;
- the production of mucus to protect the stomach;
- mechanical digestion, by the churning action facilitated by an additional layer of smooth muscle;
- the mixing food with hydrochloric acid to help eradicate pathogens and denature proteins in preparation for the action of pepsin;
- the production of chyme;
- the production of intrinsic factor.

271

Medicines management

Odansetron

Nausea and vomiting are the most common digestive system symptoms. Vomiting (emesis) occurs when the emetic or vomiting centre in the brain is activated. It can be activated as a result of irritation in the stomach. The irritation could be due to bacteria or often medication. Some medications cross the blood–brain barrier and stimulate the vomiting centre. When stimulated, the abdominal muscles and diaphragm are activated and a reverse peristalsis occurs in the stomach, leading to the ejection of the stomach contents (Marieb, 2009).

This unpleasant reaction can be treated with medications such as odansetron. Odansetron belongs to a group of medications known as anti-emetics. It acts by blocking serotonin, which promotes vomiting.

The usual adult dose is 8 mg twice daily. This can be adjusted according to need. Odansetron is often prescribed during chemotherapy, and the dose required may be increased if this is prescribed. Odansetron may also be prescribed intravenously if the patient is too nauseous to tolerate oral medication.

The most common side effects associated with odansetron are:

- constipation
- headaches
- flushing.

The side effects associated with this medication are minimal, and allergy reactions are only seen when given intravenously (Galbraith *et al.*, 2007).

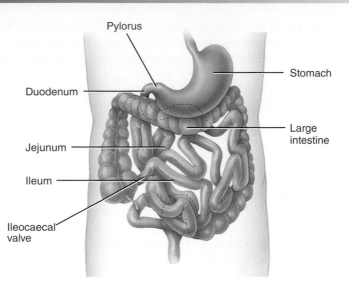

Figure 9.11　The small intestine. *Source*: Tortora and Derrickson (2009). Reproduced with permission of John Wiley & Sons.

Small intestine

The small intestine is approximately 6 m long. In the small intestine food is further broken down by mechanical and chemical digestion, and absorption of the products of digestion takes place. The small intestine is divided into three parts (see Figure 9.11):

1. The **duodenum** is approximately 25 cm long. It is the entrance to the small intestine.
2. The **jejunum** measures 2.5 m and is the middle part of the small intestine.
3. The **ileum** measures 3.5 m. It meets the large intestine at the **ileocaecal valve**. This valve prevents the backflow of the products of digestion from the large intestine back into the small intestine.

The small intestine is innervated with both parasympathetic and sympathetic nerves. It receives its arterial blood supply from the **superior mesenteric artery** and nutrient-rich venous blood drains into the **superior mesenteric vein** and eventually into the **hepatic portal vein** towards the liver.

There are four types of cell present in the mucosa of the small intestine (see Figure 9.12):

- The absorptive cell produces digestive enzymes and absorbs digested foods.
- Goblet cells secrete mucus to protect the intestine from abrasion and from the acidic chyme entering the small intestine.
- Enteroendocrine cells produce regulatory hormones such as secretin and CKK. These hormones are secreted into the bloodstream and act on their target organs to release pancreatic juice and bile.
- Paneth cells produce lysozyme, which protects the small intestine from pathogens that have survived the acid conditions of the stomach. Peyer's patches (lymphatic tissue of the small intestine) also protect the small intestine.

Partially digested food enters the small intestine and spends from 3–6 h moving through its 6 m length. The smooth muscle activity within the small intestine continues the process of

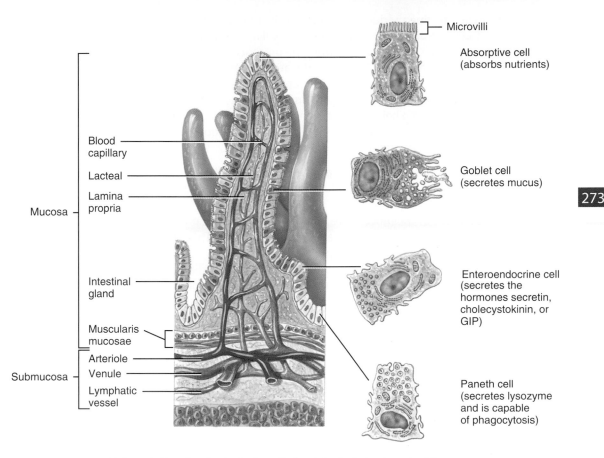

Enlarged villus showing lacteal, capillaries, intestinal glands and cell types

Figure 9.12 The cells within the villi of the small intestine. *Source*: Tortora and Derrickson (2009). Reproduced with permission of John Wiley & Sons.

mechanical digestion. There are two types of mechanical digestion in the small intestine: segmental contractions, which help to mix the various enzymes in the small intestine with the contents of the chyme, and peristalsis, which propels the food down the length of the small intestine as well as facilitating mixing.

Chemical digestion completes the breakdown of the carbohydrates, fats and proteins. Pancreatic juice from the pancreas, bile from the gallbladder and intestinal juice contribute to this.

Chemical digestion

Within the small intestine, any carbohydrates that have not been broken down by the action of salivary amylase will be broken down by pancreatic amylase.

Bile will emulsify fat and fatty acids, making it easier for lipase (also from the pancreatic juice) to break the fats into fatty acids and glycerol. Proteins are denatured by hydrochloric acid in the stomach. In the small intestine they are further acted upon by the enzymes trypsin, chymotrypsin and carboxypeptidase. The end product of protein digestion is tripeptidases, dipeptidases and amino acids.

The small intestine produce 1–2 L of intestinal juice daily. It is secreted from the cells of the **crypts of Lieberkühn** (located between the villi) in response to either acidic chyme irritating the intestinal mucosa or distension from the presence of chyme in the small intestine. Intestinal juice is slightly alkaline (pH 7.4–8.4) and watery. Intestinal juice and pancreatic juice from the pancreas mix with the acidic chyme as it enters the duodenum and increase the pH, thus preventing the corrosive action of chyme on the mucosa of the duodenum. Intestinal juice also contains mucus, which helps protect the intestinal mucosa, mineral salts and enterokinase.

The primary function of the small intestine is absorption of water and nutrients, and it has several anatomical adaptations to facilitate this:

- Permanent circular folds, called **plicae circulars**, within the mucosa and submucosa slow down the movement of the products of digestion, allowing time for absorption of nutrients to occur.
- On the surface of the mucosa are tiny, finger-like projections called **villi**. At the centre of the villi is a capillary bed and a **lacteal** (lymph capillary). This allows nutrients to be absorbed directly into the blood or the lymph.
- On the surface of the villi are cytoplasmic extensions called **microvilli**. The presence of the microvilli greatly increases the surface area available for absorption. The appearance of the microvilli resembles the surface of a brush; hence it is called the **brush border**. The brush border produces some enzymes used to further break down carbohydrates such as lactase, maltase, dextrinase and sucrase. It also produces enzymes to further break down proteins: aminopeptidase, carboxypeptidase and dipeptidase.

The absorption of nutrients occurs by diffusion or active transport. Some nutrients will be absorbed into the blood capillary and some will be absorbed into the lacteal.

Function of the small intestine

- Production of mucus to protect the duodenum from the effects of the acidic chyme.
- Secretion of intestinal juice and pancreatic juice from the pancreas increase the pH of the chyme to facilitate the action of the enzymes.
- Bile enters the small intestine to emulsify fat so that it can be further broken down by the action of lipase.
- Many enzymes are secreted to complete the chemical digestion of carbohydrates, proteins and fats.
- Mechanical digestion is by peristalsis and segmentation, and slows down to allow adequate mixing and maximum absorption.
- The small intestine is structurally designed with a large surface area for maximum absorption of the products of digestion.
- The small intestine is where the majority of nutrients, electrolytes and water are absorbed.

The pancreas

The pancreas is composed of exocrine and endocrine tissue. It consists of a head, body and tail (see Figure 9.13). The cells of the pancreas are responsible for making the endocrine and exocrine products.

- The islet cells of the **islets of Langerhans** produce the endocrine hormones **insulin** and **glucagon**. These hormones control carbohydrate metabolism.

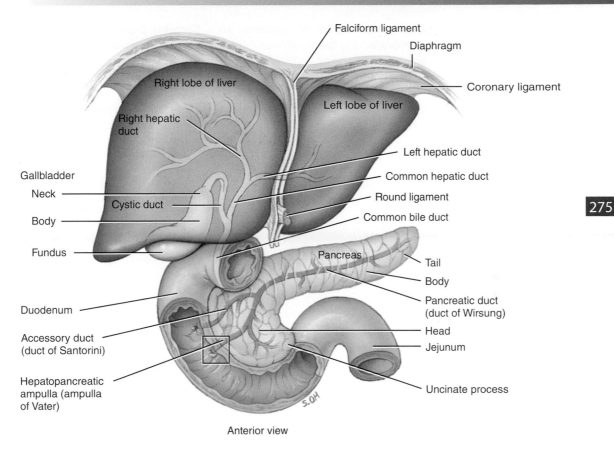

Anterior view

Figure 9.13 The liver, gallbladder and pancreas. *Source*: Tortora and Derrickson (2009). Reproduced with permission of John Wiley & Sons.

- The **acini glands** of the exocrine pancreas produce 1.2–1.5 L of **pancreatic juice** daily. Pancreatic juice travels from the pancreas via the pancreatic duct into the duodenum at the hepatopancreatic ampulla.
- The cells of the pancreatic ducts secrete bicarbonate ions, which gives pancreatic juice its high pH (pH 8). This helps to neutralise acidic chyme from the stomach, thus protecting the small intestine from damage by the acidity. Additionally, the actions of amylase and lipase are most effective at the higher pH (pH 6–8).

Pancreatic juice consists of:

- water;
- mineral salts;
- pancreatic amylase, which completes the digestion of carbohydrates;
- lipase, used in the digestion of fat;
- **trypsinogen**, **chymotrypsinogen** and **procarboxypeptidase**, which are released in an inactive form to protect the digestive system structures from the protein-digesting enzymes that they become – once they enter the duodenum they are activated by enterokinase from intestinal juice and become trypsin, chymotrypsin and carboxypeptidase respectively and are then used in the digestion of protein.

Two hormones regulate the secretion of pancreatic juice. **Secretin**, produced in response to the presence of hydrochloric acid in the duodenum, promotes the secretion of bicarbonate ions. **CKK**, secreted in response to the intake of protein and fat, promotes the secretion of the enzymes present in pancreatic juice. Parasympathetic vagus nerve stimulation also promotes the release of pancreatic juice.

In summary, the exocrine function of the pancreas is to secrete pancreatic juice into the duodenum. The actions of pancreatic juice lead to the further breakdown of carbohydrate, fat and protein.

Medicines management

Creon

Creon is a medication prescribed for patients who have cystic fibrosis or pancreatic insufficiency. It contains the following enzymes:

- amylase – for the breakdown of carbohydrate
- lipase – for the breakdown of fats
- proteases - for the breakdown of protein.

Pancreatic insufficiency can occur as a result of pancreatic cancer, pancreatic surgery and acute or chronic pancreatitis. In cystic fibrosis the ducts that transport the pancreatic enzymes become obstructed with the increased mucus production associated with this disease pathway.

The dosage of creon required will depend on the diet of the patient. If the symptoms of loose stool and weight loss persist, then the dose of creon may be increased. Creon is usually taken for life. There are some side effects associated with creon, and these include

- abdominal distension
- nausea
- vomiting
- diarrhoea
- constipation.

The tablets are enteric coated to protect them from inactivation in the stomach (Galbraith *et al.*, 2007).

NICE (2010) produces a Clinical Knowledge Summary on managing chronic pancreatitis.

The liver and production of bile

The liver is the body's largest gland. It weighs between 1 and 2 kg. It lies under the diaphragm protected by the ribs. The liver occupies most of the right hypochondriac region and extends through part of the epigastric region into the left hypochondriac region. The right lobe is the largest of the four liver lobes. On the posterior surface of the liver there is an entry and exit to the organ called the portal fissure. Blood, lymph vessels, nerves and bile ducts enter and leave the liver through the portal fissure.

The liver is composed of tiny hexagonal-shaped lobules that contain hepatocytes (see Figure 9.14). The hepatocytes are protected by Kupffer cells (hepatic macrophages). The Kupffer cells deal with any foreign particles and worn-out blood cells.

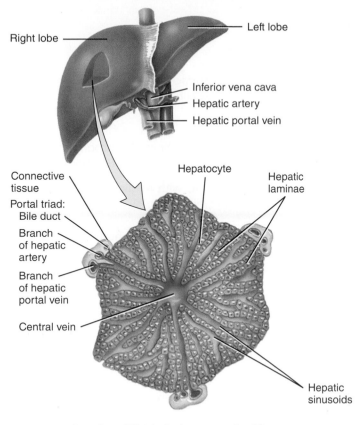

Overview of histological components of liver

Figure 9.14 Liver lobule. *Source*: Tortora and Derrickson (2009). Reproduced with permission of John Wiley & Sons.

Each corner of the hexagonal-shaped lobule has a portal triad. A branch of the hepatic artery, a branch of hepatic portal vein and a bile duct are present here. The hepatic artery supplies the hepatocytes with oxygenated arterial blood. The hepatic portal vein delivers nutrient-rich deoxygenated blood from the digestive tract to the hepatocytes. The hepatocytes' function is to filter, detoxify and process the nutrients from the digestive tract. Nutrients can be used for energy, stored or used to make new molecules. The liver sinusoids are large, leaky capillaries that drain the blood from the hepatic artery and hepatic portal vein into the central vein. This processed blood is then drained into the hepatic vein and on to the inferior vena cava.

As the blood flows towards the centre of the triad to exit at the central vein, the bile produced by the hepatocyte as a metabolic by-product moves in the opposite direction towards the bile canaliculi and on to the bile ducts. Bile then leaves the liver via the common hepatic duct towards the duodenum of the small intestine.

The liver produces and secretes up to 1 L of yellow/green alkaline bile per day. Bile is composed of:

- bile salts such as bilirubin from the breakdown of haemoglobin
- cholesterol
- fat-soluble hormones

- fat
- mineral salts
- mucus.

The function of bile is to emulsify fats, giving the fat-digesting enzymes (trypsin, chymotrypsin and carboxypeptidase) a larger surface area to work on.

Bile is stored and concentrated in the gallbladder.

The functions of the liver

Apart from the production of bile and the metabolism of carbohydrate, fat and protein (discussed further on in this chapter), the liver has many additional functions:

- detoxification of drugs – the liver deals with medication, alcohol, ingested toxins and the toxins produced by the action of microbes;
- recycling of erythrocytes;
- deactivation of many hormones, including the sex hormones, thyroxine, insulin, glucagon, cortisol and aldosterone;
- production of clotting proteins;
- storage of vitamins, minerals and glycogen;
- synthesis of vitamin A;
- heat production.

The gallbladder

The gallbladder is a small, green, muscular sac that lies posterior to the liver. It functions as a reservoir for bile. It also concentrates bile by absorbing water. The mucosa of the gallbladder, like the rugae of the stomach, contains folds that allow the gallbladder to stretch in order to accommodate varying volumes of bile. When the smooth muscle walls of the gallbladder contract, bile is expelled into the cystic duct and down into the common bile duct before entering the duodenum via the hepatopancreatic ampulla.

The stimulus for gallbladder contraction is the hormone CKK. This enteroendocrine hormone, secreted from the small intestine into the blood, is produced in response to the presence of fatty chyme in the duodenum. CKK stimulates the secretion of pancreatic juice and the relaxation of the hepatopancreatic sphincter. When the sphincter is relaxed, both bile and pancreatic juice can enter the duodenum. Figure 9.15 summarises the production and release of bile.

The large intestine

The contents of the small intestine move slowly through it by a process called segmentation. This allows time to complete digestion and absorption. Entry to the large intestine is controlled by the ileocaecal sphincter. The sphincter opens in response to the increased activity of the stomach and the action of the hormone gastrin. Once food residue has reached the large intestine it cannot backflow into the ileum (see Figure 9.15).

The large intestine measures 1.5 m in length and 7 cm in diameter. It is continuous with the small intestine from the ileocaecal valve and ends at the anus.

Food residue enters the caecum and has to pass up the ascending colon along the transverse colon, down the descending colon and out of the body via the rectum, anal canal and anus. The caecum is a descending, sac-like opening into the large intestine. The vermiform appendix is a narrow, tube-like structure that leaves the caecum but is closed at its distal end. It is composed

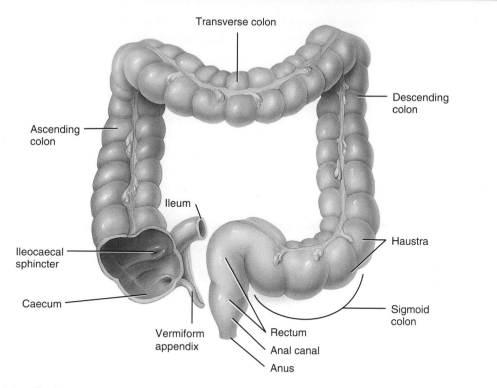

Figure 9.15   The large intestine. *Source*: Tortora and Derrickson (2009). Reproduced with permission of John Wiley & Sons.

of lymphoid tissue and has a role in immunity. Two sphincter muscles control exit from the anus. The internal anal sphincter is smooth muscle and is under the control of the parasympathetic nervous system, whereas the external anal sphincter is composed of skeletal muscle and is under voluntary control.

Clinical considerations

Appendicitis

The narrow lumen of the appendix does not allow much room for inflammation. If it becomes blocked by faecoliths (hard faecal material) or becomes twisted and kinked, this results in inflammation of the appendix. The swelling associated with this can lead to ulceration of the mucosal lining. This presents initially as central abdominal pain that eventually localises at the region of the appendix. Appendicitis can subside, but often it results in abscess formation and even rupture.

The large intestine mucosa contains large numbers of goblet cells that secrete mucus to ease the passage of faeces and protect the walls of the large intestine. The simple columnar epithelium changes to stratified squamous epithelium at the anal canal. Anal sinuses secrete mucus in response to faecal compression. This protects the anal canal from the abrasion associated with defaecation.

The longitudinal muscle layer of the large intestine is formed into bands called the taeniae coli. These give the large intestine its gathered appearance. The sac created by this gathering is called a haustrum.

The food residue from the ileum is fluid when it enters the caecum and contains few nutrients. The small intestine is responsible for some of the absorption of water, but the primary function of the large intestine is to absorb water and turn the food residue into semi-solid faeces. The large intestine also absorbs some vitamins, minerals, electrolytes and drugs. Food residue usually takes 24–48 h to pass through the large intestine; 500 mL of food residue enters the large intestine daily and approximately 150 mL leaves as faeces.

As faeces enters the rectum, the stretching of the walls of the rectum initiates the **defaecation reflex**. Acquired, voluntary control of the defaecation reflex occurs between the ages of 2 and 3 years. The external anal sphincter is under voluntary control, and, if it is appropriate to do so, defaecation can occur. Contraction of the abdominal muscles and diaphragm (the Valsalva manoeuvre) creates intra-abdominal pressure and assists in the process of defaecation. If it is not appropriate to defaecate, as it is under voluntary control, it can be postponed. After a few minutes the urge to go will subside and will only be felt again when the next mass movement through the large intestine occurs.

Faeces is a brown, semi-solid material. It contains fibre, stercobilin (from the breakdown of bilirubin), water, fatty acids, shed epithelial cells and microbes. Stercobilin gives faeces its brown colour. An excess of water in faeces results in **diarrhoea**. This occurs when food residue passes too quickly through the large intestine, so that the absorption of water cannot occur. Conversely, **constipation** occurs if food residue spends too long in the large intestine.

Medicines management

Lactulose

Lactulose belongs to a group of medications called laxatives or aperients. It is used to treat constipation. Constipation occurs as a result of a lack of fluid intake or dehydration, a lack of exercise or immobility, during pregnancy or due to a lack of dietary fibre.

People who suffer from constipation should try to increase their mobility and fluid levels. They should examine their diet to see whether additional fibre can be taken. Lactulose may also be prescribed.

The usual adult dose for lactulose is 15 mL three times a day. Lactulose acts in the large intestine and can take 48 h to have an effect. Increasing fluid intake to 2 L will also help.

Lactulose is an osmotic laxative (Galbraith *et al.*, 2007). Lactulose leads to a change in the osmotic pressure in the bowel, and therefore more water is available in the intestine. This leads to the stool having more water content, making it pass through the intestine easier.

The side effects of taking lactulose include:

- nausea
- diarrhoea
- flatulence
- abdominal discomfort.

NICE (2014b) produces a Clinical Knowledge Summary on constipation.

Digestive tract hormones

Many hormones are responsible for the activity of the digestive system. A summary of their role is contained in Table 9.1.

Nutrition, chemical digestion and metabolism

This chapter has hitherto concentrated on how the digestive tract deals with food ingested in order to break it down into its constituent parts for use by the cells of the body. This section will consider nutrition and the role of a balanced diet in health.

An adequate intake of nutrients is essential for health. Nutrition also has an important role in social and psychological well-being. If managed inappropriately, nutrition can lead to many physical and psychological illnesses. Therefore, it is important to have an understanding of the role of nutrients within the body in order to understand how a lack or excess of nutrients will lead to ill health.

The remainder of this chapter will identify the macro- and micronutrients and the food groups that provide the source of macro- and micronutrients. It will examine what the nutrients are broken down into and how the body uses these constituent parts.

Nutrients

A nutrient is a substance that is ingested and processed by the gastrointestinal system. It is digested and absorbed and can be used by the body to produce energy or become the building block for a new molecule or to participate in essential chemical reactions. Nutrients are required for body growth, repair and maintenance of cell function. Not all of food ingested can be classed as nutrients. Some non-digestible plant fibres are not nutrients but are required for healthy functioning of the digestive system.

Table 9.1 Summary of the role of the digestive system hormones

Hormone	Origin	Target	Action	Stimulus
Gastrin	Stomach	Stomach	Increases gastric gland secretion of hydrochloric acid Gastric emptying	Presence of protein in the stomach
Secretin	Duodenum	Stomach	Inhibits gastric gland secretion Inhibits gastric motility	Acidic and fatty chyme in the duodenum
		Pancreas	Increases pancreatic juice secretion Promotes cholecystokinin action	
		Liver	Increases bile secretion	
Cholecystokinin	Duodenum	Pancreas	Increases pancreatic juice secretion	Chyme in the duodenum
		Gallbladder	Stimulates contraction	
		Hepatopancreatic sphincter	Relaxes – entry to duodenum open	

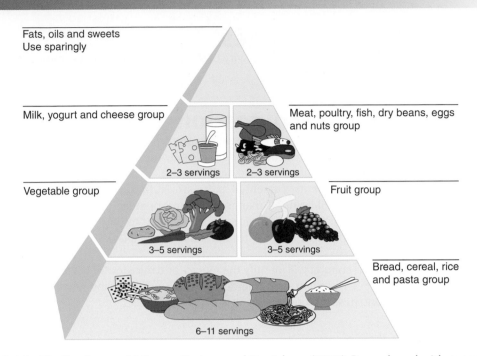

Fats, oils and sweets
Use sparingly

Milk, yogurt and cheese group

Meat, poultry, fish, dry beans, eggs
and nuts group

2–3 servings   2–3 servings

Vegetable group

Fruit group

3–5 servings   3–5 servings

Bread, cereal, rice
and pasta group

6–11 servings

Figure 9.16   The food pyramid. *Source*: Tortora and Derrickson (2009). Reproduced with permission of John Wiley & Sons.

Balanced diet

The body has the ability to break down some nutrients in order to create new molecules, but this ability is finite and there remains a group of essential nutrients that the body cannot make but are required to be ingested in the diet for homeostasis to be maintained. A balanced diet is therefore essential for health (Department of Health, 2003). The daily recommended portions of food groups required for a balanced diet are shown in the food pyramid (see Figure 9.16). Lack of a balanced diet can lead to malnourishment, and overindulgence can lead to obesity.

Snapshot

Bariatric surgery

Bariatric surgery is used as a last resort to treat those who are severely obese. The procedure works by reducing intake or the absorption of calories and is used to treat people with potentially life-threatening obesity if other treatments (e.g. lifestyle changes) have not worked. Indications include:

- a body mass index (BMI) greater than 40;
- a BMI of 35 or above and having another serious health condition that may be improved if weight is lost (e.g. type 2 diabetes or hypertension);
- other non-surgical methods have failed to maintain weight loss for at least 6 months;
- the person commits to long-term follow-up.

Weight loss surgery can help to significantly and quickly reduce excess body fat for those who meet the criteria. Bariatric surgery has to be undertaken in a specialist centre with long-term follow-up of patients. National guidelines are available concerning bariatric surgery. Contraindications include those who are unfit for surgery and those people with an uncontrolled alcohol or drug dependency.

Dietary nutrients begin life as large food molecules. They enter the digestive tract and are broken down into smaller molecules. This process is called catabolism. Digestive enzymes facilitate the breakdown of foods by a process called hydrolysis. Hydrolysis is the addition of water to break down the chemical bonds of the food molecules. Each of the three different types of food is broken down (lysed) by different enzymes.

Nutrient groups

Carbohydrates, proteins and lipids are known as the major nutrients or macronutrients. They are required in quite large quantities. Vitamins and minerals are required in much smaller quantities, but they also are crucial for the maintenance of health. They are also known as the micronutrients. There are therefore six classes of nutrients:

- water
- carbohydrates
- proteins
- lipids (fats)
- vitamins
- minerals.

283

Water

Water is essential for the action of many digestive system functions. It is required to produce the many different juices of the digestive system. As the enzymes act on the different food molecules within the diet, water is added. This process is known as hydrolysis (Cohen and Hull, 2015).

Carbohydrates

Monosaccharides, disaccharides and polysaccharides are all carbohydrates. The dietary source of carbohydrates is plants. However, the milk sugar lactose is a form of carbohydrate found in cow and human milk. Carbohydrates are found in many foods, such as bread, pasta, cereal, biscuits, vegetables and fruit.

Carbohydrates consist of carbon, hydrogen and oxygen. They can be complex, such as the polysaccharides starch and glycogen, or simple, such as the disaccharides sucrose (table sugar) and lactose (milk sugar) and the monosaccharides glucose, fructose and galactose.

Digestion of carbohydrates supplies the body with fructose, galactose and glucose. The liver converts fructose and galactose to glucose as glucose is the molecule used by the body's cells.

Digested carbohydrates are absorbed into the blood via the villi of the small intestine. They enter the hepatic portal circulation and are transported to the liver for processing. The liver is a highly metabolic organ that requires a plentiful supply of glucose to carry out its metabolic activity.

Glucose is used by the cells to produce adenosine triphosphate (ATP). Glucose plus oxygen makes ATP, carbon dioxide and water. The process of breaking down glucose is called glycolysis.

Insufficient carbohydrate intake will lead to an inability to meet the cells' energy demands. If this happens, the body will break down amino acids and lipids to create new glucose, a process called gluconeogenesis.

Excess glucose is converted to glycogen and stored in the liver. It can also be converted to fat and stored.

Fats

Dietary sources of fat include butter, eggs, cheese, milk, oily fish and the fatty part of meat. These contain saturated fat, which is mainly saturated fatty acids and glycerol. Vegetable oils and margarine are sources of unsaturated fats. The body can also create fat from excess carbohydrate and protein intake.

Fat also contains carbon, hydrogen and oxygen, but in a different combination from carbohydrates.

When fat enters the small intestine it mixes and is emulsified by bile. The action of pancreatic lipase completes the digestion of fat and it is broken down into monoglycerides, glycerol and fatty acids. The monoglycerides and some of the fatty acids enter the lacteals of the villi and are transported via the lymph to the thoracic duct and into the circulation, where they eventually reach the liver. Glycerol and the remaining fatty acids are absorbed more directly into the capillary blood and reach the liver via the hepatic portal vein.

The liver uses some of the fatty acids and glycerol to provide energy and heat. In fact, hepatocytes and skeletal muscle use triglycerides as their major energy source. Excessive triglycerides can also be stored as adipose tissue, and this can also be used as an energy store when glucose is not available to body cells.

Dietary fats make food seem tender and lead to a feeling of satisfaction with food. They are necessary for the absorption of fat-soluble vitamins. Adipose tissue protects, cushions and insulates vital organs in the body. Phospholipids are required to form the myelin sheath and cell membranes. Cholesterol is obtained from egg yolk and dairy produce but is also synthesised in the body to form steroid hormones and bile salts.

Excess fat in the diet can lead to obesity and cardiovascular disease. A lack of fat in the diet can lead to weight loss, poor growth and skin lesions.

Proteins

Dietary sources of protein include meat, eggs and milk. Beans and peas (legumes), nuts, cereals and leafy green vegetables are also sources of amino acids.

Protein digestion begins in the stomach and is completed in the small intestine. Proteins are broken down into amino acids. They are absorbed via the villi of the small intestine, where they reach the capillaries and then the hepatic portal circulation to the liver or general circulation.

Proteins are used by the body for many purposes. They are used to form muscle, collagen and elastin, necessary for body structure and tissue repair. The hormones insulin and growth hormone are required for this. Amino acids are also used to form hormones and enzymes within the body. All of the amino acids required to form a required protein must be available within the cell in order for that protein to be made. This is called the all or nothing rule. Protein can also be used as a source of energy for the body. The amino acid is broken down mainly at the liver, where the nitrogenous part of the amino acid is removed and converted first to ammonia and then to urea. Urea is excreted as a waste product in urine. The remainder of the amino acid is used to produce energy. Protein cannot be stored by the body. Any excess amino acids are converted to carbohydrate or fat to be stored as adipose tissue.

Too much protein in the diet can lead to obesity. A lack of dietary protein can lead to muscle/tissue wasting and weight loss. A lack of plasma proteins can lead to oedema.

Table 9.2 Vitamins summary

Vitamin	Source	Function	Deficiency
Fat soluble			
A, retinol	Manufactured from beta-carotene. Egg yolk, cream, fish oil, cheese, liver	Skin, mucosa integrity; bone and tooth development during growth; photoreceptor pigment synthesis in the retina, normal reproduction, antioxidant	Night blindness, dry skin and hair, loss of skin integrity, increased infection particularly respiratory, gastrointestinal and urinary
D	Manufactured by the skin. Cheese, eggs, fish oil, liver	Regulates calcium and phosphate metabolism	Rickets in children, osteomalacia in adults
E	Egg yolk, wheat germ, whole cereals, milk and butter	Antioxidant	In severe deficiency, ataxia and visual disturbances, decreased life span of red blood cells
K	Synthesised by bacteria in the large intestine. Liver, fish, fruit and leafy green vegetables	Formation of clotting proteins at the liver	Prolonged clotting times, bruising, bleeding
Water soluble			
B_1, thiamine	Egg yolk, liver, nuts, meat, legumes cereal germ	Coenzyme required for carbohydrate metabolism	Beriberi – muscle wasting, stunted growth polyneuritis and infection. Vision disturbances, confusion, unsteadiness, memory loss, fatigue, tachycardia, heart enlargement
B_2, riboflavin	Milk, green vegetables, yeast, cheese, fish roe, liver	Coenzyme required for carbohydrate and protein metabolism	Skin-cracking, particularly around the corners of the mouth, blurred vision, corneal ulcers, intestinal mucosa lesions
Folic acid	Liver, kidney, yeast, fresh leafy vegetables, eggs, whole grains	Coenzyme essential for DNA synthesis, red blood cell formation	Anaemia, spina bifida in newborn, increased risk of heart attack and stroke
Niacin, nicotinic acid	Liver, cheese, yeast, eggs, cereals, nuts, fish	Coenzyme involved in glycolysis, fat breakdown – assists with breakdown and inhibits cholesterol production	Pellagra – skin reddening to light, anorexia, nausea and dysphagia, delirium and dementia
B_6, pyridoxine	Meat, liver, fish, grains, bananas, yeast	Coenzyme involved in amino acid metabolism	Increased risk of heart disease, eye and mouth lesions. In children, nervous irritability, convulsions, abdominal pain and vomiting
B_{12} cyanocobalamin	Meat, fish, liver, eggs, milk	Coenzyme in all cells, involved in DNA synthesis. Formation and maintenance of myelin around nerves	Pernicious anaemia, peripheral neuropathy
B_5 pantothenic acid	Meat, grains, legumes, yeast, egg yolk	Coenzyme associated with amino acid metabolism and formation of steroids	Non-specific symptoms
Biotin	Egg yolk, liver, legumes, tomatoes	Coenzyme in carbohydrate metabolism	Pallor, anorexia, nausea, fatigue
C, ascorbic acid	Fruit, particularly citrus fruit, vegetables	Antioxidant, enhances iron absorption and use, maturation of red blood cells	Poor wound healing, joint pain, anaemia, scurvy

Vitamins

Vitamins are organic molecules that are required in small amounts for healthy metabolism. Essential vitamins cannot be manufactured by the body and must come from the diet, highlighting again the importance of a balanced diet. Some vitamins can be manufactured. Vitamin K is synthesised by intestinal bacteria; the skin makes vitamin D; and vitamin A is made from beta-carotene, found for example in carrots.

Many vitamins act as *coenzymes* (Seeley *et al.*, 2008). These vitamins combine with enzymes to make them functional. For example, the formation of clotting proteins requires the presence of vitamin K.

During metabolism a reaction takes place involving oxygen. Potentially harmful free radicals are formed as part of this process. Vitamins A, C and E are antioxidants that disarm free radicals and protect tissue from their potentially dangerous effects.

Vitamins are either fat soluble or water soluble. The fat-soluble vitamins combine with lipids from the diet and are absorbed in this way. Apart from vitamin K, the fat-soluble vitamins can be stored in the body; therefore, there can be problems associated with toxicity when these vitamins accumulate.

The water-soluble vitamins are absorbed with water along the digestive tract. They cannot be stored, and any excess ingested will be excreted in urine. A summary of vitamins and their functions is given in Table 9.2.

Minerals

Small quantities of inorganic compounds called minerals are required by the body for many purposes. For example, calcium gives structure and strength to tissues, and sodium forms ions essential for maintaining osmotic pressure. They also form approximately 5% of the body weight (Nair and Peate, 2013).

There are minerals that are required in moderate amounts, such as calcium and magnesium, and many others known where trace amounts are required, such as cobalt and copper. A summary of some of the minerals and their function is given in Table 9.3.

Clinical considerations

Obesity

Obesity is on the increase in Western society. Obesity occurs when more calories are taken in than are used by the body. Lack of exercise, a sedentary lifestyle and generous diet all contribute to weight gain. Obesity has serious health consequences as it predisposes people to indigestion, gallstones, hernias, cardiovascular disease, varicose veins, osteoarthritis and type 2 diabetes mellitus.

Conclusion

Digestion and nutrition play a vital role in the maintenance of health. The digestive tract processes ingested nutrients by breaking them down chemically and mechanically. Accessory structures, such as the pancreas, liver and gallbladder, have an essential role in providing the digestive tract with bile and pancreatic juice to facilitate the digestion of the macronutrients protein, carbohydrate and fat. The small intestine provides the large surface area available for the absorption of nutrients, and the liver processes the products of digestion. The large intestine

Table 9.3   Minerals summary

Mineral	Source	Function	Deficiency(D)/excess(E)
Calcium	Milk, egg yolk, shellfish, cheese, green vegetables	Bones and teeth, cell membrane permeability, nerve impulse transmission, muscle contraction, heart rhythm, blood clotting	D: osteomalacia, osteoporosis, muscle tetany. In children – rickets and retarded growth
			E: lethargy and confusion, kidney stones
Chloride	Table salt	Works with sodium to maintain osmotic pressure of extracellular fluid	D: alkalosis, muscle cramps
			E: vomiting
Magnesium	Nuts, milk, legumes, cereal	Constituent of coenzymes. Muscle and nerve irritability	D: neuromuscular problems, irregular heartbeat
			E: diarrhoea
Sodium	Table salt	Extracellular cation. Works with chloride to maintain osmotic pressure of extracellular fluid. Muscle contraction, nerve impulse transmission, electrolyte balance	D: rare – nausea
			E: hypertension, oedema
Potassium	Fruit and vegetables and many foods	Intracellular cation. Muscle contraction, nerve impulse transmission electrolyte balance	D: Rare – muscle weakness, nausea, tachycardia
			E: cardiac abnormalities, muscular weakness
Iron	Liver, kidney, beef, green vegetables	Constituent of haemoglobin	D: anaemia
			E: haemochromatosis, liver damage
Iodine	Saltwater fish, vegetables	Constituent of thyroid hormones	D: hypothyroidism
			E: thyroid hormone synthesis depressed

plays an excretory role, ridding the body of the waste products from digestion and absorbing any remaining water back into the body.

The maintenance of homeostasis is achieved through the ingestion of a balanced diet, containing a variety of elements from each of the food groups.

Without all of this activity, normal cell functioning would be at risk and this would lead to ill health. Digestive health contributes greatly to physical, psychological and social well-being.

Glossary

Absorption   Process whereby the products of digestion move into the blood or lymph fluid.

Acini glands   Produce pancreatic juice.

Amylase   Carbohydrate-digesting enzyme.

Anus   End of the digestive tract.

Bile   Fluid produced by the liver and required for the digestion of fat.

Bile duct   Tube that carries bile from the liver.

Body region   Region of the stomach.

Caecum   Beginning of the large intestine.

Canine   Type of tooth.

Carbohydrate   One of the major food groups.

Cardiac region   Region of the stomach closest to the oesophagus.

Catabolism   Process of breaking down substances into simpler substances.

Chief cells   Pepsinogen-producing cells.

Cholecystokinin   Digestive system hormone.

Chyme   Creamy, semi-fluid mass of partially digested food mixed with gastric secretions.

Deglutition   Swallowing.

Digestion   The chemical and mechanical breakdown of food for absorption.

Duodenum   First part of the small intestine.

Enamel   Covering of the tooth.

Epiglottis   Cartilage that covers the larynx during swallowing.

Faeces   Brown, semi-solid digestive system waste.

Fats   One of the major food groups.

Frenulum   Fold between the lip and gum.

Fundus   Anatomical base region of the stomach.

Gluconeogenesis   The creation of glucose from non-carbohydrate molecules.

Glycolysis   The anaerobic breakdown of glucose to form pyruvic acid.

Goblet cell   Mucus-producing cell.

Haustrum   Sac-like section of the large intestine.

Hepatocyte   Liver cell.

Hepatic portal vein   Vein that delivers dissolved nutrients to the liver.

Hepatopancreatic ampulla   The site where the bile duct and pancreatic duct meet.

Hepatopancreatic sphincter   Muscular valve that controls the entrance of pancreatic juice and bile to the duodenum.

Hyoid bone   Bone that acts as the base of the tongue.

Hydrochloric acid   Acid produced by the parietal cells of the stomach.

Hydrolysis   Addition of water to breakdown food molecules.

Hypochondriac region   Upper lateral divisions of the abdominopelvic cavity.

Ileum   The end part of the small intestine.

Ileocaecal valve   Site where the small and large intestine meet.

Ingestion   The process of taking food into the body via the mouth.

Incisors   Type of tooth.

Intestinal crypts   Also known as the crypts of Lieberkuhn – glands found in the villi of the small intestine.

Intrinsic factor   Substance required for the absorption of vitamin B$_{12}$.

Jejunum   The middle part of the small intestine between the duodenum and the ileum.

Kupffer cell   Hepatic macrophage.

Lacteal   Lymphatic capillary of the small intestine.

Lamina propria   Loose connective tissue layer of the digestive tract.

Laryngopharynx   Where the larynx and pharynx meet.

Lipase   Fat-digesting enzyme.

Liver   Accessory organ located in the abdominal cavity that has many metabolic and regulatory functions.

Liver sinusoid   Liver capillary.

Lower oesophageal sphincter   Valve between the oesophagus and stomach.

Lysozyme   Bactericidal enzyme.

Macronutrient   Food consumed in large quantities.

Mastication   Chewing.

Metabolism   Sum total of the chemical reactions occurring in the body.

Meissner's plexus   Nerves of the small intestine.

Mesenteric plexus   Digestive tract innervation.

Micronutrient   Nutrient required in small quantities.

Microvilli   Cytoplasmic extensions of the villi.

Minerals   Salts – inorganic compounds.

Molars   Type of tooth.

Mucosa   Layer of the digestive tract.

Mucous neck cells   Mucus-secreting cells of the stomach.

Muscularis mucosa   Muscular layer of the digestive tract.

Nutrient   Product obtained from the digestion of food and used by the body.

Oesophagus   Muscular tube from laryngopharynx to stomach.

Oral cavity   The first part of the digestive system.

Oropharynx   Part of the pharynx closest to the oral cavity.

Palate   Roof of the mouth.

Pancreatic duct   Duct that links the pancreas and common bile duct.

Paneth cell   Cell that produces lysozyme.

Papillae   Small mucosal projections.

Parasympathetic fibres   Autonomic nervous system nerve fibres.

Parietal cells   Hydrochloric acid-producing cell of the stomach.

Parotid glands   Salivary glands located close to the ears.

Pepsin   Enzyme required for the breakdown of protein.

Pepsinogen   Enzyme precursor of pepsin.

Peristalsis   Wave-like contractions that move food through the digestive tract.

Peritoneum   Serous membrane that lines the abdominal cavity.

Peyer's patches   Lymphatic tissue of the small intestine.

Pharyngeal phase   Second phase of swallowing.

Pharynx   Tube between the mouth and the oesophagus.

Plicae circulars   Permanent circular folds in the small intestine.

Portal fissure   Area where blood vessels and nerves enter and leave the liver.

Portal triad   Corner of liver lobule.

Premolars   Type of tooth located between the canine and molar teeth.

Propulsion   The process of moving the food along the length of the digestive system.

Proteins   Substance that contains carbon, hydrogen, oxygen and nitrogen.

Pulp cavity   Centre of the tooth.

Pyloric canal   Area where the stomach opens into the small intestine.

Pyloric region   Area of the stomach that occurs where the stomach meets the small intestine.

Pyloric sphincter   Valve that controls food movement from the stomach to the small intestine.

Rectum   Final portion of the large intestine.

Rugae   Folds or ridges found in the digestive tract.

Salivary amylase   Carbohydrate-digesting enzyme found in saliva.

Secretin   Hormone that regulates secretion of pancreatic juice.

Segmentation   Movement of chyme in the small intestine.

Serosa   Outer layer of the digestive tract.

Sphincter of Oddi   Valve that controls the movement of bile and pancreatic juice into the small intestine.

Splanchnic circulation   Blood vessels of the digestive system.

Stercobilin   Waste product of bilirubin breakdown.

Stomach   Food reservoir where the digestion of protein begins.

Sublingual glands   Salivary gland located on the floor of the mouth.

Submandibular glands   Salivary glands located below the jaw bilaterally.

Submucosa   Thick connective tissue layer of the digestive tract.

Superior mesenteric artery   Vessel that supplies the small intestine with arterial blood.

Superior mesenteric vein   Blood vessel that drains venous blood from the small intestine.

Surface mucous cells   Mucus-secreting cells of the stomach.

Stomach   Reservoir for food involved in both chemical and mechanical digestion.

Taeniae coli   Muscle bands in the large intestine.

Upper oesophageal sphincter   Controls the movement of food into the oesophagus from the oropharynx.

Uvula   Small piece of tissue that protrudes from the soft palate.

Vermiform appendix   Blind-ended tube connected to the caecum and composed of lymphatic tissue.

Villi   Tiny, finger-like projections found on the surface of the mucosa of the small intestine.

Visceral peritoneum   The innermost part of the peritoneum that is in contact with the abdominal organs.

Vitamins   Essential organic compounds require in small amounts.

Voluntary phase   The first phase of swallowing.

References

Cohen, B.J. and Hull, K.L. (2015) *Memmlers's The Human Body in Health and Disease*, 13th edn. Philadelphia, PA: Wolters Kluwer.

Department of Health (2003) *The Essence of Care: Patient-Focused Benchmarks for Clinical Governance*. London: The Stationery Office.

Galbraith, A., Bullock, S., Manias, E., Hunt, B. and Richards, A. (2007) *Fundamentals of Pharmacology. An Applied Approach for Nursing and Health*, 2nd edn. Abingdon: Routledge.

Marieb E.N. (2009) *Essentials of Human Anatomy & Physiology*, 9th edn. San Francisco, CA: Pearson Benjamin Cummings.

Marieb, E.N. and Hoehn K. (2010) *Human Anatomy and Physiology*, 8th edn. San Francisco, CA: Pearson Benjamin Cummings.

Nair, M. and Peate, I. (2013) *Fundamentals of Applied Pathophysiology. An Essential Guide for Nursing Students*, 2nd edn. Chichester: John Wiley & Sons, Ltd.

NICE (2010) *Pancreatitis – Chronic*. http://cks.nice.org.uk/pancreatitis-chronic (accessed 25 November 2015).

NICE (2014a) *Gastro-oesophageal Reflux and Dyspepsia in Adults: Investigation and Management*. NICE guidelines [CG184]. http://www.nice.org.uk/guidance/cg184 (accessed 25 November 2015).

NICE (2014b) *Constipation*. http://cks.nice.org.uk/constipation#!scenariorecommendation:4 (accessed 25 November 2015).

Seeley, R.R., Stephens, T.D. and Tate, P. (2008) *Anatomy and Physiology*, 8th edn. New York: McGraw-Hill.

Tortora, G.J. and Derrickson, B.H. (2009) *Principles of Anatomy and Physiology*, 12th edn. Hoboken, NJ: John Wiley & Sons, Inc.

Tortora, G.J. and Derrickson, B.H. (2012) *Essentials of Anatomy and Physiology*, 9th edn. New York: John Wiley & Sons, Inc.

Further reading

http://www.crohnsandcolitis.org.uk/
Crohn's & Colitis UK is a charity for those affected by inflammatory bowel disease.
https://www.nice.org.uk/guidance/cg152
Link to clinical guidelines on Crohn's disease: management in adults, children and young people.

http://www.colostomyassociation.org.uk/
The Colostomy Association is a charity for people with colostomy.
http://www.nationalsmilemonth.org/
An initiative to improve oral health and hygiene. It is organised by a charity called the British Dental Health
    Foundation.

Activities
Multiple choice questions

1. Which of these vitamins is essential for blood clotting?
   (a) vitamin A
   (b) vitamin B_{12}
   (c) vitamin E
   (d) vitamin K

2. Which mineral found in broccoli provides the body with an essential constituent of the thyroid hormone thyroxine?
   (a) iron
   (b) iodine
   (c) calcium
   (d) potassium

3. Which of these is true of fat?
   (a) it is used for the growth and repair of body cells
   (b) it is a constituent of myelin sheaths
   (c) it is essential for the transport of the water-soluble vitamins
   (d) all of the above

4. Which layer of the digestive tract is responsible for peristalsis?
   (a) mucosa
   (b) submucosa
   (c) muscularis
   (d) peritoneum

5. Which of these structures is considered an accessory organ?
   (a) salivary gland
   (b) pancreas
   (c) liver
   (d) all of them

6. Where does most of the absorption of nutrients occur?
   (a) small intestine
   (b) large intestine
   (c) stomach
   (d) oesophagus

7. Which of these is *not* a constituent of gastric juice?
   (a) hydrochloric acid
   (b) mucus
   (c) intrinsic factor
   (d) trypsinogen

8. Which enzyme is involved in the breakdown of protein?
   (a) chymotrypsin
   (b) lipase
   (c) amylase
   (d) bile
9. Where is bile produced?
   (a) the small intestine
   (b) the gallbladder
   (c) the pancreas
   (d) the liver
10. Which part of the large intestine is lymphoid tissue?
   (a) the appendix
   (b) the caecum
   (c) the ascending loop
   (d) the sigmoid colon

True or false

1. The large intestine is colonised with bacteria.
2. The first section of small intestine is called the jejunum.
3. Pancreatic juice reaches the duodenum through the cystic duct.
4. The function of bile is to emulsify fats.
5. There are 20 milk teeth.
6. The enzyme that acts on carbohydrate is lipase.
7. The sense of taste is improved when food is not dry.
8. The oesophagus contains only smooth muscle.
9. Intrinsic factor is produced by enteroendocrine cells.
10. The secretion of gastric juice is increased during the intestinal phase.

Label the diagram 1

Label the diagram using the following list of words:

Parotid gland (salivary gland), Submandibular gland (salivary gland), Oesophagus, Liver, Duodenum, Gallbladder, Jejunum, Ileum, Ascending colon, Caecum, Appendix, Mouth (oral cavity), Sublingual gland (salivary gland), Pharynx, Stomach, Pancreas, Transverse colon, Descending colon, Sigmoid colon, Rectum, Anus

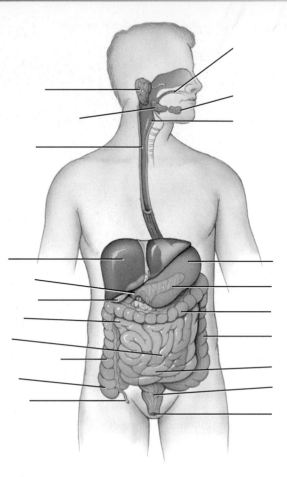

Label the diagram 2

Label the diagram using the following list of words:

Pylorus, Duodenum, Jejunum, Ileum, Ileocaecal value, Stomach, Large intestine

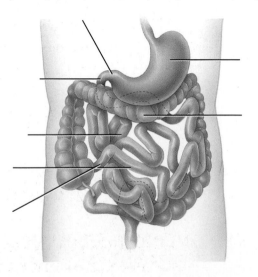

Crossword

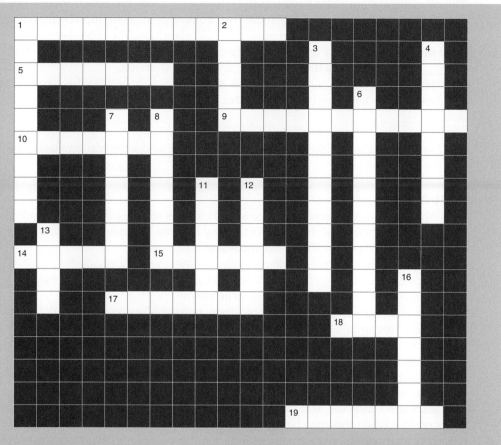

Across:

1. Another name for vitamin C (8, 4).
5. A cutting tooth (7).
9. Function of the large intestine (11).
10. Enzyme responsible for carbohydrate breakdown (7).
14. Another name for fat (5).
15. Innermost layer of the digestive tract (6).
17. Essential organic molecule (7).
18. End of the digestive system (4).
19. Passageway for air and food (7).

Down:

1. Protein is broken down into this (5, 4).
2. Food mixed with hydrochloric acid (5).
3. Describes the movement of the digestive tract (11).
4. Anti-bacterial constituent of saliva (8).
6. Another word for chewing (11).
7. Salivary gland (7).
8. Middle portion of the small intestine (7).
11. Entry to large intestine from the small intestine (6).
12. Enzyme responsible for the digestion of protein (6).
13. Made in the liver and required for the digestion of fat (4).
16. Hormone that stimulates the secretion of hydrochloric acid (7).

Fill in the blanks

The digestive system is also known as the _____ canal. The action of enzymes on ingested food is known as _____ digestion. The churning of ingested food by the muscular activity of the digestive system is known as _____ digestion. The digestive system is protected from invading pathogens by the presence of _____ in salivary amylase and _____ _____ produced by the _____ cells of the stomach.

Digestion of _____ begins in the stomach. _____ is the name of the enzyme involved in the breakdown of carbohydrates. Fat digestion relies on the presence of _____ and _____.

mechanical, lysozyme, alimentary, lipase, hydrochloric acid, chemical, amylase, parietal, protein, bile

Find out more

1. What is gingivitis and what advice would you give to help prevent this condition?
2. Oral candidiasis (oral thrush) affects many hospital in-patients. Can you suggest why this might be and discuss the treatment available?
3. What is the role of the nurse in caring for a patient with dysphagia?
4. Discuss the conditions that may lead to a patient requiring an ileostomy.
5. Differentiate between colostomy and ileostomy.
6. A 28-year-old woman has had a colostomy formed. She asks you how the colostomy would be affected should she become pregnant. How would you advise this patient?
7. Discuss how the digestive system would respond to starvation.
8. Investigate the services available to patients who have irritable bowel syndrome to help them manage everyday life.
9. A range of medications is available to minimise or eliminate digestive system conditions associated with the acid environment of the stomach. Research these medications and consider when they may be used.
10. Constipation is a very common digestive system condition. What is the role of the nurse in relation to prevention of constipation?

Test your learning

1. Where does bile and pancreatic juice enter the duodenum?
2. Which teeth are used for grinding of food?
3. What is the exocrine pancreatic product essential for?
4. What are carbohydrates broken down into?
5. List the enzymes involved in the breakdown of protein.

Conditions

The following is a list of conditions that are associated with the digestive system. Take some time and write notes about each of the conditions. You may make the notes taken from text books or other resources (e.g. people you work with in a clinical area), or you may make the notes as a result of people you have cared for. If you are making notes about people you have cared for you must ensure that you adhere to the rules of confidentiality.

Peptic ulcer	
Peritonitis	
Ulcerative colitis	
Paralytic ileus	
Obesity	
Malnutrition	

Chapter 10

The renal system

Muralitharan Nair

Test your prior knowledge

- Name the functions of the kidneys.
- List the organs of the renal system.
- Describe the components of a nephron.
- List the composition of urine.
- What is the colour of urine? Think about the destruction of the red blood cells.

Learning outcomes

After reading this chapter you will be able to:

- Describe the structure and functions of the kidney
- Describe the microscopic structures of the kidney
- Explain glomerular filtration
- List the chemical compositions of urine
- Discuss the structure and functions of the bladder

Fundamentals of Anatomy and Physiology: For Nursing and Healthcare Students, Second Edition. Edited by Ian Peate and Muralitharan Nair.
© 2017 John Wiley & Sons, Ltd. Published 2017 by John Wiley & Sons, Ltd.
Student companion website: www.wileyfundamentalseries.com/anatomy
Instructor companion website: www.wiley.com/go/instructor/anatomy

Body map

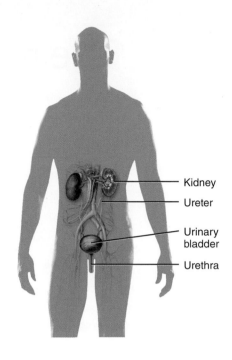

Kidney

Ureter

Urinary bladder

Urethra

Introduction

The kidneys play an important role in maintaining homeostasis. They remove waste products through the production and excretion of urine and regulate fluid balance in the body. As part of their function, the kidneys filter essential substances from the blood, such as sodium and potassium, and selectively reabsorb substances essential to maintain homeostasis. Any substances not essential are excreted in the urine. The formation of urine is achieved through the processes of filtration, selective reabsorption and excretion. The kidneys also have an endocrine function, secreting hormones such as renin and erythropoietin. This chapter will discuss the structure and functions of the renal system. It will also include some common disorders and their related nursing management and treatment.

Renal system

The renal system, also known as the urinary system, consists of:

- kidneys, which filter the blood to produce urine;
- ureters, which convey urine to the bladder;
- urinary bladder, a storage organ for urine until it is eliminated;
- urethra, which conveys urine to the exterior.

See Figure 10.1 for the organs of the renal system.

The organs of the renal system ensure that a stable internal environment is maintained for the survival of cells and tissues in the body – homeostasis.

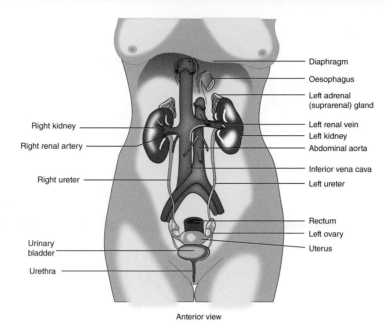

Anterior view

Figure 10.1   Organs of the renal system. *Source*: Tortora and Derrickson (2009). Reproduced with permission of John Wiley & Sons.

Kidneys: external structures

There are two kidneys, one on each side of the spinal column. They are approximately 11 cm long, 5–6 cm wide and 3–4 cm thick. They are said to be bean-shaped organs, where the outer border is convex; the inner border is known as the hilum (also known as hilus), and it is here that the renal arteries, renal veins, nerves and the ureters enter and leave the kidneys. The renal artery carries blood to the kidneys; and once the blood is filtered, the renal vein takes the blood away. The right kidney is in contact with the liver's large right lobe, and hence the right kidney is approximately 2–4 cm lower than the left kidney.

Covering and supporting the kidneys are three layers:

- renal fascia
- adipose tissue
- renal capsule.

The renal fascia is the outer layer and consists of a thin layer of connective tissue that anchors the kidneys to the abdominal wall and the surrounding tissues. The middle layer is called the adipose tissue and surrounds the capsule. It cushions the kidneys from trauma. The inner layer is called the renal capsule. It consists of a layer of smooth connective tissue that is continuous with the outer layer of the ureter. The renal capsule protects the kidneys from trauma and maintains their shape. See Figure 10.2 for the external layers.

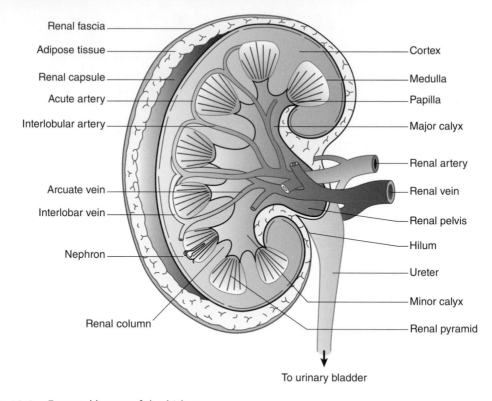

Figure 10.2   External layers of the kidney.

Clinical considerations

Renal transplant

The main role of the kidneys is to filter waste products from the blood and convert them to urine. If the kidneys lose this ability, waste products can build up, which is potentially dangerous and can be life threatening. This loss of kidney function, known as end-stage chronic kidney disease or kidney failure, is the most common reason for needing a kidney transplant.

The kidney transplant is a major surgery that could take approximately 3 h. A donor kidney, from a living person, could take 3–5 days to achieve normal function, while a cadaver donor kidney could take 7–15 days to function normally. After surgery, immunosuppressant drugs are used to suppress the immune system from rejecting the donor kidney. These medicines must be taken for the rest of the recipient's life. The most common medication regimen today is a mixture of tacrolimus, mycophenolate and prednisone.

Kidney transplant recipients are discouraged from consuming grapefruit, pomegranate and green tea products. These food products are known to interact with the transplant medications, specifically tacrolimus, cyclosporin and sirolimus; the blood levels of these drugs may be increased, potentially leading to an overdose. A healthy lifestyle after a kidney transplant goes a long way to minimising the risk of complications.

See NHS Choices (2015a).

Kidneys: internal structures

There are three distinct regions inside the kidney:

- renal cortex
- renal medulla
- renal pelvis.

The renal cortex is the outermost part of the kidney. In adults, it forms a continuous, smooth outer portion of the kidney with a number of projections (renal column) that extend down between the pyramids. The renal column is the medullary extension of the renal cortex. The renal cortex is reddish in colour and has a granular appearance, which is due to the capillaries and the structures of the nephron. The medulla is lighter in colour and has an abundance of blood vessels and tubules of the nephrons (see Figure 10.3). The medulla consists of approximately 8–12 renal pyramids (see Figure 10.3). The renal pyramids, also called malpighian pyramids, are cone-shaped sections of the kidneys. The wider portion of the cone faces the renal cortex, while the narrow end points internally, and this section is called the renal papilla. Urine formed by the nephrons flows into cup-like structures, called calyces, via papillary ducts. Each kidney contains approximately 8–18 minor calyces and two or three major calyces. The minor calyces receive urine from the renal papilla, which conveys the urine to the major calyces. The major calyces unite to form the renal pelvis, which then conveys urine to the bladder (see Figure 10.4). The renal pelvis forms the expanded upper portion of the ureter, which is funnel-shaped and it is the region where two or three calyces converge.

303

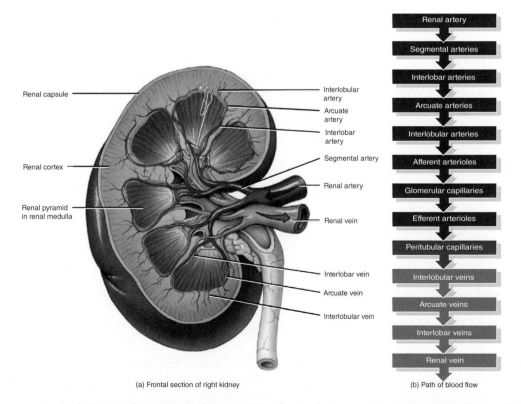

(a) Frontal section of right kidney   (b) Path of blood flow

Figure 10.3 (a, b) Internal structures showing blood vessels. *Source*: Tortora and Derrickson (2009). Reproduced with permission of John Wiley & Sons.

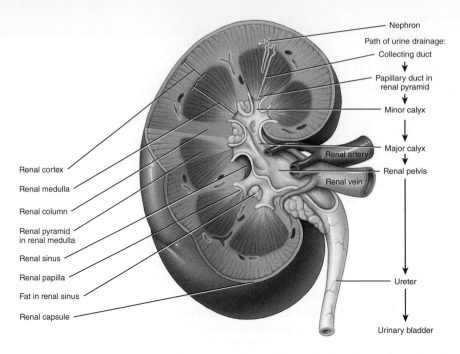

Figure 10.4 Internal structures. *Source*: Tortora and Derrickson (2009). Reproduced with permission of John Wiley & Sons.

Medicines management

Cyclosporine

Cyclosporine lowers the body's immune system. The immune system helps the body fight infections. The immune system can also fight or 'reject' a transplanted organ such as a liver or kidney. This is because the immune system treats the new organ as an invader. Cyclosporine is used to prevent organ rejection after a kidney, liver or heart transplant.

Signs of an allergic reaction include: hives; difficulty breathing; swelling of the face, lips, tongue or throat.

Some of the serious side effects include:

- urinating less than usual or not at all;
- drowsiness, confusion, mood changes, increased thirst;
- swelling, weight gain, feeling short of breath;
- blurred vision, headache or pain behind your eyes, sometimes with vomiting;
- seizure (convulsions);
- muscle pain or weakness, fast heart rate, feeling light-headed;
- signs of infection, such as fever, chills, sore throat, flu symptoms;
- pale skin, easy bruising or bleeding, unusual weakness; or
- nausea, stomach pain, loss of appetite, itching, dark urine, clay-coloured stools, jaundice (yellowing of the skin or eyes).

Call the doctor at once if the patient has any signs of kidney failure, such as urinating less than usual or not at all, drowsiness, confusion, mood changes, increased thirst, loss of appetite, nausea and vomiting, swelling, weight gain or feeling short of breath.

See RxList (2012).

Snapshot

A patient with obstructive kidney

Suresh Rama, aged 58 years, lives in a detached house with his wife Priya and their two children, Mina and Reena. Suresh is a self-employed businessman, and his wife is a school teacher. Their children go to the same school where Priya teaches.

Suresh has had a constant dull ache below his ribs on his right side for a couple of weeks. He kept this from his wife and tolerated the pain and discomfort. One day, Suresh noticed blood in his urine and broke the news to his wife and also tells her about the pain. Priya is annoyed that he kept this information from her and insisted that he sees his GP to get to the root of the problem.

Suresh makes an appointment to see his GP. Suresh goes to the surgery accompanied by his wife. After some medical history and physical examination, the GP refers Suresh to the local hospital under the care of a urologist.

Suresh is seen by the consultant urologist in the outpatient department. An ultrasound reveals a staghorn calculus of his right kidney. Suresh is admitted the following week for a right nephrectomy. Suresh made an uneventful recovery and was discharged from the hospital under the care of the community team.

If a kidney stone is not detected and treated early, it can grow into the calyces of the kidney (see Figure 10.5) and permanently damage that kidney, as in Suresh's case. If detected early, the kidney could be saved by removing the stone before it damages the kidney. If a kidney stone is too big to be passed naturally (6–7 mm in diameter or larger), it could be removed by:

- extracorporeal shock wave lithotripsy
- ureteroscopy
- percutaneous nephrolithotomy.

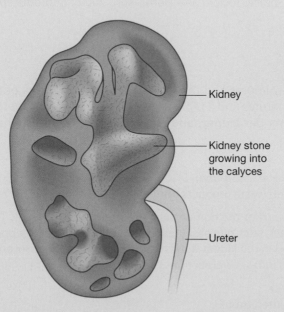

Kidney

Kidney stone growing into the calyces

Ureter

Figure 10.5 Obstructive kidney.

See NHS Choices (2014a).

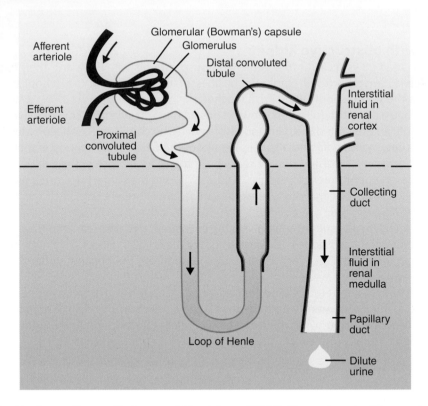

Figure 10.6 Nephron. *Source*: Tortora and Derrickson (2009). Reproduced with permission of John Wiley & Sons.

Nephrons

These are small structures and they form the functional units of the kidney. The nephron consists of a glomerulus and a renal tubule (see Figure 10.6). There are approximately over 1 million nephrons per kidney, and it is in these structures where urine is formed. The nephrons:

- filter blood;
- perform selective reabsorption;
- excrete unwanted waste products from the filtered blood.

The nephron is part of the homeostatic mechanism of the body. This system helps regulate the amount of water, salts, glucose, urea and other minerals in the body. The nephron is a filtration system located in the kidney and is responsible for the reabsorption of water and salts. The nephron is divided into several sections:

- Bowman's capsule
- proximal convoluted tubule
- loop of Henle
- distal convoluted tubule (DCT)
- the collecting ducts.

Each section performs a different function; these will be discussed in the following sections.

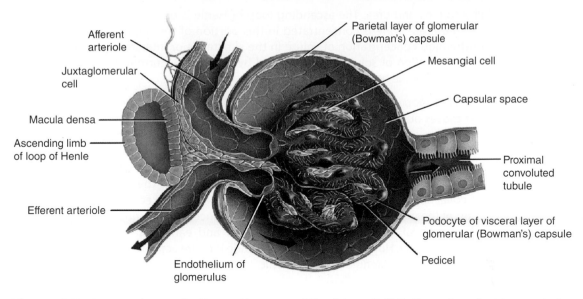

Afferent arteriole

Juxtaglomerular cell

Macula densa

Ascending limb of loop of Henle

Efferent arteriole

Endothelium of glomerulus

Parietal layer of glomerular (Bowman's) capsule

Mesangial cell

Capsular space

Proximal convoluted tubule

Podocyte of visceral layer of glomerular (Bowman's) capsule

Pedicel

307

Figure 10.7   Bowman's capsule. *Source*: Tortora and Derrickson (2009). Reproduced with permission of John Wiley & Sons.

Bowman's capsule

Also known as the glomerular capsule (see Figure 10.7), Bowman's capsule is a cup-like sac and is the first portion of the nephron. Bowman's capsule is part of the filtration system in the kidneys. When blood reaches the kidneys for filtration, it enters Bowman's capsule first, with the capsule separating the blood into two components: a filtrated blood product and a filtrate that is moved through the nephron, another structure in the kidneys. The glomerular capsule consists of visceral and parietal layers (see Figure 10.7). The visceral layer is lined with epithelial cells called podocytes, while the parietal layer is lined with simple squamous epithelium and it is in Bowman's capsule that the network of capillaries called the glomerulus (Marieb and Hoehn, 2013) is found. Filtration of blood takes place in this portion of the nephron.

Proximal convoluted tubule

From Bowman's capsule, the filtrate drains into the proximal convoluted tubule (see Figure 10.6). The surface of the epithelial cells of this segment of the nephron is covered with densely packed microvilli. The microvilli increase the surface area of the cells, thus facilitating their resorptive function. The infolded membranes forming the microvilli are the site of numerous sodium pumps. Resorption of salt, water and glucose from the glomerular filtrate occurs in this section of the tubule; at the same time, certain substances, including uric acid and drug metabolites, are actively transferred from the blood capillaries into the tubule for excretion.

Loop of Henle

The proximal convoluted tubule then bends into a loop called the loop of Henle (see Figure 10.6). The loop of Henle is the part of the tubule that dips or 'loops' from the cortex into the medulla (descending limb), and then returns to the cortex (ascending limb). The loop of Henle is divided into the descending and ascending loops. The ascending loop of Henle is much thicker than the descending portion. The main function of the loop of Henle is to generate a concentration gradient that creates a region of a high concentration of sodium in the medulla of the kidney. The descending portion of the loop of Henle is highly permeable to water and has low permeability to ions and urea. The ascending loop of Henle is permeable to ions but not to water. When required, urine is concentrated in this portion of the nephron. This is possible because of the high concentration of solute in the substance or interstitium of the medulla. This high concentration of solutes is maintained by the countercurrent multiplier. Different parts of the loop of Henle have different actions:

- The descending loop of Henle is relatively impermeable to solute but permeable to water, so that water moves out by osmosis and the fluid in the tubule becomes hypertonic.
- The thin section of the ascending loop of Henle is virtually impermeable to water, but permeable to solute, especially sodium and chloride ions. Thus, sodium and chloride ions move out down the concentration gradient; the fluid within the tubule first becomes isotonic and then hypotonic as more ions leave. Urea, which was absorbed into the medullary interstitium from the collecting duct, diffuses into the ascending limb. This keeps the urea within the interstitium of the medulla, where it also has a role in concentrating urine.
- The thick section of the ascending loop of Henle and early distal tubule are virtually impermeable to water. However, sodium and chloride ions are actively transported out of the tubule, making the tubular fluid very hypotonic.

Distal convoluted tubule

The thick ascending portion of the loop of Henle leads into the DCT (see Figure 10.6). The DCT is lined with simple cuboidal cells, and the lumen of the DCT is larger than the proximal convoluted tubule lumen because the proximal convoluted tubule has a brush border (microvilli). The DCT is an important site:

- it actively secretes ions and acids;
- it plays a part in the regulation of calcium ions by excreting excess calcium ions in response to calcitonin hormone;
- it selectively reabsorbs water;
- arginine vasopressin receptor 2 proteins are also located there;
- it plays a role in regulating pH by absorbing bicarbonate and secreting protons (H^+) into the filtrate.

The final concentration of urine, in this section, is dependent on a hormone called antidiuretic hormone (ADH). If ADH is present, the distal tubule and the collecting duct become permeable to water. As the collecting duct passes through the medulla with a high solute concentration in the interstitium, the water moves out of the lumen of the duct and concentrated urine is formed. In the absence of ADH the tubule is minimally permeable to water, so a large volume of dilute urine is formed.

Collecting ducts

The DCT then drains into the collecting ducts (see Figure 10.6). Several collecting ducts converge and drain into a larger system called the papillary ducts, which in turn empty into the minor calyx (plural: calices). From here the filtrate, now called urine, drains into the renal pelvis. This is the final stage where sodium and water are reabsorbed. When a person is dehydrated, approximately 25% of the water filtered is reabsorbed in the collecting duct. However, the cells of the collecting ducts are impermeable to water, but with the aid of the ADH and aquaporins water is reabsorbed from the collecting ducts. Aquaporins are proteins embedded in the cell membrane that regulate the flow of water. Aquaporins selectively transport water molecules in and out of the cell, while preventing the passage of ions and other solutes. Aquaporin 1 is abundant in proximal convoluted tubule and the descending thin limb of the loop of Henle, and aquaporins 2, 3 and 4 are present in the collecting ducts; however aquaporin 4 is predominantly found in the brain.

Clinical considerations

Chronic pyelonephritis

Chronic pyelonephritis is characterised by renal inflammation and fibrosis induced by recurrent or persistent renal infection, vesicoureteral reflux, or other causes of urinary tract obstruction. Chronic pyelonephritis is associated with progressive renal scarring, which can lead to end-stage renal disease.

In most patients, renal damage occurs slowly over a long period of time in response to a chronic inflammatory process or infections. This results in thinning of the renal cortex along with deep, segmental, coarse cortical scarring. Club-shaped deformity of the renal calyces occurs as the papilla(e) retract into the scar(s). One scar or several may be present, in one or both kidneys.

Some of the investigations carried out include:

- Dipstick urinalysis may show leucocytes, haematuria or proteinuria and is typically the test of choice for screening of kidney disease. It may be normal in chronic kidney disease, so should be done in conjunction with serum creatinine, which reflects the severity of renal impairment.
- Full blood count may show raised leukocytosis or normocytic, normochromic anaemia.
- Ultrasound is often recommended if renal obstruction is suspected but not confirmed by computed tomography. A kidney–ureter–bladder X-ray is less useful than computed tomography, but is a useful baseline investigation, and may show radiopaque calcifications in the renal tract.
- Urine cultures are done to detect urinary tract infection. Urine cultures are often positive for *Proteus* (60%), or less often for *Escherichia coli*, *Klebsiella*, *Staphylococcus aureus*, or mixed organisms.

Chronic pyelonephritis results in renal failure. The patient will need dialysis or a kidney transplant. Remember, recurrent attacks with acute pyelonephritis can result in chronic pyelonephritis.

See Knott (2013).

Functions of the kidney

The kidneys maintain fluid balance, electrolyte balance and the acid–base balance of the blood.

- The kidneys remove wastes and excess water (fluid) collected by, and carried in, the blood as it flows through the body. Approximately 190 L of blood enter the kidneys every day via the renal arteries. Millions of tiny filters, called glomeruli, inside the kidneys separate wastes and water from the blood. Most of these unwanted substances come from what we eat and drink. The kidneys automatically remove the right amount of salt and other minerals from the blood to leave just the quantities the body needs.
- By removing just the right amount of excess fluid, healthy kidneys maintain what is called the body's fluid balance. In women, fluid content stays at about 55% of total weight. In men, it stays at about 60% of total weight. The kidneys maintain these proportions by balancing the amount of fluid that leaves the body against the amount entering the body. When a large volume of fluid is drunk, healthy kidneys remove the excess fluid and produce a lot of urine. On the other hand, if fluid intake is low, the kidneys retain fluid and the patient does not pass much urine. Fluid also leaves the body through sweat, breath and faeces. If the weather is hot and we lose a lot of fluid by sweating, then the kidneys will not pass much urine.
- Kidneys synthesise hormones such as renin and angiotensin. These hormones regulate how much sodium (salt) and fluid the body keeps, and how well the blood vessels can expand and contract. This, in turn, helps control blood pressure.

- Kidneys produce a hormone known as erythropoietin, which is carried in the blood to the bone marrow where it stimulates the production of red blood cells. These cells carry oxygen throughout the body. Without enough healthy red blood cells anaemia develops, a condition that causes weakness, cold, tiredness and shortness of breath.
- Healthy kidneys keep bones strong by producing the hormone calcitriol. Calcitriol maintains the right levels of calcium and phosphate in the blood and bones. Calcium and phosphate balance are important to keep bones healthy. When the kidneys fail they may not produce enough calcitriol. This leads to abnormal levels of phosphate, calcium and vitamin D, causing renal bone disease. For a summary of the functions of the kidney, see Table 10.1.

Table 10.1 Summary of the functions of the kidneys

Regulation of electrolytes – help to regulate ions such as sodium, potassium, calcium, chloride and phosphate ions
Regulation of blood pH – excrete hydrogen ions into the urine and conserve bicarbonate ions, thus helping to regulate pH of blood
Regulation of blood volume – by conserving or eliminating water in the urine
Secretes renin (regulates blood pressure) and erythropoietin (production of red blood cells)
Production of calcitriol for the regulation of calcium level
Aids in regulation of blood glucose level by gluconeogenesis
Detoxification of free radicals and drugs
Excretion of waste products, such as urea, uric acid and creatinine

Medicines management

Nephrotoxic drugs

Renal impairment may be acute or chronic – both of which can result in problems with medications. Renal impairment may be the result of a variety of renal or systemic diseases, such as diabetic nephropathy or systemic lupus erythematosus. Normal ageing results in a decline in renal function due to loss of nephrons. When prescribing for elderly patients, it should therefore be assumed that some degree of renal impairment exists.

Reasons for problems with medications in renal failure include:

- failure to excrete a drug or its metabolites;
- many side effects being poorly tolerated by patients in renal failure;
- some drugs ceasing to be effective when renal function is reduced.

For example, prescribing any drug that increases potassium level is potentially very dangerous – for example, potassium supplements and potassium-sparing diuretics. Other products that contain potassium include ispaghula husk laxatives. Non-steroidal anti-inflammatory drugs (NSAIDs), even in short courses, can cause acute kidney injury as a result of renal under perfusion. Angiotensin-converting enzyme (ACE) inhibitors can also cause a deterioration in renal function.

(Continued)

However, this is a problem only in patients with compromised renal perfusion, particularly those with renal artery stenosis. Care should be taken when an ACE inhibitor and NSAID are prescribed together, as this combination may precipitate an acute deterioration in renal function.

Drugs that may cause interstitial nephritis include penicillins, cephalosporins, sulphonamides, thiazide diuretics, furosemide, NSAIDs and rifampicin.

Therefore, care should be taken when administering medications to patients with renal problems. Always check with the pharmacist or consult the British National Formulary for drug interactions before administering medications.

See Rull (2013).

Snapshot

Cystitis

Michele Watts is a 26-year-old third-year nursing student. She is married to John, who is also a third-year nursing student in the same cohort. They live in a flat, which they rent and they travel to the university for their nursing studies. They do not have any children but plan to have a family on completion of their course. Michele does not take birth-control pills; instead, she uses a coil for birth control.

Michele woke up one morning with severe lower back pain, frequency, urgency and burning sensation on urination. She noticed that her urine was slightly cloudy. Michele tells John that she had to get up twice at night with frequency and it was painful to pass urine. John decided to ring the university to inform them of their absence as he was taking his wife to see their GP.

At the surgery, the practice nurse carried out some vital signs recordings: temperature 37.5 °C, pulse 95 beats per minute, blood pressure 115/58 mmHg and respiration 23 breaths per minute. On consultations with her GP, Michele states that she has had these episodes three times in the past but has managed without any antibiotics. Now she feels that she has to urinate frequently and has difficulty starting her urine and has burning pain and cramping when voiding. The nurse does a dip stick test, which shows that she has leucocytes, blood, protein and urea.

The GP informs Michele that he would like a midstream specimen of urine (MSU) from her and gives her a course of antibiotics (Trimethoprim 200 mg BD for 3 days), informing her that when the results return and if the antibiotic is not suitable then he will change it.

Michele is encouraged to drink a lot of fluid and told to rest for a few days. Once the symptoms subside Michele can resume her studies. Her MSU results show a coliform infection and that Michele is on the right antibiotic.

Blood supply of the kidney

The role of the kidney is to filter at least 20–25% of blood during the resting cardiac output. Approximately 1200 mL of blood flows through the kidney each minute. Each kidney receives its blood supply directly from the aorta via the renal artery (see Figure 10.4), which is divided into anterior and posterior renal arteries. There are several arteries that deliver blood to the kidneys:

- renal artery – arises from the abdominal aorta at the level of first lumbar vertebra;
- segmental artery – branch of the renal artery;
- interlobar artery – branch of the segmental artery;
- arcuate artery – renal columns leading to the corticomedullary junction;
- interlobular arteries – divisions of the arcuate arteries.

Dialysis

Dialysis is the artificial process of eliminating waste (diffusion) and unwanted water (ultrafiltration) from the blood. Some patients, however, may have failed or damaged kidneys that cannot carry out the function properly – they may need dialysis. Dialysis may be used for patients who have become ill and have acute kidney injury (temporary loss of kidney function), or for fairly stable patients who have permanently lost kidney function (stage 5 chronic kidney disease).

Approximately 1500 L of blood are filtered by a healthy person's kidneys each day. We could not live if waste products were not removed from our kidneys. Patients whose kidneys either do not work properly or not at all experience a build-up of waste in their blood. Without dialysis the amount of waste products in the blood would increase and eventually reach levels that would cause coma and death.

Haemodialysis

Haemodialysis is the type of dialysis that most people are aware of. It involves inserting a needle, which is attached by a tube to a dialysis machine, into a blood vessel. Blood is transferred from the body into the machine, which filters out waste products and excess fluids. The filtered blood is then passed back into the body. Most people require three sessions a week, each lasting 4 h.

Peritoneal dialysis

Peritoneal dialysis is a less well known type of dialysis, but it is becoming more common. It involves using the lining of the abdomen (the peritoneum) as a filter. Like the kidneys, the peritoneum contains thousands of tiny blood vessels, making it a useful filtering device.

A small flexible tube called a catheter is attached to an incision in the abdomen (see Figure 10.8). A special fluid called dialysis fluid is allowed to drain into the space surrounding the peritoneum (the peritoneal cavity) via a giving set allowed to sit there for several hours while it absorbs waste products, and excess fluid from the blood and into the dialysis fluid then drained out.

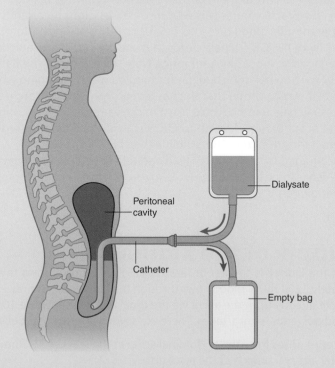

Figure 10.8 Peritoneal dialysis.

See NHS Choices (2015b).

The branches of the interlobular artery enter the nephrons as afferent arterioles. Each nephron receives one afferent arteriole, which further subdivides into a tuft of capillaries called the glomerulus. The glomerular capillaries reunite and leave Bowman's capsule as efferent arterioles. Efferent arterioles unite to form peritubular capillaries and then interlobular veins that unite to form the arcuate veins and finally into interlobar veins. Blood leaves the kidneys through the renal vein, which then flows into the inferior vena cava. The diameter of the afferent arteriole is larger than the diameter of the efferent arteriole.

Urine formation

Three processes are involved in the formation of urine:

- filtration
- selective reabsorption
- secretion.

Filtration

Urine formation begins with the process of filtration, which goes on continually in the renal corpuscles. Filtration takes place in the glomerulus which lies in Bowman's capsule. The blood for filtration is supplied by the renal artery. In the kidney the renal artery divides into smaller arterioles. The arteriole entering Bowman's capsule is called the afferent arteriole, which further subdivides into a cluster of capillaries called the glomerulus.

As blood passes through the glomeruli, much of its fluid, containing both useful chemicals and dissolved waste materials, soaks out of the blood through the membranes (by osmosis and diffusion) where it is filtered and then flows into Bowman's capsule. This process is called glomerular filtration. The water, waste products, salt, glucose and other chemicals that have been filtered out of the blood are known collectively as glomerular filtrate.

The fluid from the filtered blood is protein free but contains electrolytes such as sodium chloride, potassium and waste products of cellular metabolism; for example, urea, uric acid and creatinine (McCance *et al.*, 2010). The filtered blood then returns into circulation via the efferent arteriole and finally into the renal vein.

Selective reabsorption

Selective reabsorption processes ensure that any substances in the filtrate that are essential for body function are reabsorbed into the plasma. Substances such as sodium, calcium, potassium and chloride are reabsorbed to maintain fluid and electrolyte balance and the pH of blood. However, if these substances are in excess to body requirements, they are excreted in the urine. Only 1% of the glomerular filtrate actually leaves the body; 99% is reabsorbed into the bloodstream. The reabsorption occurs via three processes:

- osmosis
- diffusion
- active transport.

See Table 10.2 for a summary.

Blood glucose is entirely reabsorbed into the blood from the proximal tubules. In fact, it is actively transported out of the tubules and into the peritubular capillary blood. None of this valuable nutrient is wasted by being lost in the urine. Sodium (Na^+) and other ions are only partially reabsorbed from the renal tubules into the blood. For the most part, however, sodium ions are actively transported back into blood from the tubular fluid. The amount of sodium reabsorbed varies; it depends largely on how much salt we take in from the foods that we eat.

Table 10.2 Summary of filtration, reabsorption and excretion in the nephron and collecting ducts

Reabsorption	Excretion
Proximal convoluted tubule	
Water, approximately 65% Sodium and potassium, 65% Glucose, 100% Amino acids, 100% Chloride, approximately 50% Bicarbonate, calcium and magnesium Urea	Hydrogen ions Urea Creatinine Ammonium ions
Loop of Henle	
Water Sodium and potassium, approximately 30% Chloride, approximately 35% Bicarbonate, approximately 20% Calcium and magnesium	Urea
Distal convoluted tubule	
Water, approximately 15% Sodium and chloride, approximately 5% Calcium Some urea	Potassium, depending on serum values Hydrogen ions, depending on pH of blood
Collecting duct	
Bicarbonate, depending on serum values Urea Water, approximately 9% Sodium, approximately 4%	Potassium, depending on serum values Hydrogen ions, depending on pH of blood

Source: Adapted from Tortora and Derrickson (2006).

As a person increases the amount of salt intake into the body, kidneys decrease the amount of sodium reabsorption into the blood. That is, more sodium is retained in the tubules. Therefore, the amount of salt excreted in the urine increases. The process works the other way as well. The less the salt intake, the greater the amount of sodium reabsorbed into the blood, and the amount of salt excreted in the urine decreases.

Excretion

Any substances not removed through filtration are secreted into the renal tubules from the peritubular capillaries (see Figure 10.9) of the nephron (Waugh and Grant, 2014); these include drugs and hydrogen ions. Tubular secretion mainly takes place by active transport. Active transport is a process by which substances are moved across biological membranes. Tubular secretion occurs from epithelial cells lining the renal tubules and the collecting ducts. Substances secreted into the tubular fluid include:

- potassium ions (K^+)
- hydrogen ions (H^+)
- ammonium ions (NH_4^+)
- creatinine
- urea
- some hormones.

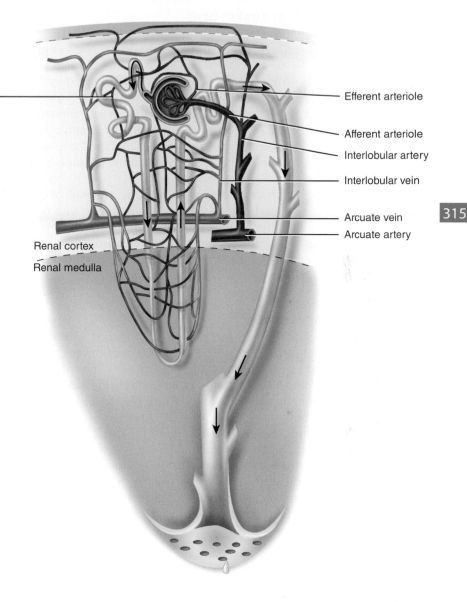

Peritubular capillary

Efferent arteriole

Afferent arteriole

Interlobular artery

Interlobular vein

Arcuate vein

Arcuate artery

Renal cortex

Renal medulla

Figure 10.9 Nephron with capillaries. *Source*: Tortora and Derrickson (2009). Reproduced with permission of John Wiley & Sons.

It is the tubular secretion of hydrogen and ammonium ions that helps to maintain the pH of blood. See Table 10.2 for a summary.

Hormonal control of tubular reabsorption and secretion

Four hormones play a role in the regulation of fluid and electrolytes:

- angiotensin II
- aldosterone
- ADH
- atrial natriuretic peptide.

Angiotensin and aldosterone

As the blood volume and blood pressure decrease, the juxtaglomerular cells secrete a hormone called renin. Juxtaglomerular cells are found near the glomerulus, and these cells synthesise, store and secrete the hormone renin. Renin acts on a plasma protein called angiotensinogen and converts it into angiotensin I. Angiotensinogen is produced by the hepatocytes of the liver. Angiotensin I is transported by the blood to the lungs. In the lung capillaries there are enzymes called ACE. ACE is predominantly found in the lung capillaries, but this enzyme is also found throughout the body. ACE converts angiotensin I into angiotensin II. Angiotensin II is a short-acting, powerful vasoconstrictor, thus increasing blood pressure. Angiotensin II promotes the reabsorption of sodium, chloride and water in the proximal convoluted tubule. It also has an effect on the release of aldosterone.

Aldosterone is a steroid hormone secreted by the adrenal glands. It serves as the principal regulator of the salt and water balance of the body and thus is categorised as a mineralocorticoid. It also has a small effect on the metabolism of fats, carbohydrates and proteins. Aldosterone is synthesised in the body from corticosterone, a steroid derived from cholesterol. Production of aldosterone (in adult humans, about 20–200 µg per day) in the zona glomerulosa of the adrenal cortex is regulated by the renin–angiotensin system.

Antidiuretic hormone

The third principal hormone is ADH, which is produced by the hypothalamus gland and is stored by the posterior pituitary gland. This hormone increases the permeability of the cells in the DCT and the collecting ducts. In the presence of ADH, more water is reabsorbed from the renal tubules; therefore, the patient will pass less urine. In the absence of ADH, less water is reabsorbed and the patient will pass more urine. Thus, ADH plays a major role in the regulation of fluid balance in the body.

The most important variable regulating ADH secretion is plasma osmolarity, or the concentration of solutes in blood. Osmolarity is sensed in the hypothalamus by neurones known as an osmoreceptors, and those neurones, in turn, stimulate secretion from the neurones that produce ADH. When plasma osmolarity is below a certain threshold, the osmoreceptors are not activated and the secretion of ADH is suppressed. When osmolarity increases above the threshold, the osmoreceptors recognise this and stimulate the neurones that secrete ADH.

Atrial natriuretic peptide

The fourth hormone involved in tubular secretion and reabsorption is atrial natriuretic peptide (ANP) hormone. ANP is a powerful vasodilator and is a protein produced by the myocytes of the atria of the heart in response to increased blood pressure. ANP stimulates the kidneys to excrete sodium and water from the renal tubules, thus decreasing blood volume, which in turn lowers blood pressure. The hormone also inhibits the secretion of aldosterone and ADH.

ANP is involved in the long-term regulation of sodium and water balance, blood volume and arterial pressure. There are two major pathways of natriuretic peptide actions: vasodilator effects and renal effects, which lead to natriuresis and diuresis. ANP directly dilates veins (increases venous compliance) and thereby decreases central venous pressure, which reduces cardiac output by decreasing ventricular preload. ANP also dilates arteries, which decreases systemic vascular resistance and systemic arterial pressure.

Medicines management

Drugs for incontinence

There are two main types of urinary incontinence:

1. *Stress incontinence* – this is when urine leaks because there is a sudden extra pressure within the abdomen and on the bladder. This pressure (or stress) is caused by things like coughing, laughing, sneezing or exercising (such as running or jumping).
2. *Urge incontinence* – this is when urine leaks before one gets to the toilet when there is an urgency to void urine.

For people with stress incontinence a medicine called duloxetine may be prescribed. It is thought to work by interfering with certain chemicals that are used in transmitting nerve impulses to muscles. This helps the muscles around the urethra to contract more strongly. It is prescribed for a month and the patient is reassessed. If the condition improves, the drug is discontinued. The most commonly reported side effects are nausea, dry mouth, fatigue and constipation. Advise the patient never to stop taking this medicine suddenly because they can get withdrawal symptoms such as dizziness, nausea and headaches.

Medicines called antimuscarinics (also called anticholinergics) are used to help treat urge incontinence. There are several different types and many different brand names. They include older medicines such as oxybutynin, tolterodine and flavoxate, as well as newer medicines such as darifenacin, fesoterodine, propiverine, solifenacin and trospium. These medicines work by blocking certain nerve impulses to the bladder that relax the bladder muscle, so increasing the bladder capacity. Antimuscarinics are prescribed for a month or so. If it is helpful, the treatment may continue for up to 6 months or so and then stopped to see how symptoms are without the medication. The most common side effect is a dry mouth, and simply having frequent sips of water may counter this. Other common side effects include dry eyes, constipation and blurred vision.

See NHS Choices (2014b).

317

Composition of urine

Urine is a sterile and clear fluid of nitrogenous wastes and salts. It is translucent with an amber or light yellow colour. Its colour is due to the pigments from the breakdown of haemoglobin. Concentrated urine tends to be darker in colour than normal urine. However, other factors, such as diet, medications and certain diseases, may affect the colour of the urine. It is slightly acidic, and the pH may range from 4.5 to 8. The pH is affected by an individual's dietary intake and state of health. Diet that is high in animal protein tends to make the urine more acidic, while a vegetarian diet may make the urine more alkaline. The volume of urine produced depends on the circulating volume of blood. ADH regulates the amount of urine passed by the individual. If the person is dehydrated, more ADH is released from the posterior pituitary gland, resulting in water reabsorption and less urine being produced. On the other hand, if the person has consumed a large amount of fluid, which increases the circulating volume, less ADH is released and more water is passed as urine.

Urine is 96% water and approximately 4% solutes derived from cellular metabolism. The solutes include organic and inorganic waste products and unwanted substances such as drugs. Normally there is no protein or blood. If these are present then the person may be suffering from a disease. See Table 10.3 for a summary of solutes.

Table 10.3   Solutes in the urine

Inorganic solutes	Organic solutes
Sodium	Urea
Potassium	Creatinine
Calcium	Uric acid
Magnesium	
Iron	
Chloride	
Sulphate	
Phosphate	
Bicarbonate	
Ammonia	

Source: Adapted from Mader (2005).

Characteristics of normal urine

The volume produced is one of the physical characteristics of urine. Other physical characteristics that can apply to urine include colour, turbidity (transparency), smell (odour), pH (acidity/alkalinity) and density.

- **Colour:** Typically yellow–amber, but varies according to recent diet, medication and the concentration of the urine. Drinking more water generally tends to reduce the concentration of urine, and therefore causes it to have a lighter colour. However, if a person does not drink a large amount of fluid, this may increase the concentration and the urine will have a darker colour. See Table 10.4 for foods, medications and illnesses that may affect colour of the urine.
- **Smell:** The smell, or odour, of urine may provide health information. For example, the urine of diabetics may have a sweet or fruity odour due to the presence of ketones (organic molecules of a particular structure). Generally, fresh urine has a mild smell, but stale urine or infected urine has a stronger odour, similar to that of ammonia.
- **Acidity:** pH is a measure of the acidity (or alkalinity) of a solution. The pH of a substance (solution) is usually represented as a number in the range 0 (strong acid) to 14 (strong alkali, also known as a 'base'). Pure water is 'neutral', in the sense that it is neither acid nor alkali; it therefore has a pH of 7. The pH of normal urine is generally in the range 4.5–8, a typical average being around 6.0. Much of the variation is due to diet. For example, high-protein diets result in more acidic urine, but vegetarian diets generally result in more alkaline urine.
- **Specific gravity:** Specific gravity is also known as 'relative density'. This is the ratio of the weight of a volume of a substance compared with the weight of the same volume of distilled water. Given that urine is mostly water, but also contains some other substances dissolved in the water, its relative density is expected to be close to, but slightly greater than, 1.000.

Table 10.4   Colours of urine

Food that changes colour of urine	
These are some of the foods that may change the colour of urine.	
Dark yellow or orange:	carrots
Green:	asparagus
Pink or red:	beetroot, blackberries, rhubarb
Brown:	fava beans, rhubarb
Medicines and vitamins that may change the colour of urine	
Yellow or yellow–green:	cascara, sulfasalazine, the B vitamins
Orange:	rifampicin, sulfasalazine, vitamin B, vitamin C
Pink or red:	phenolphthalein, propofol, rifampicin, laxatives containing senna
Green or blue:	amitriptyline, cimetidine, indomethacin, promethazine, propofol, triamterene, several multivitamins
Brown or brownish-black:	levodopa, metronidazole, nitrofurantoin, some antimalarial agents, methyldopa, laxatives containing cascara or senna
Medical conditions that may change the colour of urine	
Yellow:	concentrated urine caused by dehydration
Orange:	a problem with the liver or bile duct
Pink or red:	blood in the urine, haemoglobinuria (a condition linked to haemolytic anaemia), myoglobinuria (a condition linked to the destruction of muscle cells)
Deep purple:	porphyria, a rare inherited red blood cell disorder
Green or blue:	urinary tract infection may cause green urine if caused by *Pseudomonas* bacteria; familial hypercalcaemia, a rare genetic condition, can cause blue urine
Brown or dark brown:	blood in the urine, a liver or kidney disorder

Source: Mayo Clinic Staff (2015).

Snapshot

Mary with urinary incontinence

Mary Goldwater is a 78-year-old retired council worker. Her husband passed away with cancer of the prostate over 5 years ago. Mary has one daughter, who visits her every week to make sure that she is fine. Mary is adamant that she can cope and refuses any help from the social services. Her daughter notices a strong smell of urine in the house whenever she visits her mother. When the daughter wants to take her out, Mary is reluctant to go out and becomes very aggressive.

Concerned, the daughter asks Mary's GP to do a home visit and see if he can help her. During her GP's visit, Mary admits that she has an urine incontinence problem. She reports that when she coughs or laughs, she wets herself.

After a full assessment of Mary, her GP suggests that she should go to a care home to be looked after. After much persuasion by her GP and her daughter, Mary agrees to this.

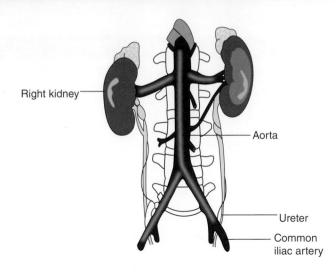

Right kidney

Aorta

Ureter

Common
iliac artery

Figure 10.10   Common iliac vessels and ureter. *Source*: Nair and Peate (2009). Reproduced with permission of John Wiley & Sons.

Ureters

The ureters are tubular organs that run from the renal pelvis to the posterolateral base of the urinary bladder. The ureters are approximately 25–30 cm in length and 5 mm in diameter (Mader, 2005). The ureters terminate at the bladder and enter obliquely through the muscle wall of the bladder. They pass over the pelvic brim at the bifurcation of the common iliac arteries (see Figure 10.10).

The ureters have three layers:

- transitional epithelial mucosa (inner layer);
- smooth muscle layer (middle layer);
- fibrous connective tissue (outer layer).

Urine is transported through the ureters via muscular movements of the urinary tract's peristaltic muscular waves. When the renal pelvis becomes laden with urine, the peristaltic wave action encourages urine to leave the body. The amount of urine in the renal pelvis determines the frequency of the peristaltic wave action, which can range from one to every few minutes to one to every few seconds. This action creates a pressure force that moves the urine through the ureters and into the bladder in small spurts.

Urinary bladder

The urinary bladder is a hollow muscular organ and is located in the pelvic cavity posterior to the symphysis pubis. In the male the bladder lies anterior to the rectum, and in the female it lies anterior to the vagina and inferior to the uterus (Mader, 2005); it is a smooth muscular sac that stores urine. Although the shape of the bladder is spherical, the shape is altered from pressure of surrounding organs. When the bladder is empty, the inner section of the bladder forms folds, but as the bladder fills with urine the walls of the bladder become smoother. As urine accumulates, the bladder expands without a significant rise in the internal pressure of the bladder. The bladder normally distends and holds approximately 350–750 mL

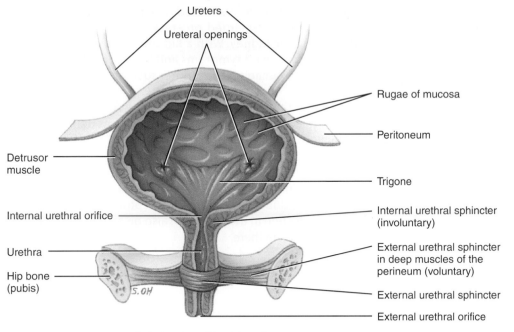

Anterior view of frontal section

Figure 10.11   Layers of the urinary bladder. *Source*: Tortora and Derrickson (2009). Reproduced with permission of John Wiley & Sons.

of urine. In females the bladder is slightly smaller because the uterus occupies the space above the bladder.

The inner lining of the urinary bladder is a mucous membrane of transitional epithelium that is continuous with that in the ureters. When the bladder is empty, the mucosa has numerous folds called rugae. The rugae and transitional epithelium allow the bladder to expand as it fills. The second layer in the walls is the submucosa, which supports the mucous membrane. It is composed of connective tissue with elastic fibres.

The inner floor of the bladder includes a triangular section called the trigone. The trigone is formed by three openings in the floor of the urinary bladder. Two of the openings are from the ureters and form the base of the trigone. Small flaps of mucosa cover these openings and act as valves that allow urine to enter the bladder but prevent it from backing up from the bladder into the ureters. The third opening, at the apex of the trigone, is the opening into the urethra (see Figure 10.11). A band of the detrusor muscle encircles this opening to form the internal urethral sphincter.

The walls of the bladder consist of muscle fibres:

- transitional epithelial mucosa;
- a thick muscular layer;
- a fibrous outer layer.

Urinary tract infection and cystitis are more common in women than men. If untreated they can result in a more serious renal problem. Urinary tract infection can be prevented by ensuring adequate intake of fluid and good personal hygiene.

The urinary tract can become blocked or obstructed (e.g. from a kidney stone, tumour, expanding uterus during pregnancy or enlarged prostate gland). The build-up of urine can lead to infection and injury of the kidney. With a kidney stone, the blockage is often painful. Other obstructions may produce no symptoms and be detected only when a blood or urine test is abnormal or when an imaging procedure, such as an X-ray or ultrasound, detects it.

Urinary tract infections, such as cystitis (an infection of the bladder), can lead to more serious infections further up the urinary tract. Symptoms include fever, frequent urination, sudden and urgent need to urinate, and pain or a burning feeling during urination. There is often pressure or pain in the lower abdomen or back. Sometimes the urine has a strong or foul odour or is bloody. Pyelonephritis is an infection of kidney tissue; most often, it is the result of cystitis that has spread to the kidney. An obstruction in the urinary tract can make a kidney infection more likely. Infections elsewhere in the body, including, for example, streptococcal infections, the skin infection impetigo or a bacterial infection in the heart, can also be carried through the bloodstream to the kidney and cause a problem there.

Urethra

The urethra is a muscular tube that drains urine from the bladder and conveys it out of the body. It contains three coats, and they are muscular, erectile and mucous; the muscular is the continuation of the bladder muscle layer. The urethra is encompassed by two separate urethral sphincter muscles. The internal urethral sphincter muscle is formed by involuntary smooth muscles, while the lower voluntary muscles make up the external sphincter muscles. The internal sphincter is created by the detrusor muscle. The urethra is longer in males than in females. Sphincters keep the urethra closed when urine is not being passed. The internal urethral sphincter is under involuntary control and lies at the bladder–urethra junction. The external urethral sphincter is under voluntary control.

Male urethra

The male urethra passes through four different regions:

- Prostatic region – passes through the prostate gland.
- Membranous portion – passes through the pelvis diaphragm.
- Bulbar urethra – located inside the perineum and scrotum, extends from the external distal urinary sphincter to the peno-scrotal junction, and is surrounded by the corpus spongiosum. It contains the opening of the ducts of the Cowper glands, and differs in length from person to person.
- Penile region – extends the length of the penis.

In the male, the urethra not only excretes fluid wastes but is also part of the reproductive system. Rather than the straight tube found in the female body, the male urethra is S-shaped to follow the line of the penis. It is approximately 20 cm long. The male urethra can be segregated into various portions: the spongy portion, the prostatic portion and the membranous portion. The spongy urethra can be subdivided into fossa navicularis, pendulous urethra and bulbous (bulbar) urethra. The proximal portion, which is also the prostatic portion, is only about 2.5 cm long and passes along the neck of the urinary bladder through the prostate gland. This section is designed to accept the drainage from the tiny ducts within the prostate and is equipped with two ejaculatory tubes (see Figure 10.12).

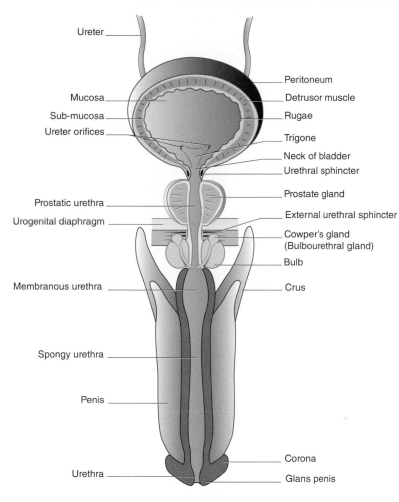

Figure 10.12   Male urethra.

Female urethra

The female urethra is bound to the anterior vaginal wall. The external opening of the urethra is anterior to the vagina and posterior to the clitoris. In the female, the urethra is approximately 4 cm long and leads out of the body via the urethral orifice. In the female, the urethral orifice is located in the vestibule in the labia minora. This can be found located in between the clitoris and the vaginal orifice. In the female body the urethra's only function is to transport urine out of the body (see Figure 10.13).

Micturition

When the volume of urine in the bladder reaches about 300 mL, stretch receptors in the bladder walls are stimulated and excite sensory parasympathetic fibres that relay information to the sacral area of the spine. This information is integrated in the spine and relayed to two different sets of neurones. Parasympathetic motor neurones (in the pons) are excited and act to contract

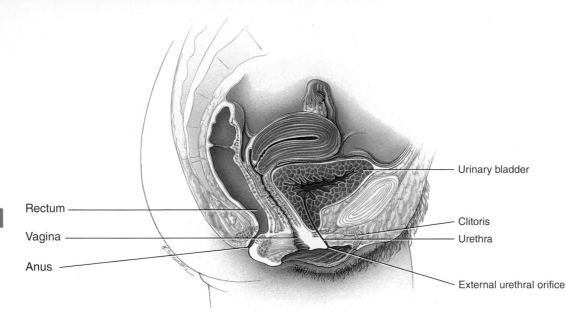

Figure 10.13 Location of female urethra. *Source*: Nair and Peate (2013). Reproduced with permission of John Wiley & Sons.

the detrusor muscles in the bladder so that bladder pressure increases and the internal sphincter opens. At the same time, somatic motor neurones supplying the external sphincter via the pudendal nerve are inhibited, allowing the external sphincter to open and urine to flow out, assisted by gravity.

A person has great control of the bladder. They can increase or decrease the rate of flow of urine, and stop and start at will (unless there are physiological problems), thus making micturition a simple reflex action.

Conclusion

The renal system consists of the kidneys, ureters, urinary bladder and the urethra. These systems collectively play an important role in maintaining homeostasis. They remove the waste products of metabolism, secrete hormones, regulate fluid balance and maintain homeostasis. Some of the functions it carries out include:

- regulating blood volume through urine production and blood pressure by releasing renin;
- regulating the electrolyte balance in the body through hormones such as aldosterone;
- maintaining the acid–base balance by regulating the secretion of hydrogen and bicarbonate ions;
- excreting waste products (e.g. urea and uric acid) and conserving valuable nutrients essential for the body.

Urine is formed by filtration, selective reabsorption and secretion. The selectivity of the glomerular filtrate is determined by the size of the opening of the filter and blood pressure. There are other factors that regulate urine production and electrolyte balance; they include hormone regulation such as ADH, aldosterone and ANP hormones and neuronal regulation through the autonomic nervous system.

The urinary bladder is a storage organ for urine and is located in the pelvic cavity. It contains three layers: the muscular, erectile and mucous layers. Urine is stored in the bladder until the person gets the urge to empty their bladder. The process of micturition is under the control of the sympathetic and parasympathetic system. During micturition, strong muscles in the bladder walls (the detrusor muscles) compress the bladder, pushing its contents into the urethra, thus voiding urine.

Glossary

Anterior   Front.

Bifurcation   Dividing into two branches.

Calyces   Small, funnel-shaped cavities formed from the renal pelvis.

Diuresis   Excess urine production.

Erythropoietin   Hormone produced by the kidneys that regulates red blood cell production.

Excretion   The elimination of waste products of metabolism.

Filtration   A passive transport system.

Glomerulus   A network of capillaries found in Bowman's capsule.

Hilum (hilus)   An indention near to the centre of the concave area of the kidney, where its vessels, nerves and ureter enter/leave.

Kidneys   Organs situated in the posterior wall of the abdominal cavity.

Nephron   Functional unit of the kidney.

Posterior   Behind.

Renal artery   Blood vessel that takes blood to the kidney.

Renal cortex   The outermost part of the kidney.

Renal medulla   The middle layer of the kidney.

Renal pelvis   The funnel-shaped section of the kidney.

Renal pyramids   Cone-shaped structures of the medulla.

Renal vein   Blood vessel that returns filtered blood into circulation.

Renin   A renal hormone that alters systemic blood pressure.

Sphincter   A ring-like muscle fibre that can constrict.

Ureter   Membranous tube that drains urine from the kidneys to the bladder.

Urethra   Muscular tube that drains urine from the bladder.

References

Knott, L. (2013) *Pyelonephritis*. http://www.patient.co.uk/doctor/pyelonephritis (accessed 26 November 2015).
Mader, S.S. (2005) *Understanding Human Anatomy and Physiology*, 5th edn. Boston, MA: McGraw-Hill.
Marieb, E.N. and Hoehn, K. (2013) *Human Anatomy and Physiology*, 9th edn. San Francisco: Pearson Benjamin Cummings.

McCance, K.L. Huether, S.E., Brashers, V.L. and Rote, N.S. (2010) *Pathophysiology: The Biological Basis for Disease in Adults and Children*, 6th edn. St Louis, MO: Mosby.

Mayo Clinic Staff (2015) *Urine Color*. http://www.mayoclinic.org/diseases-conditions/urine-color/basics/causes/con-20032831 (accessed 26 November 2015).

Nair, M. and Peate, I. (2009) *Fundamentals of Applied Pathophysiology: An Essential Guide for Nursing Students*. Oxford: John Wiley & Sons, Ltd.

Nair, M. and Peate, I. (2013) *Fundamentals of Applied Pathophysiology: An Essential Guide for Nursing and Healthcare Students*, 2nd edn. Oxford: John Wiley & Sons, Ltd.

NHS Choices (2014a) *Kidney Stones – Treatment*. http://www.nhs.uk/Conditions/Kidney-stones/Pages/Treatment.aspx (accessed 26 November 2015).

NHS Choices (2014b) *Urinary Incontinence – Non-Surgical Treatment*. http://www.nhs.uk/Conditions/Incontinence-urinary/Pages/Treatment.aspx (accessed 26 November 2015).

NHS Choices (2015a) *Kidney Transplant*. http://www.nhs.uk/conditions/Kidney-transplant/Pages/Introduction.aspx (accessed 26 November 2015).

NHS Choices (2015b) *Dialysis*. http://www.nhs.uk/Conditions/dialysis/Pages/Introduction.aspx (accessed 26 November 2015).

Rull, G. (2013) *Drug Prescribing in Renal Impairment*. http://www.patient.co.uk/doctor/drug-prescribing-in-renal-impairment (accessed 26 November 2015).

RxList (2012) *Sandimmune Patient Information Including If I Miss a Dose*. http://www.rxlist.com/sandimmune-drug/patient-avoid-while-taking.htm (accessed 26 November 2015).

Tortora, G.J. and Derrickson, B. (2006) *Principles of Anatomy and Physiology*, 11th edn. Hoboken, NJ: John Wiley & Sons, Inc.

Tortora, G.J. and Derrickson, B.H. (2009) *Principles of Anatomy and Physiology*, 12th edn. Hoboken, NJ: John Wiley & Sons, Inc.

Waugh, A. and Grant, A. (eds) (2014) *Ross and Wilson Anatomy and Physiology in Health and Illness*. Edinburgh: Churchill Livingstone.

Further reading

National Institute for Health and Care Excellence

http://www.nice.org.uk/guidance/cg73 (accessed 26 November 2015)

This guidance relates to early identification and management of chronic kidney disease in adults in primary and secondary care.

http://guidance.nice.org.uk/QS5 (accessed 26 November 2015)

This NICE quality standard defines clinical best practice within this topic area. It provides specific, concise quality statements, measures and audience descriptors to provide patients and the public, health- and social-care professionals, commissioners and service providers with definitions of high-quality care.

Cancer Research UK

http://www.cancerresearchuk.org/cancer-help/type/kidney-cancer/ (accessed 26 November 2015)

A useful website to get information about cancer. They include symptoms, causes and tests to diagnose cancer. Information about treatments (including surgery) and current research can be found on this website.

Activities

Multiple choice questions

1. The urine flows through:
    (a) the pelvis of the kidney → urethra → ureter → bladder
    (b) the bladder → pelvis of the kidney → ureter → urethra

    (c) the pelvis of the kidney → ureter → bladder → urethra

    (d) the ureter → pelvis of the kidney → urethra → bladder

2. Which of the following structures are found in the renal medulla?
   - **(a)** glomerulus
   - **(b)** Bowman's capsule
   - **(c)** loop of Henle
   - **(d)** proximal convoluted tubule

3. The kidneys produce renin when:
   - **(a)** blood pressure is low
   - **(b)** blood pressure is high
   - **(c)** pH of blood is low
   - **(d)** pH of blood is high

4. What is the name of the gland sitting above the kidneys?
   - **(a)** pancreas
   - **(b)** liver
   - **(c)** hypothalamus
   - **(d)** adrenal

5. The urinary bladder is composed of:
   - **(a)** transitional epithelium
   - **(b)** skeletal muscles
   - **(c)** cardiac muscle
   - **(d)** simple squamous epithelium

6. A patient with a urinary tract infection will probably present with:
   - **(a)** clear urine
   - **(b)** leucocytes in the urine
   - **(c)** glycosuria
   - **(d)** ketones

7. The specific gravity of urine is in the range:
   - **(a)** 1.001–1.073
   - **(b)** 1.020–1.025
   - **(c)** 1.000–1.078
   - **(d)** 1.001–1.035

8. The light yellow colour of urine results from:
   - **(a)** the pigments from the breakdown of haemoglobin
   - **(b)** breakdown of white blood cells
   - **(c)** eating too many carrots
   - **(d)** fats in the urine

9. Blood glucose is entirely reabsorbed in:
   - **(a)** the glomerulus
   - **(b)** the distal convoluted tubule
   - **(c)** the proximal convoluted tubule
   - **(d)** the collecting ducts

10. Renal calculi may develop as a result of:
    - **(a)** sarcoma of the bones
    - **(b)** drinking too much water
    - **(c)** eating too many carrots
    - **(d)** eating too much spinach

True or false

1. Urea is the end-product of nitrogen metabolism.
2. The energy for filtration of fluid in the glomeruli is generated by the heart.
3. Inulin clearance is used to estimate the renal plasma flow.
4. Creatinine is an endogenous chemical.
5. Bowman's capsule consists of endothelial cells.
6. The flow of urine down the ureter is by peristalsis.
7. Concentration of urine occurs in the bladder.
8. The muscle of the bladder wall is striated muscle.
9. Erythrocytes are present in the glomerular filtrate.
10. Renal tubular secretion occurs in the glomeruli.

Label the diagram 1

Label the diagram using the following list of words:

Renal cortex, Renal medulla, Renal column, Renal pyramid in renal medulla, Renal sinus, Renal papilla, Fat in renal sinus, Renal capsule, Nephron, Path of urine drainage: Collecting duct, Papillary duct in renal pyramid, Minor calyx, Major calyx, Renal pelvis, Ureter, Renal artery, Renal vein, Urinary bladder

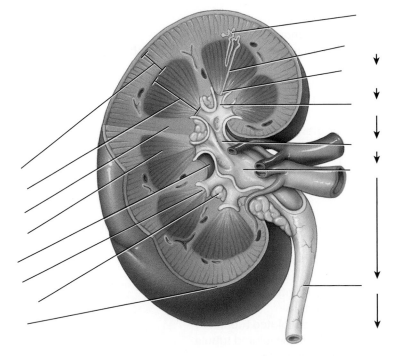

Label the diagram 2

Label the diagram using the following list of words:

Afferent arteriole, Efferent arteriole, Proximal convoluted tubule, Glomerular (Bowman's) capsule, Glomerulus, Distal convoluted tubule, Interstitial fluid in renal cortex, Collecting duct, Interstitial fluid in renal medulla, Papillary duct, Dilute urine, Loop of Henle

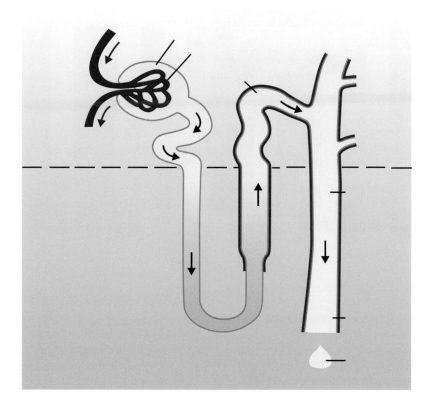

Crossword

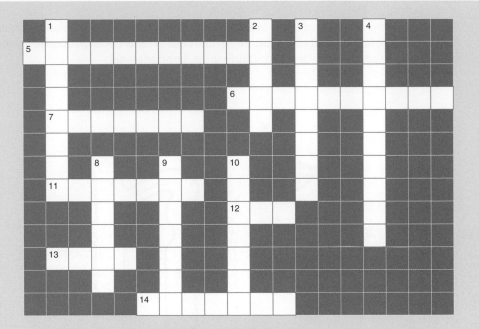

Across:

5. Hormone that regulates electrolyte balance (11).
6. One of the functions of the kidney (10).
7. Also carries sperm in man (7).
11. Gland that sits on top of each kidney (7).
12. Hormone that regulates fluid balance (3).
13. One of the waste products found in the urine (4).
14. Functional unit of the kidney (7).

Down:

1. Scanty urine output (8).
2. Hormone produced by the juxtaglomerular cells (5).
3. Inflammation of the bladder (8).
4. An invasive investigation of the bladder (10).
8. Conveys urine from the kidney to the bladder (6).
9. Outer protective layer of the kidney (7).
10. Storage organ for urine (7).

Word search

R	K	N	F	U	L	A	M	I	X	O	R	P	O	E
E	E	M	U	R	E	T	E	R	N	K	O	M	U	J
N	O	N	O	I	T	A	R	T	L	I	F	N	R	X
I	R	R	O	Z	Y	U	I	Z	Q	J	N	N	C	G
N	F	E	O	R	D	Y	R	Z	A	B	L	I	R	C
S	P	I	N	V	E	D	R	E	L	E	W	L	E	Y
E	B	Y	Y	A	P	T	J	K	T	C	F	U	A	S
C	K	Z	V	K	L	G	S	I	C	H	W	N	T	T
R	I	I	L	U	R	E	M	O	L	G	R	I	I	I
E	D	I	O	G	B	L	A	D	D	E	R	A	N	T
T	N	E	P	H	R	O	N	J	T	L	G	T	I	I
I	E	I	N	F	E	C	T	I	O	N	A	R	N	S
O	Y	T	U	B	U	L	E	M	S	T	A	F	E	L
N	L	A	T	S	I	D	G	M	I	K	K	X	G	D
D	M	A	I	R	U	T	A	M	E	A	H	T	Q	N

Renal, Glomeruli, Tubule, Kidney, Bladder, Creatinine, Secretion, Urethra, Ureter, Renin, Aldosterone, Filtration, Inulin, Proximal, Distal, Nephron, Haematuria, Cystitis, Infection

Fill in the blanks

The _____, _____, _____ and the _____ form the normal urinary system. The kidneys _____ the _____ in order to remove the wastes and _____ from the body and form the _____. This travels to the _____ via the _____. The urinary bladder _____ the urine until it is passed out of the body via the urethra.

Within the kidneys are nearly a _____ small filtering units called _____. Blood flows through _____ and intricate networks of _____ within the kidneys to the glomeruli in order to undergo the _____.

The function of the _____ is, among other things, to get rid of the _____ that result from the body's _____. One of the major _____ of the metabolism of _____ (muscle) is _____. The kidneys remove the waste products by extracting them from the blood and sending them along the _____ to the _____, from where they are _____ in the _____. If the kidney function _____, the waste products _____ in the _____ and the body. The term for this build-up is _____.

accumulate, azotaemia, bladder, blood, blood, blood vessels, by-products, excess fluids, excreted, fails, filter, filtration process, glomeruli, kidneys, kidneys, metabolism, million, protein, stores, tiny tubes, urea, ureter, ureters, ureters, ureters, urinary bladder, urinary bladder, urine, urine, waste products

Find out more

1. Describe the role of kidney in maintaining homeostasis.
2. Discuss the renin–angiotensin system.
3. What do you understand by erythropoietin doping?
4. Describe the functions of aldosterone II.
5. Explain glomerular filtration rate.
6. Explain the role of the kidneys in a person suffering from congestive cardiac failure.
7. Explain the effects of high blood pressure in a patient who is on bed rest.
8. A person with kidney disease is diagnosed as having proteinuria. The person's limbs are swollen. Explain proteinuria and why it causes swollen limbs in this person.
9. Discuss the role of the autonomic system in micturition.
10. Explain the term countercurrent at the loop of Henle.

Conditions

The following is a list of conditions that are associated with the renal system. Take some time and write notes about each of the conditions. You may make the notes taken from text books or other resources (e.g. people you work with in a clinical area), or you may make the notes as a result of people you have cared for. If you are making notes about people you have cared for you must ensure that you adhere to the rules of confidentiality.

Nephrotic syndrome	
Glomerulonephritis	
End-stage renal disease	
Polycystic renal disease	
Hydronephrosis	

Chapter 11

The respiratory system

Anthony Wheeldon

Test your prior knowledge

- List five major structures of the upper and lower respiratory tract.
- What is the main function of the respiratory system?
- Describe the physiological process of breathing – which muscles are utilised?
- How is oxygen transported to body tissue?
- What factors may increase or decrease a person's rate and depth of breathing?

Learning outcomes

After reading this chapter you will be able to:

- List the main anatomical structures of both the upper and lower respiratory tract
- Describe the events of pulmonary ventilation
- Explain how the body is able to control the rate and depth of breathing
- Discuss the principles of external respiration
- Describe how oxygen and carbon dioxide are transported around the body

Fundamentals of Anatomy and Physiology: For Nursing and Healthcare Students, Second Edition. Edited by Ian Peate and Muralitharan Nair.
© 2017 John Wiley & Sons, Ltd. Published 2017 by John Wiley & Sons, Ltd.
Student companion website: www.wileyfundamentalseries.com/anatomy
Instructor companion website: www.wiley.com/go/instructor/anatomy

Body map

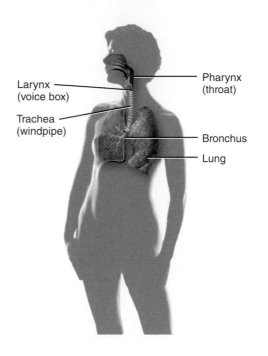

Larynx
(voice box)

Pharynx
(throat)

Trachea
(windpipe)

Bronchus

Lung

Introduction

Human cells can only survive if they receive a continuous supply of oxygen. As cells use oxygen, a waste gas, carbon dioxide, is produced. If allowed to build up, carbon dioxide can disrupt cellular activity and disturb homeostasis. The principal function of the respiratory system, therefore, is to ensure that the body extracts enough oxygen from the atmosphere and disposes of the excess carbon dioxide. The collection of oxygen and removal of carbon dioxide is referred to as respiration. Respiration involves the following four distinct processes: pulmonary ventilation, external respiration, transport of gases and internal respiration. Although all four are examined in this chapter, only pulmonary ventilation and external respiration are the sole responsibility of the respiratory system. As oxygen and carbon dioxide are transported around the body in blood, effective respiration is also reliant upon a fully functioning cardiovascular system.

Organisation of the respiratory system

The respiratory system is divided into the upper and lower respiratory tract (see Figure 11.1). All structures found below the larynx form part of the lower respiratory tract. The respiratory system can also be said to be divided into conduction and respiratory regions. The upper respiratory tract and the uppermost section of lower respiratory tract form the conduction region, in which air is conducted through a series of tubes and vessels. The respiratory region is the functional part of the lungs, in which oxygen diffuses into blood. The structures within the respiratory region are microscopic, very fragile and easily damaged by infection. For this reason, both the upper and lower respiratory tracts are equipped to fight off any invading airborne bacterial or viral pathogens.

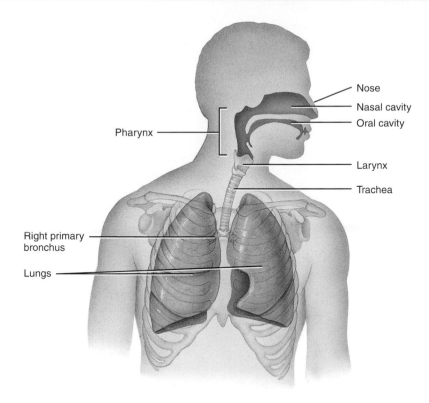

Anterior view showing organs of respiration

Figure 11.1   Major structures of the upper and lower respiratory tract. *Source*: Tortora and Derrickson (2009). Reproduced with permission of John Wiley & Sons.

The upper respiratory tract

Air enters the body via the nasal and oral cavities. The nasal cavity is divided into two equal sections by the nasal septum, a structure formed out of the ethmoid bones and the vomer of the skull. The space where air enters the nasal cavity just inside the nostrils is referred to as the vestibule. Beyond each vestibule the nasal cavities are subdivided into three air passageways, the meatuses, which are formed by three shelf-like projections called the superior, middle and inferior nasal conchae (see Figure 11.2). The region around the superior conchae and upper septum contains olfactory receptors, which are responsible for our sense of smell. The pharynx connects the nasal and oral cavity with the larynx. The pharynx is divided into three regions called the nasopharynx, the oropharynx and the laryngopharynx. The nasopharynx sits behind the nasal cavity and contains two openings that lead to the auditory (Eustachian) tubes. The oropharynx and laryngopharynx sit underneath the nasopharynx and behind the oral cavity. The oropharynx and oral cavity are divided by the fauces (see Figure 11.2). Both the oropharynx and the laryngopharynx are passageways for food and drink as well as air. To protect them from abrasion by food particles they are lined with non-keratinised stratified squamous epithelium (see Chapter 4).

As well as providing the sense of smell, the upper respiratory tract also ensures that the air entering the lower respiratory tract is warm, damp and clean. The vestibule is lined with coarse hairs that filter incoming air, ensuring that large dust particles do not enter the airways. The conchae

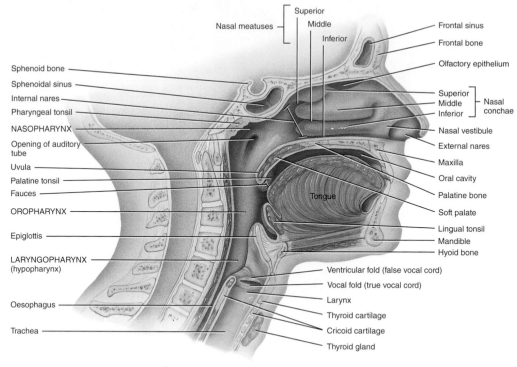

Sagittal section of the left side of the head and neck
showing the location of respiratory structures

Figure 11.2 Structures of the upper respiratory tract. *Source*: Tortora and Derrickson (2009). Reproduced with permission of John Wiley & Sons.

are lined with a mucous membrane made from pseudostratified ciliated columnar epithelium, which contains a network of capillaries and a plentiful supply of mucus-secreting goblet cells. The blood flowing through the capillaries warms the passing air, while the mucus moistens it and traps any passing dust particles. The mucus-covered dust particles are then propelled by the cilia towards the pharynx, where they can be swallowed or expectorated.

To add further protection, the upper respiratory tract is lined with irritant receptors, which when stimulated by invading particles (dust or pollen for example) force a sneeze, ensuring the offending material is ejected through the nose or mouth. The pharynx also contains five tonsils. The two tonsils visible when the mouth is open are the palatine tonsils; behind the tongue lie the lingual tonsils, and the pharyngeal tonsil or adenoid sits on the upper back wall of the pharynx. Tonsils are lymph nodules and part of the body's defence system. The epithelial lining of their surface has deep folds, called crypts. Inhaled bacteria or particles become entangled within the crypts and are then engulfed and destroyed.

The lower respiratory tract

The lower respiratory tract includes the larynx, the trachea, the right and left primary bronchi and all the constituents of both lungs (see Figure 11.3). The lungs are two cone-shaped organs that almost fill the thorax. They are protected by a framework of bones, the thoracic cage, which consists of the ribs, sternum (breastbone) and vertebrae (spine). The tip of each

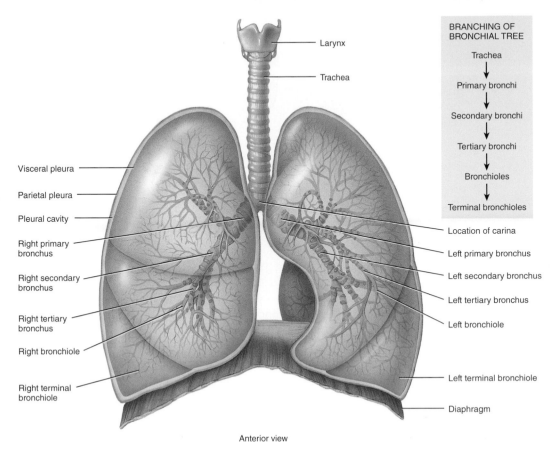

BRANCHING OF
BRONCHIAL TREE

Trachea
↓
Primary bronchi
↓
Secondary bronchi
↓
Tertiary bronchi
↓
Bronchioles
↓
Terminal bronchioles

Larynx

Trachea

Visceral pleura

Parietal pleura

Pleural cavity

Right primary
bronchus

Right secondary
bronchus

Right tertiary
bronchus

Right bronchiole

Right terminal
bronchiole

Location of carina

Left primary bronchus

Left secondary bronchus

Left tertiary bronchus

Left bronchiole

Left terminal bronchiole

Diaphragm

Anterior view

Figure 11.3 Gross anatomy of the lower respiratory tract. *Source*: Tortora and Derrickson (2009). Reproduced with permission of John Wiley & Sons.

lung, the apex, extends just above the clavicle (collarbone), and their wider bases sit just above a concave muscle called the diaphragm. The larynx (voice box) connects the trachea and the laryngopharynx. The remainder of the lower respiratory tract divides into branches of airways. For this reason, the structure of the lower respiratory tract is often referred to as the bronchial tree.

Larynx

The larynx consists of nine pieces of cartilage tissue: three single pieces and three pairs (see Figure 11.4). The single pieces of cartilage are the thyroid cartilage, the epiglottis and the cricoid cartilage. The thyroid cartilage is more commonly known as the Adam's apple and, together with the cricoid cartilage, protects the vocal cords. The cricothyroid ligament, which connects the thyroid and cricoid cartilage, is the landmark of an emergency airway or tracheostomy (McGrath, 2014). The epiglottis is a leaf-shaped piece of elastic cartilage attached to the top of the larynx. Its function is to protect the airway from food and water. On swallowing, the epiglottis blocks entry to the larynx and food and liquids are diverted towards the oesophagus, which sits nearby. Inhalation of solid or liquid substances can block the lower respiratory tract and cut off the body's supply of oxygen – this medical emergency is referred to as aspiration and necessitates the swift removal of the offending substance.

337

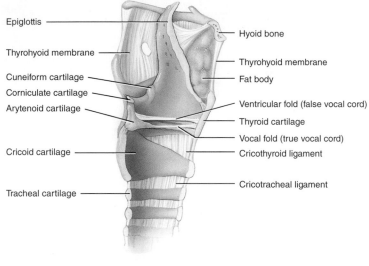

Epiglottis

Thyrohyoid membrane

Cuneiform cartilage

Corniculate cartilage

Arytenoid cartilage

Cricoid cartilage

Tracheal cartilage

Hyoid bone

Thyrohyoid membrane

Fat body

Ventricular fold (false vocal cord)

Thyroid cartilage

Vocal fold (true vocal cord)

Cricothyroid ligament

Cricotracheal ligament

Sagittal section

Figure 11.4   Anatomy of the larynx. *Source*: Tortora and Derrickson (2009). Reproduced with permission of John Wiley & Sons.

The three pairs of cartilage are the arytenoid, cuneiform and corniculate cartilages (see Figure 11.4). The arytenoid cartilages are the most significant as they influence the movement of the mucous membranes (true vocal folds) that generate the voice. Speaking, therefore, is reliant upon a fully functioning respiratory system. Many obstructive lung disorders, such as asthma, reduce a person's ability to speak a full sentence without drawing a new breath (Higginson and Jones, 2009).

Trachea

The trachea (or windpipe) is a tubular vessel that carries air from the larynx down towards the lungs. The trachea is also lined with pseudostratified ciliated columnar epithelium so that any inhaled debris is trapped and propelled upwards towards the oesophagus and pharynx to be swallowed or expectorated. The trachea and the bronchi also contain irritant receptors, which stimulate a cough, forcing larger invading particles upwards. The outermost layer of the trachea contains connective tissue that is reinforced by a series of 16–20 C-shaped cartilage rings. The rings prevent the trachea from collapsing during an active breathing cycle.

Bronchial tree

The lungs are divided into distinct regions called lobes. There are three lobes in the right lung and two in the left. The heart, along with its major blood vessels, sits in a space between the two lungs called the cardiac notch. Each lung is surrounded by two thin protective membranes called the parietal and visceral pleura (see Figure 11.3). The parietal pleura lines the wall of the thorax, whereas the visceral pleura lines the lungs themselves. The space between the two pleura, the pleural space, is minute and contains a thin film of lubricating fluid. This reduces friction between the two pleura, allowing the two layers to slide over one another during breathing. The fluid also helps the visceral and parietal pleura to adhere to each other, in the same way two pieces of glass stick together when wet.

Within the lungs the primary bronchi divide into the secondary bronchi, each serving a lobe (three secondary bronchi on the right and two on the left). The secondary bronchi split into

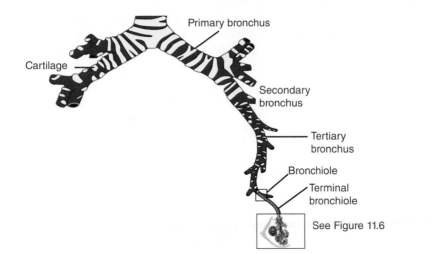

Figure 11.5 The bronchial tree. *Source*: Nair and Peate (2009). Reproduced with permission of John Wiley & Sons.

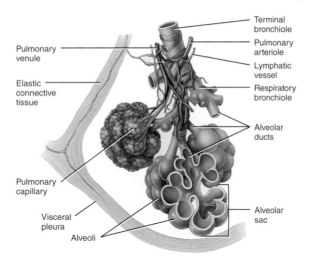

Diagram of a portion of a lobule of the lung

Figure 11.6 Microscopic anatomy of a lobule. *Source*: Tortora and Derrickson (2009). Reproduced with permission of John Wiley & Sons.

tertiary bronchi (see Figures 11.3 and 11.5), of which there are 10 in each lung. Tertiary bronchi continue to divide into a network of bronchioles, which eventually lead to a terminal bronchiole. The section of the lung supplied by a terminal bronchiole is referred to as a lobule, and each lobule has its own arterial blood supply and lymph vessels. The bronchial tree continues to subdivide, with the terminal bronchiole leading to a series of respiratory bronchioles, which in turn generate several alveolar ducts. The airways terminate with numerous sphere-like structures called alveoli, which are clustered together to form alveolar sacs (see Figure 11.6). Human lungs contain an average of 480 million alveoli (Ochs *et al.*, 2004). The transfer of oxygen from air to blood only occurs from the respiratory bronchiole onwards. The airways found between the trachea and the respiratory bronchioles form the conduction region of the lungs. The airways found beyond the respiratory bronchioles constitute the functional respiratory region of the lungs. This region accounts for two-thirds of the lungs' surface area (Tortora and Derrickson, 2009).

Snapshot

Spontaneous pneumothorax

David, a 29-year-old man, had been walking his dog in the woods near his home. After throwing a stick for his dog to chase David experienced acute pain on the left-hand side of his chest. The pain was unbearable and David found it difficult to breathe. A passer-by called an ambulance and David was taken to the accident and emergency department where he was assessed by a nurse. The nurse noticed that David's breathing was asymmetrical, with only the right-hand side of his chest rising and falling. The nurse also noted he had central cyanosis, laboured respiratory effort and a low oxygen saturation reading. An X-ray showed a pneumothorax of greater than 2 cm in width. The medical team proceeded to insert a chest drain.

David had experienced a spontaneous pneumothorax. Pneumothorax, or collapsed lung, occurs when air leaks into the pleural space and the visceral and parietal pleura separate, causing the lung to collapse. Pneumothoraces are normally caused by trauma or respiratory disease but can occur spontaneously in people who have sub-pleural blebs or bullae in the apices of the lung. Spontaneous pneumothoraces are also more likely in an individual who smokes tobacco.

See MacDuff *et al.* (2010).

Medicines management

Nebulised salbutamol

Salbutamol is a β_2 agonist bronchodilator therapy used to reverse airway constriction caused by obstructive airways diseases, such as asthma. Asthma is a chronic inflammatory airway disease in which individuals are said to have hypersensitive or hyper-responsive airways. People living with asthma experience periods of reversible inflammation and constriction in the bronchi and bronchioles, which causes breathlessness and a characteristic wheeze. When encountering a trigger (e.g. allergy, infection or stress), mast cells on the walls of the bronchi and bronchioles release a number of cytokines (chemical messengers) that cause increased mucus production and increased capillary permeability. Very soon the airways become full of mucus and fluid leaking from blood vessels and airflow becomes obstructed. β_2 agonists such as salbutamol stimulate β_2 receptor cells on the walls of the bronchi and bronchioles, causing bronchodilation.

A nebuliser forces a jet stream of air or oxygen through a liquid preparation of salbutamol, producing a salbutamol mist that the patient inhales via a special mask or pipe. While salbutamol is an effective pharmacological treatment, the nurse must be aware of the following side effects:

- tachycardia and other arrhythmias
- hand shaking and tremors
- headache
- nervous tension.

Salbutamol can also be given as an inhaler, tablet or subcutaneous or intravenous infusion. Other β_2 agonists include terbutaline, fenoterol and salmeterol.

See British Thoracic Society and Scottish Intercollegiate Guidelines Network (2014).

Medicines management

Corticosteroid therapy

Corticosteroids are potent anti-inflammatory agents that are often used to reduce bronchial hyperactivity in people living with chronic inflammatory airway diseases, such as asthma and chronic obstructive pulmonary disease. Corticosteroids reduce airway inflammation and therefore are very effective in the treatment of airway obstruction. Corticosteroids are a first-line treatment for moderate, severe and life-threatening asthma. Common corticosteroids include

- prednisolone
- hydrocortisone.

Patients taking the above corticosteroids will need careful monitoring as they may cause the following side effects:

- osteoporosis
- diabetes
- mood swings
- weight gain
- increased body hair.

Inhaled corticosteroids are used very effectively for the prophylaxis of asthma. Preparations such as beclamethasone, budesonide and fluticasone are often prescribed for patients living with asthma to be used on a daily basis to minimise the potential for exacerbation.

See British Thoracic Society and Scottish Intercollegiate Guidelines Network (2014).

Blood supply

The conduction and respiratory regions of the lungs receive blood from different arteries. Deoxygenated blood is delivered to the lobules via capillaries that originate from the right and left pulmonary arteries. Once reoxygenated, blood is sent back to the left-hand side of the heart via one of four pulmonary veins, ready to be ejected into systemic circulation (see Figure 11.7). The conduction region of the lungs receives oxygenated blood from capillaries that stem from the bronchial arteries, which originate from the aorta. Some of the bronchial arteries are connected to the pulmonary arteries, but the majority of blood returns to the heart via the pulmonary or bronchial veins.

Respiration

The process by which oxygen and carbon dioxide are exchanged between the atmosphere and body cells is called respiration. Respiration follows the following four distinct phases:

- **pulmonary ventilation** – how air gets in and out of the lungs;
- **external respiration** – how oxygen diffuses from the lungs to the bloodstream and how carbon dioxide diffuses from blood and to the lungs;
- **transport of gases** – how oxygen and carbon dioxide are transported between the lungs and body tissues;
- **internal respiration** – how oxygen is delivered to and carbon dioxide collected from body cells.

The understanding of all four processes is reliant upon the appreciation of a series of gas laws, which are summarised in Table 11.1.

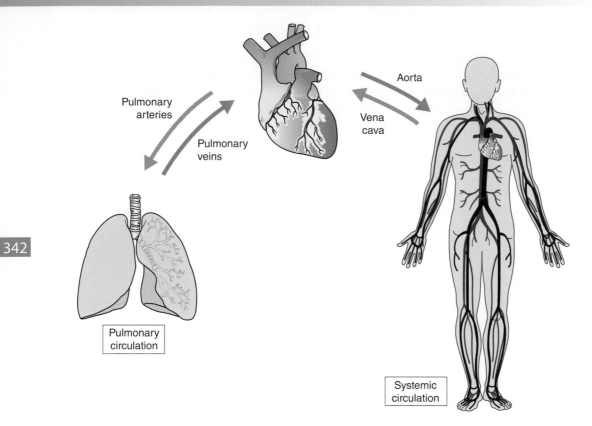

Figure 11.7   The flow of blood between the lungs, the heart and the body.

Table 11.1   Summary of important gas laws

Gas law	Summary	Clinical application
Boyle's law	At a fixed temperature the pressure exerted by gas is inversely proportional to its volume	As the thorax expands, intrapulmonary pressure falls below atmospheric pressure
Dalton's law	In a mixture of gases each gas will exert its own individual pressure, as if no other gases are present	Differences in partial pressure govern the movement of oxygen and carbon dioxide between the atmosphere, the lungs and blood
Henry's law	The quantity of gas that will dissolve in a liquid is proportional to its pressure and its solubility	Oxygen and carbon dioxide are soluble in water and are transported in blood. Nitrogen is highly insoluble and, despite accounting for 79% of the atmosphere, very little is dissolved in blood
Fick's law	The rate a gas will diffuse across a permeable membrane will depend upon pressure difference, surface area, diffusion distance and molecular weight and solubility	Helps explain how altitude, exercise and respiratory disease can influence the amount of oxygen that is diffused into blood

Source: Adapted from Davies and Moores (2003).

Pulmonary ventilation
The mechanics of breathing

Pulmonary ventilation describes the process more commonly known as breathing. In order for air to pass in and out of our lungs a change in pressure needs to occur. Before inspiration the intrapulmonary pressure, the pressure within the lungs, is the same as atmospheric pressure. During inspiration the thorax expands and the intrapulmonary pressure falls below atmospheric pressure. Because intrapulmonary pressure is now less than atmospheric pressure the air will naturally enter our lungs until the pressure difference no longer exists. This phenomenon is explained by Boyle's law and Dalton's law. Gases exert pressure, and Boyle's law states that at a fixed temperature the amount of pressure exerted by a given mass of gas is inversely proportional to the size of its container. Larger volumes provide greater space for the circulation of gas molecules, and therefore less pressure is exerted. In smaller volumes the gas molecules are more likely to collide with the walls of the container and exert a greater pressure as a result (see Figure 11.8). Dalton's law explains that in a mixture of gases each gas exerts its own individual pressure proportional to its size. For example, atmospheric air contains a mixture of gases. Each individual gas will exert its own pressure dependent upon its quantity. Nitrogen, for example, will exert the greatest pressure as it is the most abundant gas. Collectively, all the gases in the atmosphere exert a pressure, atmospheric pressure, which is 101.3 kPa (kilopascals) at sea level (see Table 11.2). On inhalation the thorax expands, intrapulmonary pressure falls below 101.3 kPa and, because air flows from areas of high pressure to low pressure, air enters the lungs (Hickin *et al.*, 2013).

A range of respiratory muscles are used to achieve thoracic expansion during inspiration (see Figure 11.9). The major muscles of inspiration are the diaphragm and external intercostal muscles. The diaphragm is a dome-shaped skeletal muscle found beneath the lungs at the base of the thorax. There are 11 external intercostal muscles, which sit in the intercostal spaces – the spaces between the ribs. During inspiration the diaphragm contracts downwards, pulling the lungs with it. Simultaneously, the external intercostal muscles pull the rib cage outwards and upwards. The thorax is now bigger than before, and intrapulmonary pressure is reduced below atmospheric pressure as a result. The most important muscle of inspiration is the diaphragm; 75% of the air that enters the lungs is as a result of diaphragmatic contraction. Expiration is a more passive process. The external intercostal muscles and the diaphragm relax, allowing the

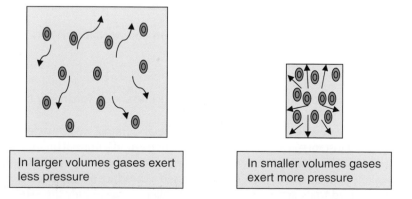

In larger volumes gases exert less pressure

In smaller volumes gases exert more pressure

Figure 11.8   Boyle's law: the volume of a gas varies inversely with its pressure.

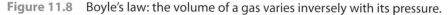

343

Table 11.2 The proportion of gases that constitute the atmosphere (partial pressures are expressed as P_{gas})

Gas	Volume (%)	Pressure (kPa)
Nitrogen (P_{N_2})	78.084	79.055
Oxygen (P_{O_2})	20.946	21.218
Carbon dioxide (P_{CO_2})	0.035	0.0355
Argon (P_{Ar})	0.934	0.946
Other gases[a]	0.001	0.001
Total atmospheric pressure (P_B)	100	101.3

Sources: Adapted from Brimblecombe (1986), Lutgens and Tarbuck (2001) and Lumb (2005).
[a] Neon, helium, methane, krypton, nitrous oxide, hydrogen, ozone, xenon.

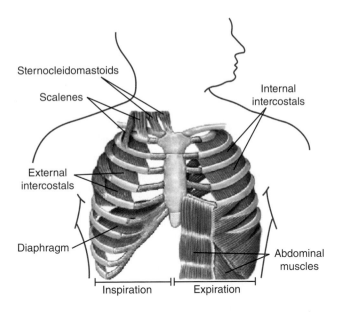

Figure 11.9 The muscles involved in pulmonary ventilation. *Source*: Nair and Peate (2009). Reproduced with permission of John Wiley & Sons.

natural elastic recoil of the lung tissue to spring back into shape, forcing air back into the atmosphere (see Figure 11.10).

Other respiratory muscles can also be utilised. The abdominal wall muscles and internal intercostal muscles, for instance, are utilised to force air out beyond a normal breath, for example, when playing a musical instrument or blowing out candles on a birthday cake. The sternocleidomastoids, the scalenes and the pectoralis can also be used to produce a deep forceful inspiration. These muscles are referred to as accessory muscles, so called because they are rarely used in normal, quiet breathing (Simpson, 2006).

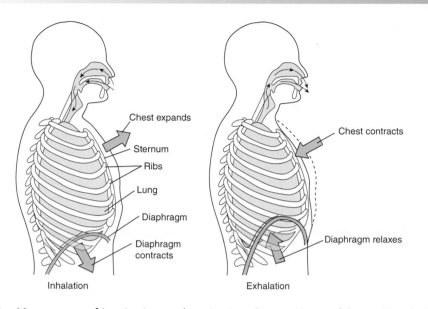

Figure 11.10   Movements of inspiration and expiration. *Source*: Nair and Peate (2009). Reproduced with permission of John Wiley & Sons.

Work of breathing

During inspiration respiratory muscles must overcome various factors that hinder thoracic expansion. The natural elastic recoil of lung tissue, the resistance to airflow through narrow airways and the surface tension forces at the liquid–air interface in the lobule all oppose thoracic expansion. The energy required by the respiratory muscles to overcome these hindering forces is referred to as work of breathing. The amount of energy expended is kept to a minimum by the ease with which lungs can be stretched. This ease of stretch is called lung compliance. Because of lung compliance, an inhalation of around 500 mL of air is achievable without any noticeable effort. Blowing a similar amount of air into a balloon would take a much greater effort. Lung compliance is aided by the production of a detergent-like substance called surfactant. Whenever a liquid and gas come into close contact with one another surface tension is generated. Surfactant reduces the surface tension that occurs where the alveoli meet pulmonary capillary blood flow in the lobule, thereby reducing the amount of energy required to inflate the alveoli. Surfactant is manufactured by type II alveolar cells, found in the alveoli.

Work of breathing is also required to overcome airway resistance. As air flows through the bronchial tree, resistance to airflow occurs as the gas molecules begin to collide with one another in the increasingly narrow airways. Despite these opposing forces, work of breathing accounts for less than 5% of total body energy expenditure. However, many lung diseases can affect lung compliance and airway resistance and, therefore, increase work of breathing. In asthma, for example, airway inflammation reduces the diameter of the airways and increases airway resistance. If the diameter of an airway is halved, resistance increases 16-fold. Lung diseases that damage lung tissue can also affect lung compliance. Any increase in airway resistance and lung compliance will inevitably increase work of breathing. In acute respiratory disease, work of breathing could account for up to 30% of total body energy expenditure (Levitzky *et al.*, 1990).

345

Volumes and capacities

Lung volumes and capacities measure or estimate the amount of air passing in and out of the lungs. Each individual has a total lung capacity (TLC), which is the total amount of air their lungs are capable of housing. Each individual's TLC will be dependent upon their age, sex and height. TLC can be subdivided into a range of potential or actual volumes of air. For example, the amount of air that passes in and out of the lungs during one breath is called the tidal volume V_T. After a normal, quiet breath the lungs will still have room for a deeper inspiration that could fill the lungs. This potential capacity for inspiration is referred to as inspiratory reserve volume (IRV). Likewise, after a normal, quiet breath, there remains the potential for a larger exhalation. This potential capacity of exhalation is referred to as expiratory reserve volume (ERV). If tidal volume increases, due to exercise for example, IRV and ERV would be reduced. Tidal volume, IRV and ERV can all be measured. However, because a small volume of air always remains in the lungs – even after maximal exhalation – TLC can only be estimated. This small volume of remaining air is called residual volume (RV). Because RV cannot be exhaled, the total amount of air that could possibly pass in and out of an individual's lungs is a combination of tidal volume, IRV and ERV, which collectively is referred to as vital capacity (see Figure 11.11).

Other important measures of lung volume include minute volume V_E, alveolar minute ventilation V_A and anatomical dead space V_D (see Table 11.3). Minute volume V_E is the amount of air breathed in each minute and is calculated by multiplying tidal volume V_T by respiration rate. In health, minute volume is around 6–8 mL per minute. However, only the air that travels beyond the terminal bronchioles will actually take part in gaseous exchange. For this reason the air present in the rest of the lungs is referred to as anatomical dead space V_D. Therefore, in order to ascertain exactly how much air is available for gaseous exchange, anatomical dead space must be accounted for. Alveolar minute ventilation V_A is calculated by subtracting anatomical dead space from minute volume, which in health would be approximately 4–6 mL per minute (Hickin *et al.*, 2013).

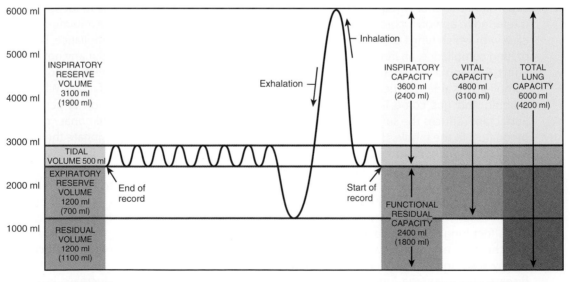

Figure 11.11 Diagrammatic description of the major lung volumes and capacities. *Source*: Tortora and Derrickson (2009). Reproduced with permission of John Wiley & Sons.

Table 11.3   Important lung volumes

Volume	Calculation
Minute volume V_E	Tidal volume (T_V) × Respiration rate e.g. 500 (T_V) × 12 = 6000 mL (V_E)
Alveolar minute ventilation V_A	[Tidal volume (T_V) – Anatomical dead space (V_D)] × Respiration rate e.g. [500 (T_V) – 150 (V_D)] × 12 = 4000 mL (V_A)

Source: Martini and Nath (2009). Reproduced with permission of Pearson Education Limited.

Clinical considerations

Spirometry and peak flow

Spirometry measures the force and volume of a maximum expiration after a full inspiration. The air the patient forces out is referred to as forced vital capacity (FVC). The volume the patient expired after 1 second is called forced expiratory volume in the first second (FEV_1). By comparing FEV_1 with FVC, the FEV_1:FVC ratio, the severity of airway obstruction can be ascertained. An FEV_1:FVC ratio of less than 80% is indicative of obstructive airways disease (Sheldon, 2005).

   Peak expiratory flow rate (PEFR), or 'peak flow', measures the extent of airway resistance. PEFR is the force of expiration in litres per minute. It measures the patient's maximum expiratory flow rate via their mouth. An inability to meet a predicted value based on age, sex and height could indicate increased airway resistance, as occurs during an asthma attack. PEFR provides a quick and simple assessment of the airways; however, regular peak flow measurements are more revealing than single arbitrary readings, and nurses should be mindful that PEFR is effort dependent (Talley and O'Connor, 2001).

Control of breathing

The rate and depth of breathing are controlled by the respiratory centres, which are found in the brainstem, within the areas called the medulla oblongata and pons (see Figure 11.12). The rate of breathing is set by the inspiratory centre of the medulla oblongata. The expiratory centre is thought to play a role in forced expiration. Also within the medulla oblongata there are specialised chemoreceptors that continually analyse carbon dioxide levels within cerebrospinal fluid. As levels of carbon dioxide rise, messages are sent via the phrenic and intercostal nerves to the diaphragm and intercostal muscles instructing them to contract. Another set of chemoreceptors found in the aorta and carotid arteries analyse levels of oxygen as well as carbon dioxide. If oxygen falls or carbon dioxide rises, messages are sent to the respiratory centres via the glossopharyngeal and vagus nerves, stimulating further contraction. Breathing is refined by the actions of the pneumotaxic and apneustic centres of the pons (see Figure 11.12). The pneumotaxic centre sends inhibitory signals to the medulla to slow breathing down, while the apneustic centre stimulates the inspiratory centres, lengthening inspiration. Both these actions fine-tune breathing and prevent the lungs from becoming overinflated. Throughout the day, whether at work, rest or play, respiration rate will change in order to meet the body's oxygen needs.

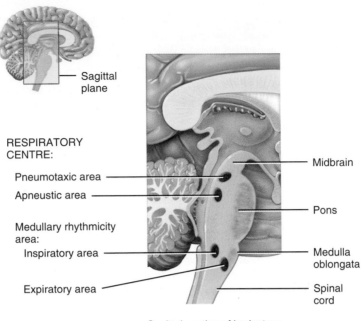

Sagittal plane

RESPIRATORY CENTRE:

Pneumotaxic area

Apneustic area

Medullary rhythmicity area:

    Inspiratory area

    Expiratory area

Midbrain

Pons

Medulla oblongata

Spinal cord

Sagittal section of brainstem

Figure 11.12 The respiratory centres of the brainstem. *Source*: Tortora and Derrickson (2009). Reproduced with permission of John Wiley & Sons.

Clinical considerations

Respiratory rate

In health, an adult's respiratory rate is normally between 12 and 16 respirations per minute. Although breathing is essentially a subconscious activity, the rate and depth of breathing can be controlled voluntarily or even stopped altogether, when swimming underwater for example. However, this voluntary control is limited, as the respiratory centres have a strong urge to keep breathing. Breathing can also be influenced by state of mind. The inspiratory area of the respiratory centres can be stimulated by both the limbic system and hypothalamus, two areas of the brain responsible for processing emotion. Fear, anxiety or even the anticipation of stressful activities can cause an involuntary increase in the rate and depth of breathing. Other factors that can influence breathing include pyrexia and pain. Because breathing is largely beyond an individual's control, any changes in respiration rate are clinically significant (Hogan, 2006).

External respiration
Gaseous exchange

External respiration only occurs beyond the respiratory bronchioles. External respiration is the diffusion of oxygen from the alveoli into pulmonary circulation (blood flow through the lungs) and the diffusion of carbon dioxide in the opposite direction. Diffusion occurs because gas molecules always move from areas of high concentration to low concentration. Each lobule of the

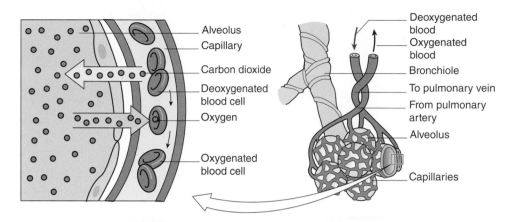

Figure 11.13   External respiration: exchange of oxygen and carbon dioxide within the lungs.

349

lung has its own arterial blood supply; this blood supply originates from the pulmonary artery, which stems from the right ventricle of the heart. The blood present in the pulmonary artery has been collected from systemic circulation and is therefore low in oxygen and relatively high in carbon dioxide. The amount (and therefore pressure) of oxygen in the alveoli is far greater than in the passing arterial blood supply. Oxygen, therefore, moves passively out of the alveoli and into pulmonary circulation and on towards the left-hand side of the heart. Because there is less carbon dioxide in the alveoli than in pulmonary circulation, carbon dioxide transfers into the alveoli ready to be exhaled (see Figure 11.13).

Factors influencing diffusion

It takes approximately 0.25 s for an oxygen molecule to diffuse from the alveoli into pulmonary circulation. However, there are various influencing factors that determine the rate by which oxygen and carbon dioxide diffuse between alveoli and pulmonary circulation. This is best explained by the use of Fick's law of diffusion, which uses an equation to determine the rate of diffusion (see Box 11.1). According to Fick's law, the rate of diffusion is determined by gas solubility/molecular weight, surface area, concentration difference and membrane thickness. The more soluble a gas is in water the easier it is for diffusion to occur. Oxygen and carbon dioxide are both soluble in water and therefore easily diffused; indeed, carbon dioxide is 20 times more soluble than oxygen. The most abundant gas in the atmosphere is nitrogen; however, nitrogen is highly insoluble in water and therefore very little diffuses into the bloodstream. The larger the surface area available for diffusion the greater the rate of diffusion will be. Large inhalations will recruit more alveoli, and a greater rate of diffusion occurs as a result. The greater the gas concentration difference between the alveoli and pulmonary circulation the faster that gas will diffuse. Because blood travelling towards the alveoli is deoxygenated there always remains a large difference in concentration of oxygen between the alveoli and pulmonary circulation. However, the rate of diffusion can be enhanced if this concentration difference is increased, by administering prescribed oxygen therapy for example. The final factor for consideration is membrane thickness. The further the distance gases have to travel the slower the diffusion will be. Conditions such as pulmonary oedema, in which fluid collects in the alveoli, result in an increased membrane thickness. The distance between alveoli and pulmonary circulation slows the rate of diffusion.

Box 11.1 Fick's law of diffusion

$$J = \frac{S}{wt_{mol}} \times A \times \frac{\Delta C}{t}$$

where

J is the rate of diffusion
S is the solubility
wt_{mol} is the molecular weight
A is the surface area
ΔC is the concentration difference
t is the membrane thickness.

Source: Hickin *et al.* (2013).

Clinical considerations

Sputum

Often, the nurse has the responsibility to examine and observe the sputum (sometimes this is called phlegm, secretions or expectorate) that a person may produce. At times the nurse is required to obtain a specimen of the person's sputum for microbiological analysis. The nurse must be able to carry out these important tasks safely and effectively. The skills required to do this include the ability to determine what is sputum and what are oral secretions (spit), the application of infection control activities and the ability to document findings accurately and report any concerns.

The production of sputum is an important part of a person's immune system. You may be required to ask the person you are caring for about their sputum production. The following questions can help generate important information:

- Is there anything that causes (provokes) you to produce sputum?
- When do you produce it?
- How often do you produce it?
- Can you describe it – what does it look like?
- Does your sputum have any particular smell?
- How much do you produce?
- The sputum you are producing at the moment, has this changed recently? If so, tell me about that.

It can be difficult for the person to provide you with answers concerning their sputum production. You can help them by asking them to measure it in relation to teaspoons, tablespoons or an egg cup. Understanding the sputum produced and describing and reporting its characteristics – for example, the consistency, the amount produced, the odour and its colour – can provide you with much information about the person you are caring for. Also note if the person producing the sputum did this with ease or difficulty, and if, after the specimen was produced, whether they became breathless or cyanotic.

If the person you are caring for needs to use a sputum pot, you must make sure that it is placed within their reach and that you offer them tissues and a receptacle to dispose of the used tissues. Disposing of sputum safely can help prevent and control infection; sputum is potentially an infectious body fluid. Care interventions include ensuring that the sputum pot is changed daily and that the lid is firmly closed when it is not in use. Used tissues and sputum pots must be carefully disposed of regardless of the care setting. Disposable, one-use-only sputum pots must be provided. Incineration is needed if sputum is infectious. Local policy and procedures must be adhered to.

Medicines management

Oxygen

Oxygen is a drug, which should be prescribed. Oxygen is used to treat hypoxaemia, not breathlessness. There is no evidence that oxygen relieves breathlessness in patients with normal or near-normal oxygen saturation readings.

The aim of oxygen therapy is to maintain a normal or near-normal oxygen saturation level and that this should be achieved on the lowest possible concentration of oxygen. The target oxygen saturation levels for acutely ill adults are 94–98% and 88–92% for those at risk of hypercapnic (excess carbon dioxide) failure – that is, patients living with chronic obstructive pulmonary disease.

Oxygen should only be administered by trained clinicians, and each patient on oxygen should have their oxygen saturations monitored regularly. For this reason it is essential that oxygen saturation reading equipment should be within easy reach of patients receiving oxygen therapy.

It is important that nurses use the correct delivery method in order to ensure the patient receives the correct prescription. Many oxygen prescriptions come in the form of a percentage. Venturi masks ensure that the patient receives the correct percentage of oxygen by mixing room air with pure oxygen. Venturi masks are available in the following concentrations – please ensure you include the correct flow rate to ensure the patient receives the correct dose:

24% – 2 L of oxygen per minute
28% – 4 L of oxygen per minute
35% – 8 L of oxygen per minute
40% – 10 L of oxygen per minute
60% – 15 L of oxygen per minute.

Simple oxygen masks do not deliver oxygen with such accuracy. They can deliver between 40% and 60% oxygen with a flow rate of 5–10 L of oxygen per minute. Flow rates of less than 5 L of oxygen per minute may lead to the build-up of carbon dioxide within the mask. Re-breather oxygen masks can deliver up to 90% oxygen and are very effective in emergency situations.

Nasal cannulae ensure a steady delivery of oxygen into the nasal cavity. Flow rates between 1 and 4 L of oxygen per minute will provide the patient with 24–40% oxygen. However, the actual volume of oxygen delivered will vary from patient to patient, as mouth breathing may dilute delivery. Flow rates greater than 4 L of oxygen per minute will provide greater concentrations of oxygen, but this may cause nasal dryness and discomfort.

Oxygen in the atmosphere is moist and humidified. Medical oxygen, on the other hand, is dry. Patients on long-term oxygen therapy may encounter nasal or oral dryness, which can cause discomfort. In such situations the medical team may consider using humidified (passed through water) oxygen.

See O'Driscoll *et al.* (2008).

Snapshot

Pulmonary tuberculosis

Leonard is a 28-year-old homeless man, who lives in a hostel in London. He was suffering with a chronic productive cough, which had lasted for most of the winter. One morning he coughed up a small amount of blood. He called into a local Urgent Care Centre, where he explained to the triage nurse that in addition to the haemoptysis he had also been experiencing night sweats.

Leonard is admitted to hospital with suspected pulmonary tuberculosis. Later, sputum samples and a chest X-ray confirm this diagnosis. He is commenced on oral rifampicin, isoniazid, pyrazinamide and ethambutol and placed in isolation.

Pulmonary tuberculosis is an infection of two phases. After the initial infection, damaged lung tissue is surrounded by a fibrous wall. Thereafter, the patient remains asymptomatic and non-contagious. On reinfection, however, the fibrous wall breaks down and the infection spreads quickly. Unless the individual is commenced on a strict antibiotic regime they will remain highly infectious. People at greatest risk of contracting tuberculosis are immunosuppressed people, people who have recently travelled to areas with high infection rates, people living in crowded conditions, homeless people and individuals who abuse drugs and alcohol.

It is essential that individuals with a diagnosis of tuberculosis adhere to their 6-month drug administration regime. Individuals taking the recommended antibiotic therapies are no longer infectious after 2 weeks. However, should an individual stop taking their medication they could develop drug-resistant tuberculosis.

See National Institute for Health and Clinical Excellence (2011).

Ventilation and perfusion

External respiration is most effective where there is an adequate supply of both oxygen and blood. In order to ensure a good enough supply of oxygen the alveoli have to be adequately ventilated. In health, an alveolar minute ventilation V_A of around 4 L is required. In order to ensure that an adequate supply of blood is reoxygenated, a plentiful supply of blood must be delivered to the lungs from the right ventricle of the heart; in other words, a pulmonary blood flow of around 5 L per minute. This ideal delivery of adequate amounts of both air and blood is referred to as the ventilation V_A:perfusion Q ratio. A normal V_A:Q ratio would be 4:5 or 0.8. Any disruption to either ventilation or pulmonary blood flow would lead to a V_A:Q mismatch and less oxygen diffusing into blood. For example, if someone hypoventilates and V_A falls below 4 L, then less blood would be reoxygenated. This would be described as a low V_A:Q ratio (i.e. 3:5 or 0.3). Another potential problem would be an inadequate pulmonary blood flow, due to an embolism for example. In such an instance, less blood is available to be reoxygenated and the V_A:Q ratio would become high (i.e. 4:3 or 1.34). In reality, however, the V_A:Q ratio differs throughout the lungs and depends upon a person's position (Margereson, 2001).

Transport of gases

Both oxygen and carbon dioxide are transported from the lungs to body tissues in blood. Both gases travel in blood plasma and haemoglobin, which is found within erythrocytes (red blood cells). Key gas transport terminology is summarised in Table 11.4.

Table 11.4   Definitions of important gas transport terminology

Gas transport term	Definition
Oxygen saturation (SaO_2)	The percentage of arterial haemoglobin carrying oxygen molecules $SpO_2 = SaO_2$ measured by a pulse-oximeter
Partial pressure of arterial oxygen (PaO_2)	The amount of oxygen dissolved in arterial blood plasma measured in kilopascals
Partial pressure of carbon dioxide ($PaCO_2$)	The amount of carbon dioxide dissolved in arterial blood plasma measured in kilopascals
Oxygen capacity	The potential space for oxygen transported by haemoglobin (Hb) per 100 mL of blood $Hb \times 1.39$ = oxygen capacity per 100 mL of blood
Arterial oxygen content (CaO_2)	The actual amount of oxygen in arterial blood carried by haemoglobin per 100 mL of arterial blood Arterial oxygen saturation (SaO_2) $\times$ oxygen capacity = oxygen content per 100 mL of arterial blood
Oxygen delivery (DO_2)	The actual amount of oxygen being delivered to body tissues based on cardiac output. Arterial oxygen content (CaO_2) $\times$ cardiac output = oxygen delivery (DO_2)
Oxygen consumption (VO_2)/oxygen extraction ratio	The amount of oxygen utilised by body tissues each minute

Transport of oxygen

The vast majority of oxygen, around 98.5%, is transported attached to haemoglobin in the erythrocyte (red blood cell). Each erythrocyte contains around 280 million haemoglobin molecules and each haemoglobin molecule has the potential to carry four oxygen molecules. The percentage of haemoglobin carrying oxygen is measured as oxygen saturation (SaO_2). The remaining 1.5% of oxygen is dissolved in blood plasma, and is often measured in kilopascals (PaO_2), which in health is around 11–13.5 kPa (82–101 mmHg). The delivery of oxygen, therefore, is also reliant upon the presence of an adequate supply of erythrocytes and haemoglobin. In health, the average male would possess between 15 and 18 g of haemoglobin for every 100 mL of blood. Each gram of haemoglobin can carry approximately 1.34 mL of oxygen. Therefore, a male with a haemoglobin of 16 g per dL would have the capacity to carry 21.44 mL of oxygen for every 100 mL of blood ($16 \times 1.34 = 21.44$). This volume of oxygen is referred to as oxygen capacity. However, it is rare for an individual's haemoglobin to be fully saturated with oxygen. The actual amount of oxygen being transported by haemoglobin is called oxygen content (CaO_2). Oxygen content is determined by oxygen saturation levels. In health, an individual's oxygen saturation level (SaO_2) would normally be between 97% and 99%. Therefore, a male with a haemoglobin of 16 g per dL and an SaO_2 of 98% would have an oxygen content of 21.01 mL (0.98×21.44). CaO_2 only provides the amount of available oxygen per 100 mL of blood. Multiplying CaO_2 by cardiac output will provide the amount of oxygen being delivered to all body tissues each minute.

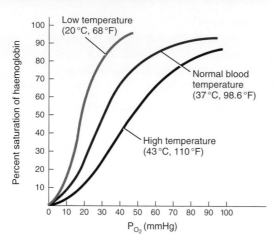

(a) Effect of temperature on affinity of haemoglobin for oxygen

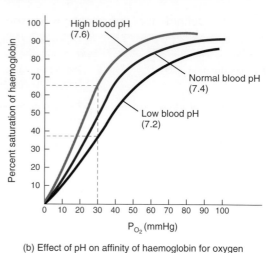

(b) Effect of pH on affinity of haemoglobin for oxygen

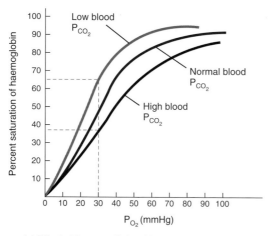

(c) Effect of P_{CO_2} on affinity of haemoglobin for oxygen

Figure 11.14   The oxyhaemoglobin dissociation curve: (a) at normal body temperature, arterial carbon dioxide levels and normal arterial blood pH; (b) with high or low arterial blood pH; (c) with high or low arterial carbon dioxide levels. *Source*: Tortora and Derrickson (2009). Reproduced with permission of John Wiley & Sons.

This volume of oxygen is called oxygen delivery (DO_2). In other words, if cardiac output is 5000 mL per minute, the aforementioned individual would have an oxygen delivery (DO_2) of 1050 mL per minute (21.01 mL per 100 mL of blood × 5000).

The relationship between oxygen attached to arterial haemoglobin (SaO_2) and oxygen dissolved in plasma (PaO_2) is described by the oxyhaemoglobin dissociation curve (see Figure 11.14). As PaO_2 falls, SaO_2 decreases in an S-shaped curve. If PaO_2 falls as low as 8 kPa (60 mmHg) SaO_2 will remain around 90%. Therefore, natural fluctuations in oxygenation, such as occur when singing, laughing and talking, will not result in dramatic reductions in oxygen saturations. The release of oxygen from haemoglobin can be increased by 2,3-diphosphoglycerate, which is released during hypoxia and high temperatures.

Clinical considerations

Measuring oxygen levels

Pulse oximeters gauge the percentage of haemoglobin carrying oxygen. This reading is called 'oxygen saturation' (SpO_2). In health, SpO_2 should be between 95 and 99%; however, tremors, anaemia, polycythaemia, cold extremities and nail varnish can all jeopardise an accurate reading. For this reason, SpO_2 should only be used in conjunction with other nursing observations (Clark *et al.*, 2006).

For a more accurate measure practitioners use an **arterial blood gas** reading. In such instances a sample of the patient's arterial blood is placed into a blood gas analyser. A printed or visual result is produced within seconds. Arterial blood gas readings provide information on pH, carbon dioxide and bicarbonate as well as oxygen. An oxygen saturation produced via blood gas analysis is referred to as SaO_2. In addition to an oxygen saturation, blood gas analysis measures the pressure exerted by the oxygen dissolved in plasma. In health, arterial oxygen should be around 11–13.5 kPa (82–101 mmHg) and is expressed as PaO_2 (partial pressure of arterial oxygen).

355

Table 11.5   The major types of hypoxia and their causes

Type of hypoxia	Cause
Stagnant or circulatory hypoxia	Heart failure, lack of cardiac output, leads to hypoxia
Haemic hypoxia	Lack of blood or haemoglobin (e.g. haemorrhage)
Histotoxic hypoxia	Poisoning (e.g. carbon monoxide inhalation)
Demand hypoxia	May occur when the demand for oxygen is high (e.g. during fever)
Hypoxic hypoxia	Hypoxia as a result of hypoxaemia

Hypoxia and hypoxaemia

Hypoxia is defined as a lack of oxygen within body tissues. Hypoxaemia is defined as a lack of oxygen within arterial blood. Naturally, hypoxaemia will lead to hypoxia as the tissues are receiving less oxygen. However, as respiration also relies on a fully functioning cardiovascular system, hypoxia can also occur even when arterial blood is fully oxygenated – see Table 11.5.

Transport of carbon dioxide

Just like oxygen, a small amount of carbon dioxide, around 10%, is transported in plasma. Carbon dioxide is also transported attached to haemoglobin, although only around 30% is transported that way. Nevertheless, haemoglobin has a greater affinity for carbon dioxide than for oxygen. Within the tissues this facilitates the release of oxygen as carbon dioxide is being created. However, as carbon dioxide levels increase (hypercapnia), the amount of oxygen binding to haemoglobin will be reduced. Any build-up of carbon dioxide will affect the oxyhaemoglobin dissociation curve by pulling the natural curve to the right, resulting in a greater risk of hypoxaemia. Conversely, a fall in carbon dioxide (hypocapnia) has the opposite effect (see Figure 11.14).

Acid–base balance

The majority of carbon dioxide is transported as bicarbonate ions (HCO_3^-). As carbon dioxide enters the erythrocyte it combines with water to form carbonic acid (H_2CO_3). H_2CO_3 then quickly dissociates into hydrogen ions (H^+) and bicarbonate ions (HCO_3). The formation of H_2CO_3 is very slow in plasma; in the red blood cell this reaction is speeded up by the presence of the enzyme carbonic anhydrase. The newly produced H^+ combines with haemoglobin, whereas HCO_3^- leaves the erythrocyte and enters blood plasma. For this reason, increased and decreased levels of H^+ can also influence the oxyhaemoglobin dissociation curve (see Figure 11.14). Within the lungs, as carbon dioxide leaves the pulmonary circulation and enters the alveoli this process is reversed. The transport of carbon dioxide as HCO_3^- is summarised by the following equation:

$$CO_2 + H_2O \leftrightarrow H_2CO_3 \leftrightarrow H^+ + HCO_3^-$$

carbon dioxide | water | carbonic acid | hydrogen ions | bicarbonate ions

Note that the arrow symbols indicate that the equation moves both ways. For example, at a tissue level the equation moves from left to right, whereas within the lungs it moves in the opposite direction.

Arterial blood pH is mainly influenced by the levels of H^+. If blood pH falls out of its optimum range of 7.35–7.45 an acid–base imbalance may occur. The respiratory system can help to maintain acid–base balance by controlling the expulsion and retention of carbon dioxide. When pH falls (acidosis), respiratory rate increases and more carbon dioxide is expelled. This results in greater amounts of hydrogen ions H^+ and HCO_3^- combining to form hydrogen ions (H+) and bicarbonate ions (HCO_3^-) combining to form carbonic acid (H_2CO_3). In other words, the above equation moves from right to left. H^+ levels are reduced, and as a result pH increases. H_2CO_3 is a weak acid and has only a minimal effect on blood pH. If blood pH rises, respiratory rate and depth may fall, resulting in the retention of carbon dioxide. The above equation will now move from left to right and more H^+ will be created.

Snapshot

Respiratory failure type 2

Mary is a 61-year-old woman living with chronic obstructive pulmonary disease. Mary had developed a chest infection that, despite a course of antibiotics prescribed by her GP, had become gradually worse over the past few days. Mary had become increasingly breathless and confused and disorientated. Concerned, Mary's daughter called for an ambulance and Mary was taken to the accident and emergency department. On admission the nurse noted that Mary had weak respiratory effort and that her oxygen saturations were less than 88%. An arterial blood gas confirmed that Mary was hypoxaemic (abnormally low oxygen levels in arterial blood) and hypercapnic (abnormally high carbon dioxide levels in arterial blood). Mary was immediately transferred to a respiratory high-dependency unit where she was commenced on non-invasive positive pressure ventilation.

The expulsion of carbon dioxide is reliant on good respiratory effort. People living with respiratory disease can experience respiratory muscle fatigue and weak respiratory effort, which leads to the build-up of carbon dioxide, a phenomenon known as respiratory failure type 2. High carbon dioxide levels can lead to confusion and disorientation and also disturb arterial acid–base balance. Indeed, patients with retained carbon dioxide are also described as having a respiratory acidosis.

Retained carbon dioxide can only be expelled through increased respiratory effort. Non-invasive ventilation seeks to enhance the rate and depth of breathing in order to expel excess carbon dioxide and correct respiratory acidosis.

See British Thoracic Society Standards of Care Committee (2002).

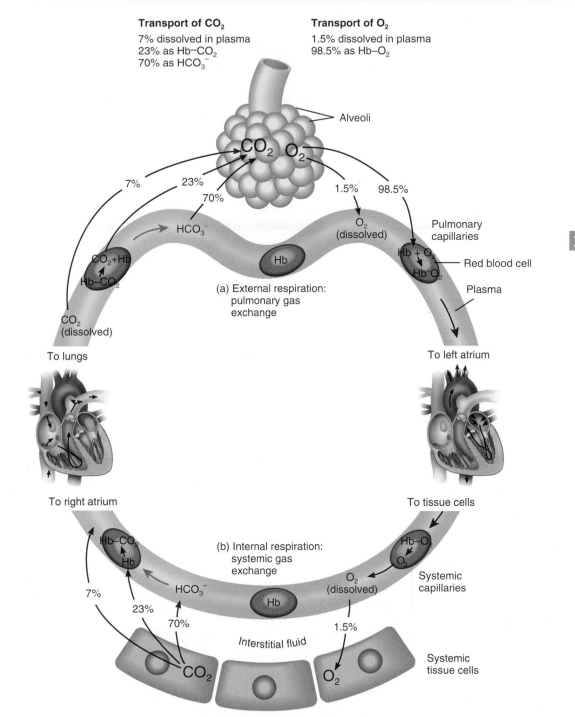

Transport of CO$_2$
7% dissolved in plasma
23% as Hb–CO$_2$
70% as HCO$_3^-$

Transport of O$_2$
1.5% dissolved in plasma
98.5% as Hb–O$_2$

Alveoli

CO$_2$ O$_2$

7%   23%
70%

1.5%   98.5%

HCO$_3^-$

O$_2$
(dissolved)

Pulmonary
capillaries

CO$_2$+Hb

Hb

Hb + O$_2$

Hb–CO$_2$

Hb O$_2$

Red blood cell

(a) External respiration:
pulmonary gas
exchange

Plasma

CO$_2$
(dissolved)

To lungs

To left atrium

To right atrium

To tissue cells

Hb–CO$_2$

Hb

(b) Internal respiration:
systemic gas
exchange

Hb–O$_2$

O$_2$

7%

HCO$_3^-$

Hb

O$_2$
(dissolved)

Systemic
capillaries

23%

70%

1.5%

Interstitial fluid

CO$_2$

O$_2$

Systemic
tissue cells

Figure 11.15 (a, b) External and internal respiration: oxygen and carbon dioxide follow their pressure gradients (Hb: haemoglobin). *Source*: Tortora and Derrickson (2009). Reproduced with permission of John Wiley & Sons.

Internal respiration

Internal respiration describes the exchange of oxygen and carbon dioxide between blood and tissue cells, a phenomenon governed by the same principles as external respiration. Cells utilise oxygen when manufacturing the cells' prime energy source, adenosine triphosphate (ATP). In addition to ATP the cells produce water and carbon dioxide. Because cells are continually using oxygen, its concentration within tissues is always lower than within blood. Likewise, the continual use of oxygen ensures that the level of carbon dioxide within tissue is always higher than within blood. As blood flows through the capillaries, oxygen and carbon dioxide follow their pressure gradients and continually diffuse between blood and tissue (see Figure 11.15). The concentration of oxygen in blood flowing away from the tissues back towards the heart is described as being deoxygenated. In reality, if measured, the oxygen saturation of venous blood would probably be around 75%. This means that only around 25% of oxygen content (CaO_2) leaves the bloodstream, leaving a plentiful supply. The actual amount of oxygen used by the tissues every minute is referred to as oxygen consumption (VO_2) or oxygen extraction ratio (see Table 11.4).

Conclusion

This chapter has examined the anatomy and physiology of the respiratory system. The respiratory system is divided into the upper and lower respiratory tracts. The lower respiratory tract consists of lung tissue and major airways. The structures within the lower respiratory tract are fragile and susceptible to infection, the main function of the upper respiratory tract therefore is the protection of the lower respiratory tract. The main function of the lower respiratory tract is the reoxygenation of arterial blood and the expulsion of excess carbon dioxide – a process called respiration. Respiration involves four distinct physiological processes: pulmonary ventilation (breathing), external respiration (gaseous exchange), transport of gases and internal respiration. Only the first two processes are the sole responsibility of the respiratory system, and effective respiration is also reliant upon a fully functioning cardiovascular system.

Glossary

Accessory muscles   Muscles not normally involved in respiration that can be utilised to increase inspiration.

Acid–base balance   The mechanisms by which the body maintains arterial blood pH between 7.35 and 7.45.

Alveolar minute ventilation   The amount of air reaching the respiratory portion of the lungs each minute.

Anatomical dead space   The portion of the airway not involved in the exchange of oxygen and carbon dioxide (also referred to as the conducting zone).

Aorta   First major blood vessel of arterial circulation. Emerges from the left ventricle of the heart.

Apex   The tip or highest point of a structure.

Apneustic centre   Area of the pons (brainstem), which influences inspiration.

Arytenoid cartilage   Cartilage tissue involved in the production of the voice.

Aspiration   The inhalation of solid or liquid substances.

Asthma   A chronic inflammatory disorder of the lungs. It causes the bronchi and bronchioles to become inflamed and constricted. As a result, airflow becomes obstructed, often resulting in a characteristic wheeze.

Bronchial artery   Artery that delivers oxygenated blood from the aorta to the bronchi and bronchioles.

Bronchial tree   The lower respiratory tract.

Bronchial veins   Veins that carry deoxygenated blood from the bronchi and bronchioles to the superior vena cava.

Bronchiole   Section of the lower respiratory tract found beyond the tertiary bronchus.

Cardiac notch   The space between the right and left lung occupied by the heart and its major blood vessels.

Carotid artery   Major artery supplying the brain, stems from the aorta.

Cartilage   Type of connective tissue that contains collagen and elastic fibres. Cartilage can stand up to both tension and compression.

Cerebrospinal fluid   Fluid found within the brain and spinal cord.

Chemoreceptors   Sensory cells sensitive to specific chemicals.

Chronic obstructive pulmonary disease   An umbrella term that encompasses chronic bronchitis, emphysema and chronic asthma – respiratory diseases which obstruct airflow.

Cilia   Hair-like extensions to the plasma membrane.

Clavicle   Anatomical term for the collarbone.

Conducting zone   Section of the airways which plays no part in the exchange of oxygen and carbon dioxide (also referred to as anatomical dead space).

Corniculate cartilage   Cartilage tissue involved in the production of the voice.

Cricoid cartilage   Ring of cartilage that forms the lower part of the larynx (voice box).

Cricothyroid ligament   Tissue that connects the thyroid cartilage and the cricoid cartilage, the main structures found in the larynx (voice box).

Cuneiform cartilage   Cartilage tissue involved in the production of the voice.

Diaphragm   Concave respiratory muscle that separates the lungs and the abdomen.

Diffusion   The passive movement of molecules or ions from a region of high concentration to low concentration until a state of equilibrium is achieved.

Embolism   Blockage of a blood vessel by a foreign substance or blood clot.

Epiglottis   Leaf-shaped piece of cartilage that sits atop the larynx.

Ethmoid bone   Sponge-like bone found in the skull. Forms part of the nasal septum.

Expectorate   To cough up and spit out mucus or sputum.

Expiratory reserve volume   The potential capacity for exhalation beyond a normal breath out.

External respiration   The process by which oxygen and carbon dioxide are exchanged between the lungs and blood.

Fauces   The opening into the pharynx from the oral cavity.

Glossopharyngeal nerve   Cranial nerve IV – nerve that communicates with tongue and pharynx. Also transmits information on oxygen and carbon dioxide levels.

359

Goblet cells   Mucus-secreting cells found in epithelial tissue.

Hypothalamus   Region of the diencephalon area of the brain. Responsible for the maintenance of homeostasis.

Hypoxaemia   A reduced amount of oxygen within arterial blood.

Hypoxia   A reduced amount of oxygen within the tissues.

Hypoventilation   Decreased ventilation – lack of air entering the alveoli.

Inspiratory reserve volume (IRV)   The potential capacity for inspiration beyond a normal breath in.

Intercostal nerves   Nerves that link the respiratory centre in the brainstem with the intercostal muscles.

Intercostal spaces   The anatomical spaces found between the ribs.

Internal respiration   The process by which oxygen is exchanged for carbon dioxide within the tissues.

Intrapulmonary pressure   The pressure exerted by all the gases present within the lungs.

Laryngopharynx   The lower section of the pharynx (throat).

Larynx   The physiological term for the voice box.

Limbic system   Part of the functional brain, which processes emotion.

Lingual tonsils   Tonsils found underneath the tongue.

Lobes   Distinct regions of the lungs. There are three lobes in the right lung and two in the left lung.

Lobule   Minute portion of lung tissue served by its own capillary.

Lower respiratory tract   All respiratory passages found below the larynx.

Lung compliance   The ease with which the lungs can be inflated.

Lymph nodules   Egg-shaped masses of lymph tissues that provide an immune response.

Lymph vessel   A vessel that carries lymphatic fluid. Part of the lymphatic system which forms part of the immune system.

Meatuses   Three passageways found within the nasal cavity.

Medulla oblongata   Area of the brainstem.

Minute volume (V_E)   The amount of air breathed in one minute.

Nasal cavity   Anatomical space within the nose.

Nasal conchae   Bones found within the nasal cavity.

Nasal septum   Structure that divides the nose into two nostrils.

Nasopharynx   The upper section of the pharynx (throat).

Non-keratinised stratified squamous epithelium   Cuboid or columnar-shaped cells that line and protect wet surfaces such as the mouth, oesophagus, epiglottis, tongue and vagina.

Oesophagus   Tubular vessel that carries food and liquid from the pharynx to the stomach.

Olfactory   Pertaining to the sense of smell.

Oropharynx   The middle section of the pharynx (throat).

Oxyhaemoglobin dissociation curve   An S-shaped curve that describes the relationship between the volume of oxygen attached to haemoglobin and the amount of oxygen dissolved in plasma.

Palatine tonsils   Tonsils found towards the rear of the oral cavity. Usually visible when the mouth is open.

Parietal pleura   Protective membrane which attaches the walls of the thorax to the lungs.

Pharyngeal tonsil   Tonsil that sits on the back wall of the pharynx. Also known as the adenoid.

Pharynx   Passageway for food and air, which links the nasal and oral cavity with the larynx. More commonly called the throat.

Phrenic nerve   Nerve that links the diaphragm to the respiratory centre in the brainstem.

Pleural space   The minute space between the visceral and parietal pleura.

Pneumotaxic centre   Portion of the medulla oblongata (brainstem) that influences inspiration.

Pons   Area of the brainstem.

Pseudostratified ciliated columnar epithelium   Covering or lining of internal body surface that contains cilia and mucus-secreting goblet cells.

Pulmonary artery   Artery that carries deoxygenated blood from the right-hand side of the heart towards the lungs.

Pulmonary oedema   A condition characterised by the leakage of fluid into the alveoli.

Pulmonary veins   Veins that carry oxygenated blood from the lungs back to the left-hand side of the heart.

Pulmonary ventilation   The process by which air enters and exits the lungs (breathing).

Pyrexia   Elevated temperature associated with fever.

Residual volume (RV)   A small amount of air that permanently remains in the lungs.

Respiratory zone   The portion of lung tissue involved in the exchange of oxygen and carbon dioxide.

Sternum   Flat bone which forms part of the thoracic cage. Protects the heart and lungs. Commonly referred to as the breastbone.

Surfactant   A detergent-like substance manufactured by cells of the alveoli, which reduces surface tension and increases lung compliance.

Systemic circulation   The flow of blood from the left ventricle and right atrium delivering oxygen to and collecting carbon dioxide from body tissues.

Thoracic cage   Framework of bones, which consists of the ribs, sternum (breastbone) and vertebrae (spine).

Thorax   The body trunk above the diaphragm and below the neck.

Thyroid cartilage   The outer wall of the larynx (voice box).

Tidal volume (V_T)   The volume of air that passes in and out of the lungs during one breath.

Tonsils   Lymph nodules found within the upper respiratory tract. They form part of the body's defence.

Total lung capacity (TLC)   The maximum amount of air that a person's lungs can accommodate.

Tracheostomy   A procedure in which an incision is made in the trachea to facilitate breathing.

Transport of gases   The process by which oxygen and carbon dioxide are delivered between the lungs and the tissues.

Upper respiratory tract   All structures of the respiratory system situated between the oral and nasal passageways and the larynx.

Vagus nerve   Cranial nerve X – major nerve in parasympathetic function. Also transmits information on oxygen and carbon dioxide levels.

Ventilation V_A: perfusion Q ratio   The ratio of blood and air delivery to the lungs every minute. Ideally 4 L of air to 5 L of blood.

Vestibule   The space inside the nasal cavity, just inside the nostrils.

Visceral pleura   Protective membrane that lines the lungs.

Vital capacity   The maximum potential for inspiration and expiration, measured in litres.

Vomer   Triangular-shaped bone that forms the base of the nasal cavity.

References

Brimblecombe, P. (1986) *Air Composition and Chemistry*, 2nd edn. Cambridge: Cambridge University Press.

British Thoracic Society and Scottish Intercollegiate Guidelines Network (2014). *SIGN 141: British Guideline on the Management of Asthma: A National Clinical Guideline*. London: BTS.

British Thoracic Society Standards of Care Committee (2002) Non-invasive ventilation in acute respiratory failure. *Thorax* **57**: 192–211.

Clark, A.P., Giuliano, K. and Chen, H. (2006) Pulse oximetry revisited: 'but his O_2 sat was normal!' *Clinical Nurse Specialist* **20**(6): 268–272.

Davies, A. and Moores, C. (2003) *The Respiratory System: Basic Science and Clinical Conditions*. Edinburgh: Churchill Livingstone.

Hickin, S., Renshaw, J. and Williams, R. (2013) *Crash Course: Respiratory System*, 4th edn. Edinburgh: Mosby.

Higginson, R. and Jones, B. (2009) Respiratory assessment in critically ill patients: airway and breathing, *British Journal of Nursing* **18**(8): 456–461.

Hogan, J. (2006) Why don't nurses monitor the respiratory rates of patients? *British Journal of Nursing* **15**(9): 489–492.

Levitzky, M.G., Cairo J.M. and Hall, S.M. (1990) *Introduction to Respiratory Care*. London: W.B. Saunders.

Lumb, A.B. (2005) *Nunn's Applied Respiratory Physiology*, 6th edn. Oxford: Butterworth-Heinemann.

Lutgens, F.K. and Tarbuck, E.J. (2001) *The Atmosphere: An Introduction to Meteorology*, 8th edn. Upper Saddle River, NJ: Prentice Hall.

MacDuff, A., Arnold, A. and Harvey, J. (2010) Management of spontaneous pneumothorax: British Thoracic Society pleural disease guideline 2010. *Thorax* **65**: ii18–ii31.

Margereson, C. (2001) Anatomy and physiology. In Esmond, G. (ed.), *Respiratory Nursing*. Edinburgh: Baillière Tindall.

Martini, F.H. and Nath, J.L. (2009) *Fundamentals of Anatomy and Physiology*, 8th edn. San Francisco, CA: Pearson Benjamin Cummings.

McGrath, B. (2014) *Comprehensive Tracheostomy Care: The National Tracheostomy Safety Project Manual*. Chichester: John Wiley & Sons, Ltd.

Nair, M. and Peate, I. (2009). *Fundamentals of Applied Pathophysiology: An Essential Guide for Nursing Students*. Oxford: John Wiley & Sons, Ltd.

National Institute for Health and Clinical Excellence (2011) *Tuberculosis: Clinical Diagnosis and Management of Tuberculosis, and Measures for its Prevention and Control*. NICE Guideline CG117. NICE, London.

Ochs, M., Nyengaard, A.J., Knudsen, L. Voigt, M., Wahlers, T., Richter, J. and Gundersen, H.J. (2004) The number of alveoli in the human lung. *American Journal of Respiratory and Critical Care Medicine* **169**: 120–124.

O'Driscoll, B.R., Howard, L.S. and Davison, A.G. (2008) Guideline for emergency oxygen use in adult patients. *Thorax* **63**(supplement VI).

Sheldon, R.L. (2005) Pulmonary function testing. In Wilkins, R.L. and Krider, S.J. (eds), *Clinical Assessment in Respiratory Care*, 5th edn. St Louis, MO: Elsevier Mosby.

Simpson, H. (2006) Respiratory assessment. *British Journal of Nursing* **15**(9): 484–488.

Talley, N.J. and O'Connor, S. (2001) *Clinical Examination: A Systematic Guide to Physical Diagnosis*, 4th edn. Oxford: Blackwell Science.

Tortora, G.J. and Derrickson, B.H. (2009) *Principles of Anatomy and Physiology*, 12th edn. Hoboken, NJ: John Wiley & Sons, Inc.

Further reading

British Thoracic Society

https://www.brit-thoracic.org.uk

The British Thoracic Society website provides a range of information and clinical guidance that is based on best available evidence. Their guidance is essential for all health professionals that wish to provide gold-standard care for their respiratory patients. British Thoracic Society guidance will also ensure that your academic work is up to date.

British Lung Foundation

https://www.blf.org.uk/Home

The British Lung Foundation website provides a wealth of information for patients with respiratory disease. By accessing this site you can gain insight into the support available for people living with lung disease, which may help you in practice and in your academic studies.

Respiratory Education UK

https://www.educationforhealth.org/REUK/

The Respiratory Education UK website has access to a range of courses and information, which you may wish to utilise for your studies. There are also quizzes and exercises, which can test your understanding.

Activities

Multiple choice questions

1. Which of the following structures is not found in the upper respiratory tract?
   (a) palatine tonsils
   (b) turbinates
   (c) carina
   (d) fauces

2. Which of the following structures is found in the respiratory zone?
   (a) alveolar ducts
   (b) terminal bronchioles
   (c) tertiary bronchus
   (d) trachea

3. Which of the following statements on pulmonary ventilation is true?
   (a) the diaphragm is responsible for 75% of thoracic expansion
   (b) expiration is dependent upon external intercostal muscle activity
   (c) intrapulmonary pressure is always greater than atmospheric pressure
   (d) the diaphragm and external intercostal muscles are two major accessory muscles

4. Which of the following statements on work of breathing is true?
    (a) increased airway diameter increases airway resistance
    (b) surfactant increases alveolar surface tension
    (c) lung disease can increase work of breathing
    (d) in health, work of breathing accounts for 50% of total body energy expenditure
5. Where are the respiratory centres?
    (a) the medulla oblongata and pons
    (b) the hypothalamus
    (c) the limbic system
    (d) cerebral cortex
6. Which of the following could increase the rate of breathing?
    (a) increased carbon dioxide levels
    (b) decreased oxygen levels
    (c) pyrexia
    (d) all of the above
7. Which of the following statements on external respiration is true?
    (a) the concentration of oxygen is greater in pulmonary circulation than in the alveoli
    (b) the concentration of carbon dioxide is greater in the alveoli than in pulmonary circulation
    (c) carbon dioxide diffuses from the alveoli into pulmonary circulation
    (d) oxygen diffuses from the alveoli into pulmonary circulation
8. Reduced levels of oxygen in blood is called
    (a) hypoxaemia
    (b) hypercapnia
    (c) hypocapnia
    (d) hypoxia
9. Which of the following can be transported attached to haemoglobin?
    (a) oxygen
    (b) carbon dioxide
    (c) hydrogen ions
    (d) all of the above
10. The amount of oxygen utilised by cells is referred to as
    (a) oxygen content (CaO_2)
    (b) oxygen delivery (DO_2)
    (c) oxygen consumption (VO_2)
    (d) oxygen capacity

True or false

1. The pharynx is found in the upper respiratory tract.
2. The trachea consists of three to five C-shaped cartilage rings.
3. The conduction region of the lungs receives oxygenated blood from capillaries that stem from the bronchial arteries, which originate from the aorta.
4. Boyle's law states that the amount of pressure exerted is inversely proportional to the size of its container.
5. If the diameter of an airway lumen is halved, resistance to airflow increases 16-fold.
6. The respiratory centres are found within the hypothalamus.

7. It takes approximately 1 min for an oxygen molecule to diffuse out of alveoli and into the pulmonary circulation.
8. Each erythrocyte contains around 280 million haemoglobin molecules.
9. Around 90% of carbon dioxide is transported in blood plasma.
10. Stagnant or circulatory hypoxia is caused by hypoxaemia.

Label the diagram 1

Label the diagram using the following list of words:

Visceral pleura, Parietal pleura, Pleural cavity, Right primary bronchus, Right secondary bronchus, Right tertiary bronchus, Right bronchiole, Right terminal bronchiole, BRANCHING OF BRONCHIAL TREE, Trachea, Primary bronchi, Secondary bronchi, Tertiary bronchi, Bronchioles, Terminal bronchioles, Location of carina, Left primary bronchus, Left secondary bronchus, Left tertiary bronchus, Left bronchiole, Left terminal bronchiole, Diaphragm, Larynx, Trachea

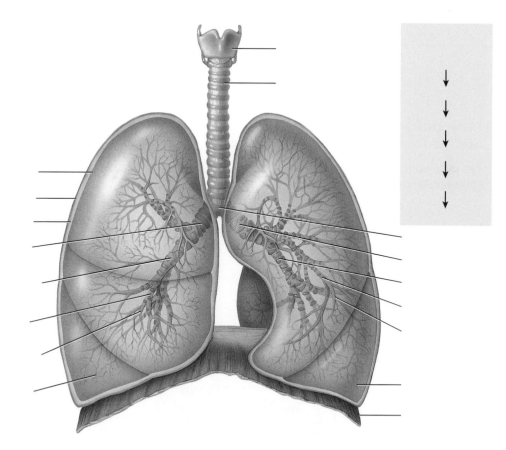

Label the diagram 2

Label the diagram using the following list of words:

Pulmonary venule, Elastic connective tissue, Pulmonary capillary, Visceral pleura, Alveoli, Terminal bronchiole, Pulmonary arteriole, Lymphatic vessel, Respiratory bronchiole, Alveolar ducts, Alveolar sac

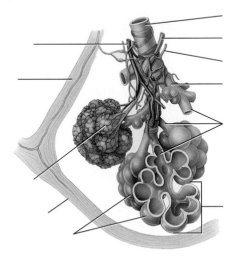

Label the diagram 3

Label the diagram using the following list of words:

Sternocleidomastoids, Scalenes, External intercostals, Diaphragm, Internal intercostals, Abdominal muscles, Inspiration, Expiration

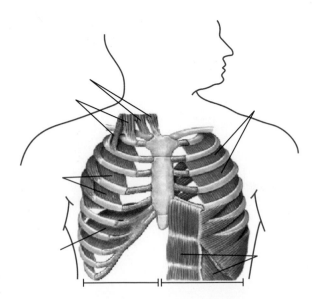

Crossword

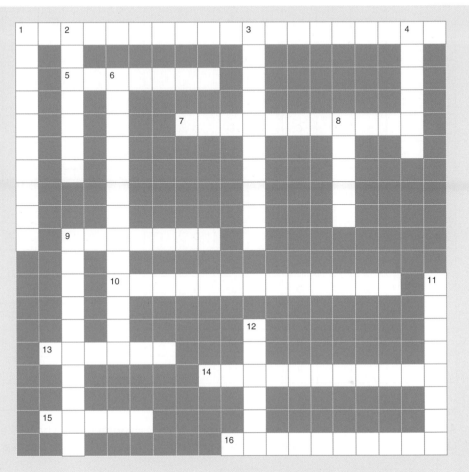

Across:

1. The process of gaseous exchange (8, 11).
5. Structure found in a lobule (7).
7. The amount of air inspired and expired during one breath (5, 6).
9. Diminished amount of oxygen in tissues (7).
10. Waste gas disposed by lungs (6, 7).
13. Voice box (6).
14. Main carrier of oxygen in blood (11).
15. _____ law of diffusion (5).
16. Fast respiration rate (10).

Down:

1. Breathing out (10).
2. Connects the larynx to the bronchi (7).
3. Reduces surface tension in alveoli (10).
4. Gas essential for life (6).
6. Total lung volume minus residual volume (5, 8).
8. Your right lung has three, your left lung has two (5).
9. Diminished amount of oxygen in blood (10).
11. Difficulty in breathing (8).
12. Protective layer of the lungs (6).

Word search

G	N	S	T	I	M	H	A	A	N	I	R	A	C	S
A	O	D	P	V	J	U	X	R	C	W	K	L	A	M
Z	I	O	I	I	Y	L	T	I	U	K	L	O	R	M
Q	T	X	O	F	R	I	A	U	Y	E	C	V	B	G
W	A	Y	O	C	F	O	D	R	P	X	L	E	O	B
S	L	G	U	P	H	U	M	G	Y	S	B	P	N	A
G	I	E	T	R	Y	N	S	E	W	N	D	O	D	I
N	T	N	E	R	F	H	M	I	T	K	X	L	I	M
U	N	E	E	D	X	I	D	T	O	R	D	Q	O	E
L	E	N	R	Y	L	F	G	H	J	N	Y	H	X	A
A	V	B	R	O	N	C	H	I	O	L	E	S	I	X
Z	R	Y	E	I	T	R	A	C	H	E	A	H	D	O
X	V	V	O	R	O	P	H	A	R	Y	N	X	E	P
R	L	S	U	R	F	A	C	T	A	N	T	U	M	Y
A	D	N	O	I	T	A	R	I	P	S	E	R	B	H

Alveoli, Bronchioles, Carbon dioxide, Carina, Diffusion, Hypoxaemia, Hypoxia, Larynx, Lungs, Oropharynx, Oxygen, Pleura, Respiration, Spirometry, Surfactant, Sputum, Trachea, Ventilation

Fill in the blanks

Lungs are divided into distinct regions called _____. The heart sits in a space called the _____, which sits between both lungs. Each lung is protected by two membranes, called the _____ and parietal _____. The lower respiratory tract starts at the _____. At a point called the _____ the airways subdivide into right and left _____, which divide again into _____. The next branch of the bronchial tree is the _____, which all lead to a network of _____. Eventually airways terminate at a _____. From this point forward this region of the airways is referred to as a _____. Within this region the airways subdivide further into _____, _____ and _____.

cardiac notch, alveolar ducts, primary bronchi, visceral, tertiary bronchi, trachea, alveoli, carina, bronchioles, lobes, lobule, secondary bronchi, pleura, terminal bronchiole, respiratory bronchioles

Find out more

1. How is a tracheostomy performed and why might a patient need one?
2. Make a list of what you consider to be the key respiratory assessments a nurse must carry out.
3. Discuss the impact breathlessness may have on an individual's psychological well-being.
4. What is the role of the nurse in respect to caring for a patient with an acute respiratory failure?
5. Discuss the role of the nurse in reducing the impact of respiratory disease in the community.
6. What advice should the nurse provide for patients prescribed bronchodilator and steroid therapy?
7. Investigate arterial blood gas readings – why might they be useful for nurses working in high-dependency or intensive-care settings?
8. What would the key nursing care interventions be when caring for a patient with a pneumothorax?
9. What is the role of the nurse and other healthcare professionals in the prevention of hospital-acquired pneumonia?
10. Discuss the role of the dietician in the care of a patient with a long-term respiratory illness.

Conditions

The following is a list of conditions that are associated with the respiratory system. Take some time and write notes about each of the conditions. You may make the notes taken from text books or other resources (e.g. people you work with in a clinical area), or you may make the notes as a result of people you have cared for. If you are making notes about people you have cared for you must ensure that you adhere to the rules of confidentiality.

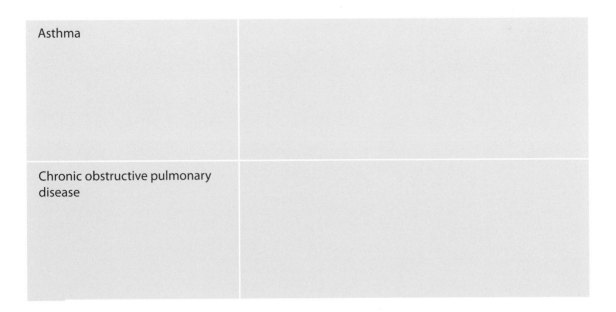

Asthma	
Chronic obstructive pulmonary disease	

Pulmonary tuberculosis

Lung cancer

Cystic fibrosis

Chapter 12

The reproductive systems

Ian Peate

Test your prior knowledge

- Where does fertilisation occur?
- What are the finger-like projections at the end of the fallopian tubes called?
- What is the name of the male reproductive organ?
- The contents of the scrotal sac sit outside of the abdominal cavity. Why?
- What is the inner layer of the uterus called?
- Describe the role and function of the hormone testosterone.
- A woman is likely to fall pregnant at what stage of the menstrual cycle?
- What is the term for surgical removal of the uterus, ovaries and fallopian tubes?
- What is the function of the prostate gland?
- What are the functions of the testes?

Learning outcomes

After reading this chapter you will be able to:

- Describe the male reproductive organs
- Describe the female reproductive organs
- Understand the role and functions of the male reproductive system
- Understand the role and functions of the female reproductive system
- Provide an overview of the role and functions of the various hormones associated with the male and female reproductive systems
- Outline the phases of the menstrual cycle

Fundamentals of Anatomy and Physiology: For Nursing and Healthcare Students, Second Edition. Edited by Ian Peate and Muralitharan Nair.
© 2017 John Wiley & Sons, Ltd. Published 2017 by John Wiley & Sons, Ltd.
Student companion website: www.wileyfundamentalseries.com/anatomy
Instructor companion website: www.wiley.com/go/instructor/anatomy

Body map

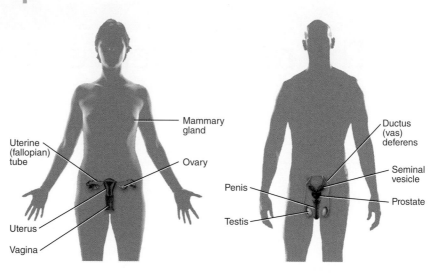

Mammary gland

Uterine (fallopian) tube

Ovary

Ductus (vas) deferens

Seminal vesicle

Penis

Prostate

Uterus

Testis

Vagina

Introduction

In men and women the reproductive systems are the only systems that differ in terms of structure and function. At certain times in a person's life the reproductive systems are the only systems that undergo specific changes.

Reproduction is one of the most important and essential attributes of living organisms; all living organisms multiply in order to form new individuals of their own kind through reproduction. One generation of living organisms gives rise to the next generation as they reproduce. Reproduction is a function essential for the life of the species (McGuinness, 2013). In humans, reproduction is sexual; this means that children are produced as a consequence of male and female mating.

Fertilisation occurs inside the body of the female; the human sexual organs are dedicated to this. The reproductive systems do not work in isolation; they work together with body systems in order to maintain homeostasis with other body systems.

Sexual reproduction usually concludes with the production of children for the continued existence of the species, as well as passing on hereditary characteristics from generation to generation. The male and female reproductive systems are responsible for contributing to the events that lead to fertilisation. When this has occurred, the female reproductive organs then take on the responsibility for developing and nurturing the human and giving birth. The testes and ovaries produce sperm and ova respectively, as well as the hormones required for the development, upkeep and performance of the organs of reproduction and other organs and tissues.

This chapter provides an overview of the structure and functions of both male and female reproductive systems. The anatomical systems of the male and female, unlike any of the other anatomical systems in the body, differ in males and females (McGuiness, 2013).

The male and female reproductive systems are made up of the reproductive organs. In the male the organs include the testes, accessory ducts, accessory glands and the penis. In the female the organs include the uterus, uterine tubes, ovaries, vagina and the vulva.

The male reproductive system

The male reproductive system, being generally outside of the body, is more obvious than the female reproductive system; there are, however, internal and external structures. Male reproductive organs, working in unison with other body systems (e.g. the neuroendocrine system), make the hormones that are essential in biological development and sexual behaviour, performance and actions. In the male these organs also include and are central to the function of the urinary system. The male reproductive system is shown in Figure 12.1.

There are a number of functions that are associated with the male reproductive system:

- to produce, maintain and transport the sperm (the male reproductive cells) and the fluid semen;
- to eject sperm from the penis;
- to manufacture and secrete the male sex hormones.

The major structures of the male reproductive system include the testes, the external genitalia, incorporating the penis, scrotum, reproductive tract and a number of ducts responsible for the transportation of the sperm from the testes to the penis and outside the body; there are also two seminal vesicles, bulbourethral glands and the prostate gland.

373

The testes

In utero the testes are developed in the abdominal cavity of the foetus. They then traverse the inguinal canal, entering the scrotal sac. The testes are suspended in the scrotal sac, hanging one on either side of the penis, and it is usual for one to hang lower than the other – this is a normal

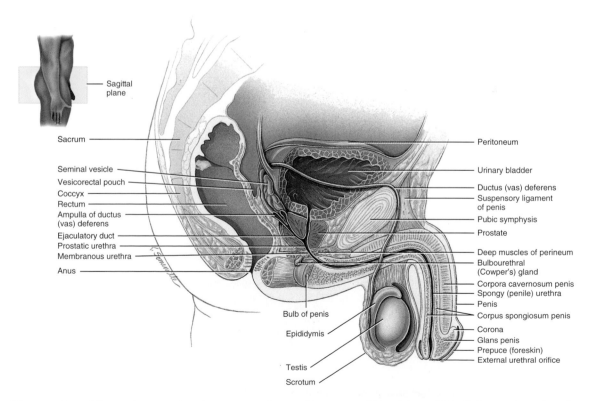

Figure 12.1   The male reproductive system. *Source*: Tortora and Derrickson (2009). Reproduced with permission of John Wiley & Sons.

finding. If sperm is to be viable it is essential that production is made at a temperature lower than the normal body temperature, and for this reason the testes in the scrotal sac are external to the body.

The key functions of the testes are to:

- produce sperm (spermatozoa);
- produce the male sex hormones (e.g. testosterone).

The testes are small oval-shaped organs measuring approximately 5 cm long and 2.5 cm wide with a layer of serous fibrous connective tissue surrounding them. There are three layers that cover the testes:

1. tunica vaginalis
2. tunica albuginea
3. tunica vasculosa.

The testes are divided into approximately 250–300 compartments or lobules. Inside each compartment is a collection of tightly coiled hollow tubes known as the seminiferous tubules. There are usually between one and four seminiferous tubules, and it is in these tubules where sperm is produced in the form of sperm stem cells (see Figure 12.2). There are spaces located

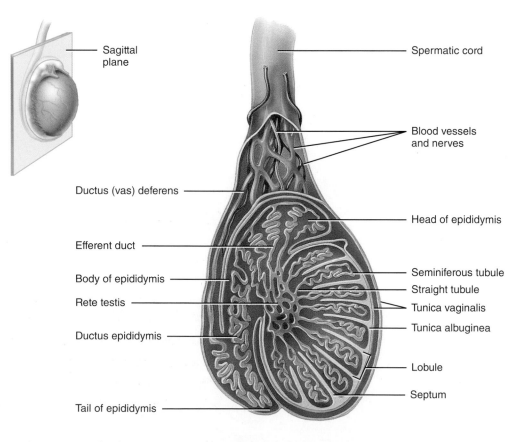

Figure 12.2   A testicle demonstrating seminiferous tubules. *Source*: Tortora and Derrickson (2009). Reproduced with permission of John Wiley & Sons.

between the tubules, and in these spaces is a cluster of cells called the Leydig cells that synthesise and secrete the hormone testosterone, as well as other androgens.

The seminiferous tubules have an outer and inner layer. The outer layer is composed of a smooth layer of muscle cells and an inner epithelial layer of cells called the Sertoli cells. Sperm cells, in their various stages of development, are stored in the spaces between the Sertoli cells. Mature sperm are found in the lumen of the seminiferous tubules. The key function of the Sertoli cells is to nurture and control the developing sperm; these cells are sometimes referred to as the nurse or mother cells and are sperm helper cells. The Sertoli cells have several functions, including phagocytosis, secretion of fluid that allows the sperm to develop and be transported, and providing a means whereby the developing sperm can be nourished.

Clinical considerations

Cryptorchidism

Undescended testes (cryptorchidism) is a common childhood condition where the child is born without both testes in the scrotal sac. In the majority of cases no action will be required, as the testes will migrate down into the scrotum during the first 3–6 months. There are, however, a small number of cases where the testes remain undescended unless treated. Cryptorchidism does not present any immediate health problems; the parent(s) should contact the GP if at any point they notice the boy's testes are not within the scrotal sac.

In utero the testes develop inside the child's abdomen prior to slowly moving down into the scrotal sac from about 2 months before birth. The exact reason why some boys are born with undescended testes is not fully understood, but risk factors that have been identified include a relationship with low birth weight, being born prematurely (before the 37th week of pregnancy) and having a family history of undescended testicles.

In most cases, the testicle(s) will move down into the scrotum naturally; if this is not the case, treatment is usually recommended (e.g. orchidopexy). Boys with undescended testicles may have problems associated with fertility, and there is also an increased risk of the boy developing testicular cancer.

Spermatogenesis

Sperm production occurs in the seminiferous tubules of the testes and is called spermatogenesis (see Figure 12.3). Spermatogenesis usually commences around puberty and continues for the rest of a man's life. It is usual for a young healthy man to be capable of producing many hundred million sperm daily.

Spermatogenesis is a complex activity, it has been estimated that it can take approximately 65–75 days to occur. Figure 12.3 highlights the fact that spermatogenesis (the life of a single sperm) begins with the spermatogonia that contains the diploid ($2n$) number of chromosomes.

The spermatogonia divide continually as a result of mitotic division to produce cells that are called primary spermatocytes with 46 chromosomes. Some spermatogonia stay close to the basement membrane of the seminiferous tubule, acting as a pool of cells poised to take part in future sperm production.

Division occurs again as a result of some spermatogonia breaking away from the basement membrane developing, differentiating and changing. Primary spermatocytes are produced with 46 chromosomes. Meiosis then occurs, with the emergence of secondary spermatocytes that now have 23 chromosomes each.

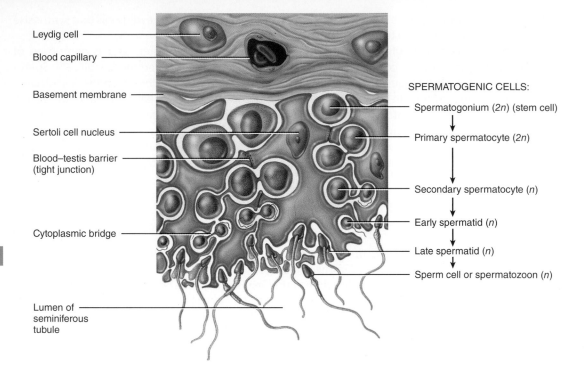

Leydig cell

Blood capillary

Basement membrane

Sertoli cell nucleus

Blood–testis barrier
(tight junction)

Cytoplasmic bridge

Lumen of
seminiferous
tubule

SPERMATOGENIC CELLS:

Spermatogonium (2n) (stem cell)

Primary spermatocyte (2n)

Secondary spermatocyte (n)

Early spermatid (n)

Late spermatid (n)

Sperm cell or spermatozoon (n)

Figure 12.3   Stages of spermatogenesis. *Source*: Tortora and Derrickson (2009). Reproduced with permission of John Wiley & Sons.

Spermatids are produced with the next stage of cell division. These then become spermatozoa or sperm cells; this stage is the final stage of spermatogenesis. The formed sperm cells have 23 chromosomes each, which is half the number required to begin human development. The remaining 23 chromosomes that are required are provided by the egg (ova) of a woman. When the sperm and ovum unite, the result of conception (conceptus) will have the required 46 chromosomes.

The sperm are released from the Sertoli cells, entering the lumen of the seminiferous tubules. The sperm are pushed along the various ducts located within the testes.

Sperm

There are approximately 300 million sperm that mature each day (Tortora and Derrickson, 2012). Each sperm cell is usually equipped with various structures that allow it to be able to penetrate the ovum. The head of the sperm cell contains a fluid that is composed of enzymes, assisting the sperm with its job of penetration, which then results in fertilisation (see Figure 12.4).

Once the sperm are formed, they travel up into the epididymis via a system of very small ducts that are known as the rete testes. These small ducts are C-shaped structures that unite from the back to the epididymis, which is positioned on the upper aspect of the testes. The crescent-shaped coiled epididymis is akin to a holding place that matures the sperm, taking on nutrients and growing for a number of weeks before travelling further. As the sperm mature further they develop the ability to move spontaneously and actively (motility).

The sperm's final stage is arrival at the vas deferens. The vas deferens emerges at the epididymis and twists up beyond the symphysis pubis and the urinary bladder. There are two vas deferens

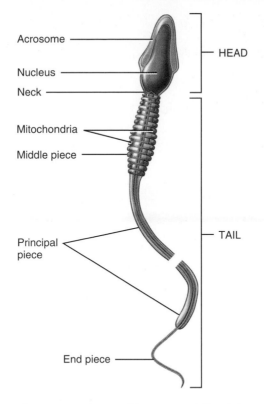

Figure 12.4 Components of a sperm. *Source*: Tortora and Derrickson (2009). Reproduced with permission of John Wiley & Sons.

arising from each testicle; they join at the back of the bladder. Each vas deferens merges with one seminal vesicle; this seminal vesicle contains the fluids necessary at the time of ejaculation. The fluids from the vas deferens and seminal vesicles are released into the ejaculatory ducts that are located within the prostate gland.

The prostate gland also secretes fluids that are found in the ejaculate. The fluid secreted is a milky alkaline fluid providing a friendly environment for sperm to survive, preparing them for survival in the acidity of the vagina. The ejaculatory ducts connect to the urethra, where the sperm will be ejaculated during orgasm as a result of sexual intercourse or masturbation. Once the sperm is ejaculated it is unusual for it to survive longer than 48 h within the female reproductive tract.

The testes and hormonal influences

The performance of the testes and their ability to function effectively are also under the influence of several hormones, the male sex hormones.

The male sex hormones are known as androgens. The majority of androgens are produced in the testes, although the adrenal cortex (located in the adrenal gland) is also responsible for producing a small amount. Testosterone is the main androgen produced by the testes. This hormone is essential for the growth and maintenance of the male sexual organs as well as the secondary sex characteristics (e.g. pitch of voice, musculature and body hair) and for effective spermatogenesis. It also encourages metabolism, growth of muscles and bone, as well as libido (sexual desire).

There is a small amount of testosterone secreted by the testes *in utero*; after birth, little testosterone is secreted until the male reaches puberty. With the onset of puberty the hypothalamus

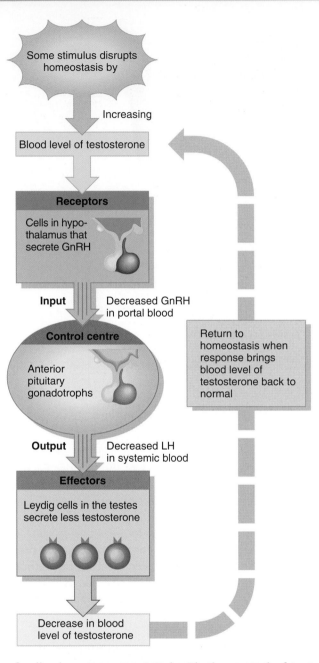

Figure 12.5   Negative feedback system associated with the control of testosterone in the blood. *Source*: Tortora and Derrickson (2009). Reproduced with permission of John Wiley & Sons.

intensifies its secretion of gonadotrophin-releasing hormone (GnRH). As GnRH is released, this stimulates the anterior pituitary gland to release and increase its discharge of luteinising hormone (LH). These hormones work on the negative feedback systems controlling the secretion of testosterone in the blood and the production of sperm (spermatogenesis) (see Figure 12.5).

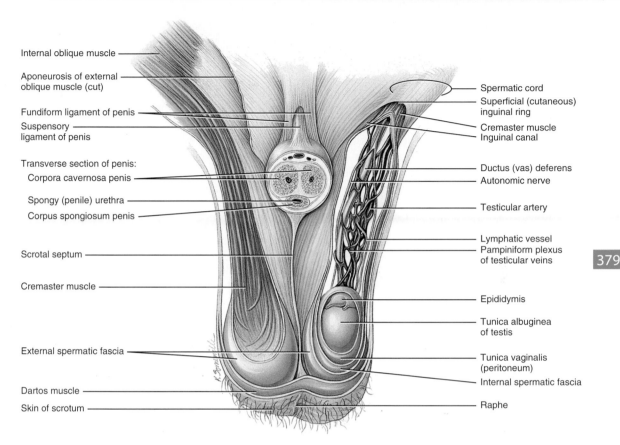

Internal oblique muscle

Aponeurosis of external oblique muscle (cut)

Fundiform ligament of penis

Suspensory ligament of penis

Transverse section of penis:
Corpora cavernosa penis

Spongy (penile) urethra

Corpus spongiosum penis

Scrotal septum

Cremaster muscle

External spermatic fascia

Dartos muscle

Skin of scrotum

Spermatic cord

Superficial (cutaneous) inguinal ring

Cremaster muscle
Inguinal canal

Ductus (vas) deferens
Autonomic nerve

Testicular artery

Lymphatic vessel
Pampiniform plexus of testicular veins

Epididymis

Tunica albuginea of testis

Tunica vaginalis (peritoneum)
Internal spermatic fascia

Raphe

379

Anterior view of scrotum and testes and transverse section of penis

Figure 12.6 The scrotum and testes. *Source*: Tortora and Derrickson (2009). Reproduced with permission of John Wiley & Sons.

The scrotum

The scrotal sac is likened to a loose bag of skin hanging between the thighs, anterior to the anus; this is a supporting structure that is suspended from the root of the penis. On the outside the scrotum usually appears as a single sac of skin that is separated into two portions by a ridge in the middle known as the raphe. From the inside the scrotum is divided into two sacs separated by a scrotal septum with a testicle in each (see Figure 12.6).

The scrotum assists with control of the temperature of the testes. The most favourable temperature for sperm production is approximately 2–3°C below core body temperature; however, too low a temperature can also impact on spermatogenesis.

Several mechanisms come into play when adjusting the position of the testes in the scrotum in relation to the body. When the temperature of the testes is too low (if the ambient temperature falls), the scrotum reacts in such a way that it contracts, bringing the testes up closer to the body. Conversely, if the testicular temperature is too high, then the scrotum relaxes, enabling the testes to descend, moving them further away from the body, exposing surface area and providing a faster dispersion of heat.

Snapshot

Testicular torsion

Anil, a 17-year-old, has been playing squash, and during the game his opponent's racquet hit him the groin with some force. This winded Anil, who fell to the ground but recovered in order to continue playing the game. After the game ended he went for a shower, and the pain in the scrotal region was excruciating. He then noticed his left testicle was swollen and very tender to touch. He vomited and his lower abdomen 'felt like is was going to bust'. He was taken to the accident and emergency department where he was examined by a nurse practitioner who tried to manually rotate what he thought was torsion of the left testicle. However, the pain was so intense that a colour Doppler examination was performed. Anil was given intramuscular pain relief and an antiemetic. The findings confirmed the nurse's diagnosis of left testicular torsion. Anil then underwent detorsion and orchidopexy.

It is important that once diagnosis has been confirmed that surgery takes place as soon as possible so as to prevent ischaemia and to preserve function and fertility. Complications of an untreated or delayed torsion include infarction of the testicle along with subsequent atrophy, infection and cosmetic deformity. There is some evidence that retention of an injured testicle can cause pathology in the contralateral testes, abnormal semen analysis and decreased fertility (Blaivas and Brannam, 2004).

The cremasteric reflex

The cremasteric reflex is a phenomenon that occurs when the body needs to lower or raise the position of the testes. The cremaster muscle is part of the spermatic cord, and when this muscle contracts, the spermatic cord becomes shorter and the testes are moved upwards towards the body. The result is that this provides slightly more heat to ensure the most favourable testicular temperature. When cooling is needed, the cremaster muscle then loosens up and the testes are subsequently moved away from the heat of the body and then cool down. It is the contraction of the dartos muscle (situated in the subcutaneous layer of the scrotum) that causes the scrotum to appear wrinkled when it is tightened up.

The penis

The penis is the male copulatory organ. The penis encloses the urethra and is a highly vascular organ. This organ is the passageway for excretion of urine as well as the ejaculation of semen. The penis has a shaft and a tip known as the glans, and in the uncircumcised male this is covered by the prepuce (also called the foreskin).

The penis is cylindrical in shape, composed of three cylindrical masses of tissues. The three columns of erectile tissue in the penis are the shaft, the corpora cavernosa and the corpus spongiosum (see Figure 12.7). The attached portion of the penis is known as the root, and the freer moving part is called the shaft or the body.

The penis is usually flaccid and hangs down, but during sexual excitation it becomes erect (an erection), swollen, engorged with blood, firmer and straighter. These changes occur as a result of blood filling the erectile tissue, permitting the penis to penetrate the vagina and deposit sperm (ejaculation) as close to the site of fertilisation as possible.

Usually, when the penile compartments become filled with blood in response to a reaction or an impulse that stimulates the parasympathetic nervous system arteriolar vasodilatation erection takes place. The erection reflex can be incited by sight, touch, pressure, sounds, smells or visions of a sexual encounter. When ejaculation has occurred the arterioles vasoconstrict and the penis becomes flaccid.

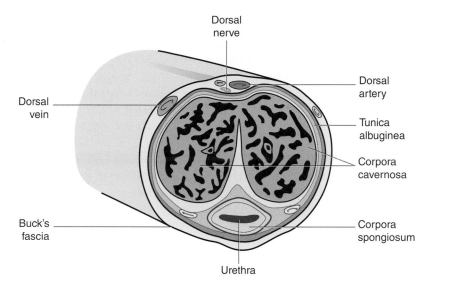

Figure 12.7   The anatomy of the penis. *Source*: Peate (2009). Reproduced with permission of John Wiley & Sons.

Medicines management

Erectile dysfunction

Erectile dysfunction occurs when a man cannot get or maintain a proper erection. There are a number of treatments for this condition. One works by preventing the action of a chemical in the body called phosphodiesterase type 5. Viagra (sildenafil) is one example; it improves the blood flow to the penis following sexual stimulation. Before taking sildenafil the prescriber needs to know if the person has:

- any disease, injury or deformity of the penis;
- any heart or blood vessel disease;
- a gastric condition that causes bleeding;
- an eye condition causing loss of vision;
- hypotension or angina;
- liver or kidney problems;
- had a stroke or a heart attack;
- sickle-cell disease;
- ever had an allergic reaction to sildenafil or to any other medicine.

Sildenafil should be taken as prescribed:
   One tablet should be taken 1 h before the man plans to have sex. The medication can be taken before or after food. Sildenafil should not be taken more frequently than once a day.

See British Society for Sexual Medicine (2013).

Epididymis

The epididymis (plural epididymides) is an approximately 4 cm long comma-shaped duct. It lies on the posterior lateral aspect of the testes. The organ is composed of a highly coiled duct. This duct leads to a larger and more muscular tube called the vas deferens; the vas deferens enters the pelvic cavity.

Within the epididymis the sperm are matured further, being prepared to become more motile so that they can eventually fertilise the ovum. It takes approximately 14 days of full maturation for this to occur (Jenkins and Tortora, 2012). Sperm is stored in the epididymis and is released via peristaltic activity as the smooth muscle contracts during sexual arousal, moving the sperm along the epididymis into the vas deferens. Sperm stored in the epididymis can remain there for several months; those sperm that are not ejaculated are eventually reabsorbed.

The vas deferens, ejaculatory duct and spermatic cord

The vas deferens (plural vasa deferentia), or the ductus deferens, as it enters the pelvic cavity is less convoluted than the epididymis; the diameter is also larger, and the length of the vas deferens is approximately 45 cm (Tortora and Derrickson, 2012). This tube contains ciliated epithelium with a thick muscle layer. The vas deferens runs from the anterior aspect of the scrotal sac as a pair of tubes via the inguinal canal into the pelvic cavity. Between the scrotal sac and the inguinal canal is a tube that the vas deferens runs through; this tube contains the blood vessels and nerves and is called the spermatic cord (Colbert *et al.*, 2012).

The vas deferens then joins the seminal vesicle to become the ejaculatory duct. This duct then passes into the prostate gland, discharging its fluid into the urethra.

The prostate gland

The function of the prostate gland is not well understood (Laws, 2006). The prostate is a single doughnut-shaped gland approximately the size of a walnut, measuring about 4 cm. It goes around the urethra under the urinary bladder and is made of 20–30 glands enclosed in smooth muscle (Marieb, 2012).

The prostate consists of three distinct zones:

- the central zone
- the peripheral zone
- the transition zone.

Secretions of the prostate gland compose approximately one-third of the volume of the semen; the fluid helps sperm motility and to maintain viability. Prostatic fluid is slightly acidic (pH 6.5). Prostatic secretions enter the urethra via a number of ducts during ejaculation.

The female reproductive system

The primary genitalia

As with the male reproductive organs, the female reproductive organs, along with the neuroendocrine system, manufacture hormones that are essential in biological development and sexual activities. The primary genitalia in the female are the ovaries, the secondary genitalia are the fallopian tubes, uterus and vagina; the vulva is the external genitalia. There are aspects of the female reproductive organs that are enclosed and integral to the function of the urinary system.

LeMone and Burke (2011) point out that the female reproductive system consists of the external genitalia:

- mons pubis
- labia
- clitoris
- vaginal and urethral openings
- glands.

The internal organs are:

- vagina
- cervix
- uterus
- fallopian tubes
- ovaries.

The breasts are also a part of the female reproductive organs. Unlike in men, the urethra and urinary meatus are not part of the reproductive organs in women; nevertheless, they are very close in proximity and, as such, health problems that may affect one can often affect the other. Figure 12.8 demonstrates the location and function of the female reproductive organs.

The female reproductive system is designed to produce ova, receive the penis during intercourse and the sperm that has been ejaculated, store, contain and nourish a foetus, and feed the

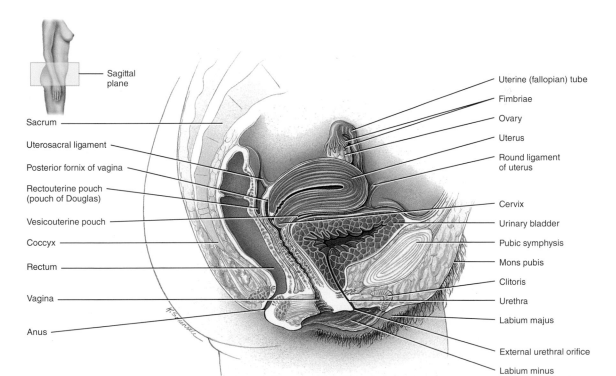

Figure 12.8   The female reproductive system. *Source*: Tortora and Derrickson (2009). Reproduced with permission of John Wiley & Sons.

newborn after birth with breast milk. Usually, each month, a woman's body (during puberty to menopause) prepares itself to become pregnant. If pregnancy does not happen then a menstrual period occurs and the cycle recommences

Medicines management

Contraception

The combined oral contraceptive pill (the pill) contains two hormones: an oestrogen and a progestogen. If taken correctly, it is a very effective form of contraception.

The pill alters the body's hormone balance so the ovaries do not ovulate. It causes the mucus made by the cervix to thicken and form a mucous plug. This makes it difficult for sperm to get through to the uterus to fertilise an egg. The pill also makes the lining of the uterus thinner. This makes it less likely that a fertilised egg will be able to attach to the uterus.

The ovaries

The ovaries are paired glands; in the adult woman they are flat, almond-shaped structures located one on each side of the uterus beneath the ends of the fallopian tubes. These glands in the female are compared to the testes in the male; the ovaries are internal organs. A collection of ligaments holds them in position, attaching the ovaries to the uterus. They are also attached to the broad ligament, and this ligament attaches them to the pelvic wall. The ovaries provide a space of storage for the female germ cells; they also produce the female hormones oestrogen and progesterone. A woman's total number of ova is present at her birth; when a girl reaches puberty she usually ovulates each month.

The ovary contains a number of small structures called ovarian follicles. Each follicle contains an immature ovum, called an oocyte. Monthly, follicles are stimulated by two hormones, the follicle-stimulating hormone (FSH) and LH, which stimulate the follicles to mature. The developing follicles are enclosed in layers of follicle cells; the mature follicles are called the Graafian follicles.

The ovarian cortex

This region lies deep and close to the tunica albuginea. The cortex contains the ovarian follicles surrounded by dense irregular connective tissue. These follicles contain oocytes in various stages of development, as well as a number of cells that feed the developing oocyte; as the follicle grows larger it secretes oestrogen.

Graafian follicles

The Graafian follicles manufacture oestrogen; this stimulates the growth of endometrium. Every month in the woman who is menstruating, one or two of the mature follicles (the Graafian follicles) release an oocyte; this is called ovulation. The remnants of a large ruptured follicle become a new structure called the corpus luteum.

Corpus luteum

The corpus luteum produces two hormones, oestrogen and progesterone, with the aim of supporting the endometrium until conception takes place or the cycle starts again. The corpus luteum gradually disintegrates and a scar is left on the outside of the ovary that is called the corpus albicans.

The outer aspect of the ovary is enveloped in a fibrous capsule that is known as the tunica albuginea; this is composed of cuboidal epithelium. The inner aspect of the ovary is divided into parts.

The ovarian medulla

The ovarian medulla contains blood vessels, nerves and lymphatic tissues surrounded by loose connective tissue. There is an unclear border between the ovarian cortex and medulla.

Figure 12.9 demonstrates the ovary during the development of oocyte.

Oogenesis

The term oogenesis relates to the development of relatively undifferentiated germ cells called oogonia (singular oogonium). Oogonia are fixed in number – between 2- to 4-million diploid (2*n*) stem cells (Stanfield, 2011) before birth, during foetal development; whereas spermatogonia are continuously regenerated at puberty, this is not the case with oogonia. All ova are ultimately derived from these clones. These oogonia develop into larger primary oocytes; the meiotic phase is not completed until the girl reaches puberty (see Figure 12.10).

Every month after puberty until menopause the two hormones FSH and LH are released by the anterior aspect of the pituitary gland and stimulate the primordial follicles. Usually only one will reach the maturity required for ovulation.

The role of the female sex hormones

Oestrogens, progesterone and androgens are produced by the ovaries in a repetitive pattern. Although oestrogens are secreted all the way through the menstrual cycle, they are at a higher level during this particular ovulation stage of the cycle.

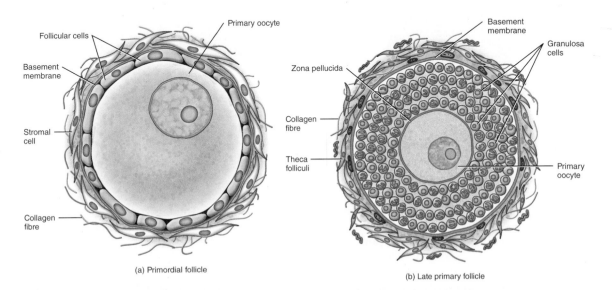

(a) Primordial follicle   (b) Late primary follicle

Figure 12.9   (a–f) The developmental sequences associated with maturation of an ovum. *Source:* Tortora and Derrickson (2009). Reproduced with permission of John Wiley & Sons.

385

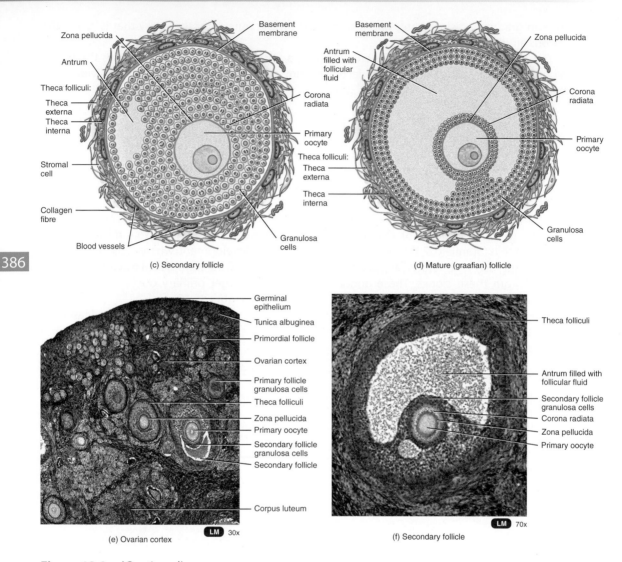

(c) Secondary follicle

(d) Mature (graafian) follicle

(e) Ovarian cortex   LM 30x

(f) Secondary follicle   LM 70x

Figure 12.9   (*Continued*)

Oestrogens are essential for the development and maintenance of secondary sex characteristics; and, working in combination with a number of other hormones, they stimulate the female reproductive organ to prepare for growth of a foetus (LeMone and Burke, 2011). Oestrogens have a key role to play in the usual structure of the skin and blood vessels. They also help to reduce the rate of bone resorption (bone breakdown), enhance increased high-density lipoproteins, decrease cholesterol levels and increase blood clotting.

The menstrual cycle

The endometrium of the uterus responds to changes in oestrogen and progesterone during the ovarian cycle when it prepares for the implantation of the fertilised embryo. The endometrium is receptive to implantation of the embryo for only a brief period every month,

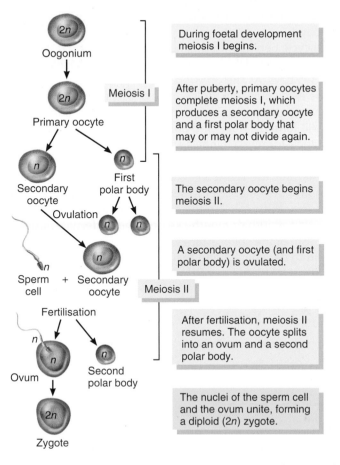

During foetal development meiosis I begins.

After puberty, primary oocytes complete meiosis I, which produces a secondary oocyte and a first polar body that may or may not divide again.

The secondary oocyte begins meiosis II.

A secondary oocyte (and first polar body) is ovulated.

After fertilisation, meiosis II resumes. The oocyte splits into an ovum and a second polar body.

The nuclei of the sperm cell and the ovum unite, forming a diploid (2n) zygote.

Figure 12.10 Oogenesis. *Source*: Tortora and Derrickson (2009). Reproduced with permission of John Wiley & Sons.

Medicines management

Atrophic vaginitis

Many women notice changes in their vagina and genital area after the menopause. These changes may include dryness (atrophic vaginitis) and discomfort during sex. These can often be improved with treatment. Treatment options include hormone replacement therapy (HRT), oestrogen cream or pessaries and lubricating gels.

HRT means taking oestrogen in the form of a tablet, gel or patches. This is often the best treatment for relieving symptoms. As with all medications, there are advantages and disadvantages of using HRT.

Sometimes a cream, pessary or vaginal tablet or ring containing oestrogen is prescribed. A pessary is inserted into the vagina using a small applicator. The ring is a soft, flexible ring with a centre containing oestrogen, releasing a steady, low dose of oestrogen, it lasts for 3 months. Oestrogen creams and pessaries can damage latex condoms and diaphragms.

If vaginal dryness is the only problem, or hormone creams are not recommended, lubricating gels may help. Three gels are available in the UK that replace moisture: Replens®, Sylk® and Hyalofemme®.

coinciding with the time when the embryo would normally reach the uterus from the uterine tube (usually 7 days).

The menstrual cycle begins with the menstrual phase and lasts from days 1 to 5. The inner endometrial layer (also called the functionalis) separates, and this is then released as menstrual fluid lasting for 3–5 days. As the growing follicle begins to produce the hormone oestrogen (days 6 to 14), the next stage, the proliferative phase, then commences. As a result of this, the functionalis layer repairs and thickens while at the same time spiral arteries multiply and tubular glands will form (LeMone and Burke, 2011). Cervical mucus alters, becoming a thin, crystalline substance, forming channels enabling the sperm to travel up into the uterus.

The final phase, lasting from days 14 to 28, is the secretory phase. As the corpus luteum produces progesterone, the rising levels act on the endometrium, resulting in an increased vascularity, changing the inner layer to secretory mucosa, stimulating the secretion of glycogen into the uterine cavity, causing the cervical mucus again to become thick, blocking the internal os (an os is a mouth or mouth-like opening). If fertilisation does not occur, hormone levels will fall. Spasm of the spiral arteries causes hypoxia (lack of oxygen) of the endometrial cells, which begin to degenerate and then slough off. As with the ovarian cycle, the process begins again with the sloughing of the functionalis layer. Figure 12.11 demonstrates the ovarian and uterine cycles.

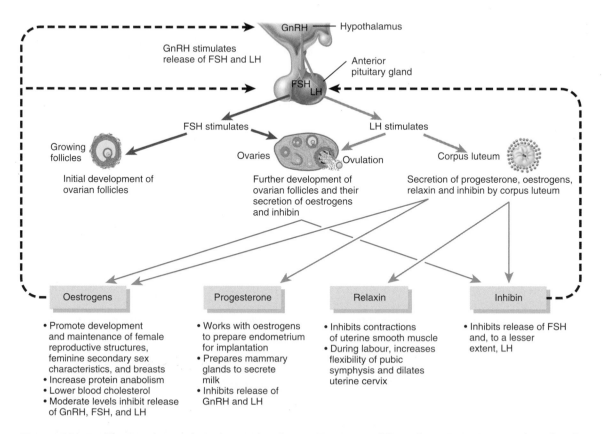

Figure 12.11   The ovarian and uterine cycles. *Source*: Tortora and Derrickson (2009). Reproduced with permission of John Wiley & Sons.

Clinical considerations

Insertion of intrauterine contraceptive device

An intrauterine device (IUD) is a small T-shaped plastic and copper device that is inserted into the uterus by a specially trained nurse or a doctor. The IUD works by preventing the sperm and egg from surviving in the uterus or fallopian tubes; it can also prevent a fertilised egg from implanting in the uterus.

There are different types of IUD; some contain more copper than others. Those IUDs with more copper are more than 99% effective. Copper changes the make-up of the fluids in the uterus and fallopian tubes. IUDs with less copper will be less effective. There are types and sizes of IUD to suit different women; they can be inserted at the GP surgery, local contraception clinic or sexual health clinic. An IUD can be inserted at any time, though it may be easier when the woman is menstruating, as the cervix is slightly open at that time.

A metal or plastic speculum is gently inserted into the vagina in order to see the cervix. The cervix is wiped with a special cleanser. Next, a small 'sound' is inserted to measure the length of the uterus. The IUD is then inserted using a very small straw. The IUD has a string attached to one end. The nurse or doctor will trim the IUD string that is coming through the cervix into the vagina. The string allows the woman to check that the IUD is in place (see Figure 12.12).

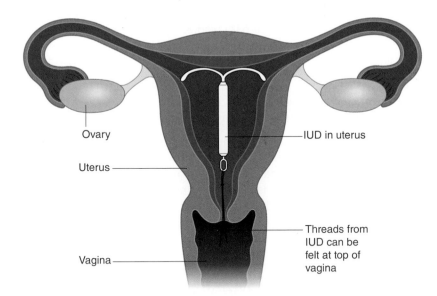

Ovary

Uterus

Vagina

IUD in uterus

Threads from IUD can be felt at top of vagina

Figure 12.12   An IUD device in situ.

The internal organs

The internal organs of the female reproductive system are the vagina and cervix, uterus, fallopian tubes and ovaries. The ovaries (discussed earlier) are the primary reproductive organs in women, as well as producing female sex hormones. The vagina, uterus and fallopian tubes act as an accessory channel for the ovaries and the growing foetus.

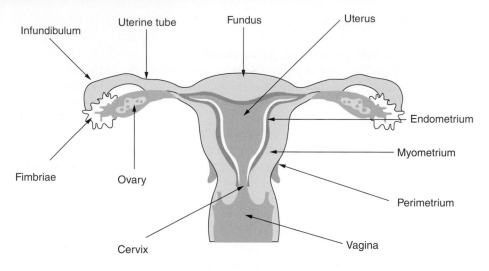

Figure 12.13 The uterus and associated structures. *Source*: Nair and Peate (2009). Reproduced with permission of John Wiley & Sons.

The uterus

This hollow organ is also known as the womb. It is a very muscular organ lying in the pelvic cavity posterior and superior to the urinary bladder; it lies anterior to the rectum (Figure 12.13 outlines the uterus and associated structures).

The uterus is approximately 7.5 cm long. There are three principal parts associated with the uterus:

- the **fundus**, a thick muscular region situated above the fallopian tubes;
- the **body**, the main portion of the uterus, joined to the cervix by an isthmus;
- the **cervix**, the narrowest part of the uterus opening out into the vagina.

As well as having three aspects or parts, the uterus also has three layers. The perimetrium is the outer serous layer, merging with the peritoneum. The middle layer is the myometrium and comprises most of the uterine wall. There are a number of muscle fibres in this layer running in a number of various directions; this arrangement allows contractions to occur during menstruation or childbirth and an increase in size as the foetus grows. The endometrium, the outermost layer, lines the uterus, and this layer is shed during menstruation. The three layers are summarised in Table 12.1.

The fallopian tubes

The paired fallopian tubes (also called the salpinges) are delicate, thin cylindrical structures approximately 8–14 cm long (Marieb, 2012). They are affixed to the uterus at one end and are supported by the broad ligaments. The lateral ends of the fallopian tubes are open and made of projections called fimbriae that drape over the ovary. The fimbriae pick up the ovum after it is discharged from the ovary.

The fallopian tubes are composed of smooth muscle and are lined with ciliated, mucus-producing epithelial cells. The actions of the cilia and contractions of the smooth muscle transport the ovum along the tubes onwards to the uterus. It is in the outer portion of the fallopian tube where the fertilisation of the ovum by the sperm usually occurs.

The term adnex is used collectively when discussing the fallopian tubes, ovaries and supporting tissues.

Table 12.1 The layers of the uterus

Layer	Comments
Perimetrium	A serous membrane enveloping the uterus; this is the outer layer. It provides support to the uterus located within the pelvis. This may also be known as the parietal peritoneum.
Myometrium	This layer is the middle layer and is composed of smooth muscle. During pregnancy and childbirth the uterus is required to stretch. and the muscular layer allows this to happen. The muscle will contract during labour, and postnatally this muscular layer contracts forcefully to force out the placenta. The contractions also help to control potential blood loss after birth.
Endometrium	The endometrium is the mucous membrane lining the inside of the uterus. The endometrium changes throughout the menstrual cycle. It becomes thick and rich with blood vessels to prepare for pregnancy. If the woman does not become pregnant then, part of the endometrium is shed, resulting in menstrual bleeding.

Source: Adapted from McGuinness (2013) and Waugh and Grant (2014).

Snapshot

Ectopic pregnancy

Alice Smethwick has undergone laparoscopic surgery for ectopic pregnancy – a right salpingectomy. Alice is at home 2 days post-procedure and experiencing abdominal discomfort; she is also complaining of neck and shoulder pain. She makes an appointment to see the practice nurse.

The practice nurse explains to Alice that the gas (carbon dioxide) that was pumped into her abdominal cavity to allow the surgeon to identify the fallopian tubes has caused the abdominal discomfort. The neck and shoulder pain experienced by some people is also related to the laparoscopy and the carbon dioxide gas. The gas irritates the diaphragm and the phrenic nerve. It is explained to Alice that this pain will go away as the gas is absorbed. She is also told that lying down can also help decrease the pain.

See National Institute of Health and Care Excellence (2012).

The vagina

The vagina is a tubular, fibromuscular structure approximately 8–10 cm in length (Jenkins and Tortora, 2012). It is the receptacle for the penis during sexual intercourse, it is an organ of sexual response and is the canal that allows the menstrual flow to leave the body and the passage for the birth of the child. The vagina is situated posterior to the urinary bladder and urethra; it is anterior to the rectum. The upper element contains the uterine cervix in an area that is known as the fornix. The vaginal walls are made of membranous folds of tissue called the rugae. These membranes are made up of mucus-secreting stratified squamous epithelial cells.

Usually, the walls of the vagina are moist and have a pH ranging from 3.8 to 4.2. This pH inhibits the growth of bacteria (it is bacteriostatic) and is maintained by the action of the hormone oestrogen and healthy vaginal microorganisms (the normal vaginal flora). Oestrogen causes the growth of vaginal mucosal cells, making them thicken and develop and increase glycogen content. The glycogen is fermented to lactic acid by lactobacilli (organisms that produce lactic acid) that usually live in the vagina, causing slight acidifying of the vaginal fluid (LeMone and Burke, 2011).

The cervix

Into the vagina projects the cervix, and this forms a pathway between the uterus and the vagina. The uterine opening of the cervix is known as the internal os, and the vaginal opening called the external os. The space between these openings, the endocervical canal, acts as a conduit for the discharge of menstrual fluid, the opening for sperm and delivery of the infant during birth. The cervix is a rigid structure, protected by mucus that alters consistency and quantity for the duration of the menstrual cycle and during pregnancy.

The external genitalia

Collectively, the external genitalia are known as the vulva. They include the mons pubis, the labia, the clitoris, the vaginal and urethral openings, and glands (LeMone and Burke, 2011).

The mons pubis is a pad of elevated adipose tissue covered with skin. It lies anteriorly to the symphysis pubis, cushioning it. After puberty, the mons is covered with coarse pubic hair.

The labia are divided into two structures. The labia majora are folds of skin and an abundance of adipose tissue covered with pubic hair; these are outermost. They begin at the base of the mons pubis and terminate at the anus. The labia minora, situated between the clitoris and the base of the vagina, are enclosed by the labia majora. They are made of skin, adipose tissue and some erectile tissues with a number of sebaceous glands. They are usually light pink and are devoid of pubic hair.

The clitoris is composed of two small erectile bodies, the corposa cavernosa and several nerves and blood vessels. The glans clitoris is the exposed portion of the clitoris and is likened to the glans penis in the male. This aspect of the external genitalia is capable of enlargement; it has a role to play in sexual excitement in the woman.

Snapshot

Genital piercing

Patient X has arrived at the sexual health clinic complaining of discharge 'down below'. The nurse takes a history from the lady and is informed that 5 days ago she had her clitoral hood pierced and yesterday she was feeling very warm, generally unwell, nauseous and she has noticed a discharge from the vulval area and her underwear is stained. The nurse examines the patient and observes a yellow discharge, redness and swelling in the vulval area.

It is likely that this patient has a bacterial infection as a result of the piercing; she may also be having an allergic reaction to the metal that has been used.

Other complications associated with genital piercings can include haemorrhage, nerve damage and thick scarring at the piercing site. There is also the risk of contracting HIV, hepatitis B and C, sexually transmitted infections or other infections. These risks can be minimised with the use of a new, sterile needle as well using a reputable piercer. Using proper jewellery made out of metals such as surgical stainless steel or titanium can reduce the risk of infection and allergic reaction.

Persons with piercings should take care when using condoms – do not use the teeth to open the packet, and avoid damaging the condom with nails, jewellery or piercings.

See British Association for Sexual Health and HIV (2012).

The breasts

The breasts are dome-shaped protrusions that differ in size between individuals; they are also sometimes called the mammary glands. They are external accessory sexual organs in the female. There are several milk-producing glands located within the breast. A hormone called prolactin controls the production of milk.

The breasts are located between the third and seventh ribs on the anterior aspect chest wall. The breasts are supported by the pectoral muscles and are provided with a rich supply of nerves, blood vessels and lymph (see Figure 12.14). A pigmented area known as the areola is situated a little below the centre of each breast and contains glands that secrete sebum – a thick substance composed of fat and cell debris (sebaceous glands), – and a nipple. The nipple is usually protruding, becoming erect in response to cold and stimulation.

The breasts are made of adipose (fat) tissue, fibrous connective tissue and glandular tissue. There are bands of fibrous tissue that support the breast and extend from the outer breast tissue to the nipple, dividing the breast into 15 to 25 lobes. The lobes are comprised of alveolar glands joined by ducts that open out on to the nipple.

393

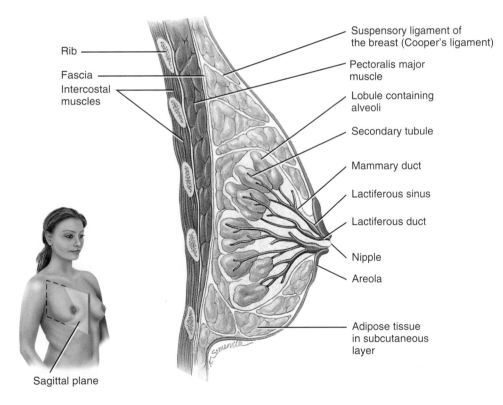

Sagittal section

Figure 12.14   The breast. *Source*: Tortora and Derrickson (2009). Reproduced with permission of John Wiley & Sons.

Conclusion

The male and female reproductive systems are complex. All living things reproduce; fundamentally, organisms make more organisms akin to themselves. Without these reproductive systems human life would end; these systems are essential for life. These systems have a number of functions; for example, the function of reproduction, producing and transporting sex cells. In the human reproductive process, two types of sex cells, or gametes, are required. The male gamete, or sperm, and the female gamete, the egg or ovum, meet in the female's reproductive system to begin the creation of a new individual. Anatomical and physiological processes are required to ensure this marvel works effectively.

Sexual reproduction, the process of producing offspring for the survival of the species and passing on hereditary traits from one generation to the next, is the key function of the male and female reproductive systems. The male and female reproductive systems contribute to the events leading to fertilisation. The female organs take on responsibility for the developing human, birth and nourishment. The systems also provide pleasure, sexual pleasure and sexual excitement; for a number of people this is an important aspect of their being.

Glossary

Adrenal cortex   The outer portion of an adrenal gland.

Androgens   Masculinising male sex hormones produced by the testes in the male and the adrenal cortex in both sexes.

Anterior   Near to the front.

Antiemetic   Anti-sickness medication.

Broad ligament   A double fold of parietal peritoneum attaching the uterus to the side of the pelvic cavity.

Canal   A channel or passageway, a narrow tube.

Connective tissue   The most prominent type of tissue in the body; this tissue provides support.

Corpus albicans   A whitish fibrous patch in the ovary formed after the corpus luteum regresses.

Corpus luteum   A yellowish body found in the ovary when a follicle has discharged its secondary oocyte.

Endometrium   The mucous membrane lining the uterus.

Foetus   The developing organism *in utero*.

Fimbriae   Finger-like structures found at the end of the fallopian tubes.

Follicle   A secretory sac or cavity containing a group of cells that contains a developing oocyte in the ovary.

Follicle-stimulating hormone   Secreted by the anterior pituitary gland; initiates the development of an ovum.

Gamete   A male or female sex cell.

Glans penis   The enlarged region at the end of the penis.

Gonad   A gland that produces hormones and gametes – in men the testes, in females the ovaries.

Gonadotrophic hormone   Anterior pituitary hormone affecting the gonads.

Haploid   Having half the number of chromosomes.

Hormone   A secretion of endocrine cells that alters the physiological activity of target cells.

Human chorionic gonadotrophin   A hormone produced by the developing placenta.

Inguinal canal   Passage in the lower abdominal wall in the male.

Inhibin   A hormone secreted by the gonads inhibiting the release of FSH by the anterior pituitary.

In utero   Within the uterus.

Isthmus   A narrow strip of tissue or a narrow passage connecting to bigger parts.

Lateral   Farthest from the midline of the body.

Leydig cell   A type of cell that secretes testosterone.

Ligament   Dense regular connective tissue.

Luteinising hormone   A hormone secreted by the anterior pituitary stimulates ovulation and prepares glands in the breast to produce milk. Stimulates testosterone secretion in the testes.

Meatus   A passage or opening.

Meiosis   A kind of cell division occurring during the production of gametes.

Menopause   The termination of the menstrual cycles.

Myometrium   The smooth muscle layer of the uterus.

Oestrogens   Feminising sex hormones produced by the ovaries.

Orchidopexy   Surgery to move an undescended testicle into the scrotum and permanently fix it there.

Oocyte   An immature egg cell.

Oogenesis   Formation and development of the female gametes.

Ovarian cycle   The ovarian cycle is a series of events in the ovaries that occur during and after the maturation of the oocyte.

Ovarian follicle   A general name for immature oocytes.

Ovary   The female gonad.

Ovulation   The rupture of a mature Graafian follicle with discharge of a secondary oocyte after penetration by sperm.

Ovum   The female egg cell.

Penis   The organ of urination and copulation.

pH   A measure of acidity and alkalinity.

Phagocytosis   The process by which phagocytes ingest and destroy microbes, cell debris and other foreign matter.

Placenta   An organ attached to the lining of the uterus during pregnancy.

Progesterone A female sex hormone produced by the ovaries.

Prolactin A hormone secreted by the anterior pituitary that initiates and maintains milk production.

Rete The network of ducts in the testes.

Scrotum The skin-covered pouch containing the testes.

Semen Fluid discharged by ejaculation.

Spermatogenesis The maturation of spermatids into sperm.

Testes The male gonads.

Testosterone Male sex hormone.

Urethra The tube from the urinary bladder to the exterior of the body that conveys urine in females and urine and semen in males.

Uterus Hollow muscular organ in the female, also called the womb.

Vagina A muscular tubular organ in the female leading from the uterus to the vestibule.

Vas deferens The main secretory duct of the testicle, through which semen is carried from the epididymis to the prostatic urethra, where it ends as the ejaculatory duct.

Vulva The female external genitalia.

References

Blaivas, M. and Brannam, L. (2004) Testicular ultrasound. *Emergency Medical Clinics of North America* **22**(3): 723–724.

British Association for Sexual Health and HIV (2012) *A BASHH Guide to Condoms*. http://www.bashh.org/BASHH/Public___patient_information/Condoms.aspx (accessed 30 November 2015).

British Society for Sexual Medicine (2013) *Guidelines on the Management of Erectile Dysfunction*. http://www.bssm.org.uk/downloads/default.asp (accessed 30 November 2015).

Colbert, B.J., Ankney, J. and Lee, K.T. (2012) *Anatomy and Physiology for Health Professionals. An Interactive Journey*, 2nd edn. Upper Saddle River, NJ: Pearson.

Jenkins, G.W. and Tortora, G.J. (2012) *Anatomy and Physiology. From Science to Life*, 3rd edn. Hoboken, NJ: John Wiley & Sons, Inc.

Laws, T. (2006) *A Handbook of Men's Health*. Edinburgh: Elsevier.

LeMone, P. and Burke, K. (2011) *Medical–Surgical Nursing. Critical Thinking in Client Care*, 5th edn. Upper Saddle River, NJ: Pearson.

Marieb, E.N. (2012) *Human Anatomy and Physiology*, 9th edn. San Francisco, CA: Pearson.

McGuiness, H. (2013) *Anatomy and Physiology. Therapy Basics*, 4th edn. London: Hodder.

Nair, M. and Peate, I. (2009) *Fundamentals of Applied Pathophysiology: An Essential Guide for Nursing Students*. Oxford: John Wiley & Sons, Ltd.

National Institute of Health and Care Excellence (2012) *Ectopic Pregnancy and Miscarriage*. NICE guideline CG154. http://www.nice.org.uk/guidance/cg154 (accessed 30 November 2015).

Peate, I. (2009) *Men's Health*. Oxford: John Wiley & Sons, Ltd.

Stanfield, C.L. (2011) *Principles of Human Physiology*, 4th edn. Boston, MA: Pearson.

Tortora, G.J. and Derrickson, B.H. (2009) *Principles of Anatomy and Physiology*, 12th edn. Hoboken, NJ: John Wiley & Sons, Inc.

Tortora, G.J. and Derrickson, B. (2012) *Essentials of Anatomy and Physiology*, 9th edn. New York: John Wiley & Sons, Inc.

Waugh, A. and Grant, A. (2014) *Ross and Wilson Anatomy and Physiology in Health and Illness*, 12th edn. Edinburgh: Churchill Livingstone.

Further reading

Family Planning Association

http://www.fpa.org.uk

The Family Planning Association is a sexual health charity, providing straightforward information, advice and support on sexual health, sex and relationships.

Prostate Cancer UK

http://prostatecanceruk.org

Prostate Cancer UK aims to help men survive prostate cancer and enjoy a better quality of life. They offer support to men and provide information, fund research, raise awareness and improve care.

Endometriosis UK

http://www.endometriosis-uk.org

A charity dedicated to providing information on endometriosis and support for those affected by endometriosis.

Activities

Multiple choice questions

1. The cell that is created by fertilisation is:
   - (a) the oocyte
   - (b) the zygote
   - (c) the sperm
   - (d) the semen
2. The sperm are stored and mature in:
   - (a) the epididymis
   - (b) the ova
   - (c) the testes
   - (d) the vas deferens
3. The primary males sex hormone is:
   - (a) testosterone
   - (b) oestrogen
   - (c) progesterone
   - (d) all of the above
4. The gland that releases a small amount of fluid prior to ejaculation is:
   - (a) the ejaculatory duct
   - (b) the prostate gland
   - (c) Cowper's gland
   - (d) the bulbourethral gland

5. The seminiferous tubules produce:
   (a) semen
   (b) inhibin
   (c) follicle-stimulating hormone
   (d) none of the above
6. The hormones that stimulate the growth of the mammary glands and the initial steps of the milk-secreting process are:
   (a) testosterone and progesterone
   (b) oestrogen and testosterone
   (c) oestrogen and progesterone
   (d) oestrogen and inhibin
7. Within the primary follicles, when do the primary oocytes develop?
   (a) as the woman reaches puberty
   (b) this varies
   (c) as the woman reaches the menopause
   (d) before the birth of the woman
8. If pregnancy does not occur, what happens to the corpus luteum?
   (a) it degenerates
   (b) it causes ectopic pregnancy
   (c) it remains and develops into a new secondary oocyte
   (d) it causes infection
9. Endometriosis can be defined as:
   (a) cancer
   (b) a sexually transmitted infection
   (c) a type of allergy
   (d) tissue from the endometrium found outside of the uterus
10. How does the contraceptive pill containing estrogen and progesterone prevent pregnancy?
   (a) it causes the endometrium to hypertrophy
   (b) it suppresses follicle-stimulating hormone and luteinising hormone, preventing ovulation
   (c) it liquefies the semen
   (d) it causes a decrease in the amount of testosterone the woman produces

True or false

1. Oxytocin combines with enzymes in semen to enhance sperm motility.
2. Erectile dysfunction and premature ejaculation are one and the same condition.
3. Ovarian follicles contain mature ova.
4. Ovulation occurs towards the cessation of the ovarian cycle.
5. The primary function of the uterus is to receive, retain and nourish a fertilised egg.
6. Vaginismus is a sexually transmitted infection.
7. The endometrium is the delicate mucosal lining of the uterus.
8. The most important risk factor for the development of testicular cancer is diet.
9. The extension of the cremaster muscle causes the penis to become erect.
10. The hormone testosterone is only detected in males.

Label the diagram 1

Label the diagram using the following list of words:

Sagittal plane, Sacrum, Seminal vesicle, Vesicorectal pouch, Coccyx, Rectum, Ampulla of ductus (vas) deferens, Ejaculatory duct, Prostatic urethra, Membranous urethra, Anus, Bulb of penis, Epididymis, Testis, Scrotum, Peritoneum, Urinary bladder, Ductus (vas) deferens, Suspensory ligament of penis, Public symphysis, Prostate, Deep muscles of perineum, Bulbourethral (Cowper's) gland, Corpora cavernosum penis, Spongy (penile) urethra, Penis, Corpus spongiosum penis, Corona, Glans penis, Prepuce (foreskin), External urethral orifice

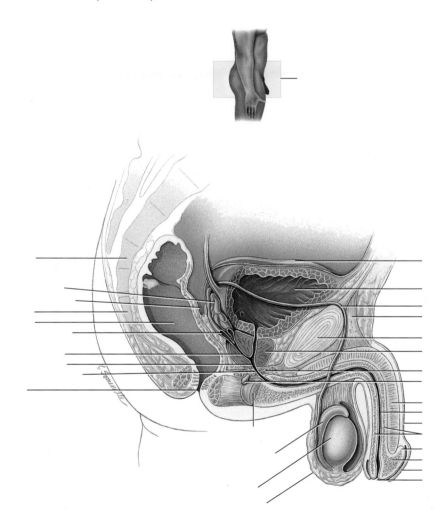

Label the diagram 2

Label the diagram using the following list of words:

Sagittal plane, Sacrum, Uterosacral ligament, Posterior fornix of vagina, Rectouterine pouch (pouch of Douglas), Vesicouterine pouch, Coccyx, Rectum, Vagina, Anus, Uterine (fallopian) tube, Fimbriae, Ovary, Uterus, Round ligament of uterus, Cervix, Urinary bladder, Pubic symphysis, Mons pubis, Clitoris, Urethra, Labium majus, External urethral orifice, Labium minus

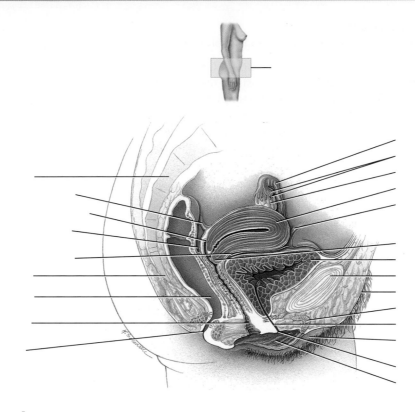

Word search

M	T	E	L	C	I	L	L	O	F	F	N	M	D	W
S	P	E	R	M	A	T	O	G	E	N	E	S	I	S
B	B	O	S	G	A	C	I	N	I	N	G	F	H	L
U	J	F	Y	T	Z	V	L	N	S	M	O	R	R	S
L	N	N	I	N	O	M	U	T	I	H	R	E	X	D
B	R	A	X	M	M	S	R	L	V	I	T	N	Q	A
O	S	C	I	R	B	U	T	E	V	S	S	U	C	N
U	S	R	E	P	A	R	S	E	A	A	E	L	Y	O
R	C	P	E	T	O	I	I	M	R	P	O	U	V	G
E	S	W	I	P	C	L	E	A	N	O	T	M	F	H
T	Y	O	Q	L	W	R	L	J	E	X	N	J	C	B
H	N	X	E	O	C	O	U	A	J	Z	O	E	L	V
R	P	S	W	F	Q	Z	C	S	F	Y	T	G	N	L
A	S	N	I	L	O	H	T	R	A	B	J	B	S	E
L	Z	A	K	B	E	V	E	S	T	I	B	U	L	E

Acini, Bartholins, Bulbourethral, Cowpers, Cremaster, Fallopian, Fimbriae, Follicle, Frenulum, Gonads, Menstruation, Oestrogen, Sperm, Spermatogenesis, Testosterone, Vesicles, Vestibule, Vulva

Fill in the blanks 1

Menstruation, or _____, is normal _____ bleeding that occurs as part of a woman's _____ cycle. Every month, the woman's body _____ for _____. If no pregnancy occurs, the _____, (also known as the _____), _____ its lining. The menstrual blood is partly _____ and partly _____ from _____ the uterus. It passes _____ of the body through the _____.

vaginal, monthly, pregnancy, lining, tissue, prepares, period, blood, womb, inside, sheds, uterus, inside, outside

Fill in the blanks 2

Menopause is a _____ of life in women that _____ the end of their _____ period. It _____ the end of _____. This means that the _____ of the women _____ producing an _____ every four _____ and there is no _____ period. Beyond _____ a woman will no _____ be able to have _____.

phase, signifies, reproductive, signifies, menstruation, ovaries, stop, egg, weeks, monthly, menopause, children, longer

Find out more

1. What does the surgical procedure circumcision entail?
2. Discuss the various methods of contraception.
3. What advice should be given to a man who is considering using Viagra for the first time?
4. What is the role and function of the nurse in respect to protecting vulnerable people?
5. How can the nurse ensure that the information provided to various communities is appropriate and informative?
6. Outline the barriers that may be encountered when conducting an assessment of a person's sexual health.
7. How may the nurse reduce the impact of the barriers identified above?
8. Describe the changes that can occur in the normal ageing process in relation to the female reproductive system.
9. List the issues a man may have to face post-prostatectomy.
10. Discuss the services and support systems available to young mums in the area where you live.

Conditions

The following is a list of conditions that are associated with the reproductive systems. Take some time and write notes about each of the conditions. You may make the notes taken from text books or other resources (e.g. people you work with in a clinical area), or you may make the notes as a result of people you have cared for. If you are making notes about people you have cared for you must ensure that you adhere to the rules of confidentiality.

Prostatitis	
Cervicitis	
Uterine cancer	
Endometriosis	
Premature ejaculation	

Chapter 13

The nervous system

Louise McErlean and Janet G Migliozzi

Test your prior knowledge

- Which other system does the nervous system work closely with?
- List the structures of the central nervous system.
- How many pairs of cranial nerves are there?
- Name the two divisions of the autonomic nervous system.
- Differentiate between sensory information and motor information.

Learning outcomes

After reading this chapter you will be able to:

- Describe the structures of the nervous system
- Describe some of the functions of each of these structures
- Describe conduction of nerve impulses
- List the functions of the neuroglial cells
- Identify the function of different areas of the brain
- Understand the structure and function of the spinal cord
- Differentiate between the sympathetic and parasympathetic nervous systems

Fundamentals of Anatomy and Physiology: For Nursing and Healthcare Students, Second Edition. Edited by Ian Peate and Muralitharan Nair.
© 2017 John Wiley & Sons, Ltd. Published 2017 by John Wiley & Sons, Ltd.
Student companion website: www.wileyfundamentalseries.com/anatomy
Instructor companion website: www.wiley.com/go/instructor/anatomy

Body map

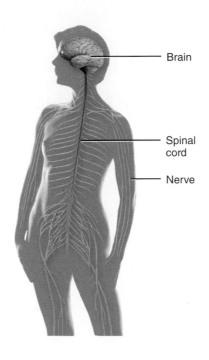

Brain

Spinal cord

Nerve

Introduction

The nervous system is a major communicating and control system within the body. It works with the endocrine system to control many body functions. The nervous system provides a rapid and short-acting response, and the endocrine system provides a slower but often more sustained response. The two systems work together to maintain homeostasis.

The nervous system interacts with all of the systems of the body. This system is large and complex. In order to facilitate understanding of the nervous system it has to be divided into smaller functional and anatomical parts. This chapter outlines the divisions of the nervous system; it discusses the structure and function of the nervous system and how it influences other structures of the body. Having such an important role in maintaining homeostasis, the nervous system possesses additional protection, and that too will be investigated.

Organisation of the nervous system

The nervous system can be divided into two parts: the central nervous system and the peripheral nervous system. The central nervous system consists of the brain and spinal cord and is the control and integration centre for many body functions.

The peripheral nervous system carries sensory information to the central nervous system and motor information out of the central nervous system. The direction of information flow to and from the nervous system is important and is shown in Figure 13.1.

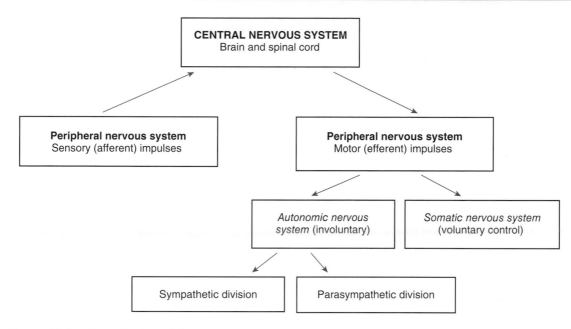

Figure 13.1   Organisation of the nervous system.

Sensory division of the peripheral nervous system

Sensory information (stimuli) is gathered from both inside and outside of the body. This sensory input is delivered to the central nervous system via the peripheral nerves. Sensory nerve fibres are also called afferent fibres. Sensory information always travels from the peripheral nervous system towards the central nervous system. There are many different kinds of sensory information, including pain, pressure, temperature, chemical levels and more. Consider the maintenance of body temperature. As warm-blooded animals, it is important that body temperature is maintained between 36.5 and 37.5 °C. Temperature receptors in the skin called thermoreceptors detect changes in temperature, and as temperature changes have the potential to cause damage to cells and tissues, this information must be relayed to the central nervous system and, if required, acted upon.

Central nervous system

The central nervous system consists of the brain and spinal cord. The central nervous system processes and integrates sensory information. The received information has to be interpreted, it can be stored to be dealt with later or it can be acted upon immediately with one or more motor responses. For example, the sensation of temperature change would be received and interpreted by the hypothalamus (a structure of the central nervous system) and an appropriate action would be initiated.

Motor division of the peripheral nervous system

The motor division of the peripheral nervous system always carries impulses away from the central nervous system, usually to effector organs. Motor nerve fibres are also called efferent fibres. There are two types of motor information. Motor information to the somatic nervous system or to the autonomic nervous system.

Somatic nervous system

The somatic nervous system is under voluntary control, and the effector (tissue or organ responding to instruction from the central nervous system) is skeletal (voluntary) muscle.

The central nervous system's response to sensory information may be to activate the somatic nervous system, eliciting a voluntary response involving skeletal muscle movement. So, from the example of temperature, if an increase in temperature is detected, then it might require the removal of a coat or the opening of a window – this is the motor response that involves the somatic nervous system. It is a voluntary activity that the person chooses to do.

Autonomic nervous system

The central nervous system's response to sensory information may be to activate the autonomic nervous system. This would lead to an involuntary action. The autonomic nervous system is responsible for involuntary motor responses. The effector may be smooth or cardiac muscle (both involuntary muscles) or a gland.

In the example of increased temperature, the involuntary response is to lose heat through the skin – so warm blood is directed to the skin when peripheral blood vessels vasodilate. Vasodilatation is an example of an involuntary autonomic nervous system response. The individual cannot control this response.

The autonomic nervous system is further divided into the sympathetic (fight or flight) and the parasympathetic (rest and digest) divisions. The autonomic nervous system will be discussed later in the chapter. A fine balance between both of these divisions is required for the maintenance of homeostasis.

Neurones

The functional unit of the nervous system is the neurone or nerve cell. It has many features in common with other cells, including a nucleus and mitochondria, but because of its vital role it is well protected and has some specialist modifications. Two specialist characteristics of neurones are:

- **irritability**, in response to a stimulus – the ability to initiate a nerve impulse;
- **conductivity** – the ability to conduct an impulse.

Neurones consist of an axon, dendrites and a cell body. Their function is to transmit nerve impulses. Nerve impulses only travel in one direction: from the receptive area – the dendrites – to the cell body, and down the length of the axon (see Figure 13.2).

Axons bundled together are called **nerves**. Neurones rely on a constant supply of oxygen and glucose. Once the neurones of the brain and spinal cord have matured after birth they will not be replaced or regenerate if they become damaged. Peripheral neurones can regenerate if the cell body is not damaged and the alignment of the neurone is not disrupted.

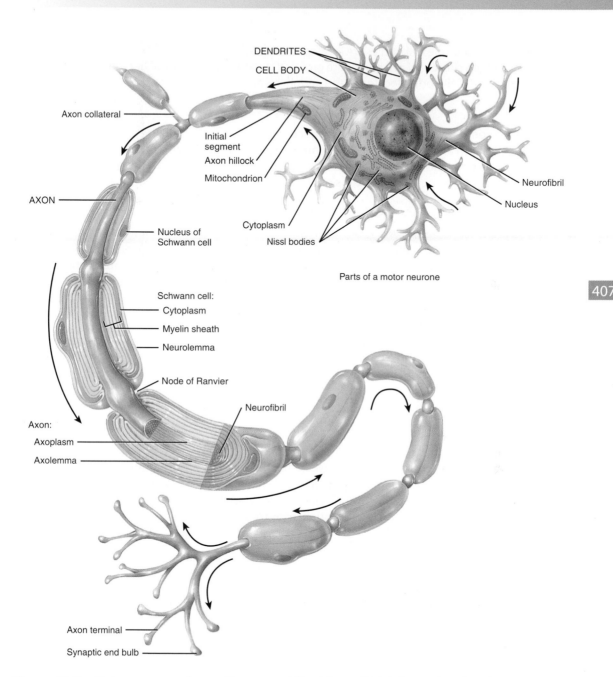

DENDRITES

CELL BODY

Axon collateral

Initial segment

Axon hillock

Mitochondrion

AXON

Nucleus of Schwann cell

Cytoplasm

Nissl bodies

Neurofibril

Nucleus

Parts of a motor neurone

Schwann cell:

Cytoplasm

Myelin sheath

Neurolemma

Node of Ranvier

Neurofibril

Axon:

Axoplasm

Axolemma

Axon terminal

Synaptic end bulb

Figure 13.2   Motor neurone. *Source*: Tortora and Derrickson (2009). Reproduced with permission of John Wiley & Sons.

Dendrites

Dendrites are short branching processes that receive information and conduct it toward the cell body. Their branching processes provide a large surface area for this function. In sensory neurones the dendrites may form the part of the sensory receptors, and in motor neurones they can form part of the synapse between one neurone and the next.

Cell body

Most of the neurone cell bodies are located inside the central nervous system and form the grey matter. When clusters of cell bodies are grouped together in the central nervous system they are called nuclei. Cell bodies located in the peripheral nervous system are called ganglia.

Axons

Each neurone has only one axon that conducts information away from the cell body. The axon can branch to form an axon collateral (see Figure 13.2). The axon will also branch at its terminal into many axon terminals. The axon delivers the impulse to another neurone or a gland or a muscle.

The axon length can vary quite significantly from very short to 100 cm long (Marieb and Hoehn, 2013).

Myelin sheath

Peripheral nerve axons and long or large axons are covered in a myelin sheath. Myelin is a fatty material whose purpose is to protect the neurone and to electrically insulate it, speeding up impulse transmission. Within the peripheral nervous system Schwann cells wrapped in layers around the neurone form the myelin sheath. The outermost part of the Schwann cell is its plasma membrane, and this is called the neurilemma. There is a regular gap (about 1 mm) between adjacent Schwann cells. The gaps are called the nodes of Ranvier. Collateral axons can occur at the node (see Figure 13.2). Some nerve fibres are unmyelinated, and this makes nerve impulse transmission significantly slower.

Clinical considerations

Multiple sclerosis

Multiple sclerosis is a disease where areas of demyelination of the white matter (myelinated fibres form white matter) can occur. Areas of demyelination are called plaques. Multiple sclerosis affects the 20–40 years age range and is most frequently seen in temperate climates. The cause is unknown but it is suspected that there may be a genetic link; viral infection has also been implicated. Neuronal damage caused by the demyelination leads to:

- skeletal muscle weakness, often progressing to paralysis
- visual disturbances
- uncoordinated movements
- burning or tingling sensations.

Multiple sclerosis can be a chronic disease characterised by periods of remission or the disease can progress rapidly, leading to death.

Sensory (afferent) nerves

The dendrites of sensory neurones are often sensory receptors, and when they are stimulated the impulse generated travels towards the spinal cord and brain. There are different types of sensory receptors:

- special senses (as discussed in Chapter 14);
- somatic sensory receptors, located in the skin, such as touch, temperature and pain;

- autonomic nervous system receptors, located throughout the body, such as baroreceptors monitoring blood pressure, chemoreceptors monitoring blood pH and visceral pain receptors;
- proprioceptors, monitoring muscle movement, stretch and pain.

Motor (efferent) nerves

Information from the central nervous system is delivered to the peripheral nervous system via the motor nerves. Information transmitted through a voluntary somatic nerve may result in skeletal muscle contraction or the information may be autonomic in nature, not under voluntary control, and may lead to smooth muscle contraction or the release of the products of a gland.

The action potential

The nervous system is a vast communicating network sending information from the internal and external environment to the central nervous system and from the central nervous system to the muscles and glands. The way that the functional unit, the neurone, achieves this is by the generation and conduction of impulses or action potentials.

Generation of the action potential occurs due to the movement of ions into and out of the neurone and the electrical charge associated with this movement.

Two principal ions are involved:

- sodium – normally found outside of the cell (principal extracellular cation);
- potassium – normally found inside the cell (principal intracellular cation).

Simple propagation of nerve impulses

When there is no impulse being transmitted the cell is in its resting state – the nerve cell membrane is said to be **polarised**. When stimulated by an impulse, the cell membrane changes its permeability and the extracellular sodium ions move into the cell – this is called depolarisation. The movement of these ions changes the electrical charge on either side of the cell membrane from more positive extracellularly to more negative extracellularly as the impulse travels the length of the axon. This activity creates the action potential. This process happens in a wave along the length of the neurone from the active part of the neurone to the resting part of the neurone, always in one direction. At the same time, potassium ions move out of the neurone into the extracellular space, returning the electrical charge associated with the polarised neurone back to more positive outside the cell and more negative inside. This is the repolarising phase. The sodium–potassium pump is activated to return sodium to the extracellular space in exchange for potassium (see Figure 13.3).

Saltatory conduction

Saltatory conduction occurs in myelinated neurones as the electrical charge associated with the nerve impulse jumps between one node of Ranvier and the next. This occurs much faster than simple propagation. Conduction is also faster when the neurone has a larger diameter.

The refractory period

When the action potential is stimulated, the neurone cannot accept another impulse or generate another action potential no matter how strong the impulse is. This is known as the refractory period.

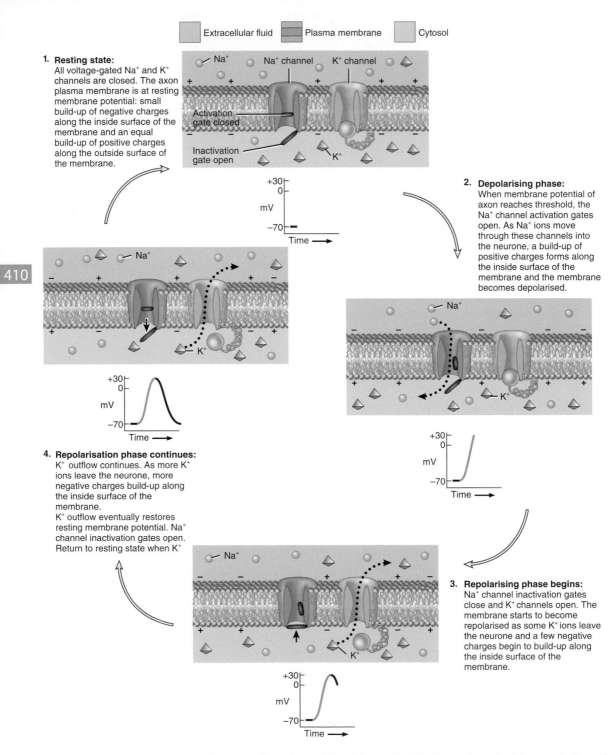

410

Figure 13.3 Action potential. *Source*: Tortora and Derrickson (2009). Reproduced with permission of John Wiley & Sons.

Neurotransmitters

Neurones do not come into contact with one another. Where one neurone ends and another begins, there is a space called the synapse. In order for communication to occur between neurones or between the neurone and a muscle or gland, a chemical messenger called a **neurotransmitter** is secreted by the neurone into the extracellular space at the synapse. Those effector cells or neurones in close proximity to the neurotransmitter will either be stimulated or inhibited by the neurotransmitter, depending upon which neurotransmitter is secreted. The action of the neurotransmitter is short-lived, and any neurotransmitter not used is absorbed by the neurone to be recycled and used again or deactivated by enzymes.

Some examples of neurotransmitters are:

- acetylcholine, released within the central nervous system and also at the neuromuscular junction;
- norepinephrine, released within the central nervous system and also at autonomic nervous system synapses;
- dopamine, released within the central nervous system and also at autonomic nervous system synapses.

411

Snapshot

An electroencephalogram (EEG) records brain activity. It is particularly useful for diagnosing conditions such as epilepsy, dementia and encephalopathy.

Electrodes are placed on the head and attached to an EEG machine. The electrical activity generated by nerve impulses is then measured. During the EEG, the patient may be asked to breathe deeply or blink several times. There are different types of EEG used to ascertain triggers that may lead to seizure activity, and these include sleep EEG, sleep-deprived EEG, ambulatory EEG and strobe lighting EEG.

The test can usually be carried out in an outpatient department (apart from sleep EEG), and the outcome could lead to a treatment plan being implemented or altered.

Neuroglia

Neuroglia (see Figure 13.4) are cells that support neurones. They are more numerous than neurones. Within the central nervous system the neuroglial cells account for more than half of the weight of the brain (Marieb and Hoehn, 2013). Neuroglia can multiply in order to support the neurones. Because of this, nervous system tumours often originate from neuroglia.

Within the peripheral nervous system, two types of neuroglia have been identified:

1. Schwann cells, responsible for forming the myelin sheath;
2. satellite cells, whose function is not known.

Within the central nervous system; four type of neuroglial cell have been identified:

1. Astrocytes are star-shaped cells which occur in large quantities between neurones and blood vessels, supporting and anchoring them to each other. They help form the **blood–brain barrier**, which gives the neurones an extra layer of protection from any toxic substances within the blood.

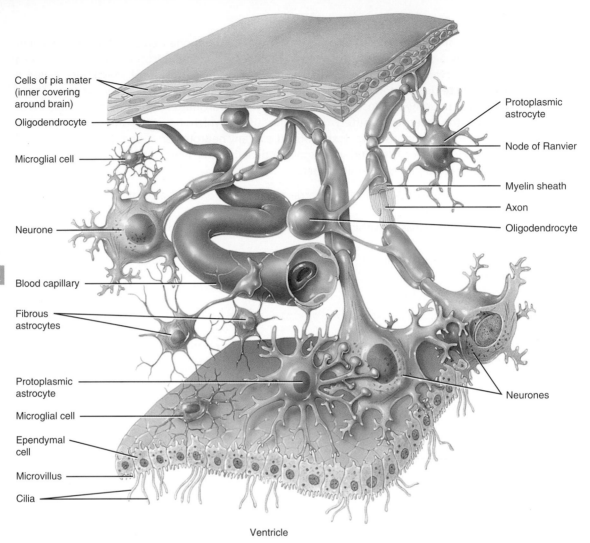

Cells of pia mater
(inner covering
around brain)

Oligodendrocyte

Microglial cell

Neurone

412

Blood capillary

Fibrous
astrocytes

Protoplasmic
astrocyte

Microglial cell

Ependymal
cell

Microvillus

Cilia

Protoplasmic
astrocyte

Node of Ranvier

Myelin sheath

Axon

Oligodendrocyte

Neurones

Ventricle

Figure 13.4   Neuroglia. *Source*: Tortora and Derrickson (2009). Reproduced with permission of John Wiley & Sons.

2. Microglia lie close to neurones and can move closer if they need to fulfil their function as nervous system macrophages. They phagocytose pathogens or cell debris.
3. Oligodendrocytes are found close to myelinated neurones. They help to form and maintain the myelin sheath.
4. Ependymal cells are often ciliated and are found lining cavities, such as the spinal cord or the ventricles of the brain. Their role is to circulate cerebrospinal fluid (CSF) (Waugh and Grant, 2014).

The meninges

Nervous tissue is easily damaged by pressure and therefore needs to be protected. The hair, skin and bone offer an outer layer of protection. Adjacent to the nervous tissue are the meninges (see Figure 13.5). The meninges cover the delicate nervous tissue, providing further protection. They also protect the blood vessels that serve nervous tissue and they contain CSF.

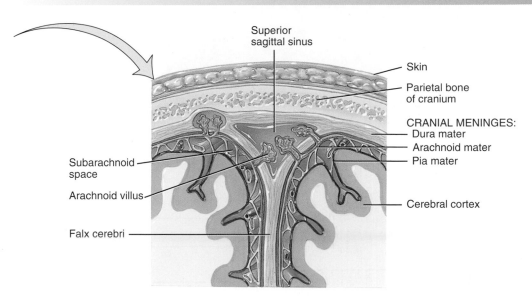

Figure 13.5 The meninges. *Source*: Tortora and Derrickson (2009). Reproduced with permission of John Wiley & Sons.

The meninges consist of three connective tissue layers:

- **Dura mater** – this layer lies closest to the bone of the skull and is a double layer of tough, fibrous, connective tissue. The outer layer is called the periosteal layer (the spinal cord lacks this layer), and the meningeal layer lies closest to the brain.
- **Arachnoid mater** – between the dura mater and the arachnoid mater there is a space called the subdural space. The arachnoid mater is a delicate serous membrane (Seeley *et al.*, 2013). The subarachnoid space is below the arachnoid mater and above the pia mater. The subarachnoid space contains **CSF** and is also home to some of the larger blood vessels serving the brain.
- **Pia mater** – this is a delicate connective tissue layer that clings tightly to the brain. It contains many tiny blood vessels that serve the brain.

Clinical considerations

Meningitis
Meningitis is inflammation of the meninges caused by either bacteria or viruses. It can be diagnosed through symptoms that include photophobia, headache, nausea and vomiting and also by a procedure called a lumbar puncture. In lumbar puncture a small amount of CSF is removed and examined in the laboratory for the presence of microbes. A lack of prompt treatment can have fatal consequences.

Cerebrospinal fluid

CSF is produced by the **choroid plexus** in the ventricles of the brain (see Figure 13.6). There is approximately 150 mL of CSF circulating around the brain, in the ventricles and around the spinal cord. The CSF is replaced every 8 h (Marieb and Hoehn, 2013). It is a thin fluid similar to plasma and has several important functions:

- it acts as a cushion, supporting the weight of the brain and protecting it from damage;
- it helps to maintain a uniform pressure around the brain and spinal cord;
- there is a limited exchange of nutrients and waste products between neurones and CSF.

413

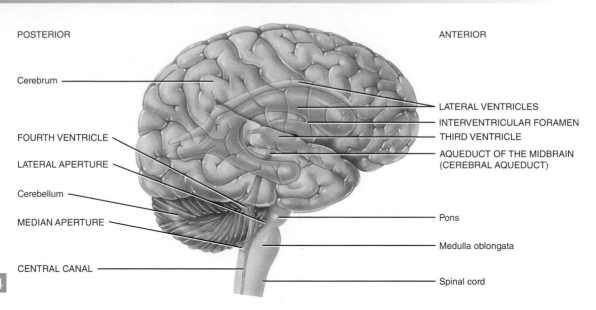

POSTERIOR   ANTERIOR

Cerebrum

LATERAL VENTRICLES
INTERVENTRICULAR FORAMEN
FOURTH VENTRICLE   THIRD VENTRICLE

LATERAL APERTURE   AQUEDUCT OF THE MIDBRAIN
                                                                           (CEREBRAL AQUEDUCT)

Cerebellum

MEDIAN APERTURE   Pons

                                                                           Medulla oblongata

CENTRAL CANAL

Spinal cord

Figure 13.6 The ventricles (right lateral view of the brain). *Source*: Tortora and Derrickson (2009). Reproduced with permission of John Wiley & Sons.

There are four ventricles in the brain: the paired lateral ventricles, one in each cerebral hemisphere; the third ventricle, situated below this; and the fourth ventricle, located inferior to the third. The third and fourth ventricles communicate via the central canal and CSF circulates through the central canal and into the spinal cord.

Any additional pressure applied to the brain caused by swelling (cerebral oedema), tumour or haemorrhage (through trauma) can lead to a reduced volume of CSF being produced.

Snapshot

Lumbar puncture is often used to diagnose conditions such as meningitis and multiple sclerosis.

A sample of CSF is removed and sent for laboratory analysis. The sample is taken by inserting a needle between the third and fourth lumbar vertebrae and the CSF is removed from the subarachnoid space. This procedure is usually carried out under local anaesthetic.

The CSF circulates around the brain and spinal cord. The pressure exerted by the CSF is known as intracranial pressure (ICP). Normal ICP is 8–20 cmH$_2$O. If the ICP is raised this could be for a variety of reasons, including cerebral oedema in the brain as might be seen in head injury, head trauma or meningitis. It could also be raised because of the additional white cells, protein or myelin within the CSF, as in multiple sclerosis.

The CSF should be colourless. Cloudy CSF may indicate the presence of infection. CSF is usually watery in viscosity. If it is more viscous then this could indicate the presence of infection or tumour. Laboratory analysis will give a more accurate interpretation than a visual inspection.

Laboratory analysis will show the amount of glucose protein and immunoglobulins, for example, present in CSF. The white cells can be analysed, and the presence of bacteria and viruses is also investigated.

There are side effects associated with lumbar puncture, and these include back pain from the site of the puncture and headache. The headache is often relieved by lying down.

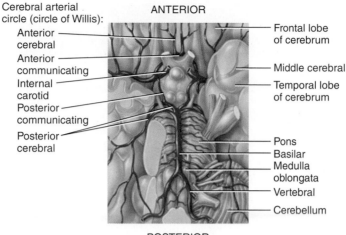

Cerebral arterial circle (circle of Willis):
- Anterior cerebral
- Anterior communicating
- Internal carotid
- Posterior communicating
- Posterior cerebral

ANTERIOR

- Frontal lobe of cerebrum
- Middle cerebral
- Temporal lobe of cerebrum
- Pons
- Basilar
- Medulla oblongata
- Vertebral
- Cerebellum

POSTERIOR

Figure 13.7   Circle of Willis. *Source*: Tortora and Derrickson (2009). Reproduced with permission of John Wiley & Sons.

The brain

The brain lies in the cranial cavity and weighs between 1450 and 1600 g (Marieb and Hoehn, 2013). It receives 15% of the cardiac output and has a system of **autoregulation** ensuring the blood supply is constant despite positional changes. The arrangement of the arteries serving the brain is unique, and they are connected to each other by a structure called the circle of Willis (see Figure 13.7). This arrangement ensures that blood pressure remains equal in both halves of the brain. Should one of the arteries serving the brain become narrowed by arterial disease or thrombus then there will be an alternative route available, maintaining the essential supply of oxygen and glucose required by the brain.

The brain can be divided into four anatomical regions. Each region contains one or more structures (see Figure 13.8):

- cerebrum
- cerebral hemispheres
- diencephalon
- thalamus
- hypothalamus
- epithalamus
- brainstem
- midbrain
- pons
- medulla oblongata
- reticular formation
- cerebellum.

Cerebrum

This is the largest brain structure. It is divided into the left and right hemispheres by the **longitudinal cerebral fissure**. Each hemisphere can be divided into lobes – occipital, frontal, parietal and temporal. The outer layer of the cerebrum is called the cerebral cortex and is made of grey

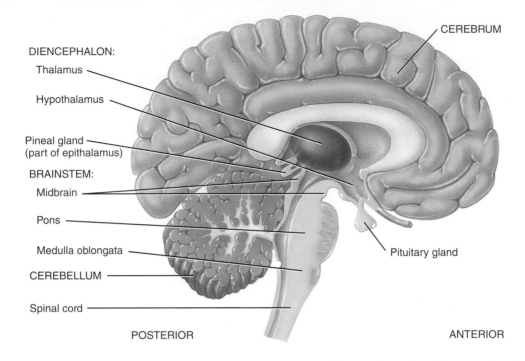

DIENCEPHALON:
Thalamus
Hypothalamus
Pineal gland
(part of epithalamus)
BRAINSTEM:
Midbrain
Pons
Medulla oblongata
CEREBELLUM
Spinal cord

CEREBRUM

Pituitary gland

POSTERIOR   ANTERIOR

Figure 13.8   The structures of the brain. *Source*: Tortora and Derrickson (2009). Reproduced with permission of John Wiley & Sons.

matter (nerve cell bodies). The layers below this are white matter (nerve fibres). The cerebral cortex is responsible for our conscious mind and consists of interneurones (the neurones that lie between sensory and motor neurones). The cerebral cortex can be divided into functional areas, which were mapped by K Brodmann in 1906 (see Figure 13.9). The circled numbers on the diagram represent important areas on Brodmann's map. While functional and structural areas of the brain have been identified, it is important to remember that the areas do not function independently from one another, and damage to one structure may have consequences for another.

The first of the functional areas is the motor area and it is subdivided as follows:

- the primary motor area – responsible for contraction of skeletal muscles;
- the premotor area – involved in fine skeletal muscle movement creating the manual dexterity associated with repetitive or learned motor movement (e.g. tying a shoelace, learning to paint);
- Broca's area – responsible for the motor movement required to produce speech;
- the frontal eye field area – controls voluntary movement of the eyes.

The second functional area is the sensory area, responsible for awareness of sensation. It can be divided as follows:

- the primary somatosensory area – receives sensory information from the skin and also from proprioceptors in skeletal muscles;
- the somatosensory association area – integrates the sensory information being relayed to the primary somatosensory area and provides information about size, texture, previous experience;
- the visual areas – the primary visual area receives information from the eye and the visual association area helps to connect this information with past visual experiences;

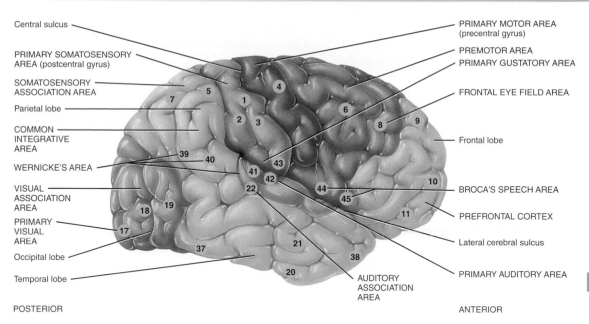

Central sulcus

PRIMARY SOMATOSENSORY
AREA (postcentral gyrus)

SOMATOSENSORY
ASSOCIATION AREA

Parietal lobe

COMMON
INTEGRATIVE
AREA

WERNICKE'S AREA

VISUAL
ASSOCIATION
AREA

PRIMARY
VISUAL
AREA

Occipital lobe

Temporal lobe

PRIMARY MOTOR AREA
(precentral gyrus)

PREMOTOR AREA
PRIMARY GUSTATORY AREA

FRONTAL EYE FIELD AREA

Frontal lobe

BROCA'S SPEECH AREA

PREFRONTAL CORTEX

Lateral cerebral sulcus

PRIMARY AUDITORY AREA

AUDITORY
ASSOCIATION
AREA

POSTERIOR   ANTERIOR

Figure 13.9 Right cerebral hemisphere. *Source*: Tortora and Derrickson (2009). Reproduced with permission of John Wiley & Sons.

- the auditory areas – associated with the interpretation of sounds;
- the olfactory area – interprets smell information received from the nose via the olfactory nerves;
- the gustatory area – interprets taste information.

There are many other association areas within the cerebrum that act as communication areas between different functional regions in the cerebrum, such as Wernicke's area, which is responsible for understanding written and spoken language and is closely associated with Broca's speech area.

Diencephalon

This part of the brain is surrounded by the cerebrum and contains three paired structures:

- Thalamus – acts as a relay station for sensory impulses going to the cerebral cortex for integration and motor impulses entering and leaving the cerebral hemispheres. It also has a role in memory.
- Hypothalamus – is closely associated with the pituitary gland and produces two hormones: antidiuretic hormone (ADH) and oxytocin. The hypothalamus has many functions and these include:
  - control of body temperature
  - control of the autonomic nervous system
  - control of fluid balance and thirst
  - control of appetite
  - associated with the limbic system dealing with emotional reactions
  - control of sexual behaviours.
- Epithalamus – this structure is linked to the pineal gland, which secretes the hormone melatonin responsible for sleep–wake cycles.

Brainstem

The structures that form the brainstem are involved in many activities that are essential for life. The brainstem is associated with the cranial nerves.

- Midbrain – conduction pathway that connects the cerebrum with the lower brain structures and spinal cord.
- Pons – also a conduction pathway communicating with the cerebellum. The pons works with the medulla oblongata to control depth and rate of respiration.
- Medulla oblongata – relay station for sensory nerves going to the cerebrum. The medulla contains autonomic centres such as the cardiac centre, the respiratory centre, the vasomotor centre and the coughing, sneezing and vomiting centre. The medulla is also the site of decussation of the pyramidal tracts – this means that the right side of the body is controlled by the left cerebral hemisphere and vice versa.

Clinical considerations

Concussion

Concussion is a minor head injury and is defined as a brief period of unconsciousness. It is also termed mild traumatic brain injury (VanMeter and Hubert, 2014). Signs and symptoms include nausea, headaches, dizziness, impaired concentration, amnesia (memory loss), extreme tiredness, and intolerance to light and noise. The symptoms usually only last for 24 h.

Cerebellum

The cerebellum coordinates voluntary muscle movement, balance and posture. It ensures that muscle movements are smooth, coordinated and precise.

The limbic system and the reticular formation

The limbic system and the reticular formation are more functional than anatomical systems as they consist of networks of neurones that can be located close to many anatomical structures.

The limbic system is located close to the cerebrum and the diencephalon. It is known as the emotional brain and is responsible for the interpretation of facial expression, helping identify fear and danger.

The reticular formation is a functional system located in the core of the brainstem and consists of a collection of neurones that have several functions:

- contains reticular activating system that is responsible for alertness;
- filters or blocks repetitive stimuli, such as background noise;
- regulates skeletal muscle activity;
- coordinates visceral activity controlled by the autonomic nervous system.

The brain is a well-protected control and integration centre that receives information from the peripheral sensory nervous system and sends motor information to the peripheral nervous system through a comprehensive network of pathways via the spinal cord.

Medicines management

Midazolam

Midazolam is a medication known as a benzodiazepine. Benzodiazepines act on central nervous system receptors and produce a sedative effect. Midazolam is thought to produce amnesia and is therefore useful in procedures that require the patient to be awake and cooperative despite the unpleasant nature of the procedure, such as endoscopy (Galbraith *et al.*, 2007). The intention is that the patient will not remember the procedure.

Midazolam is a short-acting benzodiazepine and has a half-life of 2–3 h (Galbraith *et al.*, 2007). It is available for administration via a variety of routes, including intravenous and intramuscular routes.

Midazolam has a number of side effects, and these include

- respiratory failure
- respiratory depression
- hypotension
- anaphylaxis
- convulsions
- dry mouth
- constipation
- nausea
- euphoria
- hiccups
- headache.

As benzodiazepines are addictive their use has been abused. An antagonist called flumazenil is available to reverse the effects of the medication.

Benzodiazepines should be prescribed with caution.

Medicines management

Phenytoin

John is 34 years old and suffers from seizures following his recovery from a head injury. He has been prescribed phenytoin sodium 100 mg orally three times a day for this. This medicine works during the action potential. It promotes the removal of sodium during the refractory period, thus reducing the hyperexcitability of neurones that can lead to seizure (Galbraith *et al.*, 2007). John has been advised to avoid alcohol and to maintain good oral hygiene practices, as this medicine has a known side effect of gingival hyperplasia (gum overgrowth).

The peripheral nervous system

The peripheral nervous system includes all the tissues that lie outside of the central nervous system:

- cranial nerves
- spinal nerves
- spinal cord
- autonomic nervous system.

The peripheral nervous system is subdivided into the efferent or motor system and the afferent or sensory system. The somatic sensory system serves the skeletal muscles, joints, tendons and the skin and includes the senses of vision, hearing, smell and taste (Logenbaker, 2013). The internal organs of the body are supplied by the visceral sensory system. Both the somatic and visceral sensory systems take information from peripheral sensory receptors towards the central nervous system.

Commands from the central nervous system to the skeletal muscles are carried by the somatic motor system. The autonomic motor system predominantly regulates the activity of smooth and cardiac muscles and glands (Logenbaker, 2013).

Cranial nerves

The human body contains 12 pairs of cranial nerves that emerge from the brain and supply various structures, most of which are associated with the head and neck. Figure 13.10 provides an overview of the location and function of the cranial nerves.

The 12 pairs of cranial nerves differ in their functions: some are **sensory nerves** (i.e. contain sensory fibres), some are **motor nerves** (i.e. contain only motor fibres) and some are **mixed nerves** (i.e. contain both sensory and motor nerves).

Table 13.1 provides a summary of the cranial nerves, their different components and function.

The spinal cord

The average adult spinal cord (see Figure 13.11) is between 42 and 45 cm long and extends from the medulla oblongata (lower part of the brain) to the upper part of the second lumbar vertebra. The spinal cord is enclosed within the vertebral canal, which forms a protective ring of bone around the cord. Other protective coverings include the spinal meninges, which are three layers of connective tissue coverings that extend around the spinal cord. The spinal meninges consist of

- **the pia mater** – the innermost layer;
- **the arachnoid mater** – the middle layer;
- **the dura mater** – the outermost layer, which consists of a dense, irregular connective tissue.

The spinal cord consists of a central canal and grey and white matter. The central canal and the spinal meninges contain CSF. The grey matter consists mostly of cell bodies and their dendrites, and the whiter areas consist of the axons of neurones, which carry signals up and down the cord via ascending and descending tracts. These tracts cross as they enter and exit the brain, and this explains why the right side of the brain controls the left side of the body and the left side of the brain controls the right side of the body.

The spinal cord is divided into the right and left halves by the deep **anterior median fissure** and the shallow **posterior median sulcus** (Tortora and Derrickson, 2012).

Functions of the spinal cord

The spinal cord provides a means of communication between the brain and the peripheral nerves that leave the spinal cord (Logenbaker, 2013) and has two major functions in maintaining homeostasis (Tortora and Derrickson, 2012):

- The tracts of the white matter of the spinal cord carry sensory impulses to the brain and motor impulses from the brain to the skeletal muscles and other effector muscles.
- The grey matter of the spinal cord is a site for integration of reflexes, which is a rapid, involuntary action in relation to a particular stimulus.

420

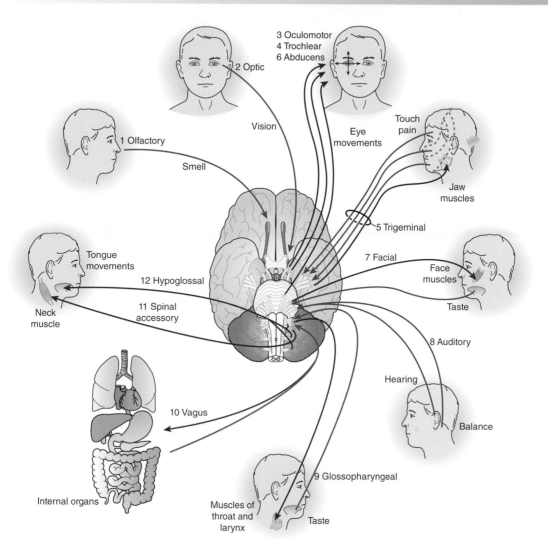

Figure 13.10   Functions of cranial nerves.

Spinal nerves

There are 31 pairs of spinal nerves attached to the spinal cord within the human body, which are named and numbered according to the region and level of the vertebral column from which they emerge (Figure 13.12).

Each nerve innervates a group of muscles (myotome) and an area of skin (dermatome), and most also innervate some of the thoracic and abdominal organs (Figure 13.13).

The spinal nerves provide the paths of communication between the spinal cord and specific regions of the body as they connect the central nervous system to sensory receptors, muscles and glands in all the parts of the body. A typical spinal nerve (Figure 13.14) has two connections to the spinal cord – a posterior root and an anterior root, which unite to form a spinal nerve at the **intervertebral foramen**. A spinal nerve is an example of a mixed nerve as it contains both sensory (posterior root) and motor (anterior root) nerves.

Table 13.1   The cranial nerves

Number	Name	Components	Location/function
I	Olfactory	Sensory	Olfactory receptors for sense of smell
II	Optic	Sensory	Retina (sight)
III	Oculomotor	Motor	Eye muscles (including eyelids and lens, pupil)
IV	Trochlear	Motor	Eye muscles
V	Trigeminal	Sensory and motor	Teeth, eyes, skin, tongue for sensation of touch, pain and temperature
VI	Abducens	Motor	Jaw muscles (chewing)
			Eye muscles
VII	Facial	Sensory and motor	Taste buds
			Facial muscles, tear and salivary glands
VIII	Vestibulocochlear	Sensory	Inner ear (hearing and balance)
IX	Glossopharyngeal	Sensory and motor	Pharyngeal muscles (swallowing)
X	Vagus	Sensory and motor	Internal organs
XI	Spinal accessory	Motor	Neck and back muscles
XII	Hypoglossal	Motor	Tongue muscles

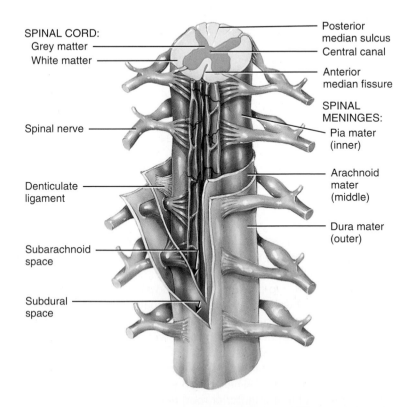

Figure 13.11   The spinal cord. *Source*: Tortora and Derrickson (2009). Reproduced with permission of John Wiley & Sons.

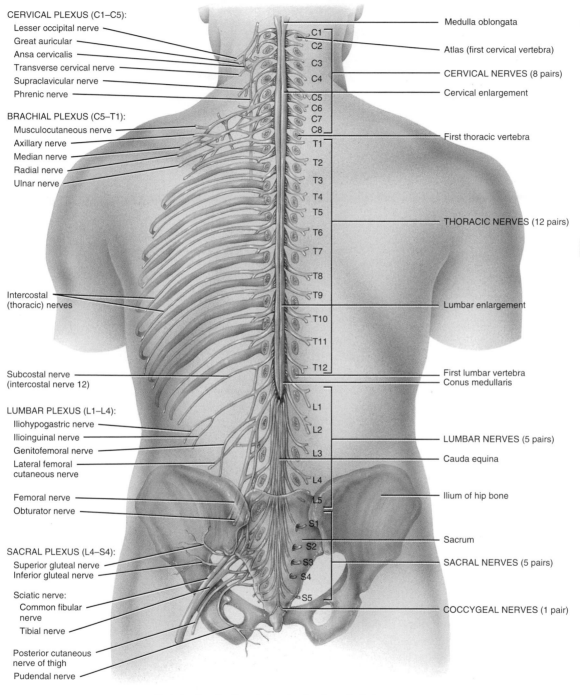

CERVICAL PLEXUS (C1–C5):
Lesser occipital nerve
Great auricular
Ansa cervicalis
Transverse cervical nerve
Supraclavicular nerve
Phrenic nerve

BRACHIAL PLEXUS (C5–T1):
Musculocutaneous nerve
Axillary nerve
Median nerve
Radial nerve
Ulnar nerve

Intercostal
(thoracic) nerves

Subcostal nerve
(intercostal nerve 12)

LUMBAR PLEXUS (L1–L4):
Iliohypogastric nerve
Ilioinguinal nerve
Genitofemoral nerve
Lateral femoral
cutaneous nerve

Femoral nerve
Obturator nerve

SACRAL PLEXUS (L4–S4):
Superior gluteal nerve
Inferior gluteal nerve

Sciatic nerve:
Common fibular
nerve
Tibial nerve

Posterior cutaneous
nerve of thigh
Pudendal nerve

Medulla oblongata

Atlas (first cervical vertebra)

CERVICAL NERVES (8 pairs)

Cervical enlargement

First thoracic vertebra

THORACIC NERVES (12 pairs)

Lumbar enlargement

First lumbar vertebra
Conus medullaris

LUMBAR NERVES (5 pairs)

Cauda equina

Ilium of hip bone

Sacrum

SACRAL NERVES (5 pairs)

COCCYGEAL NERVES (1 pair)

C1
C2
C3
C4
C5
C6
C7
C8
T1
T2
T3
T4
T5
T6
T7
T8
T9
T10
T11
T12
L1
L2
L3
L4
L5
S1
S2
S3
S4
S5

Posterior view of entire spinal cord and portions of spinal nerves

Figure 13.12 The spinal cord and spinal nerves. *Source*: Tortora and Derrickson (2009). Reproduced with permission of John Wiley & Sons.

423

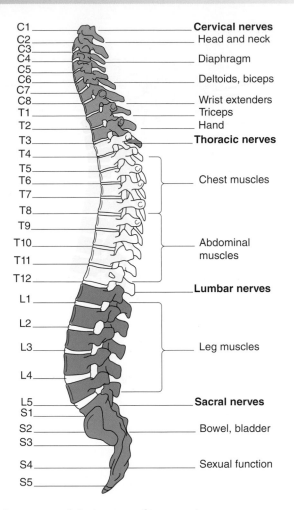

Figure 13.13   The spinal nerves and their areas of innervations.

Clinical considerations

Acute spinal cord compression

Acute spinal cord compression is a neurological emergency that requires rapid diagnosis and treatment if permanent loss of function is to be avoided. Common causes of spinal cord compression include:

- trauma (car accidents, sports injury and falls);
- tumours, both benign and malignant;
- a prolapsed intervertebral disc (L4–L5 and L5–S1 are the most common levels of disc prolapse);
- an epidural or subdural haemorrhage;
- inflammatory disease (e.g. rheumatoid arthritis);
- infection.

Signs and symptoms include sensory loss, paraesthesia, disturbance of gait, loss of power or paralysis.

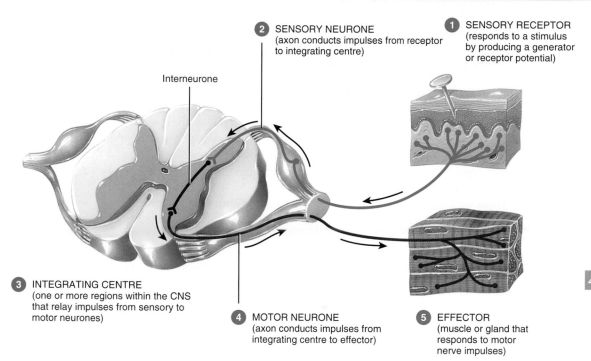

② SENSORY NEURONE
(axon conducts impulses from receptor to integrating centre)

① SENSORY RECEPTOR
(responds to a stimulus by producing a generator or receptor potential)

Interneurone

③ INTEGRATING CENTRE
(one or more regions within the CNS that relay impulses from sensory to motor neurones)

④ MOTOR NEURONE
(axon conducts impulses from integrating centre to effector)

⑤ EFFECTOR
(muscle or gland that responds to motor nerve impulses)

Figure 13.14   A typical spinal nerve (CNS: central nervous system). *Source*: Tortora and Derrickson (2009). Reproduced with permission of John Wiley & Sons.

Medicines management

Paracetamol

Paracetamol (acetaminophen) is a common over-the-counter medication used to treat mild to moderate pain and is also effective as a fever reducer. The exact mechanism of action of is not known; however, it is thought that the analgesic mechanism of paracetamol involves the metabolites of paracetamol, which act on receptors in the spinal cord and are thought to suppress the signal transduction from the superficial layers of the dorsal horn to alleviate pain (Toussaint *et al.*, 2010).

In relation to its fever-reducing properties, it has been proposed that the main mechanism of action is the inhibition of the enzyme cyclooxygenase (COX), and recent findings suggest that it is highly selective for COX-2. The COX family of enzymes is responsible for the metabolism of compounds that encourage inflammatory responses. Paracetamol is thought to reduce the oxidised form of the COX enzyme, preventing it from forming pro-inflammatory chemicals. This leads to a reduced amount of prostaglandins S, thus lowering the hypothalamic set-point in the thermoregulatory centre.

Paracetamol is used to treat many conditions, such as headache, muscle aches, arthritis, backache, toothache, colds and fevers.

Overdosage of paracetamol is particularly dangerous as it may cause liver damage, which may not be apparent for 4–6 days after ingestion. Treatment includes infusing acetylcysteine, which protects the liver. However, it is most effective if given within 8 h of ingestion, after which effectiveness declines.

425

Clinical considerations

Panic attack

A panic attack is a rush of intense psychological and physical symptoms. These symptoms of panic can be frightening and happen suddenly, often for no clear reason.

Panic attacks usually last between 5 and 20 min, and the individual may experience unpleasant psychological and physical symptoms; however, these are usually short-lived and will not cause harm (NHS Choices, 2015). Psychological symptoms can include an overwhelming sense of fear and a sense of unreality, as if the individual is detached from the world around them. Physical symptoms of panic can include sweating, trembling, shortness of breath, a choking sensation, chest pain, a feeling of nausea and palpitations.

The physical symptoms of a panic attack are caused by the body's sympathetic response to something that the individual perceives as a threat and causes the release of hormones, such as adrenaline, resulting in an increased heart rate and muscle tension.

Sufferers of panic attacks can be helped to manage their condition through learning breathing and relaxation techniques and avoiding substances such as caffeine, nicotine and alcohol (NHS Choices, 2015).

The autonomic nervous system

The autonomic nervous system plays a major role in the maintenance of homeostasis by regulating the body's automatic, involuntary functions. In common with the rest of the nervous system, it consists of **neurones**, **neuroglia** and other connective tissue. However, its structure is unique, in that it is divided into two: namely, the **sympathetic division** and the **parasympathetic division**. These two divisions have several common features (Logenbaker, 2013):

- they innervate all internal organs;
- they utilise two motor neurones and one ganglion to transmit an action potential;
- they function automatically and usually in an involuntary manner.

Sympathetic division (fight or flight)

The sympathetic division (see Figure 13.15) includes nerve fibres that arise from the 12 thoracic and first two lumbar segments of the spine; hence, it is also referred to as the **thoracicolumbar** division. The sympathetic division takes control of many internal organs when a stressful situation occurs. This can take the form of physical stress if undertaking strenuous exercise or emotional stress at times of anger or anxiety. In emergency situations, the sympathetic nervous system releases **norepinephrine**, which assists in the 'fight or flight' response (Migliozzi, 2013).

Parasympathetic division (rest and digest)

The parasympathetic division includes fibres that arise from the lower end of the spinal cord and several cranial nerves; hence, it is often referred to as the **craniosacral** division. The parasympathetic division is most active when the body is at rest; it utilises **acetylcholine** to control all the internal responses associated with a state of relaxation (Figure 13.16) and, therefore, has many opposite effects on the body to the sympathetic nervous system (Migliozzi, 2013).

Table 13.2 provides a summary of the physiological effects of the sympathetic and parasympathetic divisions of the nervous system.

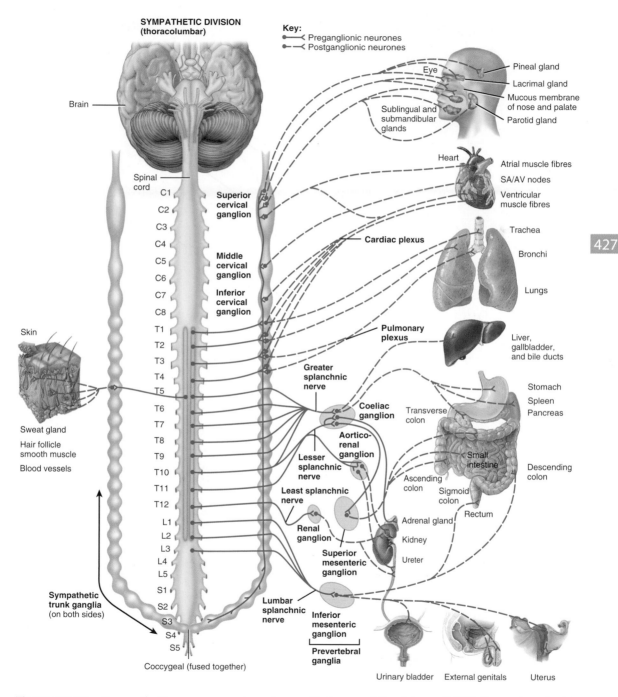

Figure 13.15   Sympathetic nervous system. *Source*: Tortora and Derrickson (2009). Reproduced with permission of John Wiley & Sons.

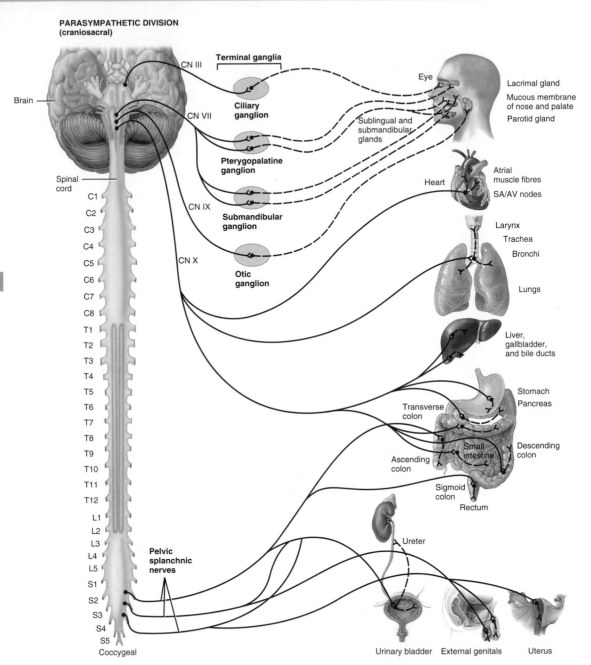

Figure 13.16 Parasympathetic nervous system. *Source*: Tortora and Derrickson (2009). Reproduced with permission of John Wiley & Sons.

Table 13.2 Effects of the parasympathetic and sympathetic divisions of the autonomic nervous system

Organ/system	Sympathetic effects	Parasympathetic effects
Cell metabolism	Increases metabolic rate, stimulates fat breakdown and increases blood sugar levels	No effect
Blood vessels	Constricts blood vessels in viscera and skin	No effect
	Dilates blood vessels in the heart and skeletal muscle	
Eye	Dilates pupils	Constricts pupils
Heart	Increases rate and force of contraction	Decreases rate
Lungs	Dilates bronchioles	Constricts bronchioles
Kidneys	Decreases urine output	No effect
Liver	Causes the release of glucose	No effect
Digestive system	Decreases peristalsis and constricts digestive system sphincters	Increases peristalsis and dilates digestive system sphincters
Adrenal medulla	Stimulates cells to secrete epinephrine and norepinephrine	No effect
Lacrimal glands	Inhibits the production of tears	Increases the production of tears
Salivary glands	Inhibits the production of saliva	Increases the production of saliva
Sweat glands	Stimulates to produce perspiration	No effect

Medicines management

Carbamazepine

Carbamazepine is an anticonvulsant primarily used in the treatment of epileptic seizures. Carbamazepine works by blocking the sodium channels of nerve cells in the brain and so reduces the increased excitability and firing activity of neurones that occur during an epileptic seizure.

Antiepileptic hypersensitivity syndrome has been associated with some antiepileptic drugs and usually starts between 1 and 8 weeks after commencing treatment, and signs and symptoms include fever, rash, lymphadenopathy liver and haematological dysfunction. If signs of hypersensitivity syndrome occur, the drug should be withdrawn immediately (Joint Formulary Committee, 2014).

Patients with epilepsy may drive a car but not larger vehicles (e.g. passenger-carrying vehicles or lorries). *Guidance from the Driver and Vehicle Licensing Agency:* However, patients are advised not to drive during medication changes or withdrawal of antiepileptic drugs, and for 6 months afterwards. Similarly, patients who have had a first or single epileptic seizure must not drive for 6 months (Joint Formulary Committee, 2014).

Conclusion

In conclusion, the human nervous system is a highly organised network of cells and structures that include the brain and cranial nerves and the spinal cord and spinal nerves, which play a major role in maintaining homeostasis. The nervous system responds to external and internal stimuli through three basic functions: the sensory, integrative and motor functions, which generate responses and create changes in bodily functions as required. Conditions affecting the nervous system can have a devastating effect on the quality of life and the functions essential for survival.

Glossary

Action potential   Conduction along a nerve or muscle cell membrane caused by a large, transient depolarisation.

Antidiuretic hormone (ADH)   Hormone that acts on the kidneys to reabsorb more water, thus reducing urine output.

Afferent fibres   Carry nerve impulses towards the central nervous system.

Arachnoid mater   Middle layer of the meninges.

Astrocyte   Neuroglial cell that helps the blood–brain barrier.

Autonomic nervous system   Involuntary motor division of the motor nervous system.

Axon   Process of a neurone that carries impulses away from the cell body.

Brainstem   Collective name given to the pons, medulla and midbrain.

Cation   An ion with a positive charge.

Central nervous system   Brain and spinal cord.

Cerebellum   Anatomical region of the brain responsible for coordinated and smooth skeletal muscle movements.

Cerebral hemispheres   Division of the cerebrum.

Cerebrospinal fluid   Fluid that surrounds the central nervous system.

Cerebrum   Large anatomical region of the brain which is divided into the cerebral hemispheres.

Circle of Willis   Part of arterial blood supply to the brain.

Cranial nerves   Twelve pairs of nerves that leave the brain and supply sensory and motor neurones to the head, neck, part of the trunk and the viscera of the thorax and abdomen.

Dendrite   Part of neurone that transmits impulses towards the cell body

Diencephalon   Anatomical region of the brain consisting of the thalamus, hypothalamus and epithalamus.

Dura mater   Tough outer layer of the meninges.

Effector   Muscle, gland or organ stimulated by the nervous system.

Efferent fibres   Carry nerve impulses away from the central nervous system.

Ependymal cells   Neuroglial cells that line the cavities of the central nervous system.

Epinephrine   Hormone produced by the adrenal medulla that is also a neurotransmitter.

Epithalamus   Part of the brain that forms the diencephalon.

Ganglia   A group of neuronal cell bodies lying outside the central nervous system.

Hypothalamus   Part of the diencephalon with many functions.

Limbic system   Part of the brain involved in emotional responses.

Lobe   A clear anatomical division or boundary within a structure.

Medulla oblongata   Part of the brainstem.

Meninges   Three layers of tissue that cover and protect the central nervous system (dura, arachnoid and pia maters).

Midbrain   Part of the brainstem that links the brainstem to the diencephalon.

Microglia   Neuroglia that has the ability to phagocytose material.

Motor area   Area located in the cerebral cortex that controls voluntary motor function.

Motor nerves   Neurones that conduct impulses to effectors which may be either muscle or glands.

Myelin sheath   Fatty insulating layer that surrounds nerve fibres responsible for speeding up impulse conduction.

Neuroglia   Cells of the nervous system that protect and support the functional unit – the neurone.

Neuromuscular junction   Region where skeletal muscle comes into contact with a neurone.

Neurone   Functional unit of the nervous system responsible for generating and conducting nerve impulses.

Nuclei   Cluster of cell bodies within the central nervous system.

Oligodendrocytes   Glial cell that helps produce the myelin sheath.

Peripheral nervous system   All nerves located outside of the brain and spinal cord (the central nervous system).

Pia mater   Innermost layer of the meninges.

Pineal gland   Part of the diencephalon that has an endocrine function.

Pituitary gland   An endocrine gland located next to the hypothalamus that produces many hormones.

Receptor   Sensory nerve ending or cell that responds to stimuli.

Refractory period   The period immediately after a neurone has fired when it cannot receive another impulse.

Reticular formation   Area located throughout the brainstem that is responsible for arousal, regulation of sensory input to the cerebrum and control of motor output.

Saltatory conduction   Transmission of an impulse down a myelinated nerve fibre where the impulse moves from node of Ranvier to node.

Sensory area   Area of the cerebrum responsible for sensation.

Sensory nerves   Neurones that carry sensory information from cranial and spinal nerves into the brain and spinal cord.

Somatic nervous system   Voluntary motor division of the peripheral nervous system.

Spinal nerves   Thirty-one pairs of nerves that originate on the spinal cord.

Synapse   Junction between two neurones or neurones and effector site.

Thalamus   Part of the diencephalon.

Ventricle   Cavity in the brain.

White matter   Myelinated nerve fibres.

References

Galbraith, A., Bullock, S., Manias, E., Hunt, B. and Richards, A. (2007) *Fundamentals of Pharmacology. An Applied Approach for Nursing and Health*, 2nd edn. Harlow: Pearson Education.

Joint Formulary Committee (2014) *BNF 68*. London: Pharmaceutical Press.

Logenbaker, S.N. (2013) *Mader's Understanding Human Anatomy and Physiology*, 8th edn. London: McGraw-Hill.

Marieb, E.N. and Hoehn, K. (2013) *Human Anatomy and Physiology*, 9th edn. San Francisco, CA: Pearson Benjamin Cummings.

Migliozzi, J.G. (2013) The nervous system and associated disorders. In Nair, M. and Peate, I. (eds) *Fundamentals of Applied Pathophysiology: An Essential Guide For Nursing And Healthcare Students*, 2nd edn. Oxford: John Wiley & Sons, Ltd.

NHS Choices (2015) *Stress, Anxiety and Depression*. http://www.nhs.uk/Conditions/stress-anxiety-depression/Pages/low-mood-stress-anxiety.aspx (accessed 1 December 2015).

Seeley, R.R., Stephens T.D. and Vanputte, C. (2013) *Anatomy and Physiology*, 10th edn. New York: McGraw-Hill.

Tortora, G.J. and Derrickson, B.H. (2009) *Principles of Anatomy and Physiology*, 12th edn. Hoboken, NJ: John Wiley & Sons, Inc.

Tortora, G.J. and Derrickson, T. (2014) *Principles of Anatomy and Physiology*, 14th edn. Hoboken, NJ: John Wiley & Sons, Inc.

Tortora, G.J. and Derrickson, B. (2012) *Essentials of Anatomy and Physiology*, 9th edn. New York: John Wiley & Sons, Inc.

Toussaint, K., Yang, X.C., Zielinski, M.A., Reigle, K.L., Sacavage, S.D., Nagar, S. and Raffa, R.B. (2010) What do we (not) know about how paracetamol (acetaminophen) works? *Journal of Clinical Pharmacy and Therapeutics* **35**(6): 617–638.

VanMeter, K.C. and Hubert, R.J. (2014). *Gould's Pathophysiology for Health Professions*, 5th edn. St Louis: Elsevier Saunders.

Waugh, A. and Grant, A. (2014) *Ross and Wilson Anatomy and Physiology in Health and Illness*, 12th edn. Edinburgh: Elsevier Churchill Livingstone.

Further reading

http://www.nice.org.uk/guidance/cg176

Link to clinical guidance on head injury: triage, assessment, investigation and early management of head injury in children, young people and adults.

http://www.nice.org.uk/guidance/cg137

Link to clinical guidance on the epilepsies. The epilepsies, the diagnosis and management of the epilepsies in adult and children in primary and secondary care.

http://www.stroke.org.uk/
The Stroke Association is a UK charity that helps those affected by stroke and their families.
http://www.parkinsons.org.uk/
Parkinson's UK is a UK charity supporting those affected by Parkinson's disease and supporting Parkinson's disease research.

Activities

Multiple choice questions

1. Which part of the brain is responsible for thinking, reasoning and intelligence?
   (a) cerebellum
   (b) hypothalamus
   (c) cerebrum
   (d) epithalamus
2. Which structures are involved in the control of respiration?
   (a) pons and medulla
   (b) thalamus and epithalamus
   (c) somatic and sensory nervous system
   (d) cerebellum and cerebrum
3. Which neuroglial cell acts as a macrophage?
   (a) oligodendrocyte
   (b) astrocyte
   (c) microglia
   (d) Schwann cell
4. Which layer of the meninges is closest to the skull bone?
   (a) dura mater
   (b) arachnoid mater
   (c) pia mater
   (d) subarachnoid space
5. Which neurotransmitter is associated with the neuromuscular junction?
   (a) dopamine
   (b) norepinephrine
   (c) acetylcholine
   (d) CSF
6. Which part of the brain is closely associated with the pituitary gland?
   (a) thalamus
   (b) epithalamus
   (c) hypothalamus
   (d) pons
7. Which is true of the autonomic nervous system?
   (a) it has two divisions – the somatic and voluntary divisions
   (b) it is housed in the cerebrum
   (c) it helps regulate heart rate and blood pressure
   (d) it does not influence any other system of the body
8. Nerves that carry impulses towards the central nervous system are:
   (a) afferent nerves
   (b) efferent nerves

      (c) motor nerves
      (d) mixed nerves

9. Sympathetic stimulation of the nervous system would lead to all but which of the following responses:
      (a) bronchioles dilate
      (b) urine output increases
      (c) heart rate increases
      (d) epinephrine (adrenaline) is released

10. Nerves that carry impulses away from the central nervous system are:
      (a) afferent nerves
      (b) efferent nerves
      (c) motor nerves
      (d) mixed nerves

True or false

1. The hypothalamus produces oxytocin.
2. Voluntary muscle movement is controlled by the afferent nervous system.
3. Ependymal cells help to circulate CSF.
4. The cranial nerves are all motor nerves.
5. There are eight thoracic nerves.
6. Sodium is the principal extracellular cation.
7. Motor nerves carry nerve impulses from the central nervous system.
8. Oligodendrocytes form the blood–brain barrier.
9. The subdural space lies between the dura mater and the pia mater.
10. The frontal eye field area controls voluntary movement of the eyes.

Label the diagram 1

Label the diagram using the following list of words:

Axon collateral, AXON, Axon, Axoplasm, Axolemma, Axon terminal, Synaptic end bulb, Nucleus of Schwann cell, Schwann cell, Cytoplasm, Myelin sheath, Neurolemma, Node of Ranvier, Neurofibril, Initial segment, Axon hillock, Mitochondrion, Cytoplasm, Nissl bodies, DENDRITES, CELL BODY, Neurofibril, Nucleus, Dendrite, Neuroglial cell, Cell body, Axon

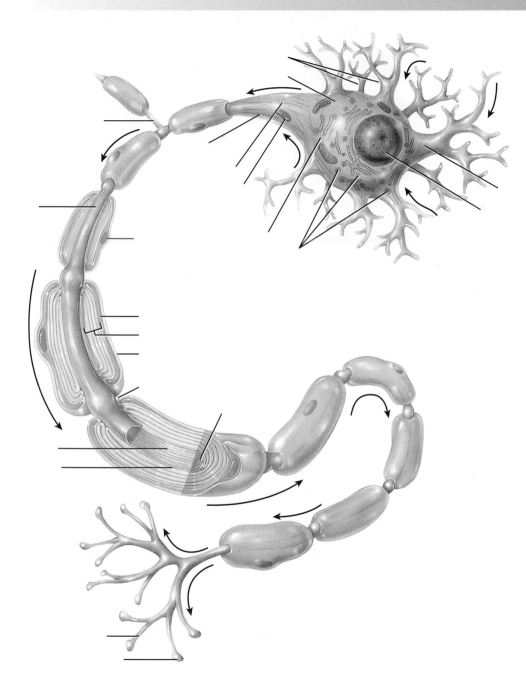

Label the diagram 2

Label the diagram using the following list of words:

DIENCEPHALON, Thalamus, Hypothalamus, Pineal gland (part of epithalamus), BRAINSTEM, Midbrain, Pons, Medulla oblongata, CEREBELLUM, Spinal cord, POSTERIOR, CEREBRUM, Pituitary gland, ANTERIOR

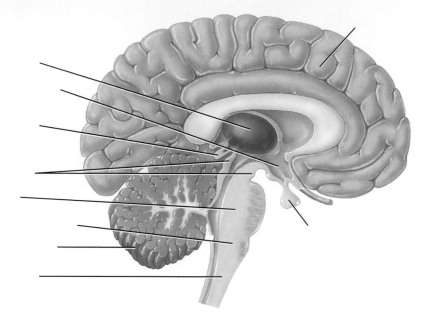

Crossword

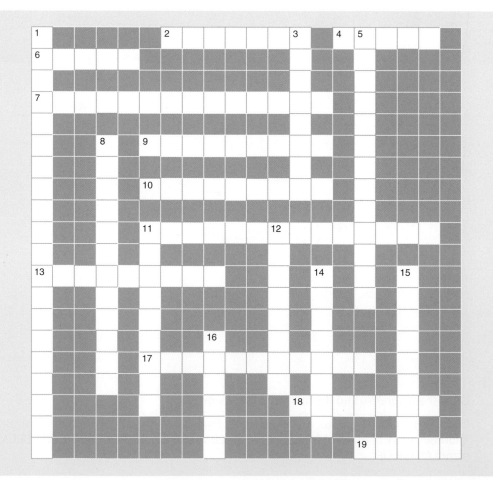

Across:

2. Cell of the nervous system (7).
4. Cranial nerve X (5).
6. Cranial nerve II (5).
7. Middle layer of the meninges (9, 5).
9. Outer layer of the meninges – closest to the skull (4, 5).
10. Star-shaped microglia (9).
11. A structure of the endocrine system that is located next to the hypothalamus (9, 5).
13. Cranial nerve I (9).
17. Describes the autonomic nervous system control (11).
18. Part of the brain that has a role in respiratory and heart rate (7).
19. One half of the central nervous system (5).

Down:

1. Voluntary part of the peripheral nervous system (7, 7, 6).
3. Name given to a nerve delivering the impulse away from the central nervous system (8).
5. Neuromuscular junction neurotransmitter (13).
8. Brain structure responsible for the autonomic nervous system (12).
11. Principal intracellular cation involved in the action potential (9).
12. Name given to a nerve delivering the impulse towards the central nervous system (8).
14. Layer of the meninges that is in contact with the brain (3, 5).
15. Nervous system phagocyte (9).
16. Principal extracellular cation involved in the action potential (6).

Find out more

1. Name the two major divisions of the nervous system.
2. Differentiate between the parasympathetic nervous system and the sympathetic nervous system.
3. Identify the functions of the neuroglia.
4. Describe the action potential.
5. Identify the functions of the different regions of the brain.
6. Describe to a patient's relative what the acronym FAST in relation to stoke means.
7. Explain the difference between stroke and transient attacks.
8. Define the term saltatory conduction.
9. What is the difference between the term afferent and efferent?
10. What is the function of brainstem?

Conditions

The following is a list of conditions that are associated with the nervous system. Take some time and write notes about each of the conditions. You may make the notes taken from text books or other resources (e.g. people you work with in a clinical area), or you may make the notes as a result of people you have cared for. If you are making notes about people you have cared for you must ensure that you adhere to the rules of confidentiality.

Multiple sclerosis	
Botulism	
Fibromyalgia	
Parkinson's disease	
Epilepsy	
Raised intracranial pressure	
Alzheimer's disease	

Chapter 14

The senses

Carl Clare

Test your prior knowledge

- Which cranial nerve is responsible for conveying information about perceived smells to the brain?
- Name the main parts of the ear involved in the sense of balance.
- What part of the tongue is involved in the sense of taste?
- Name the two substances that fill the eye chambers and help to maintain the shape of the eye.
- What is the name for short-sightedness?

Learning outcomes

After reading this chapter you will be able to:

- Describe the process by which we perceive smell
- Explain the mechanisms responsible for the perception of different tastes
- Describe the way in which human beings maintain a sense of balance
- Explore the mechanisms that lead to sound information being converted into action potentials to be relayed to the brain
- Describe the difference between rods and cones in the eye
- Explain how a visual image is focused on the retina

Fundamentals of Anatomy and Physiology: For Nursing and Healthcare Students, Second Edition. Edited by Ian Peate and Muralitharan Nair.
© 2017 John Wiley & Sons, Ltd. Published 2017 by John Wiley & Sons, Ltd.
Student companion website: www.wileyfundamentalseries.com/anatomy
Instructor companion website: www.wiley.com/go/instructor/anatomy

Introduction

The senses are usually thought of as the five senses of smell, taste, hearing, vision and touch. However, in physiology the sense of touch is excluded from the senses as it is considered a somatic sense. Thus the 'senses' is a term used to refer to the senses of:

- smell
- taste
- hearing
- sight.

Also included in this list of senses is the sense of

- equilibrium.

This chapter will explore these five senses in three sections:

- the 'chemical' senses of smell and taste;
- the senses associated with the ear: those of equilibrium and hearing;
- the sense of sight.

In all these sections there will be a review of the anatomy of the particular organs involved in these senses, followed by a discussion of the physiology of how these senses are monitored and create action potentials to be transmitted to the brain. Finally, the pathways these action potentials take to the brain will be reviewed, along with a brief discussion of the processing of this information in the brain itself.

The chemical senses

With regard to the senses, the chemical senses are the senses of smell and taste, which rely on chemoreceptors. There are two main types of chemoreceptor:

- distance chemoreceptors – for instance, the olfactory (smell) receptors;
- direct chemoreceptors – for instance, the sense of taste, which relies on the taste buds.

The sense of smell (olfaction)

In evolutionary terms the sense of smell is one of the oldest senses. The sense of smell is useful to us for the identification of food that is safe to eat and that which has gone rotten; it helps us to identify dangers such as dangerous chemicals and gives us pleasure through the smell of flowers and perfume. Olfaction (the sense of smell) is dependent on receptors that respond to airborne particles. In the nasal cavity either side of the nasal septum there are paired olfactory organs made up of two layers (Figure 14.1):

- **Olfactory epithelium** – this layer contains the olfactory receptor cells, supporting cells and regenerative basal cells (stem cells) that mature into receptor cells to replace those that die.
- **Lamina propria** – a layer of areolar tissue containing numerous blood vessels and nerves. This layer also contains the olfactory glands, which secrete a lipid-rich substance that absorbs water to form a thick mucus that covers the olfactory epithelium.

The olfactory region of each of the two nasal passages is about 2.5 cm^2 (Jenkins and Tortora, 2013) and between them they contain approximately 50 million receptor cells.

440

When air is inhaled through the nose the air in the nasal cavity is subject to turbulent flow, and this ensures that airborne smell particles (odorant molecules) are brought to the olfactory organs. Approximately 2% of the inhaled air in an average inspiration passes the olfactory organs; the act of sniffing increases this percentage by a large amount. The olfactory receptors can only be stimulated by compounds that are soluble in water or lipid and can therefore diffuse through the mucus that overlies the olfactory epithelium.

Olfactory receptors

The olfactory receptors are highly modified neurones contained within the olfactory epithelium. The tip of each receptor projects beyond the surface of the epithelium (Figure 14.1). This projection forms the base for up to 20 cilia (hair-like structures) that extend into the surrounding mucus. These cilia lie laterally in the mucus (they lie relatively flat rather than upright), thus exposing a larger surface area to any compound that is dissolved into the mucus.

Dissolved chemicals interact with odorant-binding proteins on the surface of the cilia; a local depolarisation occurs by the opening of sodium channels in the cell membrane. If enough local depolarisations occur, then an action potential is generated within the receptor cell.

Medicines administration

Flixonase

Flixonase (fluticasone propionate) is a topical glucocorticoid medicine that is commonly used for the treatment of allergic rhinitis (inflammation of the inside of the nose) and nasal polyps.

Flixonase is available as a nasal spray or nasal drops. The methods for instilling nasal drops and nasal sprays vary slightly and are detailed below.

Nasal spray technique:

- Blow the nose to clear it.
- Shake the bottle.
- Close off one nostril and put the nozzle in the open nostril.
- Tilt the head forward slightly and keep the bottle upright.
- Squeeze a fine mist into the nose while breathing in slowly. The person should not sniff hard.
- Breathe out through the mouth.
- Take a second spray in the same nostril then repeat this procedure for the other nostril if prescribed.

Nasal drops technique:

- Blow the nose to clear it.
- Shake the container.
- Tilt the head backwards.
- Place the drops in the nostril.
- Keep the head tilted and sniff gently to let the drops penetrate.
- Repeat for the other nostril if prescribed.

(Continued)

The side effects of flixonase include nose bleed (a very common side effect) and dryness or irritation of the nose or throat. Minimising the side effects of flixonase medications can be done by:

- Prescribing a nasal spray instead of drops. If nasal drops are indicated or preferred, ensure that they are used correctly.
- Prescribing the weakest potency possible, for the shortest period of time.

See National Institute for Health and Care Excellence (2015).

The olfactory pathway

The olfactory system is very sensitive, and as little as four molecules can lead to the activation of a receptor. However, activation of a receptor cell does not mean there will be awareness of the smell. There is a significant amount of convergence along the olfactory nervous pathway, and inhibition at intervening synapses can prevent the signal from reaching the olfactory cortex in the brain. However, the olfactory threshold remains very low; for instance, humans can detect very low concentrations of the chemicals added to the odourless natural gas used in the home, making it 'smell' and thus ensuring leaks are detected by the home owner.

On each side of the nose, axons leaving the olfactory epithelium receptor cells collect into 20 or more bundles that penetrate the cribriform plate of the ethmoid bone (Figure 14.2); these

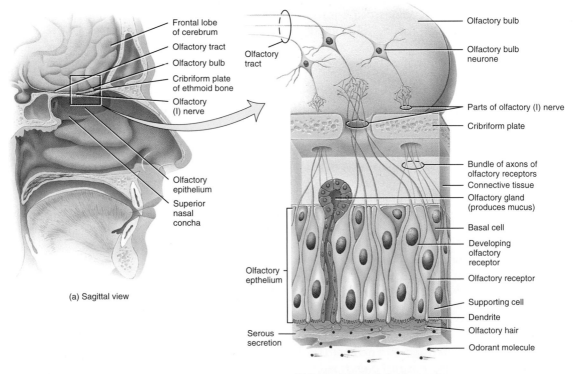

(a) Sagittal view

(b) Enlarged aspect of olfactory receptors

Figure 14.1 (a, b) Gross and microscopic anatomy of olfaction. *Source*: Tortora and Derrickson (2009). Reproduced with permission of John Wiley & Sons.

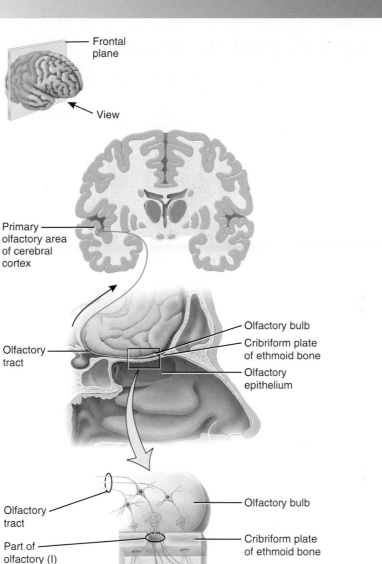

Frontal plane

View

Primary olfactory area of cerebral cortex

Olfactory tract

Olfactory bulb

Cribriform plate of ethmoid bone

Olfactory epithelium

Olfactory tract

Olfactory bulb

Part of olfactory (I) nerve

Cribriform plate of ethmoid bone

Olfactory epithelium

Olfactory receptor

Figure 14.2   Olfactory pathway. *Source*: Tortora and Derrickson (2009). Reproduced with permission of John Wiley & Sons.

bundles comprise the right and left olfactory nerves until they reach the olfactory bulbs in the brain. At the olfactory bulbs the axons converge to connect with postsynaptic (mitral) cells in large synaptic structures called glomeruli. Efferent fibres of cells elsewhere in the brain also innervate the olfactory bulb, thus allowing for the potential inhibition of the signalling pathways, for instance in central adaptation (Box 14.1).

Box 14.1   Central adaptation

Have you ever noticed that when meeting someone during the day you will smell their perfume or aftershave, but having spent some time with them you will no longer be aware of that smell? Humans tend to 'habituate' to persistent smells to the point that they are no longer perceived. This is not due to the local receptors adapting to the persistent stimuli; it is a function of central adaptation. That is, higher centres in the brain are responsible for our reduced perception of a persistent smell. The transmission of the sensory information for that particular smell is inhibited at the level of the olfactory bulb by nerve impulses from the centres in the brain.

Axons exiting from the olfactory bulbs travel along the olfactory nerves (cranial nerve I, which is a paired nerve) to reach the olfactory cortex, the hypothalamus and portions of the limbic system via the olfactory tracts. Olfactory stimulation is the only sensory information that reaches the cerebral cortex directly; all other senses are processed by the thalamus first. The fact that the limbic system and hypothalamus receive olfactory input helps to explain the profound emotional response that can be triggered by certain smells.

Olfactory discrimination

The olfactory system can make distinctions among some 2000–4000 chemical stimuli; however, there are no reasons that can be found to explain this in the structure of the receptor cells themselves. Though the epithelium is divided into areas of receptors with particular sensitivity for certain smells, it appears that the central nervous system interprets each smell by analysing the overall pattern of receptor activity (Tortora and Derrickson, 2011). It has been proposed that smell is perceived in primary odours (Haehner et al., 2013); the exact number remains a source of contention, and estimates vary from 7 to 30. Some of the smells that we perceive are not detected by the olfactory receptors at all; some of what we sense is actually pain. The nasal cavity contains pain receptors that respond to certain irritants such as ammonia, chillies and menthol. As we get older, smell discrimination and sensitivity reduce as we lose receptors compared with the total number we had when younger; and the receptors that remain become less sensitive.

Clinical considerations

Loss of the sense of smell (anosmia)

The loss of the sense of smell (known as anosmia) is normally an acquired disorder due to either trauma to the nose or brain injury, but some people are born without a sense of smell (congenital anosmia).

While appearing to be a minor problem, the loss of the sense of smell is often associated with feelings of depression and a reduced quality of life (Neuland et al., 2011).

While temporary anosmia is common with conditions such as rhinitis, the common cold and hay fever, permanent anosmia is often related to trauma, surgery and degenerative conditions such as Alzheimer's disease and Parkinson's disease.

Anosmia is noted to be an early indicator of Parkinson's disease, with 95% of patients presenting with anosmia years before motor-related symptoms appear (Haehner et al., 2011).

(Continued)

Patients with anosmia are advised to take certain safety measures:

- install smoke alarms;
- clearly mark expiry dates on food and leftovers;
- read the warning labels on chemical agents and cleaners to avoid potentially harmful gases;
- switch from gas to electric.

See NHS Choices (2015).

The sense of taste

Like the sense of smell, the sense of taste helps to protect us from poisons but also drives our appetite. There are five basic tastes:

- sweet
- sour
- bitter
- salt
- umami.

The first four tastes are already common knowledge, but the fifth was relatively unknown in the western hemisphere until recently. Umami is the taste associated with the proteins found in meat and fish (Osawa, 2012) and has been known as a concept of taste to the Japanese for many years.

The sense of taste is associated with the taste buds, which are the sensory receptor for taste and found primarily in the oral cavity. There are approximately 10,000 taste buds in the oral cavity; most are found on the tongue, but a few are on the soft palate, the inner surface of the cheeks and the pharynx and epiglottis.

Most of the taste buds are found in peg-like projections of the tongue's mucosa. These projections are known as papillae (singular is papilla) and gives the tongue its slightly rough feel. The papillae are found in four major forms (Figure 14.3):

- Fungiform – mushroom-shaped papillae found scattered over the tongue surface but most abundant at the tip and sides. They usually contain 1–18 taste buds, which are located on the top of these papillae.
- Circumvallate (otherwise known as vallate) – the largest of the papillae and found in the least number. Seven to 12 of them are found in an inverted 'V' shape at the back of the tongue. They contain approximately 250 taste buds, which are located in the side walls of these papillae.
- Foliate – 'leaf-like' papillae found on the sides of the rear of the tongue, which contain around 100 taste buds.
- Filiform – thread-like structures that contain no taste buds. They provide friction to aid the movement of food by the tongue.

Taste buds

Each taste bud is globular in structure and consists of 40–60 epithelial cells of three major types (Figure 14.4):

- Supporting cells form the greatest part of the taste bud. They help to insulate the receptor cells from each other and the epithelium of the tongue.

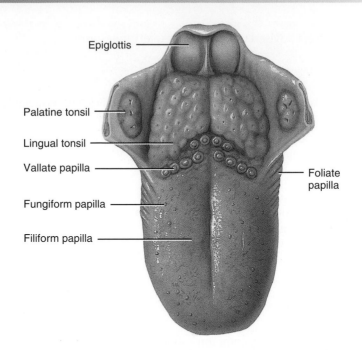

Epiglottis

Palatine tonsil

Lingual tonsil

Vallate papilla

Foliate papilla

Fungiform papilla

Filiform papilla

Figure 14.3 Tongue and the location of the papillae. *Source*: Tortora and Derrickson (2009). Reproduced with permission of John Wiley & Sons.

- Gustatory (or taste) cells – the chemoreceptor responsible for sensing taste.
- Basal cells – stem cells that mature into new receptor cells to replace those that die.

Both the supporting cells and the gustatory cells have long microvilli (protrusions of the cell membrane that increase its surface area) called gustatory hairs. These gustatory hairs project from the tip of the cell and protrude through a 'taste pore' in the epithelium to allow them to be bathed in saliva. The gustatory hairs are the sensitive portion of the gustatory cell.

Coiling around the gustatory cells are the sensory dendrites, which are the initial part of the gustatory pathway. Each afferent nerve fibre receives nerve signals from several receptor cells.

The taste receptor

The activation of the taste receptor requires the chemical compound (known as a tastant; Jenkins and Tortora, 2013) that is to be tasted to dissolve in the saliva, then diffuse into the taste pore and come into contact with the gustatory hairs. Depending on the type of taste, this has one of four potential effects (the exact mechanism that is involved in the sensing of umami is unknown):

- salt – salty taste initiates an influx of sodium into the cell;
- sour – sour taste leads to a hydrogen ion blockade of sodium and potassium channels in the cell membrane;
- bitter – bitter taste leads to an influx of calcium ions into the cell;
- sweet – sweet taste leads to an inactivation of potassium channels.

All these effects lead to the depolarisation of the cell and the release of neurotransmitters. Salt taste and sour taste have direct effects on the cell membrane. Bitter taste, sweet taste and umami exert their action on the cell by the use of messenger systems activated by G-protein-coupled receptors.

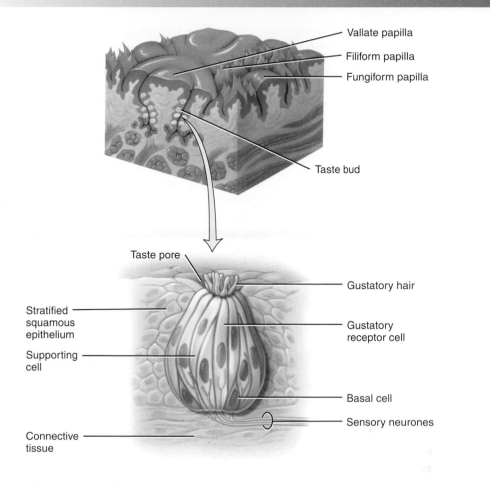

Figure 14.4   Cross-section of part of the tongue and microscopic view of a taste bud. *Source*: Tortora and Derrickson (2009). Reproduced with permission of John Wiley & Sons.

It appears that we have various sensitivities to different tastes. We are most sensitive to bitter tastes, then sour, and then sweet and salty. To an extent this makes evolutionary sense as poisons tend to taste bitter, whereas acids and food that has 'gone off' often taste sour. Thus, we are most sensitive to those tastes that may indicate something that could harm us.

It should be noted that the taste buds are not the only methods by which we experience the taste of a food. It is clear that the sense of smell is also of vital importance to how we experience taste – just think of how food tastes when your nose is blocked due to a cold; 80% of the sense of taste is actually smell. As with the sense of smell, there are also pain receptors involved with the sense of taste, and certain tastes will elicit a pain stimulus as opposed to a gustatory one.

The gustatory pathway

The release of neurotransmitters by the gustatory cells creates an action potential in related afferent nerve fibres. The sensory information from the tongue is transmitted along two cranial nerve pairs:

- chorda tympani – a branch of the facial nerve (cranial nerve VII) relays impulses from the anterior two-thirds of the tongue

- lingual branch of the glossopharyngeal nerve (cranial nerve IX) – carries the sensory information of the posterior third of the tongue.

Sensory information from the taste buds in the epiglottis and pharynx is transmitted by the vagus nerve (cranial nerve X). All the afferent fibres terminate in the solitary nucleus of the medulla. The sensory messages are then transmitted, ultimately, to the thalamus and the gustatory cortex in the parietal lobes. Afferent fibres also project into the hypothalamus and limbic system. Ultimately, many of the branches of afferent nerves that divert to various parts of the brain, apart from the cortex, are involved in the triggering of reflexes involved with digestion (for instance, salivation).

The gustatory pathway is unique among the senses because if the taste buds lose their afferent nerve fibres (for instance, they are cut) the taste bud then degenerates. As we get older we lose the sense of taste as there is a reduction in the number of taste buds; gustatory cells die and are not replaced at the same rate as they die, and those cells that remain become less sensitive.

Clinical considerations

Taste disorders

Taste disorders are relatively common in the general population and can be split into three types:

- Ageusia – the complete loss of taste. This is in fact rare.
- Hypogeusia – this is much more common and is the reduced ability to taste the five main tastes of salt, sweet, bitter, sour and umami.
- Dysgeusia – this is usually characterised as a foul, salty, rancid or metallic taste that persists in the mouth.

The causes of altered taste sensations are varied and include:

- upper respiratory and middle ear infections;
- radiation therapy for cancers of the head and neck;
- exposure to certain chemicals, such as insecticides and some medications, including some common antibiotics and antihistamines;
- head injury;
- some types of surgery to the ear, nose and throat (such as middle-ear surgery) or extraction of the wisdom teeth;
- poor oral hygiene and dental problems.

Alteration in taste can affect the appetite, and especially in the elderly can lead to a reduced food intake. The advice for improving appetite for patients with a taste disorder is:

- prepare foods with a variety of colours and textures;
- use aromatic herbs and hot spices to add more flavour – however, avoid adding more sugar or salt to foods;
- if your diet permits, add small amounts of cheese, bacon bits, butter, olive oil or toasted nuts on vegetables;
- avoid combination dishes, such as casseroles, that can hide individual flavours and dilute taste.

The senses of equilibrium and hearing

The ear is divided into three sections: external, middle and inner (see Figure 14.5).

Each of these three sections is integral in the process of hearing, and the inner ear is also essential in the maintenance of the sense of balance.

The structure of the ear

The outer ear

The outer ear consists of:

- auricle (pinna)
- external auditory canal
- tympanic membrane.

The auricle is the shell-shaped projection surrounding the external auditory canal. It is made of elastic cartilage covered with skin. The auricle can be further broken down into the rim, known as the helix, and the earlobe, which lacks supporting cartilage and so is soft. The function of the auricle is to direct sound waves into the external auditory canal.

The external auditory canal (meatus) is a short, S-shaped, narrow passage about 2.5 cm long and 0.6 cm wide, which extends from the auricle to the tympanic membrane (Figure 14.5). At the end closest to the auricle the external auditory ear canal is made of elastic cartilage; the rest of the canal is a channel through the temporal bone and thus needs no supporting cartilage. The entire canal is lined with skin with associated hairs, sebaceous (oil) glands and modified sweat

449

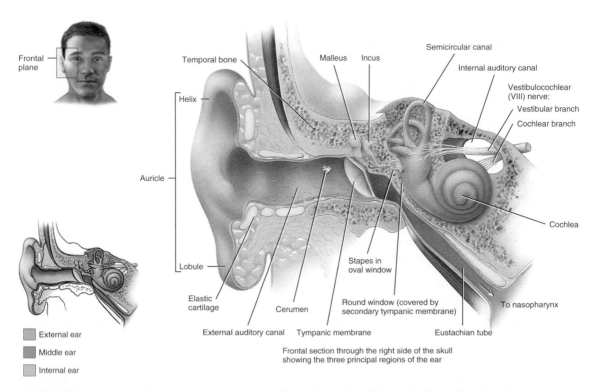

Frontal plane

Temporal bone Malleus Incus Semicircular canal
Internal auditory canal
Vestibulocochlear (VIII) nerve:
Vestibular branch
Cochlear branch

Helix

Auricle

Cochlea

Lobule

Stapes in oval window

Elastic cartilage   Cerumen   Round window (covered by secondary tympanic membrane)   To nasopharynx

External auditory canal   Tympanic membrane   Eustachian tube

External ear
Middle ear
Internal ear

Frontal section through the right side of the skull showing the three principal regions of the ear

Figure 14.5   Structure of the ear. *Source*: Tortora and Derrickson (2009). Reproduced with permission of John Wiley & Sons.

glands called ceruminous glands. The ceruminous glands secrete a yellow–brown waxy cerumen (ear wax). The purpose of the oils and the wax is to lubricate the ear canal, kill bacteria and, in conjunction with the hairs, keep the canal free of debris.

Sound waves entering the external auditory canal travel along until they reach the tympanic membrane (ear drum), a thin translucent connective tissue membrane covered by skin on its external surface and internally by mucosa, and shaped like a flattened cone protruding into the middle ear. Sound waves that reach the tympanic membrane make it vibrate, and this vibration is transmitted to the bones of the middle ear.

Snapshot

Hearing aids work by converting speech and other sounds to acoustic signals; they then amplify these. There are some hearing aids that depress lower frequency sounds and others that amplify higher frequency sounds. With advances in technology, increasingly smaller, more efficient hearing aids are now being produced. There are several different types, informally named by their placement in or around the ear: behind-the-ear, in-the-ear, or in-the-canal hearing aids. Although hearing aids can amplify sounds, they cannot make words clearer or speech any easier to understand, except by making the sounds louder.

Hearing aids can pick up the sound that is entering the ear, process it to match the hearing loss and then release the signal back into the ear instantaneously. A digital hearing aid is much more advanced than an analogue aid. It contains a silicon chip made up of millions of electrical components, continuously processing incoming sound, converting it into clearer and more audible sounds and then releasing these at the appropriate sound level into the ear. The digital hearing aid helps the user distinguish between sounds that need to be amplified and unwanted noise that needs to be reduced.

Digital hearing aids can be modified in order to work with an individual's personal degree of hearing loss and lifestyle needs. They have a number of preset programmes, which can be used in various situations; for example, quiet conversations, when at concerts, or at parties where there is much background noise. The user can watch the TV while taking part in conversations, identify where sounds are coming from, eliminate whistling and feedback while on the telephone and can link up via wireless technology to the TV, mobile telephone, computer or stereo system.

Middle ear

Otherwise known as the tympanic cavity, this is a small, air-filled cavity lined with mucosa and contained within the temporal bone. It is enclosed at both ends, by the ear drum at the lateral end and medially by a bony wall with two openings:

- oval (vestibular) window
- round (cochlear) window.

The middle ear is connected to the nasopharynx by the Eustachian (auditory) tube, a 4 cm long tube that consists of two portions:

- the section near the connection to the middle ear, which is relatively narrow and is supported by elastic cartilage;
- the section near the nasopharynx, which is relatively broad and funnel-shaped.

When open the Eustachian tube allows the passage of air, and thus ensures the equalisation of the pressures on both sides of the tympanic membrane so both are subject to the same atmospheric pressure. The Eustachian tube is normally closed at the end nearest the nasopharynx but opens during yawning and swallowing (Jenkins and Tortora, 2013). If equalisation of pressures does not happen, then the difference in pressures between the two sides can lead to reduced hearing as the tympanic membrane cannot move freely.

Within the middle ear there are three bones known as the ossicles or ossicular chain. These three bones connect the tympanic membrane with the receptor complexes of the inner ear:

- the malleus (hammer) attaches at three points to the inner surface of the tympanic membrane;
- the incus (anvil) attaches the malleus to the stapes;
- the stapes (stirrup) – the edges of the base of the stapes are bound to the edge of the oval window.

The joints between these three bones are the smallest synovial joints in the body, and each has its own tiny capsule and supporting extracapsular ligaments.

Vibration in the tympanic membrane is the first stage in the perception of sound; this vibration converts the sound waves into mechanical movement (the vibration). The ossicles act as levers and conduct the vibrations to the inner ear. They are connected in such a way that the in–out movement of tympanic vibration is converted into a rocking motion of the stapes. The ossicles collect the force applied to the tympanic membrane, amplify it and transmit it to the oval window. This amplification explains why humans can hear even very quiet noises, but can also be a problem in very noisy environments. In order to protect the tympanic membrane and the ossicular chain from violent movement resulting from extreme noises, they are supported by two small muscles:

- The tensor tympani muscle is a short ribbon of muscle connected to the 'handle' of the malleus. When it contracts, the malleus is pulled medially (towards the inner ear), stiffening the tympanic membrane.
- The stapedius muscle is attached to the stapes and pulls it, reducing the movement against the oval window.

Inner ear

The senses of equilibrium (part of the sense of balance) and hearing are provided by the receptors in the inner ear.

The inner ear is also known as the labyrinth owing to the complicated series of canals it contains. The inner ear is composed of two main, fluid-filled parts:

- bony labyrinth – a series of cavities within the temporal bone that contain the main organs of balance (the semicircular canals and the vestibule) and the main organ of hearing (the cochlea);
- membranous labyrinth – a series of fluid-filled sacs and tubes that are contained within the bony labyrinth.

Between the bony and membranous labyrinth flows perilymph, a liquid that is rather like cerebrospinal fluid; the fluid within the membranous labyrinth is known as endolymph.

As noted above, the bony labyrinth can be divided into three parts (Figure 14.6):

- The vestibule consists of a pair of membranous sacs: the saccule and the utricle. Receptors in these two sacs provide the sensations of gravity and linear acceleration.
- The semicircular canals enclose slender semicircular ducts. Receptors in these ducts are stimulated by the rotation of the head. The combination of the vestibule and the semicircular canals is known as the vestibular complex.
- The cochlea is a spiral-shaped, bony chamber that contains the cochlear duct of the membranous labyrinth. Receptors within this duct give us the sense of hearing.

451

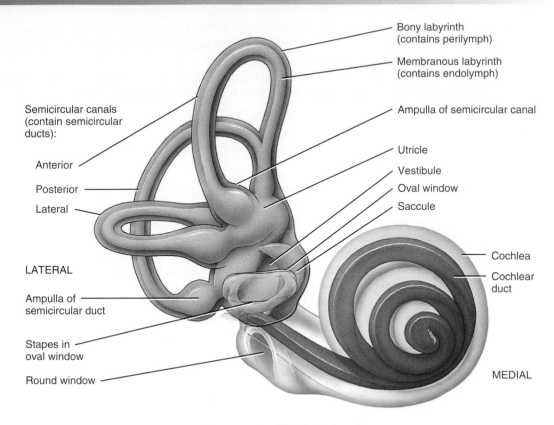

Components of the right internal ear

Figure 14.6   Inner ear. *Source*: Tortora and Derrickson (2009). Reproduced with permission of John Wiley & Sons.

Equilibrium

The sense of equilibrium is part of the sense of balance and is controlled by receptors in the semicircular ducts, the utricle and the saccule of the inner ear. The sensory receptors in the semicircular ducts are active during movement but inactive when the body is motionless. The sensory receptors in the ducts respond to rotational movements of the head. There are three of these ducts: lateral, posterior and anterior.

The ducts are continuous with the utricle. Each semicircular duct contains an ampulla, an expanded region that contains the majority of the receptors. The area in the wall of the ampulla that contains the receptors is known as the crista, and each crista is bound to a cupula – a gelatinous structure that extends the full width of the ampulla. The hair cells (receptors) are surrounded by supporting cells and are monitored by the dendrites of sensory neurones.

The free surfaces of the hair cells are covered with stereocilia, which resemble very long microvilli. Along with the fine stereocilia, the hair cell will also have one kinocilium – a single, large and thick cilium. When an external force pushes against the cilia the distortion of the plasma membrane of the hair cell alters the rate that the cell releases chemical transmitters. So, for instance, if a person moves their head to look to the left the cilia of the lateral semicircular canal are subject to pressure and thus the cell membranes are distorted, leading to an altered release of neurotransmitters and the perception of rotational movement (Figure 14.7). Any movement

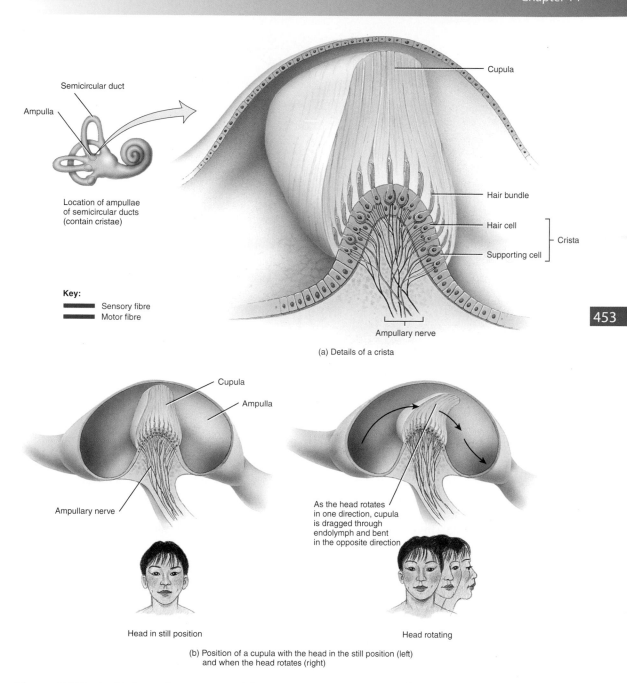

Location of ampullae
of semicircular ducts
(contain cristae)

Semicircular duct

Ampulla

Cupula

Hair bundle

Hair cell

Crista

Supporting cell

Ampullary nerve

Key:
▬▬▬ Sensory fibre
▬▬▬ Motor fibre

(a) Details of a crista

Cupula

Ampulla

Ampullary nerve

As the head rotates
in one direction, cupula
is dragged through
endolymph and bent
in the opposite direction

Head in still position

Head rotating

(b) Position of a cupula with the head in the still position (left)
and when the head rotates (right)

Figure 14.7   (a, b) Ampulla at rest and in response to movement. *Source*: Tortora and Derrickson (2009). Reproduced with permission of John Wiley & Sons.

of the head can be perceived by varying combinations of stimulation of the three ducts and their receptors.

In contrast to the semicircular canals, the utricle and the saccule provide equilibrium information whether the body is moving or stationary. The two chambers are connected by a narrow passageway that is also connected to the endolymphatic duct. The hair cells of the utricle and

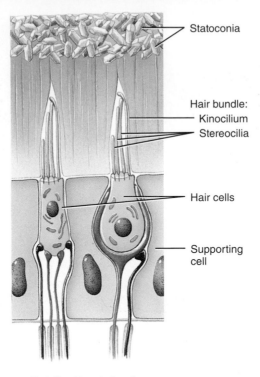

Statoconia

Hair bundle:
Kinocilium
Stereocilia

Hair cells

Supporting
cell

Details of two hair cells

Figure 14.8   Hair cells and otolith. *Source*: Tortora and Derrickson (2009). Reproduced with permission of John Wiley & Sons.

saccule are clustered in oval structures called maculae. As with the hair cells of the ampullae, the cilia of the hair cells in the utricle and saccule are embedded in a gelatine-like substance. However, the surface of this substance contains densely packed calcium carbonate crystals called statoconia. This combination of gelatine-like substance and calcium carbonate crystals is known as an otolith (Figure 14.8).

When the head is in a neutral position the statoconia sit on top of the macula. The pressure they generate is therefore downwards and the hair cell microvilli are pushed down. When the head is tilted, the pull of gravity on the statoconia shifts and the microvilli are moved to one side or the other. This distorts the cell membrane and triggers altered neurotransmitter release (Figure 14.9).

A similar type of activity happens when the body is subject to linear acceleration; for example, as a car speeds up, the otolith lags behind due to inertia. The brain would normally differentiate between the action of gravity and the action of acceleration by integrating the information from the receptors with visual information.

Pathways for the equilibrium sensations

The hair cells in the semicircular canals, the vestibule and the saccule are monitored by sensory neurones located in the vestibular ganglia. Sensory fibres from these ganglia form the vestibular branch of the vestibulocochlear nerve (cranial nerve VIII). These fibres feed into neurones within the vestibular nuclei at the boundary of the pons and the medulla oblongata in the brain.

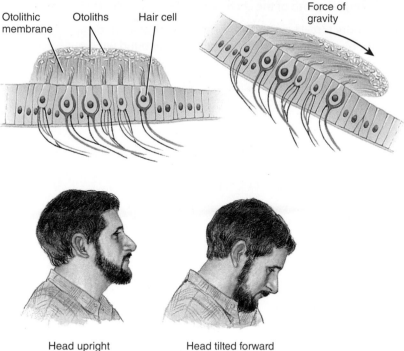

Figure 14.9 labels: Otolithic membrane, Otoliths, Hair cell, Force of gravity

Head upright   Head tilted forward

Position of macula with head upright (left) and tilted forward (right)

Figure 14.9 Action of gravity on the otolith. *Source*: Tortora and Derrickson (2009). Reproduced with permission of John Wiley & Sons.

The vestibular nuclei have four functions:

- Integrating sensory information about equilibrium received from both sides of the head.
- Relaying information to the cerebellum.
- Relaying information to the cortex.
- Sending commands to motor nuclei in the brainstem and the spinal cord. The motor commands are reflex-type commands for eye, head and neck movements, such as the movement of the eyes that occurs in response to sensations of motion.

Hearing

The sense of hearing is provided by receptors in the cochlear duct; they are hair cells similar to those of the semicircular canals and vestibule. However, their positioning within the cochlear duct and the organisation of the surrounding structures protect them from stimuli generated by anything other than sound waves.

The ossicular chains transmit and amplify pressure waves from the air into pressure waves in the perilymph of the cochlea. These waves stimulate the hair cells along the cochlear spiral:

- the **frequency** of the perceived sound is detected by the part of the cochlear duct that is stimulated;
- the **intensity** (volume) of the sound is detected by the number of hair cells that are stimulated at the particular point in the cochlea.

Within the bony labyrinth of the cochlea there are three ducts (Figure 14.10):

- the vestibular duct (scala vestibuli) connects to the oval window;
- the tympanic duct (scala tympani) connects to the round window;
- the cochlear duct (scala media) is separated from the tympanic duct by the basilar membrane.

Both the vestibular and the tympanic duct are connected at the tip of the cochlear spiral and therefore make up one continuous perilymphatic chamber (Figure 14.11).

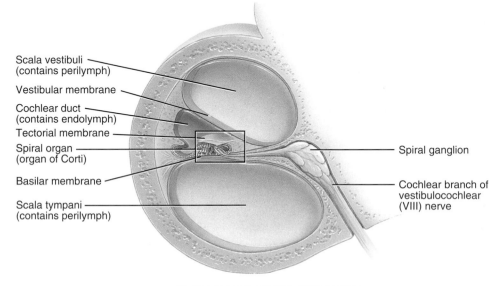

Section through one turn of the cochlea

Figure 14.10   Cross-section of the cochlea (highlighted section is shown in detail in Figure 14.12). *Source*: Tortora and Derrickson (2009). Reproduced with permission of John Wiley & Sons.

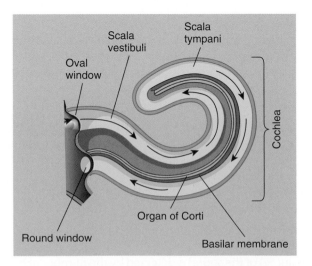

Figure 14.11   Cochlea showing the continuous nature of the vestibular and tympanic ducts.

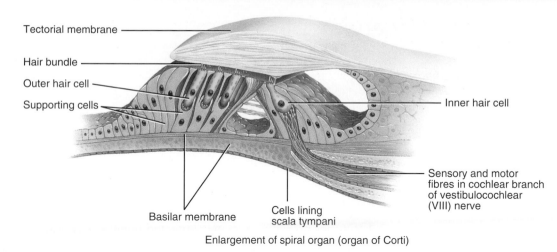

Enlargement of spiral organ (organ of Corti)

Figure 14.12   Organ of Corti. *Source*: Tortora and Derrickson (2009). Reproduced with permission of John Wiley & Sons.

Between the vestibular and the tympanic ducts is the cochlear duct; the hair cells of this duct are located in a structure called the organ of Corti (Figure 14.12). The organ of Corti sits on the basilar membrane and its hair cells are arranged in a series of longitudinal rows.

The hair cells of the organ of Corti do not have kinocilia, and their stereocilia are in contact with the overlying tectorial membrane; this membrane is attached to the inner wall of the coch-lear duct. When a portion of the basilar membrane bounces up and down in response to pres-sure waves in the perilymph the stereocilia of the hair cells are pressed against the tectorial membrane and become distorted.

The hearing process

1. Sound waves travel down the external auditory canal and arrive at the tympanic membrane.
2. Movement is created in the tympanic membrane, which leads to the movement of the ossicles and the amplification of the movement.
3. Movement of the stapes at the oval window creates pressure waves in the perilymph of the vestibular duct.
4. The pressure waves distort the basilar membrane. The location of the maximum distortion depends on the frequency of the sound, as the basilar membrane varies in width and flexibility along its length. Higher pitch sounds create maximum distortion near to the oval window and lower pitch sounds further away from the window. The amount of distortion gives sensory information as to the volume of the sound.
5. Vibration in the basilar membrane leads to vibration of the hair cell cilia against the tectorial membrane, leading to the release of neurotransmitters by the hair cells. As hair cells are arranged in rows, a soft sound may only distort a few hair cells in a single row, but more cells in more rows will be stimulated as the volume increases.
6. Information about the region of stimulation and the intensity of that stimulation is relayed to the brain via the cochlear branch of the vestibulocochlear nerve (cranial nerve VIII). The cell bodies of the neurones that monitor the hair cells of the cochlea are located in the spiral ganglia at the centre of the bony cochlea. The nerve impulses are then transmitted via the cochlear branch of cranial nerve VIII to the cochlear nuclei of the medulla oblongata and then to other centres in the brain.

Medicines management

Ototoxicity

Ototoxicity is the property of being toxic to the ear. There are over 200 drugs that can lead to oto-toxicity, tinnitus and associated hearing loss.

Many of the drugs are used in common practice, such as:

- furosemide
- gentamicin
- metropolol
- ramipril
- sodium valproate.

Patients should be informed that if they do experience any suspected tinnitus or hearing loss with a drug it is important they do not stop taking the drug until they have talked to their doctor.

Avoiding ototoxicity

Many ototoxic drugs are excreted in the urine, and thus it is best to avoid ototoxic drugs in patients with renal impairment and they should be used with caution in the elderly. Furthermore, the patient should be well hydrated to ensure good renal function.

Drugs such as gentamicin and vancomycin are normally given at set times, and the nurse should avoid giving these drugs too early as it may cause an excessive blood level. Also, blood levels of these drugs are required at regular intervals, and it is important to adhere to medical instructions regarding the administration before and after drug administration.

Furosemide toxicity is related to the speed of administration and, therefore, it is essential that the instructions for the speed of delivery of intravenous furosemide are followed.

458

Clinical considerations

Noise exposure and ear damage

As noise levels increase, the chance of damage to the ear increases. The following table gives examples of the types of noise levels at certain decibel (dB) levels and the exposure time at which damage may occur.

dB level	Maximum exposure per day	Examples
10		Breathing
20		Rustling leaves
60		Conversation
75		Typical car interior on motorway
85	16 h	City traffic (inside car)
90	9 h	Power drill, food blender
97	3 h	French horn at 10 feet

(Continued)

dB level	Maximum exposure per day	Examples
100	2 h	Farm tractor, outboard motor, jet take-off at 1000 feet
110	0.5 h	Chainsaw, pneumatic drill, car horn at 3 feet
120	0 h	Typical rock concert, loud thunderclap
125	Hearing damage occurring	Pneumatic riveter at 4 feet
132–140	Permanent hearing damage	Gunshot, very loud rock concert 50 feet in front of speakers
150–160	Eardrum rupture	Jet take off at 75 feet, gunshot at 1 foot
190	Immediate death of tissue	Jet engine at 1 foot
194		Loudest sound in air, air particle distortion (sonic boom)

The sense of sight

Vision is perhaps the sense that we value the most; we learn more about the world around us through sight than we do with any of the other senses. Without sight many of our daily tasks and pleasures would be impossible and many others would become more difficult. The sense of sight is based on the eyes, and around the eyes there are accessory structures that help to keep the eyes safe and working well (Figure 14.13):

- Eyelids (palpebrae) – a continuation of the skin. Continual blinking keeps the surface of the eye lubricated and removes dirt. The gap between them is known as the palpebral fissure.
- Eyelashes – robust hairs that help to keep foreign matter out of the eyes. They are associated with the tarsal glands. which produce a lipid-rich secretion that helps to prevent the eyelids from sticking together.

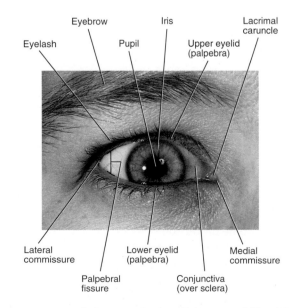

Figure 14.13   Accessory structures of the eye. *Source*: Tortora and Derrickson (2009). Reproduced with permission of John Wiley & Sons.

- Lacrimal caruncle – a small collection of soft tissue that contains accessory glands.
- Commissure – the point where the eyelids meet; there are two: the lateral and the medial.
- Conjunctiva – the epithelial cell layer that lines the inside of the eyelids and the outer surface of the eye.

Lacrimal apparatus

A constant flow of tears washes over the eyes to keep the conjunctiva moist and clean. Tears have several functions:

- reduce friction
- remove debris
- prevent bacterial infection
- provide nutrients and oxygen to parts of the conjunctiva.

The lacrimal apparatus produces, distributes and removes tears. It consists of:

- a lacrimal gland
- lacrimal canaliculi
- a lacrimal sac
- a nasolacrimal duct.

The lacrimal gland (tear gland) creates most of the content of tears (about 1 mL per day). Once the lacrimal secretions reach the eye they mix with the products of the accessory glands and the tarsal glands. This results in a mixture that lubricates the eye and reduces evaporation. The nutrient and oxygen demands of the corneal cells are supplied by diffusion from the lacrimal secretions. The secretions also contain antibacterial enzymes and antibodies to attack pathogens before they enter the body.

Blinking sweeps the tears across the ocular surface and they accumulate at the medial commissure from where they are drained by the lacrimal canaliculi into the lacrimal sac and from there into the nasal cavity through the nasolacrimal duct.

The eye

The wall of the eye

The wall of the eye has three layers (Figure 14.14):

- fibrous tunic
- vascular tunic
- neural tunic.

Fibrous tunic

The fibrous tunic is the outermost layer of the eye and consists of the sclera and the cornea; it has three main functions:

- provides support and some protection;
- is the attachment site for the extrinsic muscles;
- contains structures that assist in the focusing process.

Most of the ocular surface is covered by the sclera (the 'white' of the eye), which is made up of dense fibrous connective tissue containing collagen and elastic fibres. The surface of the sclera contains small blood vessels and nerves. The transparent cornea is continuous with the sclera and

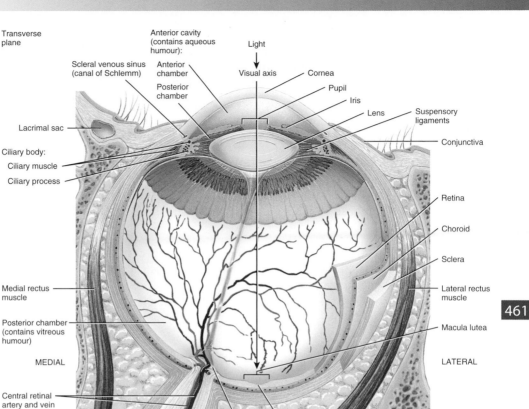

Superior view of transverse section of right eyeball

Figure 14.14 Anatomy of the eye. *Source*: Tortora and Derrickson (2009). Reproduced with permission of John Wiley & Sons.

is made up of a dense matrix of fibres laid down in such a way that they do not interfere with the passage of light.

Vascular tunic (uvea)

The vascular tunic is the middle of the three layers of the eye and contains numerous blood vessels, lymph vessels and the smooth muscles involved in eye functioning. The functions of this layer include:

- providing a structure for the blood and lymph vessels that supply the tissues of the eye;
- regulating the amount of light that enters the eye;
- secreting and reabsorbing the aqueous humour;
- controlling the shape of the lens.

The vascular tunic is made up of:

- the iris
- the ciliary body
- the choroid.

Iris

The iris is the central, coloured portion of the eye (Figure 14.13) and regulates the amount of light entering the eye by adjusting the size of the central opening (the pupil). It is formed of two layers of pigmented cells and fibres and two layers of smooth muscle (the pupillary muscles):

- pupillary constrictor muscles
- pupillary dilator muscles.

Both sets of muscles are controlled by the autonomic nervous system; activation of the parasympathetic nervous system leads to constriction of the pupil in response to bright light. Activation of the sympathetic nervous system leads to the dilation of the pupil in response to dim light levels. At its edge the iris attaches to the anterior part of the ciliary body.

Ciliary body

The greatest part of the ciliary body is made up of the ciliary muscle, a smooth muscular ring that projects into the interior of the eye. The epithelial covering of this muscle has many folds called ciliary processes. The suspensory ligaments of the lens attach to the tips of these processes.

Choroid

The choroid is a vascular layer that separates the fibrous and neural tunics. It is covered by the sclera and attached to the outermost layer of the retina. The choroid contains an extensive capillary network that delivers oxygen and nutrients to the retina.

Neural tunic (retina)

This is the innermost layer of the eye, consisting of a thin outer layer called the pigmented part and a thicker inner layer called the neural part.

- The pigmented part of the retina absorbs the light that passes through the neural part; this prevents light bouncing back through the neural part and causing 'visual echoes'.
- The neural part of the retina contains light receptors, support cells and is responsible for the preliminary processing and integration of visual information.

Organisation of the retina

Figure 14.15 shows the two types of receptor cells contained within the outermost layer of the retina (closest to the pigmented part). These receptor cells are the cells that detect light (photoreceptors).

- Rods – these photoreceptors do not discriminate between colours. They are very sensitive and enable us to see in very low light levels. Rods are mostly concentrated in a band around the periphery of the retina, and this density reduces towards the centre of the eye.
- Cones – these photoreceptors provide colour vision and give sharper, clearer images than the rods do, but they require more intense light. Cones are mostly situated in the macula lutea and particularly at its centre in an area called the fovea (Figure 14.14).

The elongated outer sections of the rods and cones contain hundreds to thousands of flattened membranous discs. In the rods the discs are separate and form the shape of a cylinder. In cones the discs are in fact folds of the plasma membrane, and the outer segment tapers to a blunt point.

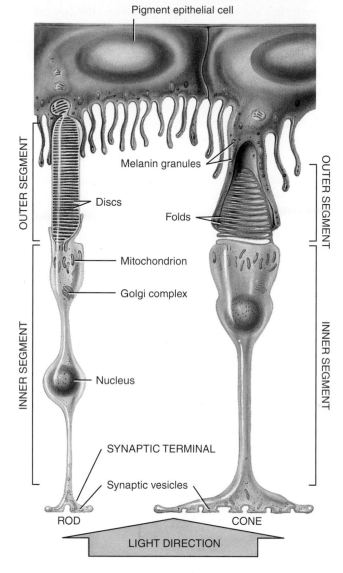

Figure 14.15   Cross-section of the retina. *Source*: Tortora and Derrickson (2009). Reproduced with permission of John Wiley & Sons.

There are three types of cones (red, blue and green), and colour discrimination is based on the integration of information received from the three types of cones. For instance, yellow is shown by highly stimulated green cones, less strongly stimulated red cones and a relative lack of stimulation of the blue cones.

A narrow connecting stalk links the outer segment to the inner segment, which is the part of the cell that contains all the usual cellular organelles. The inner segment is also the area where synapses with other cells are made and neurotransmitters are released.

The rods and cones synapse with neurones called bipolar cells, which in turn synapse within a layer of neurones called ganglion cells. At both these synapse areas there are associated cells that can stimulate or inhibit the communication between the two cells, and therefore alter the sensitivity of the retina (for instance, in response to very bright, or dim, light levels).

Axons from approximately 1 million ganglion cells converge on the optic disc, at which point they turn and penetrate the wall of the eye and proceed to the diencephalon of the brain as the optic nerve. The central retinal artery and vein pass through the centre of the optic nerve. The optic disc contains no photoreceptors, and thus this area is known as the blind spot; however, we do not notice the blind spot in our vision as involuntary eye movements keep the visual image moving and the brain can thus supply the missing information.

The chambers of the eye

The eye is divided into two main cavities: a large posterior cavity and a smaller anterior cavity. The anterior cavity is further divided into the anterior chamber and the posterior chamber (Figure 14.14).

- The **anterior cavity** is filled with a substance called aqueous humour that circulates between the anterior and posterior chambers by passing through the pupil and performing a vital role as a transport medium for nutrients and waste products. The fluid pressure created by the aqueous humour in the anterior cavity helps to maintain the shape of the eye. Aqueous humour is produced by the epithelial cells of the ciliary body and within a few hours is drained through the canal of Schlemm to the sclera to be recycled.
- The **posterior cavity** is the larger of the two cavities of the eye and is filled with a gelatinous mass known as vitreous humour. The vitreous humour helps to stabilise the shape of the eye as the activity of the extraocular muscles would otherwise distort the shape of the eye. Unlike aqueous humour, the vitreous humour is created during the development of the eye and is never replaced. A thin film of aqueous humour infiltrates the posterior chamber, bathing the retina, supplying nutrients and removing waste. The pressure it creates also helps to keep the neural part of the retina against the pigmented part; though the two are close together they are not fixed to each other, and thus this external pressure is required.

Snapshot

Using eye drops

Sarah is a 72-year-old lady who has been to see her optician for new glasses. During routine testing the optician has detected the onset of glaucoma and referred Sarah to her GP. The treatment for early open angle glaucoma is eye drops, and the GP has prescribed prostaglandin eye drops to help the flow of aqueous humour from the eye and thus reduce the pressure. At present, glaucoma cannot be cured and the treatment is dependent on early recognition to avoid permanent damage.

To use eye drops the patient should be advised to:

- wash their hands;
- ensure the eye drops are in date;
- put their head back;
- use their finger to pull down the lower eyelid;
- hold the bottle and allow a single drop to fall into the pocket made by pulling down the eyelid;
- close the eye and keep it closed for a few minutes.

Snapshot

Tonometry

Measuring intra-ocular pressure (IOP) is an important ophthalmic test, and the correct term is tonometry. Tonometry is the objective measurement of IOP and is usually based on the assessment of resistance of the cornea to indent (this is usually a blast of air). Normal IOP is between about 10 and 21 mmHg. There are several types of tonometer available; an applanation tonometer is a tool that measures the amount of force needed to temporarily flatten part of the cornea. The tonometer measures the degree of resistance provided by the cornea to gentle indentation, converting this into a figure. A drop of fluorescein/anaesthetic provides a blue light filter. The procedure does not hurt; the patient has to keep their eyes wide open. While this test is completely painless, many patients find this test very difficult.

There are contraindications to this procedure, such as trauma or corneal ulcer. Measuring IOP is quick and simple, and because of this it is routinely performed on all adults who require eye tests.

Focusing images onto the retina

In order for a visual image to be useful it must be focused onto the retina; this is the purpose of the lens of the eye. First, the light entering the eye is subject to refraction, and the lens provides the additional, adjustable refraction required to focus the image onto the retina.

Refraction

Light is refracted (bent) when it passes from one medium to another medium with a different density (Figure 14.16).

The majority of the refraction in the eye happens when light enters the cornea from the air; additional refraction occurs when light passes from the aqueous humour into the lens. The lens provides the extra refraction to focus the light onto the retina and can adjust this refraction according to the focal length.

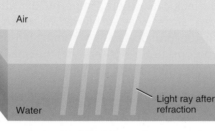

Refraction of light rays

Figure 14.16   Refraction of light passing from air (less dense) to water (dense). *Source*: Tortora and Derrickson (2009). Reproduced with permission of John Wiley & Sons.

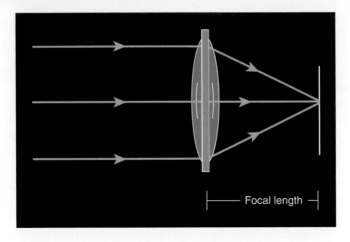

Focal length

Figure 14.17   Focal length.

466

Focal length is the distance between the focal point (e.g. on the retina) and the centre of the lens (Figure 14.17). It is dependent on:

- The distance from the object to the lens. The further away an object is, the shorter the focal length.
- The shape of the lens. The rounder the lens the more refraction occurs. A very round lens has a shorter focal length than a flatter lens.

The lens lies behind the cornea and is held in place by ligaments that are attached to the ciliary body. It is made up of concentric layers of cells that are precisely organised and are covered by a fibrous capsule. Many of the capsule fibres are elastic, and if it were not subject to external forces by the ligaments the lens would be spherical. Within the lens are lens fibres, specialised cells that have lost their nucleus and other organelles. They are filled with a protein called crystallin, which is responsible for the transparency and the focusing power of the lens.

The process of changing the shape of the lens to focus an image onto the retina is known as accommodation. The shape of the lens is altered by tension being applied to or relaxed on the suspensory ligaments by smooth muscles within the ciliary body (Figure 14.18).

Myopia, hyperopia and presbyopia

In a person who has myopia (short-sightedness) the lens is unable to focus the image onto the retina and the focus of the image falls short (Figure 14.19). With myopia, people can see objects close to them but those that are far away are blurred. Myopia is easily corrected for by the use of corrective lenses, either in the form of glasses or contact lenses.

In the person with hyperopia (long-sightedness) the image is focused onto a point behind the retina (Figure 14.20); therefore, these people can see things at a distance but not near to them.

Presbyopia is the loss of the ability to focus on close objects as the person ages; the most common theory for this is the loss of elasticity in the lens. The loss of the ability to focus on near objects occurs in everyone, but at different rates and with different effects on vision. The onset of presbyopia is most commonly noticed at 40–50 years of age. Presbyopia is treatable with corrective glasses (usually known as reading glasses, though they are corrective for all tasks that require near vision).

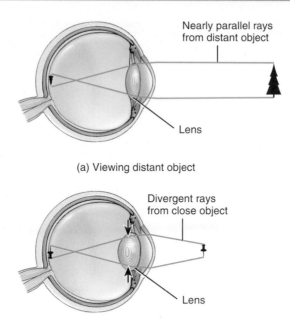

Nearly parallel rays
from distant object

Lens

(a) Viewing distant object

Divergent rays
from close object

Lens

(b) Accommodation close object

Figure 14.18 Accommodation to (a) far and (b) near objects. *Source*: Tortora and Derrickson (2009). Reproduced with permission of John Wiley & Sons.

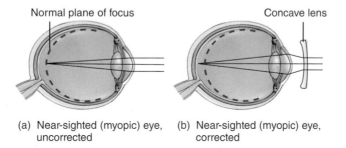

Normal plane of focus

Concave lens

(a) Near-sighted (myopic) eye,
uncorrected

(b) Near-sighted (myopic) eye,
corrected

Figure 14.19 (a) Myopic eye uncorrected and (b) corrected by a concave lens. *Source*: Tortora and Derrickson (2009). Reproduced with permission of John Wiley & Sons.

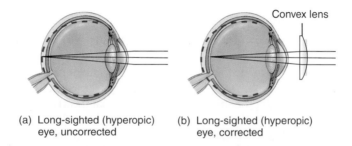

Convex lens

(a) Long-sighted (hyperopic)
eye, uncorrected

(b) Long-sighted (hyperopic)
eye, corrected

Figure 14.20 (a) Hyperopic eye uncorrected and (b) corrected by a convex lens. *Source*: Tortora and Derrickson (2009). Reproduced with permission of John Wiley & Sons.

Clinical considerations

20/20 vision

The term 20/20 vision refers to a measure of visual acuity. The meaning is that the person being tested can see the same detail from 20 feet away as a person with normal eyesight would see from 20 feet. In other words, 20/20 vision is normal vision. If a person has 20/40 vision they are only able to see detail at 20 feet that a person with normal vision can see at 40 feet. A person with a visual acuity of 20/70 can only see detail at 20 feet that a person with normal sight could see at 70 feet and so on. The visual acuity is not a direct correlation with the prescription for eyeglasses, but the prescribed glasses are intended to achieve 20/20 vision. Visual acuity is tested using a standard size Snellen chart at 20 feet and lit to a standard brightness.

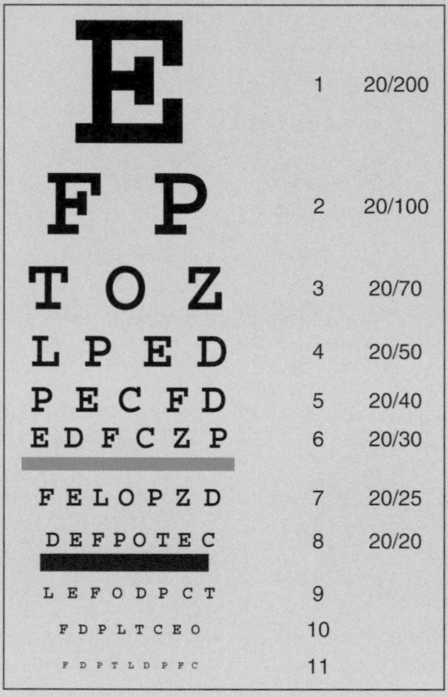

E	1	20/200
F P	2	20/100
T O Z	3	20/70
L P E D	4	20/50
P E C F D	5	20/40
E D F C Z P	6	20/30
F E L O P Z D	7	20/25
D E F P O T E C	8	20/20
L E F O D P C T	9	
F D P L T C E O	10	
F D P T L D P F C	11	

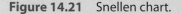

Figure 14.21   Snellen chart.

The processing of visual information

The ganglion cells that monitor the rods in the retina (M cells) supply information about the general form of an object, motion and shadows in dim light. As many as 1000 rods may pass information to one M cell. This convergence leads to a loss of specific information, and the activation of an M cell indicates that light has struck a general area rather than a specific point. This loss of specific location-based information is partially compensated for by the fact that the M cells' activity varies depending on the pattern of stimulation in their specific field (area of retina). So, for instance, an M cell would react differently to a stimulus at the edge of its receptive field than from one at its centre.

Cone cells show very little convergence; for instance in the fovea the ratio of cones to ganglion is 1 : 1 (Martini and Nath, 2009). The ganglion cells that monitor cones (P cells) are more numerous than M cells, and because there is little convergence these cells provide location-specific information. As a result of this, cones supply more precise information about a visual image than do rods.

Central processing of visual information

Once axons from the ganglion cells have exited the eye through the optic disc they proceed to the diencephalon as the optic nerves (cranial nerve II). The two optic nerves (one for each eye) reach the diencephalon at the optic chiasm. From there, half the nerves go to the lateral geniculate nucleus on the same side of the brain and the other half cross over and proceed to the lateral geniculate nucleus on the opposite side. From each lateral geniculate nucleus, visual information also travels to the occipital cortex of the cerebral hemisphere on the same side. Involuntary eye control (such as pupillary reflexes) is processed in the diencephalon and the brainstem.

Conclusion

In this chapter there has been a review of the senses:

- olfaction (smell), which is based in the olfactory receptors of the nose
- gustation (taste), which is partially based in the gustatory receptors on the tongue, but also has a large input from the olfactory receptors
- equilibrium, which is a part of the sense of balance and is based in the hair cells of the semicircular canals and the vestibule
- hearing, which is based in the hair cells in the organ of corti in the cochlea of the inner ear
- sight, which is based in the photoreceptors of the eye.

With the exception of smell, all the information generated by the senses is processed in the thalamus before being transmitted on to the higher brain centres. Some of the senses (smell and taste) also have direct input into other centres of the limbic system, such as the hypothalamus, and this is an indication of both how ancient they are in evolutionary terms and the fact that certain smells and tastes can evoke subconscious responses, such as salivation and emotions.

Glossary

Afferent: Heading towards a centre (for instance, the brain).

Ampulla   A sac-like enlargement of a canal or duct.

Anterior   Located at, or related to, the front of a structure.

Antibody   Proteins in the blood that are used by the immune system to identify and destroy pathogens.

Autonomic nervous system   The part of the nervous system that controls involuntary functions, made up of the parasympathetic and sympathetic nervous systems.

Axon   Extension of a nerve cell that conducts impulses.

Balance   The ability to control equilibrium.

Cartilage   A supporting connective tissue made up of various cells and fibres.

Cilia   Small, hair-like processes on the outer surface of some cells.

Connective tissue   Tissue that supports and binds other body tissue.

Convergence   The movement of the eyes inwards to see an object close to the face.

Efferent   Heading away from a centre.

Endolymph   The fluid in the membranous labyrinth of the inner ear.

Enzyme   A protein that increases the rate of a chemical reaction.

Equilibrium   Stability at rest or when moving.

Ethmoid bone   A bone in the skull that separates the nasal cavity from the brain.

Extrinsic   Not inherent to the process or object, external.

Focal length   The distance between the focal point (e.g. on the retina) and the centre of the lens of the eye.

Fovea (fovea centralis)   A small depression in the retina containing cones and where vision is the most acute.

Ganglion   A mass, or group, of nerve cells.

Glomeruli (glomerulus – singular)   In the olfactory pathway, a structure containing a mass of synapses.

Gustatory   Relating to the sense of taste.

Hyperopia   Long-sightedness.

Iris   The central, coloured portion of the eye.

Lacrimal   Relating to tears.

Lateral   Away from the midline of the body (to the left or right).

Ligament   Fibrous tissue that binds joints together and connects bones and cartilage.

Limbic system   A group of structures/centres in the brain associated with various emotions and feelings, such as anger, fear, sadness and pleasure.

Lipid   A group of organic compounds, including the fats, oils, waxes, sterols and triglycerides.

Medial   Towards the midline of the body.

Medulla oblongata   A part of the brainstem that contains the cardiac and respiratory centres.

Microvilli (microvillus – singular)   Protrusions of the cell membrane that increase its surface area.

Myopia   Short-sightedness.

Nasopharynx   The part of the airway that begins in the nose and ends at the soft palate.

Neurone   Nerve cell.

Olfaction   The sense of smell.

Olfactory   Pertaining to the sense of smell.

Olfactory bulb   A structure of the brain involved in olfaction, the perception of odours.

Papilla (papillae – plural)   Small, nipple-shaped projection.

Parasympathetic nervous system   Part of the autonomic nervous system.

Pathogen   An infectious agent that causes disease (for instance, bacteria or virus).

Perilymph   The clear fluid found between the bony labyrinth and the membranous labyrinth in the inner ear.

Photoreceptor   Light-sensing neurone.

Pons   Part of the brainstem, the pons contains centres that deal with sleep, swallowing, hearing, equilibrium, taste, eye movement and many other functions.

Posterior   Located at, or related to, the rear of a structure.

Presbyopia   The loss of the ability to focus on close objects as the person ages.

Pupil   The opening in the centre of the iris of the eye that allows light to enter.

Pupillary constrictor muscles   Smooth muscles contained within the iris of the eye; when stimulated they lead to the constriction of the pupil.

Pupillary dilator muscles   Smooth muscles contained within the iris of the eye; when stimulated they lead to the dilation of the pupil.

Reflex   Involuntary function or movement in response to a stimulus.

Refraction   The change of direction of light as it passes from one medium to another with a different density.

Snellen chart   Standardised chart for testing visual acuity.

Sympathetic nervous system   Part of the autonomic nervous system.

Synapse   A gap between two neurones or a neurone and an organ across which neurotransmitters diffuse to transmit a nerve impulse.

Synovial joint   A freely moving joint in which bony surfaces are covered with cartilage and connected by ligaments lined with a synovial membrane. The membrane secretes a lubricating fluid and keeps it around the joint.

Thalamus   A pair of structures in the brain that relay messages from most of the senses.

Transparent   Clear, can see through it.

Umami   The 'fifth taste', related to proteins found in meat and fish.

Visual acuity   Detailed central vision.

References

Haehner, A., Hummel, T. and Reichmann, H. (2011) Olfactory loss in Parkinson's disease. *Parkinson's Disease* **2011**: 450939. doi:10.4061/2011/450939.

Haehner, A., Tosch, C., Wolz, M., Klingelhoefer, L., Fauser, M., Storch, A., Reichman, H. and Hummel, T. (2013) Olfactory training in patients with Parkinson's disease. *PLoS ONE* **8**(4), e61680.

Jenkins, G.W. and Tortora, G.J. (2013) *Anatomy and Physiology: From Science to Life*, 3rd edn. Hoboken, NJ: John Wiley & Sons. Inc.

Martini, F.H. and Nath, J.L. (2009) *Fundamentals of Anatomy and Physiology*, 8th edn. San Francisco, CA: Pearson Benjamin Cummings.

National Institute for Health and Care Excellence (2015) *Corticosteroids – Topical (Skin), Nose, and Eyes*. http://cks.nice.org.uk/corticosteroids-topical-skin-nose-and-eyes#!scenario:1 (accessed 1 December 2015).

Neuland, C., Bitter, T., Marschner, H., Gudziol, H. and Guntinas-Lichius, O. (2011) Health-related and specific olfaction-related quality of life in patients with chronic functional anosmia or severe hyposmia. *The Laryngoscope* **121**(4): 867–872.

NHS Choices (2015) *Anosmia*. http://www.nhs.uk/Conditions/anosmia/Pages/Introduction.aspx (accessed 2 December 2015).

Osawa, Y. (2012) Glutamate perception, soup stock, and the concept of umami: the ethnography, food ecology, and history of dashi in Japan. *Ecology of Food and Nutrition* **51**(4): 329–345.

Tortora, G.J. and Derrickson, B.H. (2009) *Principles of Anatomy and Physiology*, 12th edn. Hoboken, NJ: John Wiley & Sons, Inc.

Tortora, G.J. and Derrickson, B.H. (2012) *Principles of Anatomy and Physiology,* 13th edn. Hoboken, NJ: John Wiley & Sons, Inc.

Further reading

Royal National Institute of Blind People (RNIB)

http://www.rnib.org.uk/

The RNIB is a UK-based charity offering information, support and advice to people experiencing sight loss. The website is a useful source of information, including sections on eye conditions, tests and coping with sight loss.

National Institute on Deafness and Other Communication Disorders

http://www.nidcd.nih.gov/health/Pages/Default.aspx

A useful website maintained by the United States National Institutes of Health detailing various disorders of the ear and mouth, including taste disorders, balance disorders and disorders of the ear.

ENT UK

https://entuk.org/

The website of the British Association of Otorhinolaryngologists and the British Academic Conference in Otolaryngology. This group states its aims as including promoting care, professional education and information for the public. The site has useful information on a variety of conditions of the ear and the nose.

eyeSmart

http://www.geteyesmart.org/eyesmart/index.cfm

This is a website created and maintained by the American Association of Ophthalmology (eye doctors). It contains useful sections on eye conditions, symptoms and lifestyle advice related to eye health.

Activities

Multiple choice questions

1. What percentage of inhaled air passes the olfactory organs?
   - (a) 2%
   - (b) 4%
   - (c) 5%
   - (d) 10%
2. What is the purpose of the Eustachian tube?
   - (a) to equalise the pressure between the outer ear and the nasopharynx
   - (b) to equalise the pressure between the inner ear and the nasopharynx
   - (c) to equalise the pressure between the middle ear and the nasopharynx
   - (d) to equalise the pressure between the inner ear and middle ear
3. The utricle and saccule of the ear are stimulated by:
   - (a) gravity
   - (b) linear acceleration
   - (c) rotation of the head
   - (d) vertical acceleration
4. The organ of Corti is found in:
   - (a) the vestibulocochlear duct
   - (b) the tympanic duct
   - (c) the vestibular duct
   - (d) the cochlear duct

5. Information about the volume and pitch of a sound are transmitted to the brain via a branch of which cranial nerve?
   (a) VI
   (b) VIII
   (c) IX
   (d) X
6. The eyelids are made of:
   (a) elastic cartilage
   (b) connective tissue
   (c) muscle tissue
   (d) epithelial tissue
7. The coloured part of the eye is known as:
   (a) the uvea
   (b) the cornea
   (c) the iris
   (d) the choroid body
8. Photoreceptors are found in:
   (a) the fibrous tunic
   (b) the neural part of the neural tunic
   (c) the vascular tunic
   (d) the pigmented part of the neural tunic
9. Rods are mostly found where in the retina?
   (a) centre
   (b) periphery
   (c) optic disc
   (d) fovea
10. The majority of the refraction of light in the eye happens:
    (a) when the light enters the lens of the eye
    (b) when the light enters the pupil
    (c) when the light enters the posterior cavity
    (d) when the light enters the cornea of the eye

True or false
1. The olfactory receptors are direct chemoreceptors.
2. There are five basic tastes.
3. Taste buds die if they lose their afferent nerve connections.
4. Ear wax is normally clear but gets colour from the debris it collects.
5. The stapes is bound to the round window.
6. The semicircular canals provide information when the body is moving and stationary.
7. Tears are drained into the nasal cavity.
8. Tears have no antibacterial function, they purely wash the bacteria away.
9. There are three types of cone cell in the eye.
10. The white of the eye is known as the sclera.

Label the diagram 1
Label the diagram using the following list of words:

Eyelash, Eyebrow, Pupil, Iris, Upper eyelid (palpebra), Lacrimal caruncle, Lateral commissure, Palpebral fissure, Lower eyelid (palpebra), Conjunctiva (over sclera), Medial commissure

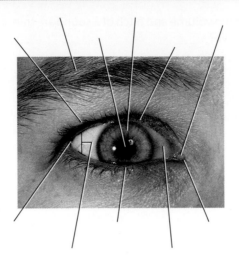

Label the diagram 2

Label the diagram using the following list of words:

Light ray before refraction, Air, Water, Light ray after refraction

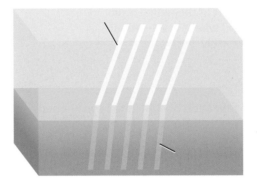

474

Word search

L	K	N	Y	N	Z	A	P	H	O	T	O	R	E	C	E	P	T	O	R
Q	A	Z	Z	M	U	M	G	N	T	G	J	X	E	O	R	O	L	P	O
S	A	C	C	U	L	E	W	H	R	Q	L	K	W	C	N	V	D	T	S
C	Y	V	R	Z	O	R	X	L	I	U	A	P	G	H	B	H	L	I	A
A	V	B	A	I	N	O	C	O	T	A	T	S	R	L	Y	J	E	C	N
M	H	K	T	G	M	P	S	A	B	Y	C	Z	X	E	Z	U	O	X	O
M	S	Q	O	S	T	A	P	E	S	X	S	J	S	A	T	M	V	N	S
L	A	S	L	C	N	D	L	A	O	A	H	R	I	B	I	G	O	R	M
G	I	M	N	L	O	F	C	K	M	G	O	D	O	R	A	N	T	J	I
V	B	U	Q	E	S	H	I	S	N	T	K	G	I	A	V	T	Y	I	A
N	R	I	Y	R	M	K	Y	P	P	A	P	I	L	L	A	E	M	D	I
F	O	L	I	A	T	E	N	E	O	W	C	K	L	K	I	Q	P	A	L
O	B	E	P	U	O	N	C	H	O	R	O	I	D	I	A	D	A	B	P
V	M	H	U	D	T	E	A	Z	B	W	S	N	R	N	C	F	N	A	A
E	A	T	F	W	R	B	P	O	O	X	E	O	L	M	J	K	I	E	B
A	H	I	W	O	Y	I	D	L	G	G	B	C	F	F	A	D	C	S	F
O	G	P	M	A	O	J	K	I	N	O	C	I	L	I	U	M	B	N	V
S	T	E	S	T	P	Z	E	J	H	B	J	X	H	D	B	E	L	J	B
N	H	E	M	R	O	F	I	R	B	I	R	C	B	Q	G	M	Q	P	T
C	I	L	I	A	W	Z	A	H	U	S	O	R	C	X	I	T	X	S	T

475

Anosmia, Cribriform, Lacrimal, Saccule, Chemoreceptors, Epithelium, Odorant, Sclera, Choroid, Foliate, Optic, Stapes, Cilia, Fovea, Papillae, Statoconia, Cochlea, Kinocilium, Photoreceptor, Tympanic

Crossword

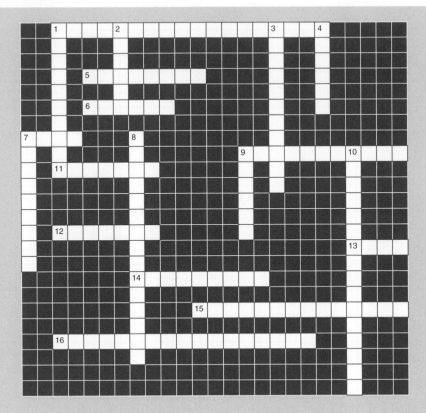

Across:

1. Structures of the inner ear that contain the ducts that respond to rotational movement of the head (12, 6).
5. The bones of the middle ear (8).
6. 'Stirrup', one of 5 across (6).
7. The adjustable focusing structure of the eye (4).
9. Epithelial cell layer that lines the outer surface of the eye (11).
11. Structure of the inner ear that contains 2 down (singular) (7).
12. Spiral-shaped bony chamber of the inner ear (7).
13. Central, coloured part of the eye (4).
14. Clear fluid found between the bony labyrinth and the membranous labyrinth (9).
15. Gel-like substance found in the posterior cavity of the eye (8, 6).
16. Reduced perception of a persistent smell (7, 10).

Down:

1. Calcium carbonate crystals found in the utricle and saccule (10).
2. Area of the wall of the ampulla of the inner ear that contains the receptors (6).
3. Retina (6, 5).
4. The 'white' of the eye (6).
7. Fibrous tissues that bind joints together (9).
8. Largest of the peg-like structures containing taste buds, found at the back of the tongue (plural) (7, 8).
9. The majority of the refraction of light in the eye happens here (6).
10. Eardrum (8, 8).

Fill in the blanks

Sound waves entering the external _____ canal travel along until they reach the tympanic membrane (_____), a thin translucent _____ tissue membrane covered by skin on its _____ surface and internally by _____, and shaped like a flattened cone protruding into the middle ear. Sound _____ that reach the tympanic _____ make it _____ and this vibration is transmitted to the bones of the middle ear.

membrane, ear drum, connective, waves, external, vibrate, mucosa, auditory

Find out more

1. What does the surgical procedure of rhinoplasty entail?
2. Discuss the procedure of ear syringing.
3. What advice should be given to a person who is experiencing an epistaxis?
4. What is role and function of the nurse in helping to stop epistaxis?
5. How can the nurse ensure that the person who has hearing problems maintains a safe environment?
6. Outline the barriers that may be encountered when conducting an assessment of a person's needs.
7. How may the nurse help to reduce the workplace hearing loss?
8. Describe how losing the sense of smell can impact on person's health and well-being.
9. List the issues a person may face with a nasal pack in place.
10. Discuss the services and support systems available to people who are blind.

Look at the diagrams

1. Which of the diagrams shows an eye with myopia?
2. Which of the diagrams shows an eye with corrected myopia (using a lens)?
3. Which of the diagrams shows an eye with hyperopia?
4. Which of the diagrams shows an eye with corrected hyperopia (using a lens)?

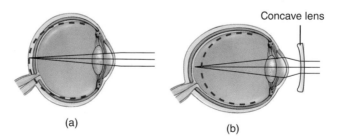

(a)   Concave lens

                                                                (b)

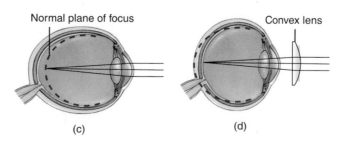

Normal plane of focus   Convex lens

(c)   (d)

Test your learning

1. Name the five basic tastes.
2. Name the three types of papillae that contain taste buds.
3. Describe the mechanism for sensing gravity and linear acceleration.

Conditions

The following is a list of conditions that are associated with the senses. Take some time and write notes about each of the conditions. You may make the notes taken from text books or other resources (e.g. people you work with in a clinical area), or you may make the notes as a result of people you have cared for. If you are making notes about people you have cared for you must ensure that you adhere to the rules of confidentiality.

Anosmia	
Ageusia	
Ménière's disease	
Otosclerosis	
Tinnitus	
Glaucoma	
Macular degeneration	
Retinal detachment	
Cataracts	
Retinopathy	

Chapter 15

The endocrine system

Carl Clare

Test your prior knowledge

- How are hormones transported in the body?
- What is meant by the 'half-life' of a hormone?
- Name one hormone released by the pituitary gland.
- Where in the body is the thyroid gland found?
- What stimulates the release of insulin?

Learning outcomes

After reading this chapter you will be able to:

- Name the endocrine glands in the body and the hormones they secrete
- Discuss the different forms of stimulus for the release of hormones
- Explain the control of hormone release by the hypothalamus
- Discuss the hormonal responses to stress
- Explain the role of insulin and glucagon in the control of blood sugar levels

Fundamentals of Anatomy and Physiology: For Nursing and Healthcare Students, Second Edition. Edited by Ian Peate and Muralitharan Nair.
© 2017 John Wiley & Sons, Ltd. Published 2017 by John Wiley & Sons, Ltd.
Student companion website: www.wileyfundamentalseries.com/anatomy
Instructor companion website: www.wiley.com/go/instructor/anatomy

Body map

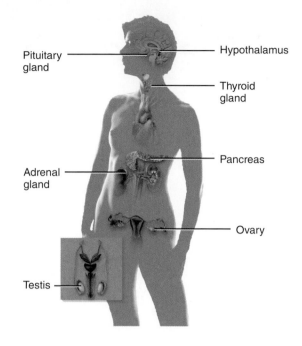

Pituitary gland

Hypothalamus

Thyroid gland

Pancreas

Adrenal gland

Ovary

Testis

Introduction

Homeostasis (from the Greek *homoios*, 'similar'; and *histēmi*, 'standing still') refers to the process of maintaining a stable internal environment. In other words, homeostasis refers to the maintenance of normal physiological balance and functioning within the body. There are two major systems in the body for maintaining homeostasis: the nervous system and the endocrine system. Table 15.1 shows the differences between these two systems.

The nervous system reacts rapidly to stimuli and effects its changes over a period of seconds or minutes; thus, it is involved in the immediate and short-term maintenance of homeostasis. Owing to its rapid onset of action, the nervous system is responsible for the control of rapid bodily processes such as breathing and movement. The endocrine system is often responsible for the regulation of longer term processes. The major functions it coordinates are

- homeostasis – maintains the internal body environment;
- storage and utilisation of energy substrates (carbohydrates, proteins and fats);

Table 15.1   Nervous system versus endocrine system

	Nervous system	Endocrine system
Speed of action	Seconds	Minutes to hours (even days)
Duration of action	Seconds to minutes	Minutes to days
Method of transmitting messages	Electrical	Chemical
Transport method	Neurones	Hormones

- regulation of growth and reproduction;
- control of the body's responses to external stimuli (particularly stress).

It should be noted, however, that though these two systems are separate they often act together and complement each other in the maintenance of homeostasis.

The endocrine system is made up of a collection of small organs that are scattered throughout the body, each of which releases hormones into the blood supply ('endo' = within, 'crine' = to secrete). These hormone-releasing organs can be split into three main categories (Jenkins *et al.*, 2007).

- Endocrine glands – organs whose only function is the production and release of hormones. These include:
  - pituitary gland
  - thyroid gland
  - parathyroid gland
  - adrenal gland.

- Organs that are not pure glands (as they have other functions as well as the production of hormones) but contain relatively large areas of hormone-producing tissue. These include:
  - hypothalamus
  - pancreas.

- Other tissues and organs that also produce hormones – areas of hormone-producing cells are found in the wall of the small intestine and the stomach.

There are no cell types, organs or processes that are not influenced by the endocrine system in some way, and while there are many hormones that we know of there are probably many more that are yet to be discovered.

The endocrine organs

Figure 15.1 shows the endocrine organs and their position within the body. Each of these organs will typically have a rich blood supply delivered by numerous blood vessels. The hormone-producing cells within the organ are arranged into branching networks around this supply. This arrangement of blood vessels and hormone-producing cells ensures that hormones enter the bloodstream rapidly and are then transported throughout the body to the target cells (see Figure 15.2).

Endocrine, paracrine, exocrine and autocrine

Many words in anatomy and physiology have a similar ending to other words used about the same processes or areas of the body (Figure 15.3). It is important to be aware of these as confusion can quickly take over.

Endocrine is usually used to refer to hormones that are secreted into the blood and have an effect on cells distant from those that released the hormone. However, many endocrine hormones are known to act locally and even on the cells that secrete them.

Paracrine refers to hormones that act locally and diffuse to the cells in the immediate neighbourhood to produce their action.

Autocrine refers to hormones that act on the cells that produce it.

Exocrine refers to glands/organs that secrete substances into ducts that eventually lead to the outside of the body (for instance, the sweat glands, the part of the pancreas that secretes digestive juices, the gallbladder).

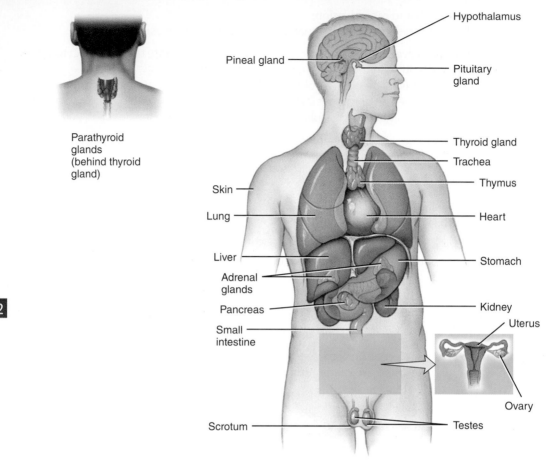

Figure 15.1   Location of the endocrine organs. *Source*: Tortora and Derrickson (2009). Reproduced with permission of John Wiley & Sons.

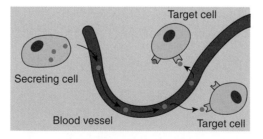

Figure 15.2   Transportation of hormones in the blood.

Hormones

Hormones are chemical messengers that are secreted into the blood or the extracellular fluid by one cell and have an effect on the functioning of other cells. Unlike the nervous system, which could be said to be based on wires (the neurones) like a telegraph, the endocrine system is like a radio broadcast. As it is with a radio broadcast, it is necessary for there to be a

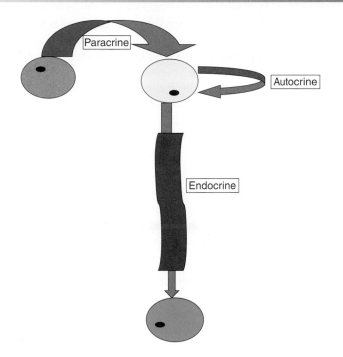

Figure 15.3   Endocrine, paracrine and autocrine.

483

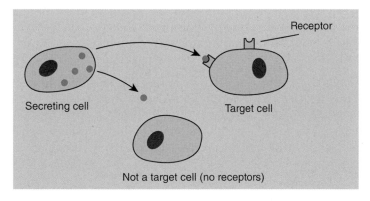

Figure 15.4   Target cell and non-target cell.

receiver in order for the hormonal message to be received and acted upon. As hormones circulate in the blood they come into contact with virtually every cell in the body, but they only exert their specific effect on those cells that have receptors for that hormone (the target cells). Like a lock and key mechanism, only the right key (hormone) can unlock a particular lock (receptor) (see Figure 15.4).

Hormone receptors are either found within the target cell or on its surface (as in Figure 15.4). The site of the receptor is dependent on the type of hormone the receptor is for. Most hormones are made from amino acids, but some are made from cholesterol (the steroid hormones).

• Amino acid-based hormones cannot cross the cell membrane, and thus their receptors are found on the cell wall. These hormones tend to exert their influence by activating enzymes and other molecules within the cell, which then affect the cell activity. This is often through a cascade of changes, with the activation of the enzyme or molecule being the first step. The best understood example of this is cyclic adenosine monophosphate.

- The steroid hormones can cross the cell membrane because they are small and lipid soluble, and thus their receptors are found within the cell itself. These hormones usually exert their effect by stimulating the production of genes within the target cell. The genes then stimulate the synthesis of new proteins.
- One exception is thyroid hormone, which is not a steroid hormone but is lipid soluble and very small and can diffuse easily across the cell membrane into the cell.

The activation of a target cell depends on the concentration of the hormone in the blood, the number of receptors on the cell and the affinity of the receptor for the hormone. Changes in these factors can happen quickly in response to a change in stimuli.

The most important factor affecting the effect of a hormone on its target cell is its concentration in the blood and/or extracellular fluid. This concentration of a hormone at the target cell is determined by three factors:

- Rate of production of the hormone – this is the most highly regulated aspect of the endocrine system.
- Rate of delivery of the hormone – for instance, the blood flow to the organ or cell.
- Rate of destruction and elimination of the hormone (half-life). Hormones with a short half-life will rapidly drop in concentration once production decreases. If the half-life of the hormone is long, then the hormone will still be present in significant concentrations for some time after its production stops.

Changes in the concentration of hormones can be a rapid mechanism of control, especially the rate of production, but longer term adjustments to target cell sensitivity to a hormone will almost certainly include changes in the numbers of receptors as well. Changes in the number of receptors are known as upregulation and downregulation.

- Upregulation is the creation of more receptors in response to low circulating levels of a hormone; the cell becomes more responsive to the presence of the hormone in the blood
- Downregulation is the reduction in the number of receptors and is often the response of a cell to prolonged periods of high circulating levels of a hormone; the cell becomes less responsive (desensitised) to a hormone.

The transportation of hormones

Most hormones are secreted into the circulating blood, though there is the exception of hormones that are released into a local circulatory system known as a portal circulation. The two portal circulations in the human body are those connecting the hypothalamus and the anterior pituitary gland and the hepatic portal circulation that merges to form the portal vein entering the liver.

The steroid hormones are mostly conveyed within the circulation by being bound to transport proteins, with less than 10% making up the 'free fraction' of the hormone (Jenkins and Tortora, 2013). In clinical placements you may have noticed that some blood tests are specifically targeted at measuring both the bound and free elements of a hormone; the most common of these are the thyroid function tests, which measure both bound thyroxine (T_4) and free T_4. Water-soluble hormones are conveyed in their free form in the blood.

Effects of hormones

Hormones typically produce one of the following changes:

- changes in cell membrane permeability and/or the cell's electrical state (membrane potential) by opening or closing ion channels in the cell membrane;
- synthesis of proteins or regulatory molecules (such as enzymes) within the cell;
- enzyme activation or deactivation;
- causing secretory activity;
- stimulation of mitosis.

Control of hormone release

The creation and release of most hormones are preceded by a stimulus that can be internal or external; for instance, a rise in blood glucose levels or a cold environment. The further synthesis and release of hormones is then usually controlled by a negative feedback system. As can be seen in Figure 15.5, the influence of a stimulus, from inside or outside the body (in this case a rise in blood glucose levels), leads to hormone release (insulin); following this, some aspect of the target organ function then inhibits further reaction to the stimulus and thus further release of the hormone by the organ.

The initial stimulus for the release of a hormone is usually one of three types, though some organs respond to multiple stimuli (Marieb and Hoehn, 2007).

- **Humoral:**   A response to changing levels of certain ions and nutrients in the blood. For example, parathyroid hormone is stimulated by falling blood levels of calcium ions.
- **Neural:**   A response to direct nervous stimulation. Very few endocrine organs are directly stimulated by the nervous system. An example is increased activity in the sympathetic nervous system that directly stimulates the release of catecholamines (adrenaline and noradrenaline) from the adrenal medulla.
- **Hormonal:**   A response to hormones released by other organs. Hormones that are released in response to hormonal stimuli are usually rhythmical in their release (that is, the levels rise and fall in a specific pattern). An example of hormonal control is the release of thyroid stimulating hormone (TSH) from the anterior pituitary gland directly stimulating the production and release of T_4 from the thyroid gland.

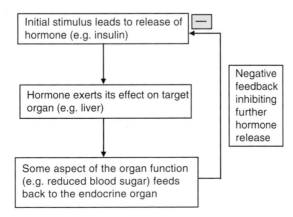

Figure 15.5   The negative feedback system. *Source*: Nair and Peate (2009). Reproduced with permission of John Wiley & Sons.

Destruction and removal of hormones

Hormones are very powerful and can have a large effect at even low concentrations; therefore, it is essential that active hormones are efficiently removed from the blood. Some hormones are rapidly broken down within the target cells. Most are inactivated by enzyme systems in the liver and kidneys and then excreted mostly in the urine, but some are excreted in the faeces.

The physiology of the endocrine organs

The hypothalamus and the pituitary gland

The hypothalamus is a portion of the brain with a variety of functions. It is a small (about 4 g), cone-like structure that is directly connected to the pituitary gland by the pituitary stalk (or infundibulum). One of the most important functions of the hypothalamus is to link the nervous system to the endocrine system via the pituitary gland. Almost all hormone secretion by the pituitary gland is controlled by either hormonal or electrical signals from the hypothalamus (Figure 15.6).

The hypothalamus receives signals from virtually all the potential sources within the nervous system but is also under negative feedback control by the hormones regulated by the pituitary gland. Thus, when there is a low level of a hormone in the blood supplying the hypothalamus this leads to the release of the appropriate releasing hormone or factor that stimulates the release of the hormone by the pituitary, which in turn stimulates the release of the appropriate hormone. As the level of the target hormone rises in the blood, this is detected by receptors in the hypothalamus and the stimulus for the release of the stimulating factor is removed, and thus release of this factor is reduced. A classic example of this system is the release of thyrotropin-releasing hormone (TRH) and the subsequent release of TSH by the anterior pituitary gland, which is described further on in this chapter.

The pituitary gland secretes at least nine major hormones and is the size and shape of a pea on a stalk. The pituitary gland is functionally and anatomically divided into two parts:

- The posterior lobe (neurohypophysis) is made up mostly of nerve fibres that originate in the hypothalamus and terminate on the surface of capillaries in the posterior lobe. The posterior lobe releases two hormones that it receives directly from the hypothalamus. In this sense it is in fact a storage area rather than a gland in the true sense of the term. The hypothalamus and the posterior pituitary are linked by a nerve bundle called the hypothalamic-hypophyseal tract.

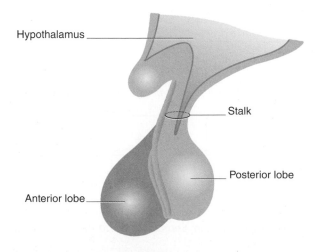

Figure 15.6 The hypothalamus and pituitary gland.

- The anterior lobe (adenohypophysis) is much larger than the posterior lobe and partly surrounds the posterior lobe and the infundibulum. It is made up of glandular tissue and produces and releases several hormones. The hypothalamus and the anterior pituitary have no direct nerve connections but do have a vascular (blood vessel) connection known as the hypothalamo-hypophyseal portal system, whereby venous blood from the hypothalamus flows to the anterior lobe. Thus, control of the anterior pituitary is by releasing and inhibiting factors (or hormones) released by the hypothalamus.

Hormones that are secreted by the posterior pituitary are the following.

- **Oxytocin:** Oxytocin has an effect on uterine contraction in childbirth and is responsible for the 'let down' response in breastfeeding mothers (the release of milk in response to suckling). In men and non-pregnant women it appears to play a role in sexual arousal and orgasm (Jenkins and Tortora, 2013).
- **Antidiuretic hormone (ADH):** Under resting conditions, large quantities of ADH accumulate in the posterior pituitary; excitation by nervous impulses leads to the release of the ADH from where it is stored into the adjacent blood vessels. The effects of ADH are that it increases water retention by the kidneys by increasing the permeability of the collecting ducts in the kidneys. The secretion of ADH is stimulated:

  - by increased plasma osmolality – increased levels of certain substances in the plasma, such as sodium;
  - by decreased extracellular fluid volume;
  - by pain and other stressed states;
  - in response to certain drugs.

487

Clinical considerations

Syndrome of inappropriate ADH secretion (SIADH)

Though relatively rare, SIADH is a potentially life-threatening condition that causes a reduced blood sodium level. The pathophysiology varies, but one type is thought to be due to changes in the ability of the hypothalamus to detect a decrease in blood osmolality, and thus ADH release is not reduced and the blood volume increases, reducing the concentration of sodium relative to the volume of blood. In the elderly it is thought that the cells of the hypothalamus increase ADH production with increasing age. Clinically detectable SIADH has many potential causes, including several commonly used medications (such as morphine, loop diuretics, angiotensin-converting enzyme inhibitors and many antidepressants), some neurological disorders, several types of cancer and hypothyroidism. It is the most common cause of hyponatraemia in critical care patients (Friedman and Cirulli, 2013) and is also common in the elderly.

The symptoms of SIADH includes loss of appetite, nausea, weakness, confusion and delirium. In the elderly the diagnosis of SIADH can be late as one of the common presenting factors is altered mental states (including confusion) which can be mistakenly ascribed to many other factors or conditions such as dementia, infection and cerebrovascular events (Nelson and Robinson, 2012).

The diagnosis of SIADH includes the detection of a low blood sodium concentration with a normal blood volume (euvolaemia).

The treatment of SIADH involves fluid restriction, thus increasing relative sodium levels in the blood by reducing blood volume and where possible treating the cause. In cases requiring urgent treatment, hypertonic saline (3% saline) can be infused to temporarily increase the blood sodium level (Gross, 2012).

Hormones released by the anterior pituitary gland

Table 15.2 summarises the range of hormones released by the anterior pituitary gland and the releasing or inhibiting hormones (or factors) from the hypothalamus that influence this release.

There are five types of pituitary cell in the anterior lobe:

- somatotropes, which secrete growth hormones;
- lactotropes, which secrete prolactin;
- thyrotropes, which secrete TSH;
- gonadotropes, which secrete luteinising hormone (LH) and follicle-stimulating hormone (FSH);
- corticotropes, which secrete adrenocorticotropic hormone (ACTH).

Growth hormone

Effects

As its name suggests, growth hormone promotes the growth of bone, cartilage and soft tissue by stimulating the production and release of insulin-like growth factor (IGF-1).

Regulation

Growth hormone release from the anterior pituitary is regulated by the release of growth-hormone-releasing hormone and growth-hormone-release-inhibiting hormone (somatostatin) by the hypothalamus. Both growth hormone and IGF-1 produce a negative feedback effect on the hypothalamus.

Table 15.2 Hormones released by the hypothalamus and the anterior pituitary gland

Hypothalamus	Anterior pituitary gland	Target organ or tissues	Action
Growth-hormone-releasing factor	Growth hormone	Many (especially bones)	Stimulates growth of body cells
Growth-hormone-release-inhibiting factor	Growth hormone (inhibits release)	Many	
Thyroid-releasing hormone (TRH)	Thyroid-stimulating hormone (TSH)	Thyroid gland	Stimulates thyroid hormone release
Corticotropin-releasing hormone (CRH)	Adrenocorticotropic hormone (ACTH)	Adrenal cortex	Stimulates corticosteroid release
Prolactin-releasing hormone	Prolactin	Breasts	Stimulates milk production
Prolactin-inhibiting hormone	Prolactin (inhibits release)	Breasts	
Gonadotropin-releasing hormone	Follicle-stimulating hormone Luteinising hormone	Gonads	Various reproductive functions

Source: Nair and Peate (2009). Reproduced with permission of John Wiley & Sons.

Prolactin
Effects
Prolactin stimulates the secretion of milk in the breast.

Regulation
Secretion is inhibited by the release of dopamine from the hypothalamus. Secretion can be intermittently increased by the release of prolactin-releasing hormone from the hypothalamus in response to the baby suckling at the breast.

Follicle-stimulating hormone and luteinising hormone (gonadotrophins)
Effects
In males, FSH stimulates sperm production. In females it leads to the early maturation of ovarian follicles and oestrogen secretion.

LH is responsible for the final maturation of the ovarian follicles and oestrogen secretion in females, and in males it stimulates testosterone secretion.

Regulation
In males and females, LH and FSH production are regulated by the release of gonadotrophin-releasing hormone (GnRH). Testosterone and oestrogen exert a negative feedback effect on the release of GnRH from the hypothalamus.

Thyroid-stimulating hormone
Effects
TSH stimulates the activity of the cells of the thyroid gland leading to an increased production and secretion of T_4 and triiodothyronine (T_3).

Regulation
TSH is produced and released in response to the release of TRH from the hypothalamus. The hypothalamus can also inhibit the release of TSH through the action of somatostatin.

Free T_3 and T_4 in the blood have a direct negative feedback effect on the hypothalamus and the anterior pituitary gland.

Adrenocorticotrophic hormone
Effects
ACTH stimulates the production of cortisol and androgens from the cortex of the adrenal gland. It also leads to the production of aldosterone in response to increased concentrations of potassium ions, increased angiotensin levels or decreased total body sodium.

Regulation

ACTH is secreted from the anterior pituitary in response to the secretion of corticotropin-releasing hormone (CRH) from the hypothalamus. Excitation of the hypothalamus by any form of stress leads to the release of CRH and the subsequent release of ACTH and then cortisol. Cortisol exerts a direct negative feedback on the hypothalamus and the anterior pituitary gland.

Snapshot

Mary is a 50-year-old lady who has been referred to the endocrinologist by her GP. Mary has been reporting increasing weight gain, especially in the face and on the back of the neck. At the same time she has noticed excessive hair growth on her face and neck. On questioning, the endocrinologist finds out that Mary has also noticed that her skin is bruising easily and she is constantly tired.

The doctor suspects that Mary has Cushing's disease, which is a disease caused by excess levels of cortisol in the body. There are several potential causes for Cushing's disease, with the most common being the long-term use of high-dose glucocorticoid medication. Mary does not take any medication normally and this leads the doctor to suspect that Mary may have a tumour that is causing the increased production of cortisol. Mary has bloods taken to measure her cortisol levels and a 24-h urine analysis is carried out; both show elevated cortisol levels.

Magnetic resonance imaging shows that Mary has a tumour of her pituitary gland, which is causing an increased production of ACTH (corticotroph adenoma).

Mary is rapidly passed on to the care of a neurosurgeon for an operation known as transsphenoidal hypophysectomy (the removal of the pituitary gland via the nasal cavity). The procedure can remove part or all of the pituitary gland (Liubinas *et al.*, 2011).

In Mary's case it was necessary to remove the whole gland. Following this procedure Mary will no longer have a pituitary gland and will no longer produce any of the pituitary hormones, including TRH and ACTH. The loss of TRH and ACTH production will mean there will be no stimulus for the thyroid gland and the adrenal glands to produce hormones, leading to the need for hormone replacement therapy for hypothyroidism and hypoadrenalism.

The thyroid gland

The thyroid gland is a butterfly-shaped gland located in the front of the neck on the trachea just below the larynx (Figure 15.7). It is made up of two lobes joined by an isthmus (a narrow strip; isthmus = neck). The upper extremities of the lobes are known as the upper poles and the lower extremities the lower poles. Each lobe is made up of hollow, spherical follicles surrounded by capillaries. This leads to an abundant blood supply; although the thyroid gland accounts for 0.4% of the total body weight, it receives 2% of the circulating blood supply.

The follicles are comprised of a single layer of epithelial cells that form a cavity that contains thyroglobulin molecules with attached iodine molecules; the thyroid hormone is created from this. One unique factor of the thyroid gland is its ability to create and store large amounts of hormone; this can be up to 100 days of hormone supply (Guyton and Hall, 2006). The thyroid gland releases two forms of thyroid hormone: T_4 and T_3; both require iodine for their creation. Iodide taken in with the normal diet is concentrated by the thyroid gland and is changed in

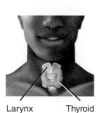

Larynx   Thyroid
          gland

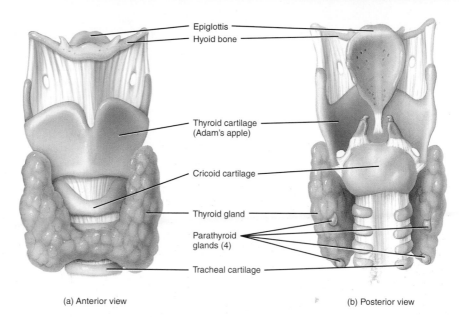

Epiglottis
Hyoid bone

Thyroid cartilage
(Adam's apple)

Cricoid cartilage

Thyroid gland

Parathyroid
glands (4)

Tracheal cartilage

(a) Anterior view   (b) Posterior view

Figure 15.7 (a, b) Position of the thyroid gland and parathyroid glands. *Source*: Tortora and Derrickson (2009). Reproduced with permission of John Wiley & Sons.

the follicle cells into iodine. This iodine is then linked to tyrosine molecules and these iodinated tyrosine molecules are then linked together to create T_3 and T_4. All the steps in thyroid hormone production are stimulated by TSH. T_4 is the primary hormone released by the thyroid gland; this is then converted into T_3 by the target cells. Most thyroid hormone is bound to transport proteins in the blood; very little is unbound (free), and T_3 is less firmly bound to transport proteins than is T_4.

Thyroid hormone affects virtually every cell in the body, except:

- the adult brain
- spleen
- testes
- uterus
- thyroid gland.

Both T_4 and T_3 easily cross the cell membrane and interact with receptors inside the cell. In the target cells, thyroid hormone stimulates enzymes that are involved with glucose oxidation. This is known as the calorigenic effect and its overall effects are:

- an increase in the basal metabolic rate;
- an increase in oxygen consumption by the cell;
- an increase in the production of body heat.

Basal metabolic rate is the amount of energy expended while at rest in a temperate environment (not hot or cold). The release of energy in this state is enough for the functioning of the vital organs. As basal metabolic rate is increased so oxygen consumption is increased, as oxygen is required in the production of energy.

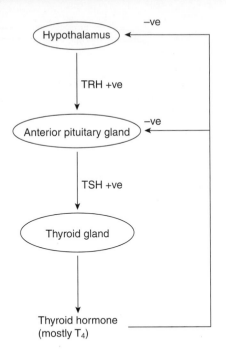

Figure 15.8   Negative feedback control of thyroid hormone production.

Thyroid hormone also has an important role in the maintenance of blood pressure as it stimulates an increase in the number of receptors in the walls of the blood vessels.

The control of the release of thyroid hormone is mediated by a negative feedback system that involves the hypothalamus and cascades through the pituitary gland (Figure 15.8).

Plasma levels of thyroid hormone are monitored in the hypothalamus and by cells in the anterior lobe of the pituitary gland. Increased levels of T_4 in the blood inhibit the release of TRH from the hypothalamus, thus reducing the stimulation for the release of TSH from the anterior pituitary gland. Thyroid hormones also have a direct negative feedback effect on the anterior pituitary gland. The effect of TSH on the thyroid gland is to promote the release of thyroid hormone into the blood; therefore, a reduction in TSH reduces the release of T_3 and T_4. A reduced level of T_4 in the blood reduces the negative feedback, and thus there is an increase in the release of TRH, which leads to an increase in thyroid gland function. Conditions that increase the energy requirements of the body (such as pregnancy or prolonged cold) also stimulate the release of TRH from the hypothalamus and therefore lead to an increase in blood levels of thyroid hormone. In these situations the stimulating conditions override the normal negative feedback system (Jenkins and Tortora, 2013). The negative feedback control of thyroid hormone can be likened to a central heating system. The hypothalamus and pituitary gland are the thermostat and the thyroid gland is the boiler. As the room temperature increases, the thermostat turns off the central heating boiler; when the temperature decreases, the thermostat turns the boiler on to increase the temperature.

The half-life of T_4 is approximately 7 days and the half-life of T_3 is 1 day. Thyroid hormones are broken down in the liver and the skeletal muscle, and while much of the iodine is recycled, some is lost in the urine and the faeces. Therefore, there is a need for daily replacement of iodide in the diet.

Clinical considerations

Hypothyroidism and hyperthyroidism

A patient's blood level of thyroid hormone can be measured. Depending on whether the thyroid gland is overactive or underactive, different levels of hormones will be shown by the test. Generally, the patient would have their free T_4 and TSH levels assessed.

	TSH	Free T_4
Hyperthyroidism	Reduced	Elevated
Hypothyroidism	Elevated	Reduced

In the case of a patient with an overactive thyroid gland (hyperthyroidism) free T_4 will often be elevated but TSH levels will be reduced as the levels of thyroid hormone will be exerting a negative feedback effect on the hypothalamus and the pituitary gland. Despite the reduced TSH levels and the negative feedback effect on the pituitary gland as well, hormone levels will remain elevated.

A patient with hypothyroidism (an underactive thyroid gland) will often present with a reduced free T_4 and an elevated TSH as the reduced hormone levels remove the negative feedback on the hypothalamus and the pituitary and thus TSH levels rise. The patient with a test results within normal ranges is called 'euthyroid'.

Sick euthyroid syndrome

During severe illness or starvation, the metabolic drive on the human body by the thyroid is reduced. The term 'sick euthyroid' is used in this condition since it represents a state of thyroid function appropriate for a sick individual; and it returns to normal with the return of good health.

T_3 is largely produced by target cell conversion of T_4. In the typical sick euthyroid patient, circulating T_3 is usually low but the total T_4 may be normal or even raised since there is reduced conversion to T_3. Conversely, T_4 may be low since the majority is carried on serum-binding proteins and their synthesis may be suppressed by severe illness. In these cases the absence of a raised TSH excludes a diagnosis of primary hypothyroidism (McDermott, 2014).

Critically ill patients with sick euthyroid syndrome are known to have increased rates of mortality, but at present the routine testing of thyroid function in the critically ill is not recommended and should only be carried out when there is clinical suspicion of hypothyroidism (Economidou *et al.*, 2011).

In addition to the thyroid epithelial cells there are C cells, which are found between the follicles and secrete calcitonin. Calcitonin is involved in the metabolism of calcium and phosphorus within the body. It decreases calcium levels in the blood by reducing the activity of osteoclasts (cells that 'digest' bone and thus release calcium and phosphorus into the blood); due to this action, calcitonin is used as a treatment for osteoporosis and may also have a future role in the treatment of osteoarthritis (Mero *et al.*, 2014). Calcitonin also inhibits the reabsorption of calcium from urine in the kidneys.

Snapshot

Holly is a 24-year-old woman who has been experiencing symptoms of lethargy, a loss of appetite, weight gain and mild depression. Initially her GP decided her symptoms were due to Holly's lifestyle and advised Holly about getting sufficient rest and exercise. As the months went by the symptoms did not improve and Holly began to lose her hair. Holly's GP took blood and sent it to the local hospital for thyroid function testing. The results showed an increase in TSH and a decrease in free T_4, suggestive of hypothyroid disease.

The GP prescribed Holly levothyroxine but warned her that it would be several weeks (if not months) before she felt completely better and in the meantime there would be a need for repeated blood tests to monitor her blood levels of T_4 to ensure that she is receiving the correct dose.

Levothyroxine is a synthetic version of the hormone T_4 and is generally free from side effects at the correct dose. Levothyroxine should be taken at the same time every day, preferably on an empty stomach. Where possible, patients are advised to take their levothyroxine an hour before breakfast.

Holly should also be counselled that before she intends to become pregnant she should discuss this with her endocrinologist. Preconception measurement of thyroid replacement levels is advised as low levels of maternal T_4 in the first trimester are associated with intellectual impairment in the baby. Levothyroxine requirements increase by about 50% in pregnancy, and the patient should be advised to increase their dose as soon as they are aware that they are pregnant (Weetman, 2013).

The parathyroid glands

The parathyroid glands (Figure 15.7) are small glands located on the back (posterior) of the thyroid gland. There are usually two pairs of glands, but the precise number varies, and some patients have been reported to have up to four pairs (Marieb and Hoehn, 2007). The cells that create and secrete parathyroid hormone (parathyroid chief cells) are arranged in cords or nests around a dense capillary network. Parathyroid hormone is the single most important hormone for the control of the calcium balance in the body. Its major target cells are in the bones and the kidneys; it

- increases intestinal calcium absorption;
- stimulates renal calcium absorption;
- stimulates osteoclast activity, and therefore reabsorption of calcium from the bones.

Physiologically, calcium is important in the transmission of nerve impulses, is involved in muscle contraction and is also required in the creation of clotting factors in the blood. The regulation of parathyroid hormone synthesis and secretion is in response to the levels of calcium in the blood, which is monitored by cells in the gland. A reduced blood calcium level leads to an increase in the synthesis and secretion of parathyroid hormone.

Calcitriol is a hormone released by the kidneys in response to a decrease in calcium ions in the blood; it is known to have some effect on parathyroid hormone secretion and inhibits the release of calcitonin. It also promotes the absorption of calcium from the gut and the reabsorption of calcium from the renal tubules. Parathyroid hormone is a known stimulus for the release of calcitriol, but when calcitriol levels achieve a high enough level its effect changes to that of inhibiting the release of parathyroid hormone. This prevents an uncontrollable increase in calcium in the blood.

Snapshot

Peter is a 74-year-old gentleman with chronic renal failure. He has been persistently reporting severe bone and joint pains. Blood tests have shown that Peter has high levels of parathyroid hormones but low levels of calcium. Peter has secondary hyperparathyroidism related to his renal disease.

The destruction of the kidney can lead to a loss of the creation and release of calcitriol, and thus a reduction in the blood levels of calcium. In response to this the parathyroid gland increases the production and release of parathyroid hormone and becomes hypertrophied (hypertrophy is the enlargement of an organ).

The clinical treatment of secondary hyperparathyroidism is focused on the prevention of osteoporosis by the administration of calcium and an active form of vitamin D. Vitamin D is required to aid the absorption of calcium from the intestines. Normally, vitamin D is converted into an active form by the kidneys, but in kidney failure this cannot happen; thus, the patient has to take an active form of vitamin D.

If the parathyroid glands do not respond to the increase in calcium levels and blood levels of parathyroid hormones remain high, surgery may be considered to remove the parathyroid glands. Research has been undertaken to trial a calcimimetic drug to mimic the effect of calcium on the parathyroid glands and thus reduce the production of parathyroid hormone and reduce the need for surgery (Ballinger *et al.*, 2014).

The adrenal glands

The adrenal glands are complex, multifunctional organs whose secretions are essential for the maintenance of homeostasis. The two adrenal glands are found on the top of each of the two kidneys (Figure 15.9). The right gland is roughly triangular in shape, and the left, which is commonly the larger of the two, is crescent-shaped. Both glands are encased in a connective tissue capsule and embedded in an area of fat. Adrenal glands are very vascular (have a rich blood supply from many blood vessels).

Functionally, each adrenal gland is actually two glands and is comprised of two major regions (Figure 15.10):

- adrenal medulla
- adrenal cortex.

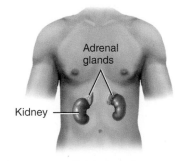

Figure 15.9   Position of the adrenal glands. *Source*: Tortora and Derrickson (2009). Reproduced with permission of John Wiley & Sons.

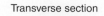

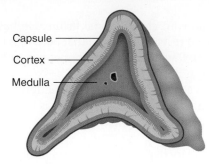

Figure 15.10   Cross-section of an adrenal gland. *Source*: Nair and Peate (2009). Reproduced with permission of John Wiley & Sons.

Adrenal medulla

The adrenal medulla is the inner part of the adrenal gland; it makes up about 30% of the total mass of the adrenal gland. The function of the adrenal medulla is the secretion of catecholamines:

- adrenaline
- noradrenaline
- dopamine.

The adrenal medulla is mostly a modified, densely innervated, sympathetic ganglion made up of granule-containing cells. Within the adrenal medulla approximately 90% of the cells secrete adrenaline and the remaining 10% secrete noradrenaline. It is unclear which cells secrete dopamine at this time.

The effects of the catecholamines are many and varied:

- they stimulate the nervous system;
- they have metabolic effects – for instance, glycogenolysis in the liver and skeletal muscle;
- they increase metabolic rate;
- they increase heart rate;
- they increase alertness – though adrenaline frequently evokes anxiety and fear;
- noradrenaline causes significant, widespread, vasoconstriction;
- adrenaline causes vasoconstriction in the skin and viscera but vasodilatation in skeletal muscles.

Although adrenaline and noradrenaline are essential for normal bodily functioning, adrenaline and the noradrenaline secreted by the adrenal medulla are not essential and serve only to intensify the effects of sympathetic nervous stimulation.

Secretion of catecholamines from the adrenal medulla is initiated by sympathetic nervous activity controlled by the hypothalamus and occurs in response to

- pain
- anxiety
- excitement
- hypovolaemia
- hypoglycaemia.

The medulla receives its blood supply from the adrenal cortex rich in corticosteroids. These regulate the production of the enzymes that convert noradrenaline to adrenaline. Thus, an increase in corticosteroid production leads to an increased conversion of noradrenaline to adrenaline. With emergency stimulation of the hypothalamus there is a responding diffuse medullary

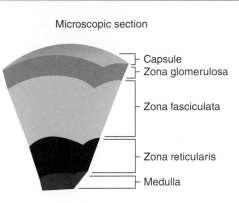

Microscopic section

Capsule
Zona glomerulosa

Zona fasciculata

Zona reticularis

Medulla

Figure 15.11   Cross-section of the adrenal cortex. *Source*: Nair and Peate (2009). Reproduced with permission of John Wiley & Sons.

activity preparing for fight or flight. Catecholamines have a very short half-life in the blood of less than 2 min as they are rapidly degraded by blood-borne enzymes.

Adrenal cortex

The outer part of each adrenal gland is made up of three distinct functional layers (Figure 15.11). Each layer is involved in the production of steroid-based hormones (known collectively as the corticosteroids):

- zona glomerulosa – produces the mineralocorticoids;
- zona fasciculata – produces the glucocorticoids;
- zona reticularis – this zone is also involved in the production of glucocorticoids but also produces small amounts of adrenal sex hormones (the gonadocorticoids).

Mineralocorticoids

Mineralocorticoids are the group of hormones whose main function is the regulation of the concentration of the electrolytes in the blood. There are several known mineralocorticoids, but the most common is aldosterone, which accounts for 95% of all the mineralocorticoids synthesised and is also the most potent.

The effect of aldosterone is to reduce the excretion of sodium in the urine by regulating the reabsorption of sodium from the urine in the distal portion of the renal tubules. Sodium is in effect exchanged for potassium and hydrogen, which results in the renal excretion of potassium and acidic urine. Aldosterone also has an effect on the levels of water in the body and several other ions (including potassium, bicarbonate and chloride) due to the fact that their regulation is coupled to the regulation of sodium in the body. The control of aldosterone secretion is primarily related to the blood concentrations of sodium (Na^+) and potassium (K^+), the mean arterial blood pressure and blood volume. Increased concentrations of potassium, reduced blood concentrations of sodium and a reduction in blood pressure and/or blood volume all stimulate the release of aldosterone, while the opposite inhibits release (Figure 15.12). High blood levels of potassium are also known to have a direct effect on the adrenal cortex in the stimulation of aldosterone production and secretion.

There are several mechanisms that regulate the release of aldosterone. The primary control mechanism is the production of angiotensin II by the renin–angiotensin system in response to reduced blood pressure in the kidneys or reduced sodium delivery to the distal tubules of the kidneys. Raised levels of potassium and reduced levels of sodium in the blood are also known to

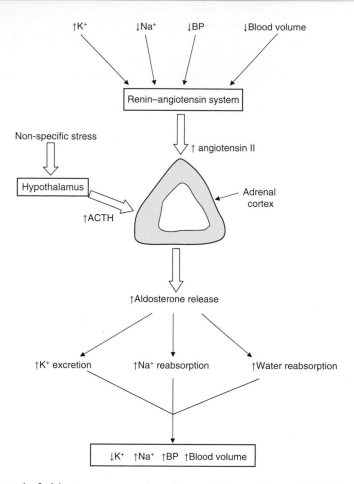

Figure 15.12 Control of aldosterone secretion. *Source*: Nair and Peate (2009). Reproduced with permission of John Wiley & Sons.

have a direct effect on the adrenal cortex and stimulate the release of mineralocorticoids. However, in response to a severe, non-specific stressor, hypothalamic release of CRH stimulates the increased release of ACTH. This increase in ACTH stimulates a slight increase in the release of aldosterone, leading to a slight increase in blood volume and pressure, which will help to maintain delivery of oxygen and nutrients to the tissues.

Glucocorticoids

There appears to be no cell within the body that does not have receptors for the glucocorticoid hormones. The glucocorticoid hormones have several effects:

- they influence the metabolism of most body cells;
- they promote glycogen storage in the liver;
- during fasting they stimulate the generation of glucose;
- they increase blood glucose levels;
- they are involved in providing resistance to stressors;
- they potentiate the vasoconstrictor effect of catecholamines;

- they decrease the permeability of vascular endothelium;
- they promote the repair of damaged tissues by promoting the breakdown of stored protein to create amino acids;
- they suppress the immune system;
- they suppress inflammatory processes.

The glucocorticoid hormones include:

- cortisol (hydrocortisone)
- cortisone
- corticosterone.

Only cortisol is secreted in any significant amounts. Cortisol is normally released in a rhythmical pattern, with most being released shortly after the person gets up from sleep and the lowest amount being released just before, and shortly after, sleep commences.

Cortisol release is stimulated by ACTH from the anterior pituitary gland. ACTH releases cholesterol from the cytoplasm in the cells, which is then converted and modified to create the steroid hormones. ACTH secretion is regulated by the release of CRH from the hypothalamus. Increasing levels of cortisol have a negative feedback effect on both the hypothalamus and the pituitary gland, inhibiting further release of both CRH and ACTH. However, this negative feedback system can be overridden by acute physiological stress (for instance, trauma, infection or haemorrhage) and mental stress. The increase in sympathetic nervous system activity in response to an acute stress triggers greater CRH release, and thus there is a significant increase in subsequent cortisol production (Figure 15.13).

499

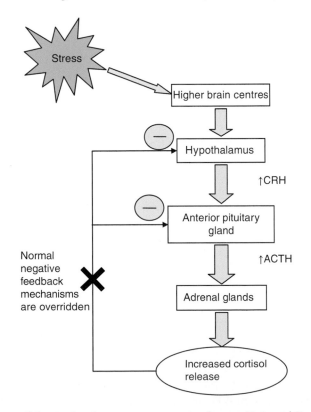

Figure 15.13   Response of the endocrine system to stress. *Source*: Nair and Peate (2009). Reproduced with permission of John Wiley & Sons.

Clinical considerations

Glucocorticoid steroids and inflammatory diseases

Synthetic glucocorticoid steroid hormones are used widely in healthcare for the suppression of inflammation in diseases such as arthritis, ulcerative colitis and acute severe asthma. However, after taking glucocorticoid steroids such as prednisolone for a significant length of time (except in asthma inhalers), steroid treatment should be gradually reduced, not stopped suddenly. Trials have shown that a short-term (5 days) course of high-dose prednisolone (60 mg) led to some suppression of ACTH production in children, but this did not require a tapering dose of steroids to prevent hypoadrenalism. However, it is felt that these patients should be counselled as to the potential symptoms of hypoadrenalism and to seek medical aid if these symptoms did appear (Crowley *et al.*, 2014).

The constant intake of synthetic steroids for long-term treatment of inflammatory disease leads to a reduction in the production of steroids by the adrenal cortex (probably due to reduced CRH and ACTH secretion because of negative feedback to the hypothalamus and pituitary gland), and suddenly stopping steroid treatment may leave the patient with reduced levels of glucocorticoid steroids in their blood and may lead to a life-threatening hypoadrenal crisis. Thus, the patient will be advised to take a gradually reducing dose of steroids to allow the hypothalamus, pituitary gland and adrenal glands to respond to the reducing blood levels of steroids.

The need for adherence to the prescribed regimen of any course of steroid medication and advice on what to do in the event of gastrointestinal disease preventing the patient taking their steroids must be impressed on the patient. The patient should also carry a blue 'steroid card' at all times detailing the dose and type of steroid taken so that healthcare professionals can respond appropriately, even when the patient is unconscious.

Pancreas

The pancreas is an elongated organ and is found next to the first part of the small intestine. The pancreas is composed of two different types of tissues. The majority of the pancreas is made up of exocrine tissue and the associated ducts. This tissue produces and secretes a fluid rich with digestive enzymes into the small intestine. Scattered throughout the exocrine tissue are many small clusters of cells called islets of Langerhans (islets). These islets are the site of the endocrine cells of the pancreas. Each islet has three major cell types, each of which produces a different hormone:

- alpha cells, which secrete glucagon;
- beta cells, the most abundant of the three cell types and which secrete insulin;
- delta cells, which secrete somatostatin.

The different cell types within each islet are distributed in a set pattern, with the beta cells being the central portion of the islet, surrounded by alpha and delta cells. The islets are highly vascularised, ensuring rapid transit of the hormones into the bloodstream. Although the islets only account for 1–2% of the mass of the pancreas they receive about 10–15% of the pancreatic blood flow. The pancreas is innervated by the parasympathetic and sympathetic nervous systems, and it is clear that nervous stimulation influences the secretion of insulin and glucagon.

Medicines management

Type 2 diabetes

George is a 56-year-old gentleman who has recently been diagnosed with type 2 diabetes. For the last few months he has noticed that he feels increasingly thirsty and is also constantly tired. George has been reluctant to go to the GP as he does not feel that there is anything really wrong with him and he does not like to bother the doctor anyway. During a routine health screening the practice nurse carries out a dipstick test on George's urine and it is found that there is a significant level of glucose in it. The diagnosis is made of type 2 diabetes; in addition to being educated about lifestyle and dietary changes, George is prescribed metformin.

Metformin is an oral antidiabetic drug that is normally used as the first-line drug in the treatment of type 2 diabetes. It works by reducing the amount of glucose produced by the liver. In order to try to prevent the development of gastrointestinal side effects the GP has decided to start George on a relatively low dose of metformin and then to slowly increase the dose. If George is unable to tolerate metformin due to gastrointestinal side effects, current guidelines suggest a trial of extended absorption metformin (National Institute for Health and Care Excellence, 2009).

Insulin

Insulin is well known for its effect in reducing the blood glucose levels. It does this by:

- Facilitating the entry of glucose into muscle, adipose tissue and several other tissues. Note that the brain and the liver do not require insulin to facilitate the uptake of glucose.
- Stimulating the liver to store glucose in the form of glycogen.

However, as well as its effects on glucose, insulin is known to have an effect on protein and mineral metabolism. Finally, insulin has an effect on lipid metabolism. As has been noted, insulin promotes the synthesis of glycogen in the liver. As glycogen accumulation in the liver rises to higher levels (5% of the total liver mass), further glycogen synthesis is suppressed. Further uptake of glucose is then diverted by insulin into the production of fatty acids, and insulin inhibits the breakdown of fat in adipose tissue and facilitates the production of triglycerides from glucose for further storage in these tissues.

From a whole-body perspective, insulin has a fat-sparing effect in that it promotes the use of glucose instead of fatty acids and stimulates the storage of fat in the adipose tissue.

The stimulation of insulin synthesis and secretion is primarily a response to a rise in blood glucose levels, but rises in blood levels of amino acids and fatty acids also have a stimulating effect. Some neural stimuli, for instance the sight and smell of food, also increase insulin secretion. The pancreas is innervated by the sympathetic and parasympathetic nervous systems, and nervous stimulation clearly influences the secretion of insulin (and glucagon).

As blood glucose levels fall there is a corresponding fall in the production and secretion of insulin. When insulin levels in the blood fall, glycogen synthesis in the liver reduces and enzymes that break down glycogen become active. The half-life of insulin is approximately 5 min and it is destroyed in the liver.

Medicines management

Insulin

There are more than 20 types of insulin available in four basic forms. Insulin types have three important factors to be considered when prescribing and using them:

1. how soon they start working (onset);
2. when they work the hardest (peak time);
3. how long they last in the body (duration).

The decision as to which insulin to prescribe a patient is based on multiple factors, including the patient's lifestyle and blood sugar levels.

On the ward, insulin is usually stored in the fridge, but cold insulin increases the pain of the injection and slows down the insulin absorption, so for better injection comfort and insulin efficiency it is advisable to take the insulin out of the refrigerator a minimum of 1 h prior to injection.

Insulin pens

Patients should be advised not to store insulin pens in the fridge (especially with the needle attached). Refrigerating a fluid leads to it contracting and warming it up causes it to expand. This is especially dangerous with cloudy insulins. Taking cloudy insulin from the fridge and allowing it to warm in a pen with needle attached can lead to the leakage of either the insulin or the inert carrier fluid, thus changing the strength of the insulin preparation. Leakage into the needle also leads to the formation of insulin crystals, which can block the needle and change the injection pressure or the amount injected.

Taking a pen (and needle) from the warm and putting it into the fridge leads to the contraction of the fluid and the development of air bubbles. Air bubbles are compressible and lengthen injection time. Even after the standard 10 s count, insulin can still be leaking from the needle when it is withdrawn.

Unopened pen cartridges are stored in a fridge, but once inserted into an insulin pen the pen should be kept out of the fridge. The insulin can be stored at room temperature for 30 days (Strachan and Frier, 2013).

Premixed insulins

When a patient (or nurse) is going to administer a cloudy, or premixed, insulin it is important that the pen or vial is rotated end over end 10 times (not shaken), otherwise the insulin may not be mixed correctly (Frid *et al.*, 2010). Research has shown that patients are often confused about this technique, and the actual mixing of insulin by patients has a large variation that may be affecting glycaemic control (Brown *et al.*, 2004).

Clinical considerations

Hypoglycaemia

Hypoglycaemia is a constant worry in the patient with diabetes, and as many hypoglycaemic episodes are associated with exercise, the fear of hypoglycaemia prevents many patients with diabetes from undertaking regular exercise (Younk *et al.*, 2011). This is unfortunate, as exercise is one of the cornerstones in the prevention of diabetes-related complications and also aids in the control of diabetes by aiding weight loss and promoting vascular health (reducing heart attack and stroke risk).

(*Continued*)

502

Current guidelines suggest that the promotion of exercise in patients with both type 1 and type 2 diabetes should be associated with guidance on the management of blood sugar level changes associated with exercise. The patient should take their blood sugar before and after exercise and again several hours later. Patients with either very high or very low blood sugars should avoid exercising until the blood sugar has normalised (Kourtoglou, 2011). The patient may be advised to either omit the insulin dose prior to exercise or consume a carbohydrate load (such as a carbohydrate drink) before exercise (American Diabetes Association, 2010).

Any patient with diabetes who is considering exercise as part of their diabetes management should be encouraged, but they should always be advised to consult with their endocrinologist first for advice on the intensity and timing of exercise.

Glucagon

Glucagon has an important role in maintaining normal blood glucose levels, especially as the brain and neurones can only use glucose as a fuel.

Glucagon has the opposite effect on blood glucose levels to insulin (Figure 15.14); it:

- stimulates the breakdown of glycogen stored in the liver;
- activates hepatic gluconeogenesis (the creation of glucose from substrates such as amino acids);
- has a minor effect enhancing triglyceride breakdown in adipose tissue – providing fatty acid fuel for most cells, and thus conserving glucose for the brain and neurones.

503

The production and secretion of glucagon are stimulated in response to a reduction in blood glucose concentrations and elevated blood levels of amino acids (for instance, after a protein-rich meal). It has also been found that glucagon levels in the blood rise in response to exercise, but it is unclear whether this is a response to the exercise itself or a response to the reduced blood glucose levels that exercise creates.

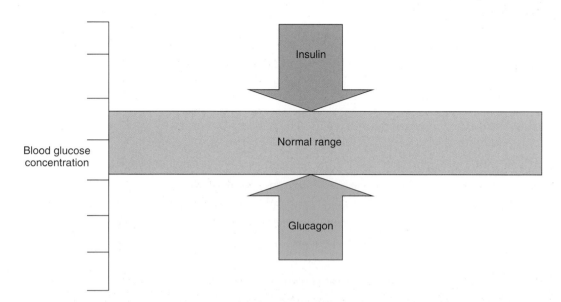

Figure 15.14   Effects of insulin and glucagon on blood glucose concentrations.

Glucagon production and secretion are inhibited when there is increased glucose levels in the blood; however, it is unknown whether this is a direct effect of the glucose levels or a response to rising levels of insulin, as insulin is known to inhibit the release of glucagon.

Somatostatin

Somatostatin is actually released by a broad range of tissues. Its physiological effect in the pancreas is to inhibit the release of insulin and glucagon; it does this in a paracrine fashion; that is, the hormone is released and has its effect locally. The exact mechanism of control of this hormone is unknown.

Conclusion

This chapter has introduced the reader to the endocrine system, a diverse system that is one of the two bodily systems necessary for the maintenance of haemostasis. While often working in close conjunction with the nervous system, the endocrine system is often responsible for the control of longer term processes. The major functions of the endocrine system are based on four main areas:

- the maintenance of homeostasis (especially electrolyte levels and fluid balance);
- metabolism;
- growth and development;
- responses to stress.

The secretion of hormones can be stimulated by nervous impulses, hormones or changes in the body levels of ions and nutrients; and further regulation of hormone release is then often controlled by negative feedback loops. Hormones can only have an effect on a cell if that cell has a receptor for the hormone; however; there appears to be virtually no cell within the body that is not affected by the endocrine system.

Glossary

Amino acid   Chemical compound that is the basic building block of proteins and enzymes.

Carbohydrate   A group of compounds (including starches and sugars) that are a major food source.

Catecholamines   A collective term for adrenaline, noradrenaline and dopamine.

Cortex   The outermost layer of an organ.

Corticosteroids   Steroid hormones released by the adrenal cortex, further divided into glucocorticoids and mineralocorticoids.

Cortisol   The major glucocorticoid steroid released by the adrenal gland.

Cytoplasm   The part of the cell enclosed within the cell membrane.

Downregulation   The reduction in the number of hormone receptors of a cell, often the response of a cell to prolonged periods of high circulating levels of a hormone.

Electrolytes   A group of chemical elements or compounds that includes sodium, potassium, calcium, chloride and bicarbonate.

Fatty acids   Dietary fats that have broken down into elements that can be absorbed into the blood.

Free T$_4$ Thyroxine in the blood that is not bound to proteins.

Ganglion   A mass, or group, of nerve cells.

Gland   Any organ in the body that secretes substances not related to its own, internal, functioning.

504

Glucocorticoids   A group of hormones that exert their major effect on the metabolism of carbohydrates.

Gluconeogenesis   Creation of new glucose from non-carbohydrate substrates.

Glycogen   A carbohydrate (complex sugar) made from glucose.

Glycogenolysis   Breakdown of glycogen to create glucose.

Hormonal stimulation   Stimulation of a gland that produces a change in the activity of that gland in response to hormones released by other organs.

Hormone   Chemical substance that is released into the blood by the endocrine system, and has a physiological control over the function of cells or organs other than those that created it.

Humoral stimulation   Stimulation of a gland that produces a change in the activity of that gland in response to changing levels of certain ions and nutrients in the blood.

Hyperglycaemia   High blood levels of glucose.

Hypoglycaemia   Low blood levels of glucose.

Hypovolaemia   Low levels of fluid in the circulation.

Ion   An atom or group of atoms that carry an electrical charge.

Lipids   A group of organic compounds, including the fats, oils, waxes, sterols and triglycerides.

Medulla   The most internal part of an organ.

Mineralocorticoids   A group of hormones released by the adrenal glands that exert their effect on the electrolytes and water balance in the body.

Neural stimulation   Stimulation of a gland that produces a change in the activity of that gland in response to direct nervous activity.

Osmotic   The movement of water through a semi permeable barrier from an area of low concentration of a chemical to an area of high concentration of a chemical.

Osteoclasts   A type of cell that breaks down bone tissue and thus releases the calcium used to create bones.

Substrate   A molecule on which an enzyme acts.

Triglycerides   A form of fatty acid having three fatty acid components.

Upregulation   The increase of hormone receptors of a cell, usually in response to low circulating levels of a hormone.

References

American Diabetes Association (2010) Standards of medical care in diabetes – 2010. *Diabetes Care* **33**(Supplement 1): S11–S61.

Brown, A., Steel, J.M., Duncan, C., Duncan, A. and McBain, A.M. (2004) An assessment of the adequacy of suspension of insulin in pen injectors. *Diabetic Medicine* **21**(6): 604–608.

Ballinger, A.E., Palmer, S.C., Nistor, I., Craig, J.C. and Strippoli, G.F.M. (2014) Calcimimetics for secondary hyperparathyroidism in chronic kidney disease patients. *Cochrane Database of Systematic Reviews* **12**: CD006254. doi: 10.1002/14651858.CD006254.pub2.

Clare, C. (2009) The endocrine system and associated disorders. In Nair, M. and Peate, I. (eds), *Fundamentals of Applied Pathophysiology: An Essential Guide for Nursing Students*. Oxford: John Wiley & Sons, Ltd; pp. 318–348.

Crowley, R.K., Argese, N., Tomlinson, J.W. and Stewart, P.M. (2014) Central hypoadrenalism. *Journal of Clinical Endocrinology & Metabolism* **99**(11): 4027–4036.

Economidou, F., Douka, E., Tzanela, M., Nanas, S. and Kotanidou, A. (2011) Thyroid function during critical illness. *Hormones* **10**(2): 117–124.

505

Frid, A., Hirsch, L., Gaspar, R., Hicks, D., Kreugel, G., Liersch, J. and Strauss, K. (2010) New injection recommendations for patients with diabetes. *Diabetes & Metabolism* **36**: S3–S18.

Friedman, B. and Cirulli, J. (2013) Hyponatremia in critical care patients: frequency, outcome, characteristics, and treatment with the vasopressin V2 receptor antagonist tolvaptan. *Journal of Critical Care* **28**(2): 219.e1–219.e12.

Gross, P. (2012) Clinical management of SIADH. *Therapeutic Advances in Endocrinology and Metabolism* **3**(2): 61–73. doi: 10.1177/2042018812437561.

Guyton, A.C. and Hall, J. (2006) *Textbook of Medical Physiology*, 11th edn. Philadelphia, PA: Elsevier Saunders.

Jenkins, G.W., Kemnitz, C.P. and Tortora, G.J. (2007) *Anatomy and Physiology: From Science to Life*. Hoboken, NJ: John Wiley & Sons, Inc.

Jenkins, G. and Tortora, G.J. (2013) *Anatomy and Physiology: From Science to Life*, 3rd edn. Singapore: John Wiley & Sons.

Kourtoglou, G.I. (2011) Insulin therapy and exercise. *Diabetes Research and Clinical Practice* **93**: S73–S77.

Liubinas, S.V., Porto, L.D. and Kaye, A.H. (2011) Management of recurrent Cushing's disease. *Journal of Clinical Neuroscience* **18**(1): 7–12.

McDermott, M.T. (2013) *Endocrine Secrets*, 6th edn. Philadelphia, PA. Elsevier Health Sciences.

Marieb, E.N. and Hoehn, K. (2007) *Human Anatomy and Physiology*, 7th edn. San Francisco, CA: Pearson Benjamin Cummings.

Mero, A., Campisi, M., Favero, M., Barbera, C., Secchieri, C., Dayer, J.M. and Pasut, G. (2014) A hyaluronic acid–salmon calcitonin conjugate for the local treatment of osteoarthritis: chondro-protective effect in a rabbit model of early OA. *Journal of Controlled Release* **187**: 30–38.

Nair, M. and Peate, I. (2009) *Fundamentals of Applied Pathophysiology: An Essential Guide for Nursing Students*. Oxford: John Wiley & Sons, Ltd.

Nelson, J.M. and Robinson, M.V. (2012) Hyponatremia in older adults presenting to the emergency department. *International Emergency Nursing* **20**(4): 251–254.

National Institute for Health and Care Excellence (2015) *Type 2 Diabetes in Adults: Management*. NICE Guideline NG28. http://www.nice.org.uk/guidance/ng28 (accessed 3 December 2015).

Strachan, M.W. and Frier, B.M. (2013) *Insulin Therapy: A Pocket Guide*. London. Springer.

Tortora, G.J. and Derrickson, B.H. (2009) *Principles of Anatomy and Physiology*, 12th edn. Hoboken, NJ: John Wiley & Sons, Inc.

Weetman, A. (2013) Current choice of treatment for hypo- and hyperthyroidism. *Prescriber* **24**(13–16): 23–33.

Younk, L.M., Mikeladze, M., Tate, D. and Davis, S.N. (2011) Exercise-related hypoglycemia in diabetes mellitus. *Expert Review of Endocrinology & Metabolism* **6**(1): 93–108. doi:10.1586/eem.10.78.

Further reading

British Thyroid Foundation

http://www.btf-thyroid.org/
The British Thyroid Foundation is a charity dedicated to helping people with thyroid disorders and their families. The website includes video stories of patient journeys and quick reference guides about thyroid diseases.

Addison's Disease Self Help Group

http://www.addisons.org.uk/
The Addison's Disease Self Help Group is a charity that aims to provide information about Addison's disease to patients, families and professionals. There are many publications on the site, including a guide specifically aimed at nurses.

Diabetes UK

http://www.diabetes.org.uk/
Diabetes UK is the country's leading charity for people with diabetes. As well as providing information for patients and their families it is also a pressure group, campaigning both for better diabetes care and funding diabetes research.

Activities
Multiple choice questions

1. The receptors for amino acid-based hormones are found:
   (a) on the cell wall
   (b) inside the cell
   (c) inside the cell nucleus
   (d) none of the above

2. What stimulates the release of glucagon from the pancreas?
   (a) high levels of blood glucose
   (b) high levels of amino acids in the blood
   (c) high levels of calcium in the blood
   (d) high levels of sodium in the blood

3. Where in the body are the adrenal glands?
   (a) in the chest
   (b) behind the thyroid gland
   (c) next to the stomach
   (d) on top of the kidneys

4. The concentration of a hormone at the target cell is determined by:
   (a) the rate of hormone production
   (b) the rate of delivery of the hormone
   (c) the half-life of the hormone
   (d) all of the above

5. Adrenaline and noradrenaline are released in response to stimulation from:
   (a) the parasympathetic nervous system
   (b) the sympathetic nervous system
   (c) the enteric nervous system
   (d) somatic nervous system

6. The connection between the hypothalamus and the anterior pituitary gland is:
   (a) lymphatic
   (b) neural
   (c) vascular
   (d) humoral

7. The average person has how many parathyroid glands?
   (a) 2
   (b) 4
   (c) 6
   (d) 8

8. Thyroid hormone requires what to be produced?
   (a) amino acids
   (b) iodine
   (c) lipids
   (d) proteins

9. Which cells in the pancreas produce insulin?
   (a) alpha
   (b) beta
   (c) delta
   (d) gamma

10. ACTH is secreted by:
   (a) the posterior pituitary gland
   (b) the anterior pituitary gland
   (c) the hypothalamus
   (d) the adrenal gland

True or false

1. Antidiuretic hormone is released from the anterior pituitary gland.
2. Gonadotropes secrete luteinising hormone.
3. Follicle-stimulating hormone stimulates sperm production.
4. Bound T_4 in the blood has a negative effect on T_4 release.
5. The thyroid gland can store T_4 for up to 100 days.
6. Iodine is required for the production of thyroid hormone.
7. Calcitriol is released by the kidneys.
8. Aldosterone accounts for 75% of mineralocorticoids.
9. Alpha cells in the pancreas secrete glucagon.
10. Insulin promotes fat breakdown.

Label the diagram 1

Label the diagram using the following list of words:

Parathyroid glands (behind thyroid gland), Pineal gland, Skin, Lung, Liver, Adrenal glands, Pancreas, Small intestine, Scrotum, Hypothalamus, Pituitary gland, Thyroid gland, Trachea, Thymus, Heart, Stomach, Kidney, Uterus, Ovary, Testes

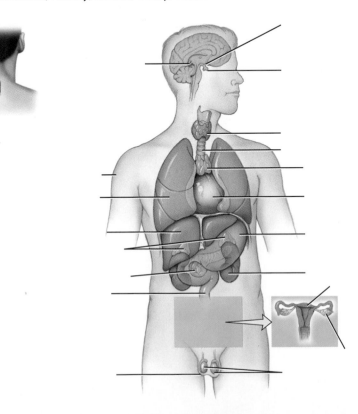

Label the diagram 2

Label the diagram using the following list of words:

Larynx, Thyroid gland, Epiglottis, Hyoid bone, Thyroid cartilage (Adam's apple), Cricoid cartilage, Thyroid gland, Parathyroid glands (4), Tracheal cartilage

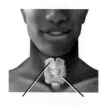

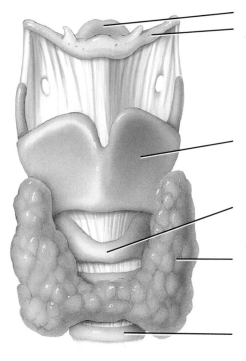

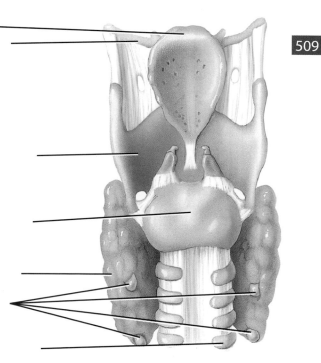

Label the diagram 3

Label the diagram using the following list of words:

↑K⁺, ↓Na⁺, ↓BP, ↓Blood volume, Renin angiotensin system, Non-specific stress, ↑angiotensin II, Hypothalamus, ↑ACTH, Adrenal cortex, ↑Aldosterone release, ↑K+ excretion, ↑Na+ reabsorption, ↑Water reabsorption, ↓K⁺, ↑Na⁺, ↑BP, ↑Blood volume

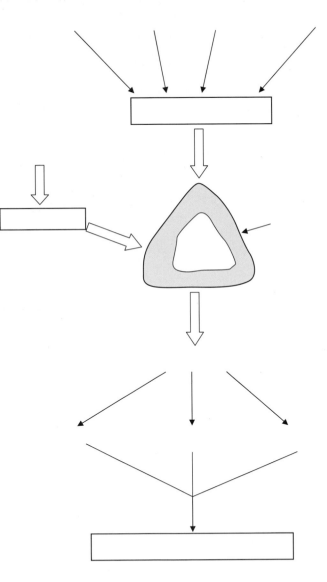

Word search

B	Z	S	X	T	U	E	F	I	L	F	L	A	H	C	P	N	J	H	H
A	J	B	B	G	W	J	T	O	F	K	G	Y	P	H	H	E	O	G	C
G	L	Y	C	O	G	E	N	G	U	O	L	H	S	T	U	U	Q	R	R
L	O	J	I	E	S	Z	O	X	C	N	A	C	S	H	R	R	O	A	O
U	Q	R	V	W	E	X	O	C	R	I	N	E	A	Q	D	A	L	V	A
C	S	A	U	S	N	N	T	M	Y	M	D	N	T	D	G	L	I	E	A
A	R	F	V	H	I	H	O	W	L	A	G	B	S	U	M	H	T	S	I
G	A	V	N	C	X	G	U	R	E	K	K	L	G	A	K	P	B	U	N
O	F	I	V	H	O	H	I	S	E	B	I	O	E	T	E	R	C	E	S
N	H	V	O	Y	R	A	T	I	U	T	I	P	Q	K	O	P	G	M	U
W	H	I	I	J	Y	R	P	D	V	H	S	A	I	U	H	I	R	J	L
A	I	L	Q	K	H	K	B	C	H	Y	P	O	D	Q	E	N	O	S	I
N	P	C	O	R	T	I	S	O	L	P	C	W	D	F	B	F	T	R	N
T	M	O	J	I	D	S	C	R	E	E	E	B	O	L	P	M	P	R	A
O	N	R	H	U	R	L	D	T	C	R	K	U	B	J	A	L	E	J	S
M	R	T	Q	G	B	E	S	E	C	K	Q	R	B	A	C	M	C	L	K
L	P	E	H	T	B	T	P	X	B	J	N	I	M	M	U	N	E	S	L
H	R	X	C	I	E	N	T	M	U	Q	V	A	C	F	X	C	R	B	G
A	L	O	R	E	T	S	E	L	O	H	C	E	D	E	U	Z	P	T	B
N	O	R	S	M	A	S	T	R	E	S	S	W	W	Y	F	O	U	D	G

Aldosterone, Cortisol, Graves, Insulin, Pituitary, Amino, Exocrine, Half-life, Islet, Receptor, Beta, Gland, Hypo, Isthmus, Secrete, Cholesterol, Glucagon, Hyper, Lobe, Stress, Cortex, Glycogen, Immune, Neural, Thyroxine

Fill in the blanks

The influence of a _____, from inside or outside the _____, leads to the release of a _____ that has an effect on the stimulus; following this, some aspect of the _____ organ function then _____ further reaction to the stimulus and thus further release of the hormone by the organ.

Target, stimulus, inhibits, hormone, body

Find out more

1. What effect does insulin have on lipid metabolism?
2. What is the most common form of thyroid hormone?
3. Name three cell types in the pancreas?
4. What gland is often referred to as the size of a pea?
5. What differentiates diabetes insipidus from diabetes mellitus?

Conditions

The following is a list of conditions that are associated with the endocrine system. Take some time and write notes about each of the conditions. You may make the notes taken from text books or other resources (e.g. people you work with in a clinical area), or you may make the notes as a result of people you have cared for. If you are making notes about people you have cared for you must ensure that you adhere to the rules of confidentiality.

Addison's disease	
Cushing's disease	
Diabetes insipidus	
Diabetes mellitus	
Graves' disease	

Chapter 16

The immune system

Peter S Vickers

Test your prior knowledge

- How do the T-helper and T-suppressor cells work together in order to help control the immune system?
- Which cells are involved in humoral immunity?
- What is the role of immunoglobulin E (IgE) in fighting infections?
- List the organs of the lymphatic system.
- What do we mean by phagocytosis?

Learning outcomes

After reading this chapter you will be able to:

- Describe and discuss the development of white blood cells and their roles in immunity
- Explain how the immune system works to protect us from infections
- List all the various physical, mechanical and chemical barriers that the human body possesses to prevent infectious organisms from entering the body
- Explain the process of phagocytosis
- Understand how inflammation works to protect us once the body has been damaged in some way or has been infected
- Describe and discuss cellular immunity
- Describe and discuss humoral immunity
- Explain the body's response to infection and the rationale for immunisations

Fundamentals of Anatomy and Physiology: For Nursing and Healthcare Students, Second Edition. Edited by Ian Peate and Muralitharan Nair.
© 2017 John Wiley & Sons, Ltd. Published 2017 by John Wiley & Sons, Ltd.
Student companion website: www.wileyfundamentalseries.com/anatomy
Instructor companion website: www.wiley.com/go/instructor/anatomy

Body map

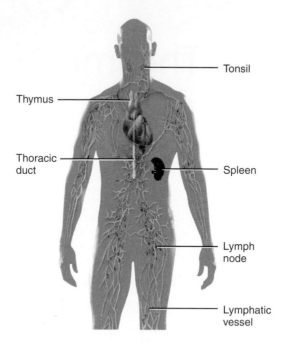

Thymus

Thoracic
duct

Tonsil

Spleen

Lymph
node

Lymphatic
vessel

Introduction

The body is constantly under attack from organisms out to destroy it. This may sound dramatic, but it is true. Infectious microorganisms, toxins and pollutants are some of the harmful substances from which it has to defend itself. Fortunately, the body has evolved and developed many defences to repel and destroy these harmful substances – this is what we call the immune system.

Immunology – the study of the **immune system** – is a relatively new branch of bioscience and medicine. Although some of the mechanisms and components of immunity, such as antibodies and blood cells, have been known for some time, it is actually only relatively recently (over the past 30 years) that much research has been undertaken into the immune system.

The rapid development of human immunodeficiency virus (HIV) and acquired immunodeficiency syndrome (AIDS) in the 1980s was the trigger for much of this research, and we now know that the immune system is a complicated and wonderful system that underpins so much of our understanding of disease and disease process, and not only those diseases caused by infectious microorganisms, but also many others, including cancer, arthritis, stress, and so on.

This chapter will show what the body's immunological defences consist of and how they work together to give the body an opportunity of surviving the continuous and continuing assaults by microorganisms, toxins and other pollutants to which it is subjected.

Blood cell development

The blood cells that form a major part of the immune system are the white blood cells. All our blood cells are descended from multipotent stem cells, which have the ability to switch to different types of cells, and, in terms of the immune system, develop into two major branches of white blood cells.

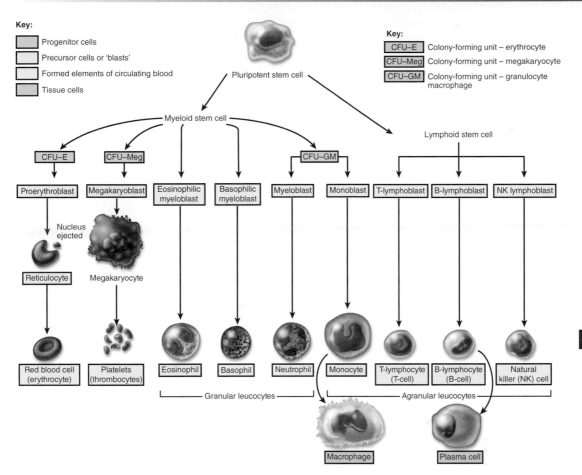

Figure 16.1 The development of blood cells. *Source*: Tortora and Derrickson (2009). Reproduced with permission of John Wiley & Sons.

One branch will develop into the **myeloid** family of cells, which include the neutrophils and monocytes, while the other branch will develop into the **lymphoid** family of cells, which is made up of lymphocytes.

Figure 16.1 shows the development of the white blood cells from the initial multipotent stem cell.

It can be seen from the family tree of blood cells that the myeloid family includes the macrophages (consisting of monocytes and tissue macrophages) and granulocytes (consisting of neutrophils, eosinophils and basophils). The lymphoid branch of white blood cells gives us T-lymphocytes and B-lymphocytes (with many of the B-lymphocytes developing into plasma cells). In addition, the myeloid branch also provides us with megakaryocytes (leading to platelets) and erythroid cells, which develop into erythrocytes (i.e. red blood cells). Red blood cells and platelets are discussed in Chapter 7.

Because it is the white blood cells that are concerned primarily with the immune system, in this chapter we are not interested in red blood cells, although they are important to the immune system because they carry oxygen to the other cells of the immune system, such as the skin cells.

Similarly, platelets do play a very important role in the defence of the body in terms of helping to seal off any breaks in the skin and, by doing so, prevent any more infectious organisms getting into the body. However, in this chapter, platelets will only be discussed in terms of the process of inflammation.

All the white blood cells commence initially in the bone marrow as stem cells, but, as they slowly mature through their various stages, they are to be found in different places around the body, including:

- the blood and lymph circulation
- the thymus
- the spleen
- the tonsils and other lymph nodes.

They also are found in all the mucosal membranes, such as the lining of the mouth and the gastrointestinal tract.

Blood cells: a brief glossary (Vickers, 2007: 9)

B-lymphocytes	These lymphocytes arise in the bone marrow and differentiate into plasma cells, which in turn produce **immunoglobulins** – also known as antibodies.
Bone marrow	The site in the body where most of the cells of the immune system are produced as immature (stem) cells.
Immunoglobulins	Immunoglobulins – also known as **antibodies** – are highly specialised protein molecules, and their job is to connect with, and hold on to, foreign **antigens**, so that they cannot escape destruction by other cells of the immune system.
Monocytes	These white blood cells are also **phagocytes** and are found in the blood. However, they have the ability to migrate into tissues, where they are known as macrophages.
Plasma cells	These cells develop from B-lymphocytes and produce the **immunoglobulins**.
Platelets	Blood cells that have an important role to play in the clotting of blood.
Polymorpho-nuclear leucocytes	These white blood cells are also known as **phagocytes**, and are found in the blood.
Red blood cells	These cells carry oxygen from the lungs to the tissues.
Stem cells	These cells have the potential to differentiate and mature into the different cells of the immune system.
Thymus	An organ located in the chest that instructs immature T-lymphocytes to become mature T-lymphocytes, which are then able to help fight infections.
T-effector lymphocytes	Also known as **T-cytotoxic** lymphocytes. These lymphocytes have the ability to produce chemicals that can kill foreign cells and microorganisms, as well as helping in the process of inflammation.
T-helper lymphocytes	While in the thymus, these specialised lymphocytes develop the ability to help other lymphocytes to mount an immune response.
T-lymphocytes	T-lymphocytes arise in the bone marrow but migrate to the thymus where they mature, and also learn to differentiate between 'self' and 'non-self' matter.
T-suppressor lymphocytes	These are specialised lymphocytes that can suppress the helper T-lymphocytes and help to regulate the immune system by turning off the immune system response, so reducing the potential damaging effects of an overactive immune system.

Organs of the immune system

The main organs of the immune system are all part of the lymphatic system. These organs of the immune system consist of:

- the thymus
- the spleen
- the lymph nodes
- the lymphoid tissues scattered throughout the gastrointestinal, respiratory and urinary tracts.

The thymus

The **thymus** is situated in the chest (Figure 16.2), and in babies it is a large organ (relative to size). It shrinks (atrophies) with age.

Within the thymus, certain blood stem cells mature and differentiate into various **T-cell lymphocyte** subclasses. In addition, they also acquire the ability to recognise and differentiate 'self' cells from 'non-self' cells.

'Self' cells originate and belong to the individual with that thymus, while 'non-self' cells come from outside of the individual such as viruses and bacteria; so think of the thymus as a school for T-cell lymphocytes in which the cells take part in learning experiences as they mature and in which they also are guided to different careers for when they leave the 'school'.

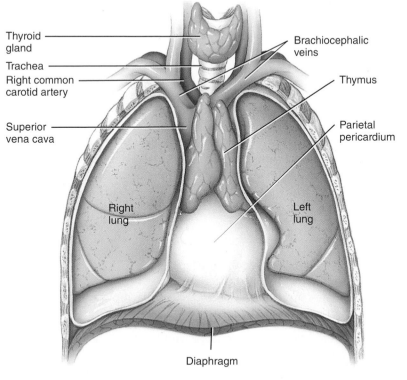

Thymus of adolescent

Figure 16.2 Position of the thymus within the body. *Source*: Tortora and Derrickson (2009). Reproduced with permission of John Wiley & Sons.

Even though the thymus starts to atrophy at puberty, T-cells will continue to develop in the thymus throughout an individual's life (Delves and Roitt, 2000; Vickers, 2005, 2007).

The lymphatic system

The lymphatic system is a specialised system of **lymph vessels** (similar to blood vessels) and **lymph nodes**. The lymphatic vessels contain a fluid called **lymph**, which drains into the organs of the lymph system from nearby organs. This lymph originates from plasma leaking from the blood capillaries.

Lymphocytes migrate from the blood system by passing through the walls of the smallest venous capillaries in the lymph node. Lymphocytes spend only a few minutes in the bloodstream during each circuit of the body, but, in contrast, spend several hours in the lymphoid system.

The lymphatic system can be thought of as a parallel system to the blood circulatory system, but it does not have a pump like the heart, which pumps blood around the body. Instead, the lymph is agitated around the body by a combination of the smooth muscular walls of the lymph vessels and the flexing and relaxing of striated muscle as an individual moves around.

The peripheral lymphatic system (Figure 16.3) is made up of lymphatic vessels and lymphatic capillaries, as well as encapsulated organs (i.e. organs that are situated within their own 'capsule').

These include:

- spleen
- tonsils
- lymph nodes.

In addition, the lymphatic system includes unencapsulated (not bound by a capsule, but more diffuse) **lymphoid tissue** in the gastrointestinal tract, the urogenital tract and the lungs.

The lymph vessels and capillaries form a network throughout the body and connect the tissues of the body to the lymphoid organs, such as the **spleen**, and the lymph nodes.

Lymphatic capillaries have some anatomical similarities to blood capillaries in that their walls consist of a layer of **endothelial cells**. However, lymphatic capillary walls do not have a basement membrane. This lack of a basement membrane allows substances of relatively large molecular size, such as plasma proteins, to enter the lymphatic capillaries between the cells of the capillary walls.

Lymph flows through the vessels by means of:

- muscle contraction in the limbs (arms and legs);
- the pulsing of arteries (caused by the beating of the heart);
- negative intrathoracic pressure (which draws up the lymph, as from a vacuum);
- the rhythmic contraction of the lymphatic vessels themselves.

The lymph eventually flows into two large lymph ducts. One of them is called the thoracic duct, and this receives lymph from:

- the lower limbs
- the digestive tract
- the left arm
- the left side of the thorax, head and neck.

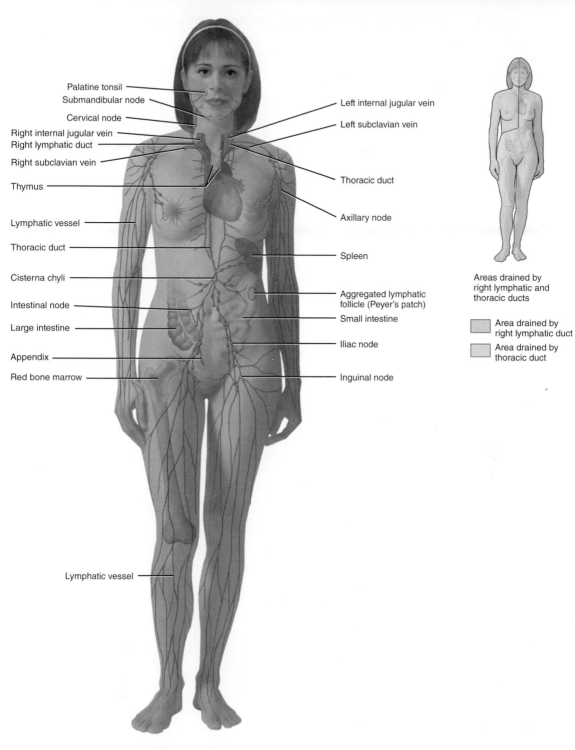

Palatine tonsil

Submandibular node

Cervical node

Right internal jugular vein

Right lymphatic duct

Right subclavian vein

Thymus

Lymphatic vessel

Thoracic duct

Cisterna chyli

Intestinal node

Large intestine

Appendix

Red bone marrow

Left internal jugular vein

Left subclavian vein

Thoracic duct

Axillary node

Spleen

Aggregated lymphatic follicle (Peyer's patch)

Small intestine

Iliac node

Inguinal node

Lymphatic vessel

Areas drained by right lymphatic and thoracic ducts

Area drained by right lymphatic duct

Area drained by thoracic duct

519

Figure 16.3 Principal components of the lymphatic system. *Source*: Tortora and Derrickson (2009). Reproduced with permission of John Wiley & Sons.

The other large lymph vessel, the right lymphatic duct, receives lymph from:

- the right arm
- the right side of the head, neck and thorax.

The two lymph ducts then empty into the great veins in the neck, thus restoring fluid and proteins to the venous circulation.

Lymph nodes

Lymph enters the lymph nodes from the afferent lymphatic vessels and from there it goes to the **trabeculae**. Afferent means 'leading towards'; therefore, in the case of lymph nodes, afferent vessels are those vessels that lead **towards** the lymph node.

The lymph node is made up of a mesh of cells – just like a net. The lymph at this stage contains **antigens** from infected cells and tissues. This lymph passes through this mesh in the lymph node and the antigens are trapped – like fish in fishing nets (Figure 16.4).

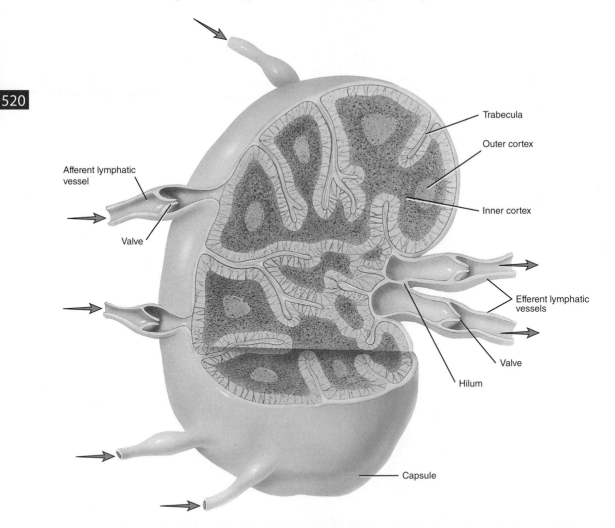

Figure 16.4   Structure of a lymph node. *Source*: Nair and Peate (2009). Reproduced with permission of John Wiley & Sons.

Antigens entering the body at any point are rapidly swept along the lymph vessels towards a lymphoid organ or lymph node.

Within the lymph node, **B-cell lymphocytes** are located in the primary lymphoid follicles as well as the secondary lymphoid follicles (which contain the germinal centres), and it is inside these germinal centres that the B-cells proliferate after encountering their specific antigen and its co-operating T-cell. The B-cells that are found at the centre of the secondary lymphoid follicles are actively dividing, while those at the periphery are antibody forming.

In addition, large numbers of **phagocytic macrophages** and plasma cells producing antibodies are found in the **medulla** of the gland. Macrophages and other antigen-presenting cells spend most of their lives migrating through the tissues until they encounter antigens. These are then **phagocytosed** (engulfed by phagocytes and 'eaten') and transported to the nearest lymph node.

Macrophages in the lymph node also encounter trapped antigens within the meshwork of reticular cells, and they phagocytose the dead cells and bacteria. The lymph that has destroyed the antigens in the lymph nodes then leaves through the efferent lymphatic vessel. Efferent means 'to lead away from'.

Clinical considerations

Secondary immunodeficiencies

Secondary immunodeficiencies are those disorders that, due to another illness, age, injury, environmental poisons or treatment, result in an increased susceptibility to infection. Indeed, almost all serious illnesses are associated with some impairment of one or more components of the immune system.

Most people are aware of one particular secondary immunodeficiency, namely AIDS caused by the HIV, but there are many other causes of secondary immunodeficiencies.

One of the major causes of immunodeficiency globally is protein deficiency due to malnutrition or to such disorders as Kwashiorkor disease. In developed countries, apart from HIV, the major causes of secondary immunodeficiencies are iatrogenic (i.e. caused by medical personnel/ treatment). These particularly include immunodeficiencies that occur following steroid or cytotoxic drug therapy for various diseases.

Someone with a secondary immunodeficiency will have a susceptibility to opportunistic infections, anorexia, diarrhoea and an increased risk of cancer.

Secondary immunodeficiencies are associated with a multitude of factors, of which we only have time to look at a very few. These include:

- infections – for example, HIV, hepatitis, measles, mumps, TB, congenital rubella, cytomegalovirus and infectious mononucleosis (glandular fever);
- medications – for example, steroids, cytotoxic drugs and immunosuppressive drugs, and even antibiotics, as well as so-called recreational drugs, such as alcohol, cocaine and heroin;
- stress – including psychological and physical stress;
- malnutrition;
- cancers;
- autoimmune diseases;
- ageing;

(Continued)

- environmental chemicals – for example, polychlorinated biphenyls and dioxin;
- burns and other traumas;
- pregnancy;
- anaesthesia and surgery (stress);
- radiation.

The treatment of secondary immunodeficiencies consists of removing or treating the cause (if at all possible) and supportive therapy. For example, if an infection is the cause, then the relevant antimicrobial drugs need to be given. If there is an iatrogenic cause, such as drugs or surgery, once these are stopped and recovery is under way the immune system will usually right itself. Similarly, if other diseases are causing the immunodeficiency, then they have to be tackled. If malnutrition is the cause, then the solving of the problem leading to malnutrition needs to take place.

Along with the elimination of the cause, supportive therapy is required to help to boost the immune system and to prevent infections. Drugs and nutrition, changes of lifestyle, and occasionally isolation may be necessary.

Secondary immunodeficiencies are often transient, and supportive therapy is usually only necessary until the cause has been dealt with and the immune system starts to recover. Unfortunately, however, there are some secondary immunodeficiencies to which this does not apply. The best known of these is AIDS, although if a cure were ever found for it then it, in turn, would become a transient immunodeficiency.

Lymphoid tissue

As well as lymphatic vessels, the lymphatic system contains lymphoid tissue. This consists of lymph glands (i.e. lymph nodes), which are approximately the size and shape of a broad bean, and lymphoid tissue, which is found in specific organs, particularly:

- the spleen
- the bone marrow
- the lungs
- the liver
- other lymphoid tissue.

The spleen

The spleen is situated just behind the stomach and is about the size of a fist. It collects antigen from the blood for presentation to phagocytes and lymphocytes, and also collects, and disposes of, dead red blood cells.

To sum up the lymph system (Vickers 2005, 2007):

- The lymphoid system enables lymphocytes to protect the tissues and vessels of the body from infectious microorganisms.
- It holds them in antigen 'traps' in the lymph nodes and other lymphoid organs, and it brings them into close proximity with other immune cells.
- This is essential for the cell-to-cell communication that is necessary to recruit, direct and regulate a coordinated immune response.
- Lymph glands are the major centres for lymphocyte proliferation and antibody production, as well as for filtering the lymph.

Types of immunity

There are two major types of immunity in humans: the **innate** and the **acquired**.

Innate immunity is the immunity we possess at birth, so it is innate in all of us. On the other hand, **acquired immunity** is not present at birth; instead, it is something that we acquire as we go through life.

Innate immunity is the oldest type of immunity and is present in all creatures, whereas the second type of immunity, acquired immunity, is only found in more developed organisms, such as humans.

Another name for **innate immunity** is **non-specific immunity**. This means that these defences come into action no matter what infectious or non-self organism is trying to attack us; therefore, they are non-specific. Similarly, **acquired immunity** is also known as **specific immunity** because it responds to known specific organisms.

The innate immune system

Many parts of the body, as well as the white blood cells, combine to make up the innate immune system.

It is possible to categorise the innate immune system into four groups, although some parts may use more than one class of defence:

- physical barriers
- mechanical barriers
- chemical barriers
- blood cells.

Physical barriers

These include the **skin** and **mucosal membranes**. The skin acts as a physical barrier to prevent infectious organisms and other matter from getting to the more 'at risk' and undefended organs within our body. However, not only is skin a physical barrier, it is also a chemical barrier, in that sweat produced from the skin is **bactericidal** (dangerous for bacteria). However, skin also has weak spots, namely the various orifices that connect the internal body to the outside, such as the mouth, nose, urethral opening and anus.

Mechanical barriers

In this category are included **cilia**, **coughing**, **sneezing** and **tears**.

- **Cilia** are the tiny hairs found in the nose. They are constantly moving and they move dirt, microorganisms and mucus away to the adenoids (made of lymphatic tissue) where they can be dealt with.
- **Sneezing and coughing** work quite simply by expelling any microorganisms or irritants out of the body and into the external atmosphere. So, if someone has a cold or a cough and sneezes or coughs, millions of viruses are expelled into the atmosphere, which means that there are fewer viruses in that person's body to cause even worse problems. This is very effective for the infected person, but means that there are all these viruses in tiny droplets suspended in the air, just waiting for someone else to come along and breathe them in, thereby becoming infected themselves.
- **Tears** are also a mechanical barrier. When someone cries, the tears wash any dirt particles or microorganisms away from their eyes (like a windscreen washer in a car). Tears are also a chemical barrier because they contain a bactericidal enzyme known as lysozyme. Lysozyme will crop up quite a lot in the section on the innate immune system.

Chemical barriers

Chemical barriers include **tears**, **breast milk**, **sweat**, **saliva**, **acidic secretions**, including **stomach acid**, and **semen**.

Most of these secretions contain either bactericidal enzymes, such as lysozyme, or antibodies. In addition, bacteria cannot survive in acidic secretions.

Blood cells

As well as the previously mentioned defences, the innate system includes certain blood cells, namely **leucocytes** (white cells) and **thrombocytes** (platelets).

The white cells involved in the innate immune system are known as

- **neutrophils**, which make up 60% of the leucocytes in the body;
- **monocytes** and **tissue macrophages**, which make up a total of 3% of leucocytes;
- **eosinophils**, which only make up 1% of leucocytes;
- **basophils**, which also make up only 1% of leucocytes.

The **neutrophils**, **eosinophils** and **basophils** are also known as **granulocytes**, because when seen through a powerful microscope they appear to be full of little granules (or grains). In fact these granules are vacuoles, or empty spaces, within the cells, and are very important when looking at one particular function of these white cells, namely **phagocytosis**.

Blood cells of the immune system

These, as mentioned previously, are the white blood cells. There are three main activities of the white blood cells:

- **Phagocytosis** – this is the destruction of infectious organisms/non-self matter by engulfing and then ingesting them/it. This will be explained a little later in this chapter.
- **Cytotoxity** – **cyto** means cell and **toxicity** means poisonous or, in immunological terms, 'lethal to'. So cytotoxicity is the action that some types of white cell take in killing infectious organisms by damaging their cell membranes (see also complement system).
- **Inflammation** – white cells are very much involved in the response of body tissue to infection and injury.

There are many other roles that white cells take within the immune system, and these will be discussed throughout this chapter, but for now we will concentrate on the three roles above.

Phagocytosis

The cells that make up our innate immunity have two major functions: they are either **phagocytes** or **mediator cell**s.

The **phagocytes** are cells that actually devour the infectious organisms that have managed to get through the other innate immune defences previously mentioned.

There are two types of phagocytes: **mononuclear phagocytes** and **polymorphonuclear phagocytes**.

Mononuclear phagocytes include monocytes and macrophages. They are called **mononuclear** because the nuclei of the cells are single round blobs (or spheres) when looked at through a microscope; in other words, they have a clearly defined single nucleus; **neutrophils**, on the other hand, make up the polymorphonuclear phagocytes.

When looked at through a microscope, the nuclei of neutrophils are seen as a blob which can take many shapes, hence **poly** (many) **morpho** (shape) **nucleocyte** (cell nucleus) – in other words, polymorphonucleocyte.

The role of a phagocytic cell is to **phagocytose**, or consume, any infectious organism or non-self matter that overcomes the external barriers. This process is known as **phagocytosis**, and it works as follows.

- **Stage 1.** A bacterium approaches a phagocyte – in this case a neutrophil (Figure 16.5). It is held in place by **opsonins – complement factors** or **antibodies (immunoglobulins)**. Opsonins prepare the bacterium for being digested by the phagocyte by firmly holding the bacterium to the phagocyte so that it cannot escape.
- **Stage 2.** As the bacterium approaches the neutrophil, the neutrophil recognises that it is 'non-self' matter and it sends out **pseudopodia** (false arms) and starts to surround the bacterium (Figure 16.6).
- **Stage 3.** Once surrounded by the phagocyte, the bacterium comes into contact with the vacuoles (as mentioned above). A vacuole completely surrounds the bacterium and kills it, and then breaks it up by means of bactericidal enzymes such as lysozyme. The phagocyte

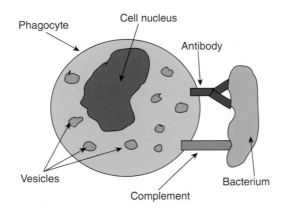

Figure 16.5   Phagocytosis (stage 1).

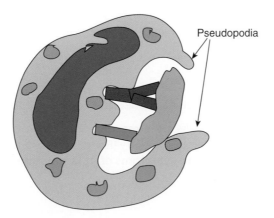

Figure 16.6   Phagocytosis (stage 2).

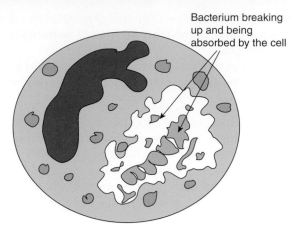

Bacterium breaking
up and being
absorbed by the cell

Figure 16.7   Phagocytosis (stage 3).

then uses what it can from the bacterium for its own functions (growth, nutrition, etc.) and ejects the parts that it cannot use. This is the process of phagocytosis (Figure 16.7).

As well as bacteria, phagocytes also remove pus and other infected matter, as well as any other non-self matter that has found its way into the body.

Cytotoxicity

Cytotoxicity is the process of damage to or death of cells. Many substances are toxic to cells, including certain chemicals, components of the immune system, viruses and bacteria, and some types of venom (e.g. from certain snakes).

Within the immune system, T-cells that can kill other cells are known as cytotoxic T-cells, and produce proteins that play a role in the destruction of target cells. Cytotoxic T-cells (Tc cells) work by programming their target cells (often cells that have been infected by viruses, or even cancerous/pre-cancerous cells) to undergo apoptosis – otherwise known as cell suicide.

Inflammation

Inflammation is the body's immediate reaction to tissue injury or damage. This can be caused by

- physical trauma
- intense heat
- irritating chemicals
- infection by viruses, fungi or bacteria (Marieb and Hoehn, 2013).

The inflammatory process involves the movement of white cells, complement and other plasma proteins into a site of infection or injury (Roitt and Rabson, 2000).

There are four **cardinal signs and symptoms of inflammation** at the site of the injury:

- swelling (also known as oedema)
- pain
- heat
- redness.

There may also be:

- nausea
- sweating
- raised pulse
- lowered blood pressure
- possibly loss of consciousness.

These last symptoms and signs are the body's response to pain and shock, but in terms of immunology, the first four signs and symptoms are the important ones, and that is why they are known as the 'four cardinal signs of inflammation'.

According to Nairn and Helbert (2007), inflammation can be defined clinically as the presence of swelling, redness and pain. Although inflammation does cause pain and other problems, it actually has beneficial properties and effects. These are:

- the prevention of the spread to nearby tissues of infectious microorganisms and other damaging agents;
- the disposal of killed pathogens and cell debris;
- preparation for repair of the damage (Marieb and Hoehn, 2013).

Following injury or other damage to the body, three processes occur at the same time:

- **Mast cell degranulation. Mast cells** are tissue cells that contain granules in their cytoplasm. These granules contain, among other substances, **serotonin** and **histamine**, which are released into the tissues during the process of degranulation. These substances cause some of the signs and symptoms of inflammation, but they also work with the other two processes to provide the complete inflammatory signs and symptoms.
- **The activation of four plasma protein systems.** These systems are the complement system, the clotting system, the kinin system and immunoglobulins. The complement system consists of more than 30 proteins that are found in blood plasma and on cell surfaces. It works very closely with antibodies, and indeed is so called because the proteins in the system are seen to 'complement' antibodies in the destruction of bacteria (Walport, 2001). The complement system activates and assists the inflammatory and immune processes and plays a major role in the destruction of bacteria. The clotting system traps bacteria that have entered the wound and also interacts with platelets to stop any bleeding. The kinin system helps to control vascular permeability, while immunoglobulins help in the destruction of bacteria.
- **The movement of phagocytic cells** to the area in order to phagocytose bacteria or any other non-self debris in the wound (Figure 16.8).

Complement factors stimulate the mast cells to release histamine and other chemicals, which in turn can increase the permeability of blood vessels (Tortora *et al.*, 2014).

Other factors involved in vascular permeability are:

- **cytokines** (cell messengers), which promote inflammation and also attract white blood cells to the affected area (Marieb and Hoehn, 2013);
- **kinins** and **prostaglandins**, which are chemical messengers released from damaged and stressed tissue cells, phagocytes and lymphocytes.

All these factors – histamine, complement, cytokines and kinins – as well as having their own specific individual inflammatory roles, cause the small blood vessels in the area that has been damaged to dilate so that more blood is able to flow into the region surrounding the damaged area. This causes the redness and heat associated with inflammation (Marieb and Hoehn, 2013).

527

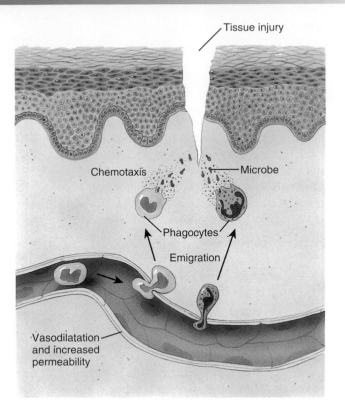

Figure 16.8   Phagocytes migrate from blood to the site of tissue injury. *Source*: Tortora and Derrickson (2014). Reproduced with permission of John Wiley & Sons.

Clinical considerations

Rheumatoid disease

Rheumatoid disease is caused by an autoimmune reaction (the body's immune system attacking the body's own cells). It is one of the commonest chronic inflammatory conditions in developed countries. Some inflammatory cytokines have a major role to play in the pathogenesis of this disease. Rheumatoid arthritis is a common cause of disability, with one-third of patients likely to be severely disabled. The joint changes, which almost certainly represent an autoimmune reaction, consist of:

- inflammation
- erosion of cartilage and bone.

Autoimmune diseases

Specific examples of autoimmune diseases include such diverse conditions as rheumatoid arthritis, type 1 diabetes mellitus, multiple sclerosis and systemic lupus erythromatosus (lupus). Autoimmune

(Continued)

diseases affect 3% of the Western population and are found to be more common in people living in the more northerly latitudes. Almost all autoimmune diseases are more common in women; and they are rare in childhood, with the onset usually occurring between puberty and retirement. In addition, there tend to be clusters in families – not necessarily of the same disease, but of a tendency to an autoimmune disease.

Drug treatment

The drugs most frequently used in rheumatoid disease are disease-modifying anti-rheumatoid drugs (DMARDS), as well as non-steroidal anti-inflammatory drugs. These drugs reduce the symptoms of rheumatoid disease, but do not prevent the progress of the disease. Other drugs that are used with this disease include:

- some immunosuppressants (drugs that suppress the immune system to try to prevent it attacking the body's own cells);
- steroids;
- anticytokine drugs – these are newer drugs and they have more specific action against the disease processes of rheumatoid disease.

Included within the category of DMARDs are a variety of drugs with different chemical structures and mechanisms of action. They can improve symptoms and reduce disease activity in rheumatoid arthritis. This can be measured by a reduction in:

- the number of swollen and tender joints
- the pain score
- the disability score.

However, there are doubts as to whether or not they halt the long-term progress of the disease.

Snapshot

The nurse's role(s) in assessing the needs of a patient with multiple sclerosis

Multiple sclerosis (MS) is an autoimmune disorder in which the myelin sheath that surrounds and protects the nerve fibres is damaged by the body's own immune system. This, in turn, leads to the damage of the underlying nerve fibres.

The signs and symptoms of MS are many and varied and depend upon which part of the central nervous system is affected, but potential symptoms can include problems with vision and balance, dizziness, fatigue, bladder and bowel problems, speech and swallowing difficulties, stiffness and/ or spasms, and tremors, as well as memory, cognitive and emotional problems. It is also important for the nurse to know that there are different types of MS, namely, new, relapsing, progressive and advanced forms of MS.

Consequently, the role of the nurse is to ensure that they have a good knowledge of the signs, symptoms, cause and effects of MS, as well as knowledge of the patient. This knowledge

(Continued)

will allow the nurse to help to provide explanations, initiate education of patients and families as to MS, its treatment and prognosis, and to take part in (or refer for) counselling for both the patients and their families.

To be able to take on this role of guiding the patient and family through all the vagaries of this disease, nurses first of all must make a comprehensive assessment of the individual patient, looking at such areas as physical, cognitive, emotional, sensory effects and coping strategies, along with any problems concerning bowel and bladder functioning (and any sexual issues that may arise). These assessments must continually be updated throughout the course of the patient's life with MS in order to ensure that the best physical, psychological, emotional and social care is always available and relevant for that patient and family. To that end, nurses need to have a knowledge and understanding of how various MS drugs work, and, with the medical team, ensure that the drug regimen is the most suitable for that patient in order to minimise the patient's MS symptoms and to ensure as good a quality of life as is possible. This will help to ensure that there is a better chance of patient compliance with the drug and other therapeutic regimens. Within this category, nurses must be aware of how any individual patient's condition responds to the therapies, as well as any side effects that may arise.

The nurse must also become an advocate for follow-up with the appropriate interdisciplinary health and social/psychological team that may be available.

Above all, the nurse needs to know the individual patients (and families) and to allow them to retain as much autonomy as possible in managing this disease, its effects and therapies, and to always keep in mind that this is a life-long condition for which – at the moment – there is no cure, for be assured that the patients and families will always be aware of this fact.

These chemicals also increase the permeability of the capillary walls, which allows blood cells and protein-rich fluid to seep into the surrounding tissues, which leads to **oedema** – the third of the classic signs of inflammation. Oedema performs three functions that are important to the healing of damaged tissue:

- the dilution of harmful substances in the area to make them less concentrated;
- the movement into the area of large quantities of oxygen and the nutrients necessary for the repair of any damage;
- the entry of clotting proteins to help seal off the damage (Marieb and Hoehn, 2013).

That leaves **pain** as the remaining classic sign of inflammation. Pain is caused partly by the pressure on the nerve endings as a result of the oedema in the tissues and partly by the release of bacterial toxins (Marieb and Hoehn, 2013).

Summary of inflammation

The timetable of a typical inflammatory response to tissue in injury is as follows.

- Arterioles near the injury site constrict briefly.
- This vasoconstriction is followed by vasodilatation, which increases blood flow to the site of the injury (**redness and heat**).
- Dilatation of the arterioles at the injury site increases the pressure in the circulation.

(Continued)

- This increases the **exudation** of both plasma proteins and blood cells into the tissues in the area.
- Exudation then causes **oedema** and **swelling**.
- The nerve endings in the area are stimulated, partly by pressure (**pain**).
- The clotting and kinin systems, along with platelets, move into the area and block any tissue damage by commencing the clotting process.
- White blood cells – phagocytes and lymphocytes – move into the area and start to destroy any infectious organisms in the vicinity of the trauma.
- These phagocytes and protein cells, along with the substances they produce, kill any bacteria or other microorganisms in the vicinity and remove the debris that results from the battle between the microorganisms and the immune system – this includes exudates and dead cells (pus).
- All these parts of the immune and blood systems remain in the area until tissue regeneration (repair) takes place – this is known as resolution.

Medicines management

New therapies: adalimumab

Adalimumab is a synthetic drug, and is basically a fully human anti-tumour necrosis factor alpha monoclonal antibody. In effect, it is a drug that is based upon the normal immune system. It is derived from synthetic antibodies that are programmed to target tumour necrosis factor alpha (TNFα). TNFα is a normal part of the human immune system, which, following an infection, allows for an increasing inflammatory reaction within the body as well as helping to mobilise the various cells of the immune system (e.g. lymphocytes) to fight the invading infectious microorganism.

Adalimumab is used as part of the drug therapy for people with autoimmune diseases such as rheumatoid arthritis. In an autoimmune condition, the body's own immune system attacks the body cells and tissues, because circulating levels of TNFα remain constantly high, whether or not there is an infection, and it is these high levels of TNFα that cause the immune cells to malfunction and so attack the body's own cells. Adalimumab blocks this TNFα production and consequently reduces the physical effects of rheumatoid arthritis, psoriasis and other autoimmune disorders.

531

The acquired immune system

Acquired immunity is the immunity that we acquire as we go through life – the acquired immune system is barely functioning when we are born, but is reliant upon the mother's own acquired immune system giving protection *in utero* – some of which (mainly certain immunoglobulins) remain within the infant for a short time post-natally. Another name for the acquired immune system is the specific immune system, because it is aimed at specific infectious organisms. It is very much based upon the white blood cells known as lymphocytes.

There are two types of acquired immunity: cell-mediated immunity and humoral immunity.

Cell-mediated immunity (T-cell lymphocytes)

This type of immunity is known as cell-mediated immunity because the cells themselves destroy any invading antigens.

T-cell lymphocytes originate in the bone marrow, but then, at a certain stage in their development, leave the bone marrow as immature lymphocytes. These immature lymphocytes find

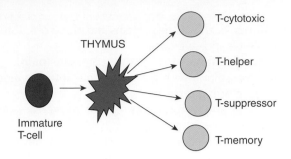

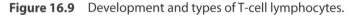

Figure 16.9 Development and types of T-cell lymphocytes.

their way to the thymus, where they fully develop. In addition, they learn to recognise our own cells and so do not destroy these, but do destroy invading cells; for example, bacteria and viruses (see Figure 16.11). The thymus is situated in the chest. In babies it is a large organ (relative to size), but atrophies with age.

T-cell lymphocytes have different functions to perform within the acquired immune system, and the functions that they perform are dependent upon the differentiation they undergo within the thymus (Figure 16.9). Different types of T-cells carry different receptors on their surfaces, and these are known as clusters of definition (CDs) – so-called because the way in which these receptors are organised on the cell surface defines their role and function.

There are four classes of T-cell lymphocytes:

- T-cytotoxic lymphocytes
- T-helper lymphocytes
- T-suppressor lymphocytes
- T-memory lymphocytes.

The major functions performed by the T-cell lymphocytes are:

- cytotoxicity (cell destruction)
- control of the immune system
- memory.

Cytotoxicity (cell destruction)

This function is performed by the T-cytotoxic lymphocytes that possess CD8 glycoprotein on their membrane. These cells mediate the direct cellular killing of target cells (Rote and Crippes Trask, 2006). The target cells may be virally infected cells, tumours or 'non-self' grafts, such as kidney transplants.

The T-cytotoxic lymphocytes bind to the target cell and release toxic substances into the target cell, which are capable of destroying it. If the target cell is a virally infected cell, that cell is destroyed, as are the viruses that have infected it. In this way the viruses are unable to go on to invade other cells.

Control of the immune system

This is a task undertaken by the T-helper and T-suppressor lymphocytes working together.

T-helper cells are coated with CD4 proteins and they stimulate the immune system – both the acquired immune system and many parts of the innate immune system – to proliferate in response to infectious organisms (or other antigens) present in the body. There are two types of T-helper cell: type 1 T-helper cells and type 2 T-helper cells.

The body is usually very efficient at stimulating immune activity in response to an invasion by antigens, but there is a need for balances and checks to prevent the overstimulation of immuno-logical activity, and this function is performed by the T-suppressor cells.

While many studies have identified T-suppressor cells, there appears to be no unique receptor marker for T-suppressor cells, and so immune suppression may actually be a task performed by a combination of T-helper and T-cytotoxic cells by means of a negative feedback mechanism (Male, 2013).

Memory

A special quality that the acquired immune system possesses is the ability to remember anti-gens – or, more specifically, the antigen receptors that have been previously detected by the immune system, and so produce a group of lymphocytes which can stimulate the parts of the immune system that are able to counter these antigens immediately if that antigen is detected in future infections. T-memory lymphocytes are responsible for a rapid response to further attacks by specific infectious microorganisms (Rote and McCance, 2014). This process is known as the secondary immune response and will be explained towards the end of this chapter (Figures 16.10 and 16.11).

Memory cells are long-lived and there is always a constant number of T-memory cells for a given antigen in circulation (Murphy, 2014).

533

Humoral immunity (B-cell lymphocytes)

This second type of acquired immunity (which involves B-cell lymphocytes) is known as humoral immunity because the components effective in the immune system are soluble in fluids (and so is called humoral immunity from the old English term 'humours').

B-cell lymphocytes originate and mature within the bone marrow.

As with the T-cell lymphocytes, the B-cells need to undergo a maturation process in which they have to survive a negative selection process. This is an attempt to ensure that the antigen receptors on their surface membrane do not display self-reactivity (i.e. do not react against our own cells) (Nairn and Helbert, 2007).

During this process, those B-cell lymphocytes that are autoreactive to the host cells and tissues are destroyed, leaving only non-autoreactive naive lymphocytes behind, which will then be able to go on to the next stage of maturation and selection (Figure 16.10). This is a very important process, because if there should be any self-reactivity of the B-cells, as with T-cell self-reactivity, then autoimmunity may be the result.

The actual mechanism of the B-cell negative selection process within the bone marrow is similar to that process which is undergone by T-cells during their maturation and differentiation within the thymus (Figure 16.11). However, in addition, B-cells undergo a positive selection process in which those lymphocytes that are able to respond to non-self antigens are preserved, while those that are not are left to die. The B-cells that have survived this negative selection find their way to the peripheral lymphoid organs, where they may encounter actual non-self antigens for which they have specificity. It is thought that more than 10^8 (100,000,000) different antigens may be recognised by the B-cell lymphocytes.

Mature B-cells are of two types: B-memory cells (with a similar role to play as the T-memory cells) and antibody-secreting plasma cells.

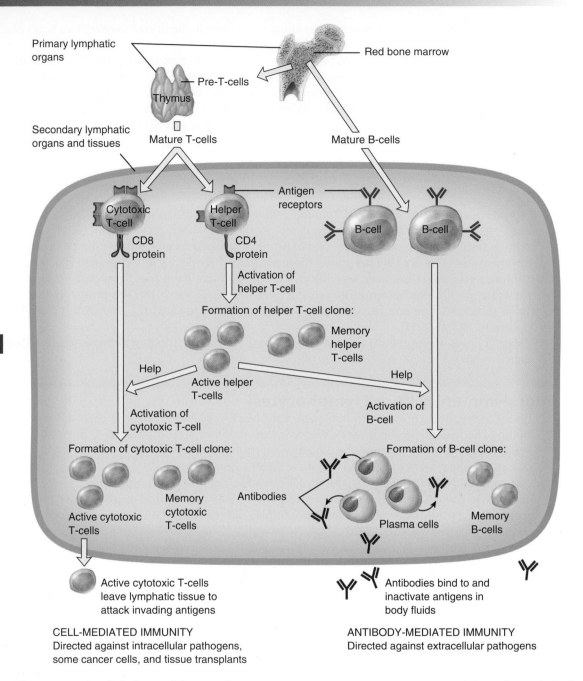

Figure 16.10 Cellular and humoral immune responses. *Source*: Tortora and Derrickson (2009). Reproduced with permission of John Wiley & Sons.

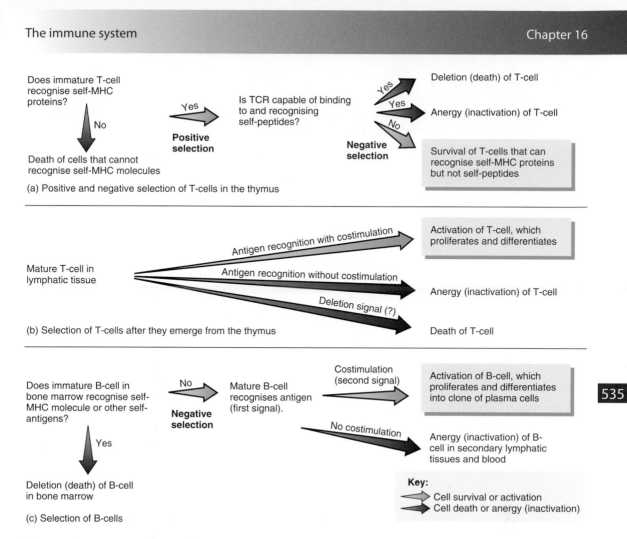

Figure 16.11 (a–c) Process of teaching T-cells and B-cells to recognise pathogens (infectious organisms). *Source*: Tortora and Derrickson (2009). Reproduced with permission of John Wiley & Sons.

Immunoglobulins (antibodies)

The antibodies secreted by the plasma cells are also known as **immunoglobulins**, and their role is to act as mediators in the destruction of non-self antigens. These immunoglobulins are not responsible for the actual killing. Instead, they assist other components of the immune system in destroying non-self antigens.

There are five classes of immunoglobulin:

- IgG
- IgA
- IgM
- IgE
- IgD.

Immunoglobulin G

This is the most important class of immunoglobulins involved in the secondary immune response. It makes up about 75% of total serum immunoglobulin (Seymour *et al.*, 1995), and it divides into four subclasses, namely IgG1, IgG2, IgG3 and IgG4.

Because it has a low molecular weight (i.e. it is very small), IgG is found within both the intra-vascular and extravascular areas of the body. This means that it can reach all parts of the body, and therefore its effects are far reaching. In particular, it plays a major role against blood-borne infective organisms as well as those invading the tissues.

The low molecular weight also means that IgG can cross the placental barrier to give a high degree of temporary passive immunity to the newborn child. This is important, because although maternal IgG disappears by the age of 9 months, by then the infant is hopefully producing its own IgG.

IgG helps the immune system in several ways (Seymour *et al.*, 1995; Vickers, 2005; Nairn and Helbert, 2007; Delves *et al.*, 2011):

- it is important for activating the complement system;
- it can bind to macrophages, and so enhance phagocytosis;
- it binds to the T-cytotoxic cells and helps them in destroying infected cells;
- it binds to platelets and helps with the inflammatory response.

Immunoglobulin A

There are two types of IgA: 'serum' and 'secretory'. Serum IgA has similar roles to IgG.

Secretory IgA (SIgA) is most important because it is the major immunoglobulin found in external body secretions, such as saliva, breast milk, colostrum, tears, nasal secretions, sweat and the secretions of the respiratory tract and gastrointestinal tract.

As its name suggests, SIgA has a secretory component, which allows for the easy transfer of SIgA across the epithelial cells into various bodily secretions. It also helps to protect the IgA from the proteolytic (destruction of protein) attack mounted by enzymes that are themselves secreted by bacteria.

The main function of SIgA is to prevent antigens crossing the epithelium. In addition, SIgA can activate the complement system.

SIgA plays an important role in the protection of the host's body against respiratory, urinary and bowel infections. Also, because it is present is such large quantities in colostrum and breast milk, it performs a vital role in the prevention of neonatal gut infections – this is one of the reasons why breastfeeding is so heavily promoted (Seymour *et al.*, 1995; Vickers, 2005; Nairn and Helbert, 2007; Delves *et al.*, 2011).

Immunoglobulin M

IgM is the predominant antibody involved in the primary immune response (see 'Primary immune response' section), as well as being involved in the early stages of the secondary immune response.

It is very effective in activating the classic pathway of the complement system.

Because of its large size, IgM is restricted almost entirely to the intravascular (within blood vessels) spaces, and it is also often involved with any response by the immune system to complex, blood-borne infectious microorganisms (Seymour *et al.*, 1995; Vickers, 2005; Nairn and Helbert, 2007; Delves *et al.*, 2011).

Immunoglobulin E

Only very small amounts of IgE are found in the body – in normal circumstances it makes up less than 0.01% of the total serum immunoglobulins, but is also found on the surfaces of mast cells and basophils because it has a very high avidity (binding potential) to tissue mast cells and circulatory basophils, and it is the binding of IgE to receptors on these cells in the presence of antigen that can trigger an allergic reaction.

This allergic reaction consists of:

- the activation of the mast cell
- the degranulation of the cell
- the release of mediators such as histamine.

Degranulation of the mast cell and release of histamine helps to cause an acute inflammatory response, which leads to the classic signs of allergic reactions, such as those seen in hay fever and asthma. IgE is also responsible for sensitising cells on mucosal surfaces, such as the conjunctival, nasal and bronchial mucosa. This gives rise to other symptoms of an allergy, including rhinitis and conjunctivitis (Seymour *et al.*, 1995; Vickers, 2005; Nairn and Helbert, 2007; Delves *et al.*, 2011).

The main role of IgE in helping to maintain good health is that it can bind onto helminths and other intestinal worms and so lead to their destruction. Allergic reactions and autoimmune diseases are less common in areas where worm and parasitic infestation is rife. In more developed societies, where helminth infestation is rare, it is thought that the IgE then turns its attention to the cells of the body, and allergy/autoimmunity is a response to this.

537

Medicines management

New therapies: nematode therapy

As mentioned in the main text, IgE is a major factor in allergic reactions. However, it is known that allergic reactions (eczema, food allergies, etc.) are not as prevalent in countries where there is a high parasitic infestation, particularly in terms of intestinal nematodes and helminths, and particularly hookworm or ascaris. At the same time, in more developed countries with high levels of hygiene and general cleanliness, allergies are very much on the increase. It is this dichotomy that has persuaded researchers to think about helminth therapy to alleviate allergies (Cooper, 2004; Zaccone *et al.*, 2006). Indeed, there have been trials where patients with allergies have swallowed hookworm larvae (the maximum tolerated number being 10) and have reported improvements – although not enough to significantly improve allergic symptoms. However, because the treatment made some subjects 'feel better', they opted to remain in the treatment once the trial had ended. Although not proven as such, further trials may well take place in the future, and hookworm therapy may become one of the standard therapies for allergies.

Immunoglobulin D

The first thing to say is that little is known about the functions of IgD. However, we do know that it is chiefly found on B-cell surface membranes and that it acts as a receptor molecule, but work is ongoing in trying to decipher and understand this particular immunoglobulin.

Role of immunoglobulins

According to Delves *et al.* (2011), the primary function of an antibody is to bind our phagocytes and other elements of the immune system to antigens by attaching to **epitopes** (or receptors) on the surface of the antigen (Figures 16.12 and 16.13); thus, the main functions of antibodies are to protect the host by (Rote and McCance, 2014):

- neutralising bacterial toxins;
- neutralising viruses;

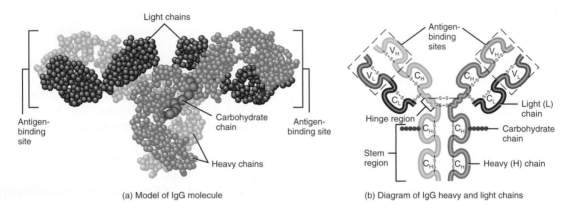

(a) Model of IgG molecule

(b) Diagram of IgG heavy and light chains

Figure 16.12 (a, b) Model of an antibody (IgG). *Source*: Tortora and Derrickson (2014). Reproduced with permission of John Wiley & Sons.

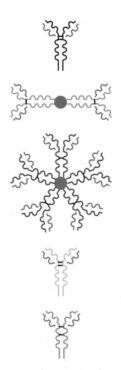

Figure 16.13 Model of an antigen showing the epitopes (receptors). *Source*: Tortora and Derrickson (2014). Reproduced with permission of John Wiley & Sons.

- opsonising bacteria – opsonins are molecules that bind to non-self matter and to receptors on phagocytes, in this way acting as a bridge between the two and holding the non-self matter bound to the phagocytes (Male, 2013);
- activating components of the inflammatory response.

Antibodies rarely act in isolation. Instead, they join with other components of the immune system to destroy the infecting organisms.

A second role of the immunoglobulin is the neutralisation of bacterial toxins. These toxins are produced by the bacteria and make them more pathogenic (harmful), thus causing more harm to the host. When this happens, the immunoglobulins function as antitoxins.

Similarly, the immunoglobulins neutralise viruses by binding to the viral surface receptors, so preventing them from binding to the host's cells, allowing the viruses then to be phagocytosed and so preventing the viruses from infecting cells of the body.

Immunoglobulins also activate components of the inflammatory response.

Medicine management

New therapies: immunoglobulin therapy

Immunoglobulin therapy uses purified immunoglobulins (antibodies) taken from the blood of volunteer donors. It can be administered intramuscularly, intravenously or subcutaneously. It is particularly important for people with antibody or combined immunodeficiencies, and has become essential for the management of these conditions. Immunoglobulin therapy has been available for patients with immunodeficiencies for many years, but in recent years the therapy has been found to be important for many other medical conditions, so that, no matter in what ward or clinic – or even at home – that a nurse is working, you will likely encounter this therapy at some time.

What is new about this therapy is that it can also be used for a huge number of medical conditions – and the list is growing continuously. The following are just a very few of the conditions for which immunoglobulin therapy may be useful, or which are under review.

Immunological conditions:

Antibody deficiency	HIV
Combined immunodeficiency (T- and B-cells)	
Complement deficiencies	

Haematological/oncological conditions:

Various types of leukaemia	Aplastic anaemia
Haemophagocytic syndrome	
Idiopathic thrombocytopaenia purpura	

Infectious conditions:

Rheumatic fevers	Lyme disease
Recurrent otitis media	Chronic sinusitis

Neurologic conditions:

Alzheimer's disease	Encephalopathy
Epilepsy	Multiple sclerosis
Myeloma	

(*Continued*)

539

Rheumatologicical diseases:

Rheumatoid arthritis   Scleroderma

Kawasaki disease   Systemic lupus erythematosus

Other conditions:

Asthma   Atopic dermatitis

Cystic fibrosis   Diabetes mellitus

Sepsis and septic shock   Transplant rejection

Recurrent pregnancy loss or miscarriage

Snapshot

Skills in practice education of patients with hypogammaglobulinaemia to self-administer subcutaneous immunoglobulin therapy at home

For chronic conditions, such as hypogammaglobulinaemia (low or absent B-lymphocytes leading to a lack of antibodies), the ability to self-treat at home leads to a better quality of life for the patient and family – because the patient is taking control of their condition and also there is less disruption to the patient's (and family's) lifestyle, as well as being more cost effective in terms of the healthcare professional's time. This then allows for more new or difficult (with regard to treatment) patients to be seen and monitored in a clinical setting. However, for this to be able to happen, some form of home therapy management needs to be put into place, and the first and most important is the ability of the nurse to teach the methods of subcutaneous treatment as well as monitoring of the ongoing treatment at home along with support of the patient and family. This requires the nurse to set up a teaching/training course once the patient has been deemed to be coping well with hospital/clinic-based treatment and after being assured that the patient (and/or a family member) has the desire, cognitive ability and manual dexterity to carry out this procedure at home. This is a new skill for many nurses, and will require time and expertise to accomplish.

Protocols will have to be written and then agreed by the hospital/clinic before training can begin for this procedure to be undertaken by the patient/family at home.

First of all there is the home visit to ensure that the home environment and facilities available are suitable for this procedure to be carried out at home.

For training in self-administration of subcutaneous immunoglobulins, there are three steps during the training sessions for each patient – may also include the family of the patient:

1. Nurse demonstration of the procedure.
2. The procedure carried out by the patient with the help of the nurse.
3. The patient carrying out self-administration on their own – validated by the nurse observing.

The whole training period can last for several weeks until the nurse is assured that the patient can safely cope at home.

Arrangements will need to be made for regular checks by the nurse on the situation to ensure that no problems occur, such as regular checks on the ongoing ability of the patient/family to carry out this procedure safely, as well as setting up a system of being able to be contacted to deal with questions or emergences if/as they arise at home.

Natural killer cells

There is a further type of lymphocyte, which appears to express only the earliest markers of T-cell differentiation. These are known as **null cells** or **NK (natural killer) cells**. The NK cells do not bind antigen, nor are they induced to proliferate by contact with an antigen. Rather, they bind to chemical changes on the surfaces of virally infected cells or malignant cells, rather than antigen receptors (Rote and McCance, 2014).

Although they are lymphocytes, these cells are usually classified within the innate immune system.

Primary and secondary response to infection

Finally, we will examine the immune system's response to infections. The one thing that really marks out the acquired immune system as special is its ability to 'remember' previous encounters with an antigen. Without this ability, each time an individual came into contact with a particular antigen there would be a risk of a serious, possibly fatal, illness. This immune memory is crucial because it allows the body to mount an immediate immune response to an antigen without waiting for the immune system to work out a way of destroying that antigen each time it infects us.

How does the immune system gain this memory of a specific antigen? There are two immune responses: the primary and secondary responses. The primary response occurs when the immune system first comes into contact with a new antigen (such as an infectious organism), and the secondary response occurs with all subsequent encounters with that same antigen.

Primary immune response

With the primary immune response, there is always a long time period before a response can be made. This is known as the 'lag' phase because the response lags some way behind the encounter with the antigen (Figure 16.14). During this time there are no detectable

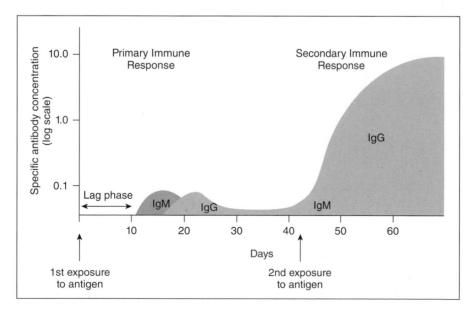

Figure 16.14   Antibody responses to an infection.

antibodies produced by the mature B-cell lymphocytes, but the immune system is working out how to destroy the antigen.

In the case of the primary immune response, the lag phase can take anything from 5 to 10 days before there has been sufficient production of antibodies to make a difference. During this period, the host can become very sick and may even die.

The major immunoglobulin class produced at this stage is IgM, and only small amounts of IgG are produced, but hopefully enough to destroy the antigen.

At the same time as the antigen is being destroyed, the memory cells are retaining a memory of this specific antigen and how to defeat it, and this memory will stay with the host for a long time. Each time the host is infected by that same antigen, the memory cells are reinforced.

Clinical considerations

Hand washing

Hand washing is the single most important measure in preventing cross-infection. The technique employed involves thoroughly cleaning, rinsing and drying both hands. Hands are the principal route by which cross-infection occurs.

There have been many concerted efforts to enforce stricter hand washing policies in all health and social care settings; effective hand washing remains an essential public health initiative. Hand washing is an essential aspect of any caregiver's repertoire of skills, and these skills must be mastered in order to provide all people with a safe environment. Those people with immunological deficiencies are at a particular risk of infection; and as such, attention to scrupulous hand washing techniques must be carried out at all times.

All healthcare providers should strive to make hand washing an automatic behaviour that is performed by all in homes, schools and other environments. Families and carers who come into contact with those people with an immunological deficiency must adhere to effective hand washing. The key aim of effective hand washing is to prevent the spread of microorganisms between people or between other living things and people. Inanimate objects and surfaces, such as contaminated cutlery or clinical equipment, may put the health and well-being of an immunologically compromised person at risk.

Using the correct hand washing technique not only saves lives but can also save money. Poor hand washing practices can lead to urinary tract infections, bloodstream infections, respiratory infections and infection of incisional wounds. These infections are caused by the transfer of microorganisms from staff and families to vulnerable people, which could be prevented by using the correct hand washing procedures.

In all healthcare environments hand washing is mandatory and must be carried out using established policies and procedures. There are a number of practices associated with hand hygiene – for example, using alcohol hand rubs and the act of physically washing the hands. The consequences of failing to use the correct procedure are many; the impact this can have on the health and well-being of the person you are caring for can be devastating.

Secondary immune response

If, at a later date, the same antigen infects the body again, because of the memory T-cell lymphocytes, the body is capable of mounting a secondary immune response that is much quicker. Because the memory cells are carrying their memory of this antigen, production of antibodies can take place very quickly, so that there is a very short lag phase.

542

In a secondary immune response, the major antibody class produced is IgG, although occasionally IgA or IgE may be produced depending upon the nature of the antigen and its route of entry (Nairn and Helbert, 2007). IgG is produced in huge quantities very quickly, and therefore the response is very rapid and effective – often, the antigen is destroyed before any signs and symptoms appear.

Immunisations

Immunisation, or vaccination, is either the process of transferring antibodies to an individual who is lacking them (passive immunisation) or the process of inducing an immune reaction in an individual (active immunisation). Immunisations induce the primary response by exposing the immune system to a vaccine that includes an infectious organism which is either inactivated (killed) or attenuated (weakened) so that it is no longer infectious but still possesses the receptors that can stimulate the immune system.

Passive immunisation

In passive immunisation, the individual is actually injected with the antibodies. There are two types of passive immunisation, which are natural and very common:

- The mother transfers IgG antibodies across the placenta to the foetus. Whatever organisms the mother is immune to, the newborn baby will also be immune to them.
- During breastfeeding, when the mother passes IgA antibodies to the baby in her colostrum and milk.

Passive immunisation is also short-lived and lasts only as long as it takes for these antibodies to be cleared from the body. This type of immunisation will not normally provoke an immune response in the recipient; therefore, there will be no immunological cover for subsequent exposure to that particular antigen.

Active immunity

Active immunity is the process of presenting antigen to the immune system to induce an immune response to it. This is the type of immunity that takes advantage of the primary and secondary responses to immunity and is the basis for all the immunisations/vaccinations that we have throughout our lives.

A vaccine has to be able to stimulate both T- and B-cell lymphocytes to provide an immune response. If a vaccine is effective, it provides common immunity to a population.

Conclusion

This completes the chapter on the immune system. As you have learned, it is a very complex system, with each of the many components interacting with others to provide us with the protection that we need to survive in this very dangerous world. But, above all, hopefully you will be amazed and awestruck at its ability to fulfil its major role: that of keeping us safe from infections and other potential harm that could befall us.

What you must remember is that immunology is a dynamic subject. Research in the specialty is continually bringing us new knowledge, not only of the anatomy and physiology of the immune system, but also of disorders affected by it and of new therapies.

There is now so much progress being made in immunology that it is impossible to predict the future. But then, this is what makes immunology such an exciting specialty with which to be involved.

Glossary

Acquired immunity   Immunity that is acquired throughout life by coming into contact with many different infectious agents.

Active immunity   Immunity developed inside the body as a result of encountering infectious agents.

Antibodies   Also known as **immunoglobulins**, antibodies can recognise and attach to infectious agents and so provoke an immune response to these infectious agents. They are also **opsonins**.

Antigens   Anything that provokes an antibody response.

Atopy   A type of hypersensitivity that is linked to **immunoglobulin** E.

Bactericidal   The ability to kill bacteria.

Basophils   White blood cells that take part in the process of phagocytosis. Also involved in allergic/atopic reactions.

B-cell lymphocytes   Blood cells from which antibodies (immunoglobulins) develop. Part of the humoral immune system.

Cell-mediated immunity   The type of acquired immunity generated by the T-cell **lymphocytes**.

Clotting system   The clotting of blood to reduce blood loss. Also involving **thrombocytes** (platelets).

Complement factors   A group of proteins that are involved in many of the immune processes (e.g. phagocytosis and inflammation). They are also **opsonins**.

Cytokines   Chemical messengers that affect the behaviour of other cells, including cells of the immune system.

Cytotoxicity   The process by which infectious microorganisms are killed or damaged (cyto = cell, toxicity = dangerous to).

Eosinophils   White blood cells involved in the destruction of parasitic worms, but also linked to hypersensitivity.

Epitopes   The parts of a cell that can bind to other cells (i.e. cell receptors).

Granulocytes   White blood cells that take part in the process of phagocytosis.

Humoral immunity   Another name for antibody immunity. This is the part of the **acquired immune** system that relies upon antibodies to help in the destruction of infectious agents.

Hypersensitivity   A heightened immune response that can cause allergies and atopic diseases.

Immunisation   The process of either transferring antibodies to someone (i.e. passive immunisation) or inducing an immune reaction naturally but safely (i.e. active immunity).

Immunity   The body's response to infection, damage or other diseases.

Immunoglobulins   Also known as antibodies.

Inflammation   The body's immediate reaction to tissue injury or damage.

Innate immunity   The immunity with which we are born.

Kinins   A specialist group of plasma proteins (i.e. proteins that circulate within blood plasma) and have a role to play in the process of inflammation.

Kinin system   The system in which kinins operate in order to activate and help inflammatory cells, such as neutrophils, to function properly as well as being involved in making the blood vessels more permeable to allow cells of the immune system to get to the area of inflammation or damage.

Leucocyte   Another term for a white blood cell (leuco = white, cyte = cell).

Lymph   A colourless liquid derived from blood.

Lymph nodes   Nodules within the lymphatic system that contain mesh traps which are able to trap antigens in order for them to be destroyed by antibodies and other components of the immune system.

Lymph vessels   These are similar to blood vessels, but they carry lymph, antigens (e.g. bacteria), antibodies and other components of the immune system, from the site of infection towards **lymph nodes**.

Lymphatic system   This shadows the blood system, but is very much involved in immunity. It consists of lymph vessels that contain **lymph** (which transports antigens and antibodies) and also lymph nodes and other lymphatic tissues (such as the tonsils and the spleen).

Lymphocyte   The major white blood cell of the acquired immune system.

Macrophage   Also known as a tissue macrophage, it is a white blood cell that takes part in the process of phagocytosis within the tissues as opposed to within the blood circulation.

Mast cells   Cells of connective tissue that are involved in the activation of the inflammatory response (inflammation).

Medulla   The central part of an organ.

Monocyte   A type of phagocytic white blood cell (known as a tissue macrophage once it migrates into the tissues).

Neutrophils   White blood cells that take part in the process of phagocytosis.

NK cells   Natural killer cells are a class of lymphocytes that are not specific to certain infectious agents and so are often classed with innate immunity as opposed to acquired immunity.

Null cells   Another name for the NK cells.

Oedema   A scientific term for swelling.

Opsonins   Substances that bind antigens to phagocytic cells, and so enhance the process of phagocytosis (e.g. complement factors and antibodies).

Passive immunity   The process of transferring **antibodies** to someone who is vulnerable to infections and cannot make their own active immunity.

Phagocyte   White blood cells that are able to ingest and destroy infectious microorganisms and other non-self matter, and include, among others, neutrophils and macrophages.

Phagocytosis   The ingestion and destruction of infectious microorganisms and other non-self matter by specialised cells (phagocytes).

Plasma cells   Cells that develop from B-cell **lymphocytes** and that produce antibodies.

Platelet   See **thrombocyte**.

Primary response   The immune response that occurs when we first come into contact with a new infectious agent.

Prostaglandins   Fatty acids that function as part of the inflammatory process (inflammation).

Pseudopodia   (Literal meaning = 'false arms'). These are finger-like projections that emerge from cells and, within immunity, they are very important in the process of phagocytosis.

Secondary response   The immune response that, following a successful primary immune response to a specific infectious agent, occurs every time we encounter that same specific infectious agent.

Spleen   Part of the lymphatic system, it functions to fight infections and to filter and clean blood. In addition, it serves as a blood reservoir.

T-cell lymphocytes　White blood cells that have many functions, including control of the acquired immune system and killing viruses. The major component of the cell-mediated immune system.

Thrombocyte　Another name for a platelet; it is important in the **clotting** process

Thymus　The organ of the body where T-cell lymphocytes mature, distinguish between self and non-self cells and differentiate into various types of T-cells that each have different functions within the acquired immune system.

Tonsils　Lymph tissue that is situated within the oral region (the mouth) and helps to protect the respiratory and gastrointestinal tracts from infections.

Trabeculae　Connective tissue strands that help to form part of the framework of organs, so giving them rigidity.

References

Cooper, P.J. (2004) Intestinal worms and human parasites. *Parasite Immunology* **26**(11–12): 455–467.

Delves, P.J. and Roitt, I.M. (2000) The immune system: part 1. *New England Journal of Medicine* **343**: 137–149.

Delves, P.J., Martin, S.J., Burton, D.R. and Roitt, I.M. (2011) *Roitt's Essential Immunology*, 12th edn. Oxford: Blackwell Science.

Male, D. (2013) *Immunology: An Illustrated Outline*, 5th edn. London: Garland Science Publishing.

Marieb, E.N. and Hoehn, K. (2013) *Human Anatomy and Physiology*, 9th edn. San Francisco, CA: Pearson Benjamin Cummings.

Murphy, K. (2014) *Janeway's Immunobiology*, 8th edn. New York: Garland Publishing.

Nair, M. and Peate, I. (2009) *Fundamentals of Applied Pathophysiology: An Essential Guide for Nursing Students*. Oxford: John Wiley & Sons, Ltd.

Nairn, R. and Helbert, M. (2007) *Immunology for Medical Students*, 2nd edn. St Louis, MO: Mosby.

Roitt, I.M. and Rabson, A. (2000) *Really Essential Medical Immunology*. Oxford: Blackwell Science.

Rote, N.S. and Crippes Trask, B. (2006) Adaptive immunity. In McCance, K.L. and Huether, S.E. (eds), *Pathophysiology: The Biologic Basis for Disease in Adults and Children*, 5th edn. St Louis: Mosby; pp. 211–248.

Rote, N.S. and McCance K.L. (2014) Adaptive immunity. In: McCance, K.L. and Huether, S.E. (eds), *Pathophysiology: The Biologic Basis for Disease in Adults and Children*, 7th edn. St Louis, MO: Elsevier.

Seymour, G.J., Savage, N.W. and Walsh, L.J. (1995) *Immunology: An Introduction for the Health Sciences*. Roseville, NSW: McGraw-Hill.

Tortora, G.J. and Derrickson, B.H. (2014) *Principles of Anatomy and Physiology*, 14th edn. Hoboken, NJ: John Wiley & Sons, Inc.

Tortora, G.J., Funke, B.R. and Case, C.L. (2014) *Microbiology: An Introduction*, 8th edn. San Francisco, CA: Pearson Benjamin Cummings.

Vickers, P.S. (2005) Acquired defences. In Montague, S. Watson, R. and Herbert, R.A. (eds), *Physiology for Nursing Practice*. Edinburgh: Elsevier; pp. 685–724.

Vickers, P.S. (2007) Section 1: Anatomy and physiology of the immune system. In *Immunology/ Immunodeficiencies – Antibody Deficiency*. CD ROM, Baxter (pp. 3–51).

Walport, M.J. (2001) Complement: part 1. *New England Journal of Medicine* **344**(14): 1058–1066.

Zaccone, P., Fehervari, Z., Phillips, J.M., Dunne, D.W. and Cooke, A. (2006) Parasitic worms and inflammatory diseases. *Parasitic Immunology* **28**(10): 515–523.

Further reading

INGID (International Nursing Group for Immunodeficiencies)

www.ingid.org

Contains excellent learning/teaching materials and information on immunology and immunodeficiencies.

UK Primary Immunodeficiency Network (UKPIN)

http://www.ukpin.org.uk/
Combines doctors, researchers and nurses.

European Federation of Immunology Societies (EFIS)

http://www.efis.org/
An umbrella organisation for all European immunology societies.

Immune Deficiency Foundation (IDF)

http://www.primaryimmune.org/
American immune deficiency organisation – much excellent information.

Allergy UK

www.allergyuk.org
Offers support and advice to adults and children on all allergies and intolerances, including allergic
conditions such as eczema, dermatitis, asthma, and so on.

Activities

Multiple choice questions

1. The two branches of white blood cells that form a major part of the immune system are:
   (a) lymphoid and myeloid
   (b) lymphoid and megakaryocytes
   (c) megakaryocytes and erythrophils
   (d) myeloid and macrophages

2. Immunoglobulins are produced by:
   (a) antibodies
   (b) plasma cells
   (c) T-cell lymphocytes
   (d) platelets

3. The specific immune system is also known as:
   (a) lymphatic immunity
   (b) mechanical immunity
   (c) innate immunity
   (d) acquired immunity

4. The spleen is the organ in which:
   (a) T-cells mature
   (b) immune cells learn to recognise 'non-self' cells
   (c) lymph nodes develop
   (d) dead red blood cells are disposed of

5. Immunoglobulin E:
   (a) triggers allergic reactions
   (b) activates the complement system
   (c) enhances phagocytosis
   (d) protects the body against respiratory infections

6. Natural killer (NK) cells are:
   (a) antibodies
   (b) erythrocytes
   (c) lymphocytes
   (d) opsonins

7. The primary response to infection:
   (a) builds on a memory of past infections
   (b) mainly concerns IgG antibodies
   (c) is a passive process
   (d) mainly concerns IgM antibodies
8. Immunisation is another name for:
   (a) immunoglobulin production and development
   (b) antibodies
   (c) vaccination
   (d) maturation of lymphocytes
9. Cytotoxicity is the process of:
   (a) cell memory
   (b) cell suppression
   (c) cell destruction
   (d) cell development
10. T-helper cells are:
   (a) coated with CD8 glycoproteins
   (b) coated with CD4 proteins
   (c) cytotoxic cells
   (d) inflammatory cells

True or false

1. Phagocytes are red blood cells.
2. The thymus is where immature T-cells mature.
3. Another name for an antibody is an immunoglobulin.
4. White blood cells are descended from omnipotent stem cells.
5. Macrophages include monocytes and granulocytes.
6. One branch of T-cells develop into plasma cells.
7. The spleen is a lymphatic organ.
8. The right lymphatic duct receives lymph from the right arm.
9. The lymphoid system enables lymphocytes to protect tissues from infections.
10. Sneezing is a physical barrier within the immune system.

Label the diagram

From the following list of words, complete the labelling of the diagram of the first stage of phagocytosis:

Antibody, cell nucleus, complement, phagocyte, vesicles

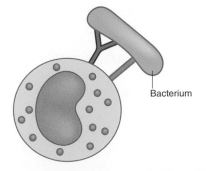

Bacterium

Fill in the blanks

Granulocytes are divided into three types; namely, neutrophils, _____ and basophils. These cells are called granulocytes because, under a high-powered microscope, they appear to be full of little _____. These, however, are actually _____ (or empty spaces) within the cells, and they are very importantly involved in the process of _____, which is the destruction of _____ organisms, such as _____ and viruses. They work by first of all _____ them and then they ingest them, so destroying the organisms and, at the same time, also providing the cell with _____.

bacteria, engulfing, eosinophils, granules, infectious, nutrition, phagocytosis, vacuoles

Word search

Find the following words within the grid:

cilia, cytotoxicity, IgM, inflammation, lymphocyte, NK cell, node, phagocytosis, platelets, spleen, tears, thymus

P	H	A	G	O	C	Y	T	O	S	I	S	Z
L	X	V	N	W	Y	G	E	T	C	N	I	Y
A	J	K	E	X	T	D	N	Y	A	F	H	G
T	U	U	E	D	O	N	T	D	B	L	M	O
E	G	X	L	N	T	Y	H	L	M	A	R	N
L	Y	M	P	H	O	C	Y	T	E	M	R	T
E	W	A	S	T	X	Y	M	C	X	M	S	G
T	S	R	N	Z	I	T	U	D	N	A	R	N
S	C	E	P	T	C	Y	S	T	X	T	F	P
F	R	A	I	L	I	C	V	V	L	I	G	M
J	S	R	A	E	T	S	Q	U	A	O	L	W
K	R	Q	U	I	Y	V	E	Q	U	N	V	X
N	T	U	L	L	E	C	K	N	K	C	E	L

Find out more

1. What are the immunisation schedulers for your country?
2. Find out the differences, in terms of cause, symptoms and treatment, between rheumatoid arthritis and osteoarthritis.
3. Explore the different methods of immunoglobulin therapy for people with primary immunodeficiency disorders
4. Look at what medical conditions are treated by immunoglobulin therapy, other than primary immunodeficiencies.
5. What is anaphylaxis and how is it treated?

6. What are the differences between bacteria and viruses, and what are the differences between how these infectious conditions treated?
7. What is the normal treatment for a patient diagnosed with pulmonary tuberculosis (TB)?
8. Find out about and discuss the isolation policy for the hospital/healthcare centre, etc., that you are working in or have worked in as part of your nurse education.
9. How can nurses prevent infectious disease in hospitals and other healthcare institutions, as well as the home?
10. Find more out about the link between stress (physical, social, and psychological) and the immune system.

Conditions

The following is a list of conditions that are associated with the immune system. Take some time and write notes about each of the conditions. You may make the notes taken from text books or other resources (e.g. people you work with in a clinical area), or you may make the notes as a result of people you have cared for. If you are making notes about people you have cared for you must ensure that you adhere to the rules of confidentiality.

Septicaemia	
Myasthenia gravis	
Pernicious anaemia	
Skin allergy	
Hay fever	
Coeliac disease	
Multiple sclerosis	
Tuberculosis	

Chapter 17

The skin

Ian Peate

Test your prior knowledge

- Name the layers of the skin.
- Describe the role of the skin in health.
- What are three key functions of the skin?
- How does the skin provide or help to provide the body with various defence mechanisms?
- Why is ultraviolet light sometimes harmful to the skin?
- What is the role of the skin in relation to thermoregulation?
- Discuss skin changes as the body ages.
- What is melanin?
- How does skin regenerate?
- How does pigment add to skin colour?

Learning outcomes

After reading this chapter you will be able to:

- Discuss the anatomy and physiology of the skin
- Describe the various functions of the skin
- Discuss the structure and growth of the appendages
- Explain how the skin functions as a homeostatic mechanism
- Outline the factors that determine skin colour

Fundamentals of Anatomy and Physiology: For Nursing and Healthcare Students, Second Edition. Edited by Ian Peate and Muralitharan Nair.
© 2017 John Wiley & Sons, Ltd. Published 2017 by John Wiley & Sons, Ltd.
Student companion website: www.wileyfundamentalseries.com/anatomy
Instructor companion website: www.wiley.com/go/instructor/anatomy

Body map

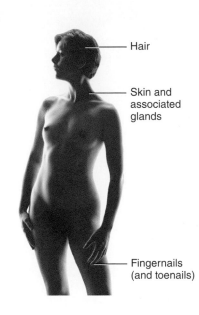

Hair

Skin and
associated
glands

Fingernails
(and toenails)

Introduction

The skin, sometimes referred to as the integumentary system, protects the body in a number of ways; without skin and its protective mechanisms the human being would not survive. The skin is often the only organ of the body that is on show all of the time, and because of this the skin can reveal how we feel emotionally; for example, we may blush. It can also reveal how we are from a physiological perspective; for example, it can appear cyanosed. The skin is the organ that is the most commonly exposed to disease or infection. The skin is almost entirely waterproof.

The skin has a number of homeostatic elements; for example, it can regulate body temperature and is often spoken of as the skin with appendages. The appendages are modifications of the skin. LeMone and Burke (2011) suggest that the average adult has 2 m^2 of skin, which weighs approximately 4.1 kg. The skin is twice as heavy as the brain. There are about 4.5 m of blood vessels, 3.6 m of nerves, 2.6 million sweat glands, 1500 sensory receptors and over 3 million cells that are continuously dying and being replaced. The skin receives nearly one-third of all blood that flows through the body (Rizzo, 2006).

The skin plays a vital role in health and well-being. Any disturbance in skin can lead to physical and or psychological problems, and this in turn has the ability to impact on a person's quality of life. Just as a house needs bricks and mortar to act as a framework, the house would be of little value if it were not waterproof. Using this analogy, the house also needs shelter from the environment, and in the human this job is carried out by the skin. The skin provides a defensive barrier, defending the body from the elements and safeguarding against pathogens. It also offers a number of other functions. The skin is made up of a superficial epidermis and a deeper structure called the dermis. Prior to discussing the functions of the skin, the next section will outline the structure of the skin.

Snapshot

Acne vulgaris

Acne vulgaris is a disorder of the pilosebaceous follicles located in the face and upper trunk. At puberty, androgens increase the production of sebum from enlarged sebaceous glands; these become blocked and infected, causing an inflammatory reaction.

Karl is 15 years of age and has acne vulgaris. This has impacted his self-confidence, and his father reports that he has become withdrawn so much that he dreads going to school as his classmates tease him. Acne can cause severe psychological problems, undermining the person's self-assurance and self-esteem at a vulnerable time in their life.

Follicles that are impacted and distended by incompletely desquamated keratinocytes and sebum are known as comedones. These can be open (blackheads) or closed (whiteheads). The inflammation causes papules, pustules and nodules to appear.

Acne is a mild and self-limiting condition; however, teenagers like Karl are very sensitive about it, and because of this it is essential to be empathetic as well as providing advice and reassurance. In Karl's case the condition was ongoing and he required referral to a dermatologist, who instigated topical and systemic treatment.

The structure of skin

According to Shier *et al.* (2013), the skin is one of the more versatile organs of the body. The skin is composed of two distinct regions: the dermis and the epidermis. The subcutaneous facia (sometimes referred to as the hypodermis) lies under the dermis (Colbert *et al.*, 2012); these masses of loose connective and adipose tissue attach to the skin and organs beneath; they are not part of the skin.

The epidermis

The superficial and thinnest aspect of the skin, the epidermis is the area of skin that can most commonly be seen. While the skin covers the whole of the body, there are several regional distinctions, and these are associated with flexibility, distribution and type of hair, density and types of gland, pigmentation, vascularity, innervations and thickness (Jenkins *et al.*, 2013). The thinnest part of the skin can be found on the eyelids; here, it is just 0.5 mm in thickness, whereas at the heel it is 4.0 mm thick.

The epidermis is made up of epithelium, called keratinised stratified squamous epithelium, and contains four key cell types (Figure 17.1):

- keratinocytes
- melanocytes
- Langerhans cells
- Merkel cells.

Keratinocytes

These cells are organised in four layers. They are responsible for producing a protein called keratin. Keratin is a tough, fibrous protein that aids in the protection of the skin and tissues below from the heat, microorganisms and chemicals. The keratinocytes are also responsible for the

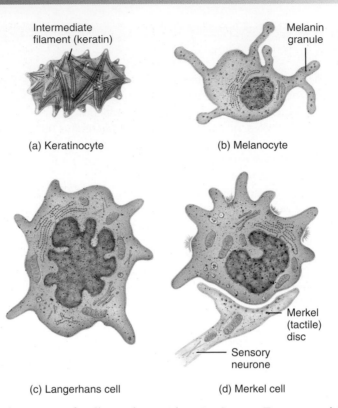

Figure 17.1 (a–d) The types of cells in the epidermis. *Source*: Tortora and Derrickson (2009). Reproduced with permission of John Wiley & Sons.

production of the water-resistant properties of the skin, and act as a type of sealant that reduces water entry as well as water loss; they also prevent the entry of foreign matter.

Melanocytes

The developing embryo produces the pigment melanin from the melanocytes. Melanocytes are most profuse in the epidermis of the penis, nipples, the areola, face and limbs. Melanocytes have long, slender projections that extend between the keratinocytes and have the ability to transfer melanin granules. Melanin is responsible for the natural colour of a person's skin, and it helps to defend it from the damaging effects of the sun.

When skin has been exposed to a great deal of sun the melanocytes multiply the quantity of melanin in order to absorb more ultraviolet rays. This activity makes the skin darker, giving it a suntanned appearance. A suntan indicates that the skin has been harmed and is attempting to defend itself.

All people have about the same number of melanocytes; those people with brown or black skin have the same number of melanocytes but they make more of the pigment melanin. It is the amount of melanin produced and how it is distributed that results in a variation of skin colour. These people have more natural protection from the harmful ultraviolet rays of the sun. Moles (sometimes called naevi) are a group or a cluster of melanocytes that lie close together. The majority of people with white skin have approximately 10–50 moles on their skin.

Snapshot

Skin biopsy

A skin biopsy is a procedure in which a sample of skin tissue is removed, processed and then examined under a microscope; it is usually performed to diagnose skin cancer. There are several methods that may be used to obtain a skin sample; the method chosen will depend on the size and location of the abnormal area of skin (the skin lesion). When the specimen has been taken it is placed in a solution (e.g. formaldehyde) and sent to the laboratory for processing and examination.

An assessment of the patient is carried out prior to a skin biopsy being performed. There is no special preparation required before having the biopsy. A consent form will need to be signed.

The skin is cleaned and a marker may be used to outline the edges of the skin sample. The procedure is undertaken using sterile conditions. A local anaesthetic is injected and the procedure performed; in some cases sutures will not be needed (e.g. a shave biopsy). The biopsy site is then covered with a sterile dressing. In a punch biopsy there may be a need for sutures, depending on the size of biopsy. In excision biopsy, pressure may be applied to the site until the bleeding stops; sutures will be required to close the wound.

After the procedure, specific instructions are given to the patient on how to care for the biopsy site. The biopsy site should be kept clean and dry until it heals completely. The clinic or hospital where the biopsy took place should be contacted if the patent experiences excessive bleeding or drainage through the bandage. If there is increased tenderness, pain, redness or swelling at the biopsy site then the dermatology nurse or doctor should be contacted.

Langerhans cells

These cells are part of the immune system and arise from the red bone marrow (see Chapter 5 for a discussion on the red bone marrow). These cells migrate from the bone marrow to the epidermis and make up a small part of the epidermal cells. The Langerhans cells regulate immune reactions in the skin as a defence against microorganisms that invade it (Lewis and Roberts, 2009); these cells are very fragile when exposed to the sun.

The Langerhans cells process microbial antigens (they help to stimulate lymphocytes); their role is to assist other cells of the immune system in response to and recognition of microorganisms and destroy the invading microbes.

Merkel cells

A Merkel cell has the ability to have contact with a flattened process of a sensory neurone (a synaptic contact); this is a structure called a tactile disc (sometimes this is called a Merkel disc). The Merkel cells and the tactile discs (the least numerous of cells on the epidermis) are capable of detecting touch sensations (Tortora and Derrickson, 2011).

Layers of the epidermis

Just as there are two distinct layers of skin – the dermis and epidermis – there are also a number of distinct layers of keratinocytes. These layers are developed over time and form the epidermis. These layers are called strata and are microscopically visible (see Figure 17.2).

The superficial and deeper levels of the skin are:

- the stratum basale
- the stratum spinosum
- the stratum granulosum

- the stratum lucidum
- the stratum corneum.

These are now discussed separately, and Table 17.1 provides an overview of the layers of the epidermis.

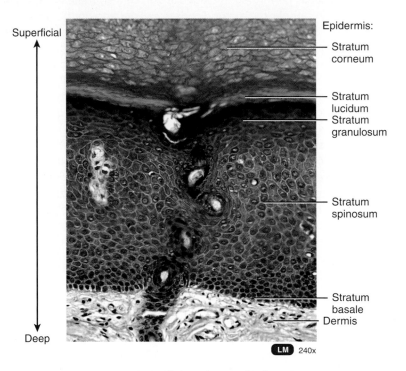

Figure 17.2 A microscopic perspective of the skin with the various strata. *Source*: Tortora and Derrickson (2009). Reproduced with permission of John Wiley & Sons.

Table 17.1 The layers of the epidermis

Layer	Location	Description
Stratum basale (sometimes called the basal cell layer)	The deepest layer	Cuboidal cells that are arranged as a single row; these divide and grow. The stratum basale also contains melanocytes
Stratum spinosum	Above the stratum basale and below the stratum granulosum	These keratinocytes are tightly packed, flat and have spine-like projections
Stratum granulosum	Under the stratum corneum	Flattened cells arranged in approximately three to five layers. Protect the body from losing fluid and also protect from harm. Compact brittle cells as they lose their nucleus
Stratum lucidum	When present, situated between the stratum corneum and the stratum granulosum	These cells are not present on the soles and palms. The cells have no nucleus and are tightly packed
Stratum corneum	The most superficial of layers	Several layers of keratinised, dead epithelial cells. These cells are flattened and have no nucleus

Clinical considerations

Personal hygiene

One of the most important aspects of the role and function of the nurse is to help people to wash themselves when they are unable to do so. Washing is often seen as a basic nursing task; however, the nurse should consider this is a skilled activity that requires much thought and assessment of the person being cared for.

Understanding the anatomy and physiology of the skin and the complexities associated with this body system can help you to help the people you care for. When helping a person to maintain personal hygiene you should ensure that you use soaps and other toiletries that will not damage or potentially damage skin integrity. This will include ensuring that the person is not allergic to any of the products that have been chosen to wash and cleanse the skin. As far as is possible you should always ask the person if they are allergic to any toiletries or other skin products, as some people are allergic to some of the chemicals found in soaps and cleansing products. This element of care provision requires you to be able to assess an individual's needs.

You should bear in mind that when using some kinds of soap this can have the same effect on the skin as swimming in the sea, the lather worked up by the soap when it is on the skin has a higher concentration of glycerine and this can then draw out water from the epidermis. The product that has been chosen to clean the skin may have a harmful effect on the person's skin and can potentially lead to the development of some skin conditions; for example, dermatitis and eczema.

Stratum basale

The stratum basale rests on the basement membrane and is the deepest layer of the epidermis; this layer provides a definite border between the dermis and epidermis. This is made up of a single row of columnar keratinocytes. The cells (stem cells or mother cells) of the epidermis originate from this deep layer. New cells are being constantly produced; they are continually dividing (the constant regeneration of the skin), slowly pushing older cells (called daughter cells) up through the other layers of the epidermis until they reach the surface.

Stratum spinosum

Above the stratum basale lies the stratum spinosum. The keratinocytes in this layer have spine-like projections (spinosum means thorn-like or prickly). The keratinocytes are tightly packed here. This tight packing arrangement provides strength and flexibility to the skin.

Stratum granulosum

As the layers move towards the superficial level, the next layer is the stratum granulosum. There are between three and five layers of flattened keratinocytes in this aspect of the skin. These cells contain granules (hence the name stratum granulosum) that form a water-resistant lipid (lamellar granules), protecting the body from losing excess fluid and at the same time guarding against the entry of microbes. The flattening of the cells occurs as a result of pressure from below. The cells here undergo apoptosis; they lose their nucleus prior to dying, becoming compact and brittle as they move slowly up towards the surface; this process is known as keratinisation. The skin is now becoming tougher and stronger, getting ready to perform its protective function. This layer lies below the stratum lucidum.

Stratum lucidum

Lying below the stratum corneum is the stratum lucidum, also known as the clear layer. There are five layers of flat dead cells here; this layer is not found on all aspects of the body, only on areas of thick skin; for example, the heels. The cells have no nucleus and are tightly packed, providing a barrier to fluid loss.

Stratum corneum

This is the outer layer of the epidermis and is made up of a number (about 25) of scale-like layers that are dead and overlap with each other; the chief component of these dead cells is keratin; most of the fluid within these cells has been lost. The cells of the lower layers are composed of approximately 70% water, whereas this layer is made up of 20% fluid (Rizzo, 2006). These cells are very tough and horny. The surface is covered in lipids, which provide a protective barrier; this layer provides structural strength. Constant friction means that this layer is being continuously rubbed off (sloughed off).

There are other important functions associated with this layer, and these are in relation to a physical barrier to light and heat waves, microorganisms, chemicals and injury. The stratum corneum becomes thicker when it is exposed to strong sunlight, providing a barrier to ultraviolet rays. If the ultraviolet rays do reach the dermis, they will destroy the protein content of the skin, and this can lead to cancer of the skin.

558 The dermis

The deepest part of the skin is called the dermis and lies directly below the epidermis; it is predominantly composed of dense connective tissue that contains collagen and elastic fibres. Embedded within the dermis are:

- blood vessels
- nerves
- lymph vessels
- smooth muscles
- sweat glands
- hair follicles
- sebaceous glands.

The elastic system associated with the dermis supports the components above, as well as allowing the skin to flex with movement and to return to its normal shape when at rest. The dermis can be divided into two layers:

- the papillary aspect
- the reticular aspect.

The surface area of the dermis is much increased as a result of the projectile-like papillary layers; the papillary layers connect the dermis to the epidermis. The fingerprints arise from this layer. The deeper aspect of the dermis is attached to the subcutaneous layer. Figure 17.3 shows the epidermis, the dermis and the subcutaneous layer.

The papillary and reticular aspects

This aspect of the dermis, according to Tortora and Derrickson (2012), accounts for one-fifth of the total dermal layer, the superficial layer. The ridges caused by the papillary aspect are also known as friction ridges. These friction ridges can help the hand or foot grasp by increasing friction.

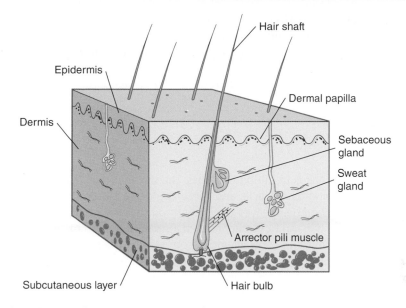

Figure 17.3 Three layers of skin: the epidermis, the dermis and subcutaneous layer. *Source*: Nair and Peate (2009). Reproduced with permission of John Wiley & Sons.

There is a capillary network within the papillary aspect. The dermal papillae also contain Meissner's corpuscles, and these are tactile receptors or touch receptors. The nerve endings here are sensitive to touch, as well as to sensations associated with warmth, coolness, pain and itching.

Attached to the subcutaneous layer are irregular, dense, connective tissues containing fibroblasts and collagen bundles, and coarse elastic fibre forms the reticular aspect. Other sensory receptors are found in this layer, for example, the Pacinian receptors for deep sensory pressure. This layer also contains sweat glands, lymph vessels, smooth muscle and hair follicles; these are called the accessory structures and are discussed next.

The accessory skin structures

The accessory structures are also known as the appendages. The following accessory structures of the skin will be outlined in this section of the chapter:

- hair
- skin glands
- nails.

The hair

Hair can be found on most surfaces of the body apart from the palms, soles and lips; the amount, its distribution, the colour and texture differ depending on location, gender, age and ethnic group. There are different types of hair, and the earliest type is distinctive at approximately the fifth month of foetal development. Known as lanugo, it is a very fine, downy, non-pigmented hair and covers the body of the foetus. Just prior to birth the lanugo of the eyelashes, eyebrows and scalp is shed and replaced by coarse hair, longer in length and heavily pigmented.

The hair can play a part in a person's distinctive appearance. The colour of the hair is influenced by the melanocytes that are found within the hair bulb. A progressive decline in melanin results in hair that is grey in colour. Hair growth is determined by genetic and hormonal factors.

Hairs are growths of dead keratin; each hair is a thread of keratin and is formed from cells at the base of a single follicle (Timby, 2012). There are a number of functions associated with hair:

- sexual
- social
- thermoregulation
- protection.

The primary role of hair is to inhibit heat loss. The whole of the skin surface has hair follicles; every pore is an opening to a follicle, and these are located deep in the dermis on top of the subcutaneous layer. When heat leaves the body through the skin it becomes trapped in the air between the hairs. Each gland has attached to it a small collection of smooth muscle known as the arrector pili. These muscles contract and become erect in response to cold, fear and emotion. The contraction of the muscle can be seen on the skin in the form of 'goose bumps'.

Hair on the head can protect the scalp from the damaging effects of the sun. The hair on the eyelashes and eyebrows guards the eyes from foreign particles entering, and the hair situated in the nostrils helps to protect against the inhalation of foreign material (e.g. insects).

Sebaceous glands accompany the hair follicles, and sebum (a liquid substance) is exuded by these glands, supplying lubrication to the skin and at the same time ensuring that the skin and hair are waterproof as well as removing waste (e.g. old dead cells). Sebum is a slightly acidic substance and has antibacterial and antifungal properties (Page, 2006). The distribution of the sebaceous glands differs. They are foremost on the scalp, face, upper torso and anogenital region, and these glands are at their most active during puberty. Lawton (2006) and Page (2006) point out that the manufacture of sebum is influenced by sex hormone levels. Figure 17.4 shows a pilosebaceous unit; this is made up of the follicle, the hair shaft, the sebaceous gland and the arrector pili.

The base of the onion-shaped bulb – the follicle – contains blood vessels, providing nourishment for the developing hair.

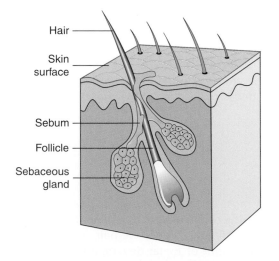

Hair
Skin surface
Sebum
Follicle
Sebaceous gland

Figure 17.4   A pilosebaceous unit. *Source*: Nair and Peate (2009). Reproduced with permission of John Wiley & Sons.

Skin glands

There are a number of glands located within the skin; these can be thought of as mini-organs of the skin, which have a number of functions to fulfil. The sweat glands are coiled tubes composed of epithelial tissue and open out to pores that are located on the skin surface (see Figure 17.5). All of the glands have separate nerve and blood supplies; each secretes a slightly acidic fluid made up of water and salts.

There are two kinds of sweat gland: eccrine and apocrine.

Eccrine glands

Reaction to heat and fear and the production of secretions by the eccrine glands occur in response to activity of the sympathetic nervous system. These types of gland are located all over the body; there are however sites on the body where they are more numerous; for example, the forehead, axillae, soles and palms.

The primary function of the eccrine glands is associated with thermoregulation. This is accomplished through the cooling effect of the evaporation of sweat on the surface of the skin. During hot weather, stress, exercise and pyrexia these glands produce more sweat.

Apocrine glands

The apocrine glands are also coiled; there are not as many of these in comparison with the eccrine glands, and they are found in more localised sites, for example, the pubic and axillary areas, the nipples and perineum. The exact function of the apocrine glands is not fully understood. These glands are not fully active until the person reaches puberty; they are larger, deeper and produce thicker secretions than the eccrine glands. During periods of stress and when in a heightened emotional state these glands produce more sweat.

There are a number of modified types of apocrine glands (specialised types); for example, those that are seen on the eyelids, the cerumen-producing (ear wax) glands of the external auditory canal, and the milk-producing glands of the breasts.

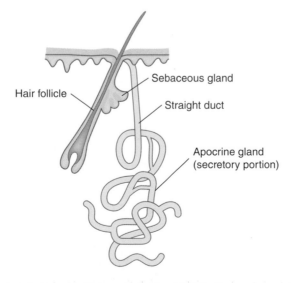

Figure 17.5 A sweat gland. *Source*: Nair and Peate (2009). Reproduced with permission of John Wiley & Sons.

The apocrine glands first develop on the soles and palms and then gradually appear all over the body. It is understood that they secrete pheromones; these are released into the external environment, enabling communication through the sense of smell with other members of the species, and this can provoke a number of reactions, including a sexual arousal reaction. A viscous material is excreted that results in body odour when activated by surface bacteria.

Nails

The nails provide a protective covering for the ends of the fingers and the toes. Nails are tightly packed, dead, hard, keratinised epidermal cells that form a clean, solid covering over the digits (see Figure 17.6).

The horn-like structure of the nails is a result of the concentrated amount of keratin present; there are no nerve endings in nails. Lawton (2006) notes that the nails act as a counterforce to the fingertips, the fingertips have numerous nerve endings, permitting a person to receive information about objects that are touched.

The majority of the nail body is pink, a result of the blood capillaries lying underneath. The white crescent present at the proximal ends of the nail is known as the lunula and is formed by air mixed with keratin matrix. The size of the lunula varies with individuals. The cuticle (also called the eponychium) is stratum corneum extending over the proximal end of the nail body.

Fingernails grow faster than toenails; as a person ages, the growth of nails slows. Nail growth varies, on average they grow at a rate of 0.01 cm per day (1 cm per 100 days). Four to six months is required for fingernails to regrow completely; it takes toenails between 12 and 18 months for total regrowth. There are a number of factors that will influence the growth; for example, the age of the individual, the time of year, the amount of exercise undertaken, as well as hereditary factors (Haneke, 2006). The growth of nails can be delayed by trauma and inflammation; changes in the integrity of the nails can be caused by injury or infection. In some cases, evidence of systemic diseases can be identified by the condition of the nails, for example, chronic cardiopulmonary disease or fungal infection (Timby, 2012).

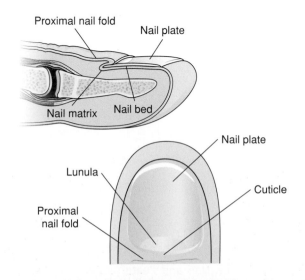

Figure 17.6   The nail. *Source*: Nair and Peate (2009). Reproduced with permission of John Wiley & Sons.

Capillary nail bed refill (also called the nail blanch test)

This test is performed on the nail beds as an indicator of tissue perfusion.

An explanation of the test is given to the patient; the nurse should explain that there will be minor pressure to the bed of the nail and this should not cause discomfort. Nail polish should be removed prior to taking the test.

Gently, pressure is applied to the nail bed until it turns white, indicating that the blood has been forced from the tissue (blanching). Once the tissue has blanched, pressure is removed. While the patient holds their hand above their heart, the nurse measures the time it takes for blood to return to the tissue. Return of blood is indicated by the nail turning back to a pink colour. If there is a good blood flow to the nail bed, a pink colour should return in less than 2 seconds after pressure is removed.

Any abnormalities must be reported to the person in charge. The outcome of the test should be documented in the person's notes.

The functions of the skin

A fundamental understanding of the structure of the skin allows the reader to begin to understand the numerous functions of the skin. These functions include:

- sensation
- thermoregulation
- protection
- excretion and absorption
- synthesis of vitamin D.

Sensation

There are several receptor sites on the skin that have the ability to sense change in the external environment in respect to temperature and pressure; these receptors throughout the skin are made up of a wide and varied range of nerve endings. The messages picked up in the skin are then usually transferred to the brain. Chapter 14 considers the senses in more detail.

Sensations that arise in the skin are known as cutaneous sensations; other sensations are those associated with vibration and tickling and irritations. There are some areas of the body that have more sensory receptors than others; for example, the lips, genitalia and tips of the fingers. The sensation of pain can signify actual or potential tissue injury.

Use of topical steroids

Topical steroids are used in addition to emollients (moisturisers) for treating skin conditions such as eczema. Topical steroids reduce skin inflammation. Topical steroids are creams, ointments and lotions containing steroids; they work by reducing inflammation in the skin. Steroid medicines that reduce inflammation are also known as corticosteroids.

(Continued)

They are generally grouped into four categories, depending on their strength: mild, moderately potent, potent and very potent. There are various brands and types in each category. Hydrocortisone cream 1%, for example, is a commonly used steroid cream and is classified as a mild topical steroid. The greater the strength, the more effect it has on reducing inflammation but the greater the risk of side effects with continued use. Creams are usually best to treat moist or weeping areas of skin. Ointments are usually best to treat areas of skin that are dry or thickened. Lotions may be useful to treat hairy areas, such as the scalp.

It is usual to use the lowest strength topical steroid first. Hydrocortisone 1%, for example, is often used, particularly when treating children. If there is no improvement after 3–7 days, a stronger topical steroid may be prescribed. For severe cases a stronger topical steroid may be prescribed from the outset. Occasionally, two or more preparations of different strengths are used at the same time, for example, a mild steroid for the face and a moderately strong steroid for patches of eczema on the thicker skin of the arms or legs. A very strong topical steroid is often needed for eczema on the palms and soles of the feet of adults as these areas have thick skin.

In most cases, a course of treatment for 7–14 days is enough to clear a flare-up of eczema. In some cases, a longer course is needed. Many people with eczema may require a course of topical steroids to clear a flare-up. The frequency of flare-ups and the number of times a course of topical steroids is needed is dependent on patient needs.

Short courses of topical steroids are usually safe and cause no problems. Problems may arise if topical steroids are used for long periods, or if short courses of stronger steroids are repeated often. Side effects associated with mild topical steroids are uncommon. Side effects from topical steroids can either be local or systemic.

Thermoregulation

The skin has a role to play in homeostasis through thermoregulation, helping to keep the temperature of the body within narrow ranges, adapting and adjusting as a person engages in a number of different activities. Effective thermoregulation is essential for survival; temperature changes can influence alteration in enzyme function and, as such, can impact on the chemical make-up of cells. The skin acts as a temperature regulator through a range of complex and integrated activities.

Changes in the size of blood vessels in the skin can help to regulate temperature. As body temperature rises, so the blood vessels dilate – this is known as vasodilatation; this is a multifaceted bodily defence mechanism that is attempting to get hot blood from the deeper tissues beneath to the surface of the skin for cooling down: the surface of the skin is cooler, as heat radiates away from the body. As this is happening, the sweat glands secrete water onto the surface of the skin. Evaporation occurs and, as a result of this, so too does cooling.

The opposite will occur when the person is in a cold environment. The blood vessels constrict – vasoconstriction – and blood stays closer to the core of the body, preserving heat.

The hair (as previously described) plays an important part in thermoregulation. Pockets of air are trapped in the hair when the arrector pili are stimulated to contract, making the hairs stand up. The trapped air causes insulation to occur, insulating the surrounding environment on the skin from the cooler atmosphere.

Medicines management

Transdermal patches

Transdermal drug administration (skin patch) provides consistent, continuous drug delivery through the skin into the bloodstream. When applying the medication the nurse should follow the manufacturer's instructions and:

- Follow the 'five rights' of drug administration.
- Provide privacy, perform hand hygiene and explain the procedure.
- Use gloves. If applicable, remove the old patch and dispose of it per local policy.
- Select a new site for the patch on a flat surface, such as the chest, back, flank, or upper arm. Rotate sites throughout therapy.
- Ensure the skin is intact, non-irritated and non-irradiated.
- Avoid hairy areas if possible, or shave/cut excessive hair.
- If the site needs to be cleaned prior to application, use only clear water; let the skin dry completely.
- Remove the patch from its pouch and peel half of its protective liner.
- Place the adhesive side on the skin, and then peel off the other half of the liner. Press the skin patch firmly with the palm of your hand for at least 30 seconds, making sure it adheres to the skin, particularly at the edges.
- Remove gloves, and perform hand hygiene.
- Document the medication administration according to policy.

Protection

There are many ways in which the skin protects the body, and a number of these have already been discussed, for example, the skin's ability to protect by the production of melanin against the harmful effects of ultraviolet light. Through its ability to intensify normal cell replacement when needed and the ability to shed dead skin and cause the migration of cells, the skin maintains the integrity of the body. Wound healing is an example of the skin's protective mechanism.

By eliminating waste products through the pores on the skin (and there are over 2 million of these), the skin can help to protect the body from a build-up of poisonous substances. The skin also has the ability to prevent body fluids from escaping, preventing dehydration and helping to regulate the amount of fluid through the content and volume of sweat produced. As a water-proof barrier, the skin can also ensure that harmful fluids in the environment are prevented from entering the body.

Clinical considerations

Dehydration

Many people in a number of care environments are prone to dehydration. The older person is particularly at risk, and your role is to prevent and to identify dehydration and to take actions to remedy any deficits; you will be required to assess, plan, implement and evaluate care.

Undertaking a safe and effective assessment of needs requires you to use a variety of skills: you will be required to observe, measure and ask questions (Lapin, 2014). The skin can tell you much about

(Continued)

the people you care for. You can make a diagnosis of dehydration by observing the skin of those in your care, although this is not and should not be used as the sole diagnostic tool. The classic signs of dehydration in older people include loss of skin recoil (also described as loss of skin turgor), increased thirst, reduced urinary output, tachycardia and hypotension; the person may also be confused.

The skin may lack its normal elasticity and revert to its usual position slowly when gently pinched up into a fold if lack of skin turgor is present. Normally, the skin springs right back into position in a hydrated person. Care must be taken not to harm the person when trying to make an assessment and diagnosis.

Sebum (an oily substance) secreted by the skin contains bacterial chemicals that have the ability to destroy surface bacteria. When sweat is produced, the acidic pH has the potential to hamper the proliferation of bacteria. Phagocytic macrophages present in the dermis have the ability to ingest and destroy viruses and bacteria that have penetrated the surface of the skin.

Excretion and absorption

Some elements of secretion and absorption have already been mentioned in respect to the skin's function in protecting the person. The skin has the ability to excrete substances from the body; sweat is composed of water, sodium, carbon dioxide, ammonia and urea. Jenkins *et al.* (2013) point out that the body (despite its almost waterproof nature) can excrete approximately 400 mL of water daily; those who lead a less active lifestyle will lose less, and a more active person will lose more.

The skin also has the ability to absorb substances from the environment. Materials are absorbed from the external environment into the body cells, and some of these substances when absorbed are toxic, for example, heavy metals such as lead and mercury. There are some therapeutic and non-therapeutic medications that can be absorbed through the skin. A number of fat-soluble vitamins – A, D, E and K – oxygen and carbon dioxide are also absorbed.

Medicines management

Administration of medicines

There are some medications that you may be asked to administer via the skin. These include ointments, lotions, creams and gels. The application of medicines via the skin through an adhesive patch is also used in a number of care areas. All of these medicines are subject to the same rules and regulations associated with the administration of any medicine. Medicines applied to skin are often needed to treat skin conditions, and they are known as topical medications; they are administered externally onto the body as opposed to being ingested or injected.

Lotions are used to protect, soften and soothe and can provide relief from itching. Ointments are oil-based, and body heat causes them to melt after application; often, these medications are used to fight infection or relieve inflamed tissue. Gloves must be used when applying these medicines; they must be applied in thin, even layers unless the prescription states otherwise (Nair, 2014).

Most skin medications are provided for use in tubes; one tube must only be used for one person in order to prevent cross-infection. There are some skin medicines that must be sterile for use; when this is the case, after application, the leftover medication must be discarded.

When you are applying the medication you must take care that you do not increase discomfort by using too much pressure or rubbing areas that are inflamed or causing the person pain.

Synthesis of vitamin D

The skin is actively involved in the production and synthesis of vitamin D. For vitamin D to synthesise effectively, activation of a precursor molecule in the skin by ultraviolet rays in the sunlight (ultraviolet radiation) is required. Enzymes present in the kidneys and liver alter the molecules, producing calcitriol. Calcitriol (a hormone) assists in the absorption of calcium present in food in the intestines into the blood.

Conclusion

The skin is an exceptional organ, and is also known as the integumentary system. There are a variety of diseases or injuries that can easily be observed on the surface of the skin; for example, a skin rash, the presence of jaundice or cyanosis. It is the largest organ in the body in weight and surface area. The skin has the ability to reveal how we feel and what emotional state we may be in: humans blush, sweat and tremble. No other organ in the body is as easily looked over or palpated as the skin; the skin is also more easily exposed to injury, for example, infection and trauma.

This organ is the interface between the external and internal environments. The skin contributes to the homeostasis of the body, and the physical changes noted can point to homeostatic imbalance. The skin is also composed of the accessory structures, for example, the nails and a number of glands; these are sometimes called the appendages.

The skin has the ability to allow a person to experience pleasure, pain and other stimuli from the external environment.

567

Glossary

Absorption   Intake of fluids or other materials by cells of the skin.

Apocrine   A type of gland found in the skin, apocrine glands in the skin and eyelids are sweat glands.

Apoptosis   Death of cell as signalled by the nuclei in a normally functioning cell.

Arrector pili   A microscopic muscle attached to hair follicles.

Calcitonin   A hormone that participates in calcium metabolism.

Cerumen   Ear wax secreted by ceruminous glands.

Collagen   A protein that is the main component of connective tissue.

Cutaneous   Relating to the skin.

Cyanosis   A bluish discolouration of the skin and mucous membranes.

Dermatitis   Inflammation of the skin.

Enzyme   A substance that accelerates chemical reactions.

Erythema   Redness.

Excretion   The process of elimination of waste products from the body.

Extrinsic   Originates externally.

Fascia   A fibrous membrane covering, supporting and separating muscles.

Hair   A thread-like structure produced by the hair follicles emerging from the dermis.

Homeostasis   The ability to maintain a constant internal environment.

Hyperkeratosis　Excess keratins are produced, resulting in thickening of the skin.

Innervation　Related to the supply of nerves.

Integumentary　The external covering of the body, relating to the skin.

Intrinsic　Originates internally.

Keratin　A tough, insoluble protein found in the hair and nails and other keratinised areas of the body.

Keratinise　To convert into keratin.

Lanugo　Fine, downy hair covering the foetus.

Lunula　The moon-shaped white area at the base of nails.

Melanin　Pigment found in some parts of the body, for example, the skin and hair.

Metabolism　A set of chemical reactions in the body required to maintain life.

Nail　A hard plate that is mainly composed of keratin.

Organ　A structure that is composed of two or more kinds of tissue with a specific function and a recognised shape.

Organism　A total living form.

Pathogen　A disease-producing microbe.

Phagocytosis　The act of destroying and ingesting microbes by phagocytes.

Pheromones　Chemicals that trigger an innate behavioural response in another.

Prognosis　A prediction about how a patient's disease will progress.

Proliferation　A rapid and repeated reproduction of new cells.

Pruritus　Itching.

Sebum　An oily substance made of fat and the debris of fat-producing cells produced by the sebaceous glands.

Stratum　A layer.

Tactile　Pertaining to touch.

Thermoreceptor　A sensory receptor that has the ability to detect changes in heat.

Thermoregulation　Ability to regulate temperature.

Vasoconstriction　Reduction in the diameter of blood vessels.

Vasodilatation　Increase in diameter of blood vessels.

References

Colbert, B.J., Ankney, J. and Lee, K.T. (2012) *Anatomy and Physiology for Health Professionals: An Interactive Journey*, 2nd edn. Upper Saddle River, NJ: Pearson.

Haneke, E. (2006) Surgical anatomy of the nail apparatus. *Dermatology Clinic* **24**(3): 291–296.

Jenkins, G.W., Kemnitz, C.P. and Tortora, G.J. (2013) *Anatomy and Physiology: From Science to Life*, 3rd edn. Hoboken, NJ: John Wiley & Sons, Inc.

Lapin, M. (2014) The nursing process. In Peate, I., Wild, K. and Nair, M. (eds), *Nursing Practice, Knowledge and Care*. Oxford: John Wiley & Sons, Ltd; chapter 6, pp. 111–129.

Lawton, S. (2006) Anatomy and function of the skin. Part 4 – appendages. *Nursing Times* **102**(34): 26–27.

LeMone, P. and Burke, K. (2011) *Medical–Surgical Nursing. Critical Thinking in Client Care*, 5th edn. Upper Saddle River, NJ: Pearson.

Lewis, K. and Roberts, R. (2009) Skin integrity. In Mallik, M., Hall, C. and Howard, D. (eds), *Nursing Knowledge and Practice. Foundations for Decision Making*, 3rd edn. Edinburgh: Baillière Tindall; pp. 337–362.

Nair, M. (2014) The principles of medicine administration and pharmacology. In Peate, I., Wild, K. and Nair, M. (eds), *Nursing Practice, Knowledge and Care*. Oxford: John Wiley & Sons, Ltd; chapter 1, pp. 383–408.

Nair, M. and Peate, I. (2009) *Fundamentals of Applied Pathophysiology: An Essential Guide for Nursing Students*. Oxford: John Wiley & Sons, Ltd.

Page, B.E. (2006) Skin disorders. In Alexander, M.F., Fawcett, J.N. and Runciman, P.J. (eds), *Nursing Practice, Hospital and Home: The Adult*, 3rd edn. Edinburgh: Churchill Livingstone; pp. 525–552.

Rizzo D.C. (2006) *Delmar's Fundamentals of Anatomy and Physiology*, 2nd edn. New York: Thomson.

Shier, D., Butler, J. and Lewis, R. (2013) *Hole's Anatomy and Physiology*, 13th edn. Boston, MA: McGraw-Hill.

Timby, B.K. (2012) *Fundamental Nursing Skills and Concepts*, 10th edn. Philadelphia, PA: Lippincott.

Tortora, G.J. and Derrickson, B.H. (2009) *Principles of Anatomy and Physiology*, 12th edn. Hoboken, NJ: John Wiley & Sons, Inc.

Tortora, G.J. and Derrickson, B. (2012) *Principles of Anatomy and Physiology*, 13th edn. Hoboken, NJ: John Wiley & Sons, Inc.

Further reading

British Skin Foundation

http://www.britishskinfoundation.org.uk/SkinInformation/AtoZofSkindisease/Eczema.aspx
This organisation has a number of aims. They fund research to further understanding of the different types of skin disease, fundraise, campaign for change, institutionally and behaviorally for the good of those who have skin disease. They raise awareness and work with the community to encourage people to share their experience with one another so they do not have to suffer in silence.

Psoriasis Association

https://www.psoriasis-association.org.uk
The Psoriasis Association works to help people whose lives are affected by psoriasis and psoriatic arthritis. They do this through research, information and raising awareness.

Cancer Research UK

http://www.cancerresearchuk.org
Cancer Research UK provides information concerning cancer, including statistics. They work in order to beat cancer and develop strategy.

Activities
Multiple choice questions

1. How often (approximately) are the epidermal cells replaced? Every:
   (a) 30 days
   (b) 42 days
   (c) 15 days
   (d) 28 days

2. The skin is thickest on:
   (a) the lips
   (b) the earlobes
   (c) the hands
   (d) the nose

3. What is the name of the pigment that makes skin different colours?
   (a) melaena
   (b) melatonin
   (c) melonite
   (d) melanin

4. Hair follicles are made of:
   (a) sebum
   (b) sweat
   (c) keratin
   (d) muscle

5. The outermost layer of the skin is called:
   (a) the dermis
   (b) the epidermis
   (c) the muscularis
   (d) the subcutaneous

6. The skin does all of these except:
   (a) absorb sugar
   (b) protect the body
   (c) provide the sense of touch
   (d) help to thermoregulate

7. The word used when the skin has no melanin is:
   (a) aged
   (b) exhausted
   (c) eczema
   (d) albino

8. In what aspect of the skin are the cells that divide to form new cells?
   (a) the medulla
   (b) the follicle
   (c) the basal layers of the epidermis
   (d) the sebaceous glands

9. What will eventually happen to the cells of the epidermis?
   (a) they are reabsorbed
   (b) they become scars
   (c) they become infected
   (d) they die off and flake

10. The structures in the dermis that produce oil are called:
    (a) the sebaceous glands
    (b) the Merkel cells
    (c) the Meissner corpuscle
    (d) lamellar granules

True or false

1. Skin is the largest organ of the body.
2. Total healing of body piercings takes between 2 and 4 months.
3. Nerve endings tell the body when things are too hot.
4. Blood vessels bring sweat to the skin.
5. The skin's natural oil is called serum.
6. Goosebumps are caused by the pilomotor reflex.
7. The thickest part of the skin is to be found at the heels.
8. The hypodermis is also known as the epidermis.
9. Innervation relates to blood supply.
10. The Merkel cells are the least numerous of the epidermal cells.

Label the diagram 1

Label the diagram using the following list of words:

Superficial, Deep, Epidermis, Stratum corneum, Stratum lucidum, Stratum granulosum, Stratum spinosum, Stratum basale, Dermis

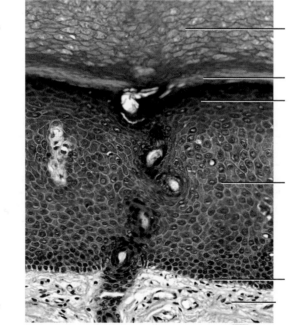

LM 240x

Label the diagram 2

Label the diagram using the following list of words:

Hair, Skin surface, Sebum, Follicle, Sebaceous gland

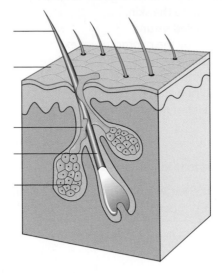

Word search

In the grid below there are 22 words that you will have seen in this chapter. Can you find them all?

S	N	G	S	E	V	R	E	N	C	L	H	T
U	I	L	I	P	R	O	T	C	E	R	R	A
B	N	A	S	S	K	I	N	S	L	U	W	E
C	A	N	R	I	A	H	Q	I	L	O	V	W
U	L	D	E	J	M	K	C	M	T	D	P	S
T	E	B	N	E	A	R	T	R	H	O	B	O
A	M	A	O	L	L	F	E	E	I	O	L	K
N	A	S	M	C	U	P	A	D	N	W	O	C
E	L	A	R	I	N	H	C	T	I	U	O	I
O	E	L	O	T	U	D	U	C	T	P	D	H
U	M	B	H	U	L	A	Y	E	R	S	E	T
S	U	O	E	C	A	B	E	S	O	L	I	P

Subcutaneous, Melanin, Pilosebaceous, Gland, Basal, Hormone, Nerves, Cuticle, Lunula, Itch, Duct, Layer, Epidermis, Skin, Hair, Dermis, Cell, Thin, Odour, Blood, Arrectorpili, Fat

Fill in the blanks

The skin has _____. The outer layer is called the _____ and the inner layer is the _____. The dermal layer contains hair _____, sebaceous _____, small blood vessels called _____ and a pigment called _____ that helps to protect against _____ light. The skin has a number of functions, and one of those functions is related to heat control; this is called _____. The skin can also protect from _____ invading the body. The skin is the _____ organ of the body. When a person becomes hot the blood vessels on the _____ of the skin _____. _____ when released helps a person to _____ down.

The epidermis is situated on the _____ of the skin and is made from _____ of _____ with a basal layer. This layer drives through _____. The newly divided cells gradually _____; this can take about _____. As the cells gradually _____ they become _____, and _____, the outermost layer of _____, is being _____ eroded by _____. The keratin and _____ from the sebaceous _____ assist in making the skin _____.

1–2 months, capillaries, cell division, cells, cool, dermis, die, dilate, epidermis, follicles, glands, largest, layers, melanin, microorganisms, move towards the surface, outside, surface, sweat, thermoregulation, two layers, ultraviolet, flattened, keratin, flat dead cells, continually, friction, oil, glands, waterproof

Find out more

1. What are the names of the touch receptors?
2. Where does nail growth originate?
3. Describe the anatomical and physiological changes that occur when a person experiences goosebumps.
4. Name three potential complications of body piercing.
5. What procedures can be used to remove tattoos?
6. What is needed to activate vitamin D and why?
7. What is the role and function of the arrector pili?
8. Describe what happens to the skin when vasodilatation occurs.
9. Outline the processes involved as skin repairs itself after being damaged.
10. How does the skin and renal system work together to maintain homeostasis?

Conditions

The following is a list of conditions that are associated with the skin. Take some time and write notes about each of the conditions. You may make the notes taken from textbooks or other resources (e.g. people you work with in a clinical area), or you may make the notes as a result of people you have cared for. If you are making notes about people you have cared for you must ensure that you adhere to the rules of confidentiality.

Allergy	
Skin cancer: • Malignant melanoma • Basal cell carcinoma (BCC) • Squamous cell carcinoma (SCC)	
Eczema	
Psoriasis	

Burns:
  • First degree
  • Second degree
  • Full thickness	

Pressure sores	

Normal values

Haematology
Full blood count
Haemoglobin (males) 13.0–18.0 g dL^{-1}
Haemoglobin (females) 11.5–16.5 g dL^{-1}
Haematocrit (males) 0.40–0.52
Haematocrit (females) 0.36–0.47
MCV 80–96 fL
MCH 28–32 pg
MCHC 32–35 g dL^{-1}
White cell count (4–11) $\times$ 10^9 L^{-1}

White cell differential
Neutrophils 1.5–7 $\times$ 10^9 L^{-1}
Lymphocytes 1.5–4 $\times$ 10^9 L^{-1}
Monocytes 0–0.8 $\times$ 10^9 L^{-1}
Eosinophils 0.04–0.4 $\times$ 10^9 L^{-1}
Basophils 0–0.1 $\times$ 10^9 L^{-1}
Platelet count 150–400 $\times$ 10^9 L^{-1}
Reticulocyte count (25–85) $\times$ 10^9 L^{-1} or 0.5–2.4%

Erythrocyte sedimentation rate
Westergren
Under 50 years:
    Males 0–15 mm/1st hour
    Females 0–20 mm/1st hour
Over 50 years:
    Males 0–20 mm/1st hour
    Females 0–30 mm/1st hour

Plasma viscosity 1.50–1.72 mPa s^1 (at 25 °C)

Coagulation screen
Prothrombin time 11.5–15.5 s
International normalised ratio <1.4
Activated partial thromboplastin time 30–40 s
Fibrinogen 1.8–5.4 g L^{-1}
Bleeding time 3–8 min

Fundamentals of Anatomy and Physiology: For Nursing and Healthcare Students, Second Edition. Edited by Ian Peate and Muralitharan Nair.
© 2017 John Wiley & Sons, Ltd. Published 2017 by John Wiley & Sons, Ltd.
Student companion website: www.wileyfundamentalseries.com/anatomy
Instructor companion website: www.wiley.com/go/instructor/anatomy

Coagulation factors
Factors II, V, VII, VIII, IX, X, XI, XII 50–150 IU dL^{-1}
Factor V Leiden Present or not
Von Willebrand factor 45–150 IU dL^{-1}
Von Willebrand factor antigen 50–150 IU dL^{-1}
Protein C 80–135 IU dL^{-1}
Protein S 80–120 IU dL^{-1}
Antithrombin III 80–120 IU dL^{-1}
Activated protein C resistance 2.12–4.0
Fibrin degradation products <100 mg L^{-1}
D-dimer screen <0.5 mg L^{-1}

Haematinics
Serum iron 12–30 µmol L^{-1}
Serum iron-binding capacity 45–75 µmol L^{-1}
Serum ferritin 15–300 µg L^{-1}
Serum transferrin 2.0–4.0 g L^{-1}
Serum B$_{12}$ 160–760 ng L^{-1}
Serum folate 2.0–11.0 µg L^{-1}
Red cell folate 160–640 µg L^{-1}
Serum haptoglobin 0.13–1.63 g L^{-1}

Haemoglobin electrophoresis
Haemoglobin A >95%
Haemoglobin A2 2–3%
Haemoglobin F <2%

Chemistry
Serum sodium 137–144 mmol L^{-1}
Serum potassium 3.5–4.9 mmol L^{-1}
Serum chloride 95–107 mmol L^{-1}
Serum bicarbonate 20–28 mmol L^{-1}
Anion gap 12–16 mmol L^{-1}
Serum urea 2.5–7.5 mmol L^{-1}
Serum creatinine 60–110 µmol L^{-1}
Serum corrected calcium 2.2–2.6 mmol L^{-1}
Serum phosphate 0.8–1.4 mmol L^{-1}
Serum total protein 61–76 g L^{-1}
Serum albumin 37–49 g L^{-1}
Serum total bilirubin 1–22 µmol L^{-1}
Serum conjugated bilirubin 0–3.4 µmol L^{-1}
Serum alanine aminotransferase 5–35 U L^{-1}
Serum aspartate aminotransferase 1–31 U L^{-1}
Serum alkaline phosphatase 45–105 U L^{-1} (over 14 years)
Serum gamma glutamyl transferase 4–35 U L^{-1} (<50 U L^{-1} in males)
Serum lactate dehydrogenase 10–250 U L^{-1}
Serum creatine kinase (males) 24–195 U L^{-1}

Serum creatine kinase (females) 24–170 U L^{-1}
Creatine kinase MB fraction <5%
Serum troponin I 0-0.4 μg L^{-1}
Serum troponin T 0–0.1 μg L^{-1}
Serum copper 12–26 μmol L^{-1}
Serum caeruloplasmin 200–350 mg L^{-1}
Serum aluminium 0-10 μg L^{-1}
Serum magnesium 0.75–1.05 mmol L^{-1}
Serum zinc 6–25 μmol L^{-1}
Serum urate (males) 0.23–0.46 mmol L^{-1}
Serum urate (females) 0.19–0.36 mmol L^{-1}
Plasma lactate 0.6–1.8 mmol L^{-1}
Plasma ammonia 12–55 μmol L^{-1}
Serum angiotensin-converting enzyme 25–82 U L^{-1}
Fasting plasma glucose 3.0–6.0 mmol L^{-1}
Haemoglobin A1 C 3.8–6.4%
Fructosamine <285 μmo L^{-1}
Serum amylase 60–180 U L^{-1}
Plasma osmolality 278–305 mosmol kg^{-1}

Urine
Albumin/creatinine ratio (untimed specimen) <3.5 mg mmol^{-1} (males)
 <2.5 mg mmol^{-1} (females)

Lipids and lipoproteins
Target levels will vary depending on the patient's overall cardiovascular risk assessment
Serum cholesterol <5.2 mmol L^{-1}
Serum LDL cholesterol <3.36 mmol L^{-1}
Serum HDL cholesterol >1.55 mmol L^{-1}
Fasting serum triglyceride 0.45–1.69 mmol L^{-1}

Blood gases (breathing air at sea level)
Blood H$^+$ 35–45 nmol L^{-1}
pH 7.36–7.44
PaO$_2$ 11.3–12.6 kPa
PaCO$_2$ 4.7–6.0 kPa
Base excess ±2 mmol L^{-1}

Carboxyhaemoglobin
Non-smoker <2%
Smoker 3–15%

Immunology/rheumatology
Complement C3 65–190 mg dL^{-1}
Complement C4 15–50 mg dL^{-1}
Total haemolytic (CH50) 150–250 U L^{-1}
Serum C-reactive protein <10 mg L^{-1}

Serum immunoglobulins

IgG 6.0–13.0 g L^{-1}
IgA 0.8–3.0 g L^{-1}
IgM 0.4–2.5 g L^{-1}
IgE <120 kU L^{-1}
Serum β_2-microglobulin <3 mg L^{-1}

Cerebrospinal fluid

Opening pressure 50–180 mmH_2O
Total protein 0.15–0.45 g L^{-1}
Albumin 0.066–0.442 g L^{-1}
Chloride 116–122 mmol L^{-1}
Glucose 3.3–4.4 mmol L^{-1}
Lactate 1–2 mmol L^{-1}
Cell count ≤5 mL^{-1}

Differential

Lymphocytes 60–70%
Monocytes 30–50%
Neutrophils None
IgG/ALB ≤0.26
IgG index ≤0.88

Urine

Glomerular filtration rate 70–140 mL min^{-1}
Total protein <0.2g/24 h
Albumin <30 mg/24 h
Calcium 2.5–7.5 mmol/24 h
Urobilinogen 1.7–5.9 µmol/24 h
Coproporphyrin <300 nmol/24 h
Uroporphyrin 6–24 nmol/24 h
δ-Aminolevulinate 8–53 µmol/24 h
5-Hydroxyindoleacetic acid 10–47 µmol/24h
Osmolality 350–1000 mosmol kg^{-1}

Faeces

Nitrogen 70–140 mmol/24 h
Urobilinogen 50–500 µmol/24 h
Fat (on normal diet) <7 g/24 h

Answers

Chapter 1

Multiple choice questions
1. (c); **2.** (b); **3.** (d); **4.** (b); **5.** (a); **6.** (a); **7.** (c); **8.** (d); **9.** (d); **10.** (b)

True or false
1. False – an ion is an atom with a positive or negative electrical charge
2. True
3. True
4. True
5. False – it is a chemical property
6. False – it is a compound of sodium and chloride
7. False – following a chemical reaction, there are the same number of atoms/molecules, but in different combinations
8. True
9. False – lipids are organic substances
10. True

Fill in the blanks 1
Homeostasis is the body's attempts to maintain a stable internal environment. To do this, it has to be able to change in response to both external (e.g. environmental temperature) and internal stimuli (e.g. blood pressure changes). Various mechanisms are utilised by the body to maintain homeostasis, including receptors to sense external and internal environmental changes. Receptors then send out messages to the homeostatic control centre, which determines the particular value – for example the correct temperature or blood pressure required for the essential functioning of the body. This then sends a message to the body's effectors, which, in turn, cause the body's internal environment to counteract the effects of the various stimuli/changes.

Fundamentals of Anatomy and Physiology: For Nursing and Healthcare Students, Second Edition. Edited by Ian Peate and Muralitharan Nair.
© 2017 John Wiley & Sons, Ltd. Published 2017 by John Wiley & Sons, Ltd.
Student companion website: www.wileyfundamentalseries.com/anatomy
Instructor companion website: www.wiley.com/go/instructor/anatomy

Word search 1

A	C	O	Z	E	J	I	R	O	N	K	P	A
N	A	J	O	Z	Y	O	F	Q	I	U	R	N
A	T	O	M	I	P	N	E	U	T	R	O	N
T	O	J	M	O	R	T	I	O	N	B	T	L
O	C	H	E	R	L	S	N	T	R	H	O	E
M	A	Y	B	G	S	E	D	A	H	A	N	Y
Y	E	D	A	A	H	T	C	Q	O	J	E	K
E	N	R	Y	N	E	X	T	U	R	N	I	P
P	R	O	T	E	I	N	S	A	L	T	C	H
S	I	G	P	L	I	P	I	D	F	E	V	L
U	V	E	B	L	Y	I	F	R	U	K	L	O
Z	E	N	Y	E	L	E	M	E	N	T	O	X
E	S	S	T	I	M	A	B	L	E	Q	U	E

Fill in the blanks 2

An ion is an atom or molecule in which the total number of electrons is not equal to the total number of protons. Hence the atom or molecule has a net positive or negative electrical charge.

Word search 2

P	O	L	A	R	B	O	N	D	S	U	Z	K
P	H	R	E	M	O	Z	I	A	X	Y	N	X
S	A	Y	G	O	N	I	L	A	K	L	A	V
T	M	A	S	S	T	T	Q	U	E	R	G	H
C	H	R	M	I	G	M	E	R	C	U	R	Y
A	O	V	O	U	O	H	Z	W	R	D	O	D
L	O	V	T	X	E	L	E	I	P	U	S	R
C	S	I	A	O	R	S	O	D	I	U	M	O
I	N	F	V	L	T	I	O	G	L	X	A	G
U	Q	A	Y	Z	E	I	N	L	Y	A	Z	E
M	E	T	A	L	X	N	Z	A	S	I	O	N
P	W	S	R	E	A	C	T	I	O	N	G	H
Q	U	E	R	T	Y	U	I	O	P	L	K	J

Chapter 2

Multiple choice questions

1. (b); **2.** (d); **3.** (b); **4.** (d); **5.** (a); **6.** (c); **7.** (b); **8.** (a); **9.** (a); **10.** (a).

True or false

1. False
2. False
3. True
4. True
5. True
6. False
7. True
8. False
9. False
10. False

Circle the word or term

1. Centrioles
2. Mitochondria
3. Lysosomes
4. Smooth ER
5. Cilia

Word search

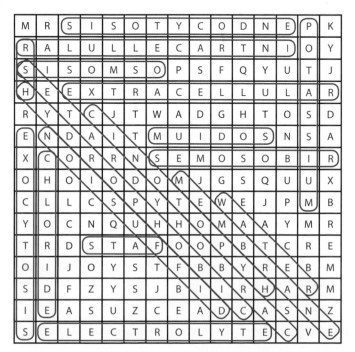

Chemical symbols

Potassium	K^+
Sodium	Na^+
Bicarbonate	HCO_3^-
Chloride	Cl^-
Organic phosphate	PO_4^{3-}
Sulfate	SO_4^{2-}
Calcium	Ca^{2+}

Fill in the blanks 1

Plasma is the only major fluid compartment that exists as a real fluid collection all in one location. It differs from interstitial fluid (ISF) in its much higher protein content and its high bulk flow (transport function). Blood contains suspended red and white cells so plasma has been called the ISF of the blood. The fluid compartment called the blood volume is interesting in that it is a composite compartment containing ECF (plasma) and ICF (red cell fluid).

Fill in the blanks 2

Electrolytes are vital to one's health and survival. They are positively and negatively charged particles (ions) that are formed when mineral or other salts dissolve and separate (dissociate) in water. Since electrolytes carry a charge, they can conduct electrical current in water, which itself in its pure form is a poor conductor of electricity. This characteristic of electrolytes is important because the current enables electrolytes to regulate how and where fluids are distributed throughout the body, which includes keeping water from floating freely across cell membranes.

Chapter 3

Multiple choice questions

1. (a); **2.** (c); **3.** (b); **4.** (b); **5.** (d); **6.** (b); **7.** (d); **8.** (c); **9.** (b); **10.** (c).

True or false

1. False – it is DNA that is carried within a chromosome
2. True
3. True
4. False – two chromatids are joined by a centromere, not the other way round
5. True
6. False – the synthesis of amino acids/protein is stopped by a termination codon
7. False – Huntington's disease is an example of autosomal dominant inheritance
8. False – **generally**, autosomal recessive disorders are more serious than autosomal dominant disorders (although there are some exceptions)
9. True
10. False – **statistically** there would be a 50% chance of having an affected child

Fill in the blanks

During protein synthesis all the genetic instructions for making proteins are found in DNA. The first stage of protein production involves the transcription of this information into RNA, which, in turn, is translated into a corresponding sequence of amino acids that join together to form protein molecules.

Word search

D	Y	N	A	S	T	P	O	B	J	E	C	T
T	N	U	X	V	Z	R	U	Q	M	N	V	E
L	R	A	M	I	N	O	A	C	I	D	W	L
P	R	A	E	D	I	T	R	O	T	O	R	O
N	T	Z	N	C	O	E	T	G	O	S	T	P
P	L	Y	D	S	N	I	E	V	S	C	I	H
T	W	Y	E	Y	L	N	R	G	I	O	R	A
C	E	L	L	T	E	A	R	S	S	P	E	S
N	H	Y	C	O	D	A	T	E	A	E	I	E
P	G	R	E	C	E	S	S	I	V	E	R	N
L	N	V	N	T	V	S	O	Z	O	X	R	G
A	Q	U	A	E	S	A	H	P	A	N	A	T
V	L	P	R	T	Y	O	I	Y	J	W	C	Y

Chapter 4

Multiple choice questions

1. (c); **2.** (a); **3.** (b); **4.** (a); **5.** (b); **6.** (c); **7.** (a); **8.** (c); **9.** (b); **10.** (a).

True or false

1. True
2. False
3. False
4. True
5. True
6. True
7. False
8. False
9. True
10. True

Crossword

Across

1. Simple cuboidal
3. Reticular
5. Osteoblasts
8. Ground substance
11. Elastic
13. Hyaline
14. Dense
15. Collagen

Down

1. Skeletal
2. Pseudostratified
4. Adipose
6. Stratified
7. Mucous
9. Serous
10. Cartilage
12. Loose

Word search

A	C	N	Q	C	E	R	D	O	O	L	B	T	E	Y
P	O	O	O	I	A	D	I	P	O	S	E	L	U	B
L	N	I	L	K	J	R	H	G	F	D	C	S	O	E
M	N	T	N	L	B	V	T	C	X	S	Z	N	A	L
Q	E	P	W	E	A	R	T	I	U	Y	E	U	I	A
R	C	R	J	K	L	G	E	M	L	P	O	M	E	S
A	T	O	H	G	F	N	E	D	S	A	U	A	N	T
L	I	S	B	V	I	C	S	N	X	I	G	Z	A	I
U	V	B	N	L	M	E	A	Q	L	Q	W	E	R	C
D	E	A	A	I	R	S	U	E	U	Y	T	R	B	E
N	O	Y	P	B	U	L	H	K	J	A	H	G	M	F
A	H	B	I	O	V	T	C	X	Z	A	M	S	E	D
L	N	F	R	M	I	Q	W	E	R	T	Y	O	M	U
G	L	E	P	P	A	R	E	O	L	A	R	O	U	I
J	S	H	E	G	L	A	D	I	O	B	U	C	F	S

Fill in the blanks

Muscle tissue contains long muscle fibres whose primary function is to generate force. It is found where there is a need for movement and maintenance of posture. Skeletal muscle is found adjacent to the skeleton and is said to be striated or stripy in appearance and voluntary in action. Smooth muscle, on the other hand, is involuntary and non-striated. As its name suggests, cardiac muscle is only found in the heart and provides the driving force of contraction.

Chapter 5

Multiple choice questions

1. (b); **2.** (c); **3.** (c); **4.** (d); **5.** (a); **6.** (d); **7.** (a); **8.** (d); **9.** (c); **10.** (b).

True or false

1. True
2. False
3. True
4. False
5. False
6. False
7. False
8. False
9. True
10. False

Word search

O	P	C	H	T	S	A	L	B	O	E	T	S	O	W	J
N	E	A	R	B	E	T	R	E	V	R	F	I	T	O	I
O	L	T	D	I	O	M	H	T	E	O	P	P	I	P	E
T	A	A	K	L	U	C	O	B	O	N	E	N	O	A	R
E	S	L	I	N	S	Y	S	R	S	C	T	Y	D	T	U
L	R	F	R	C	R	O	O	S	S	E	O	U	S	E	T
E	A	E	P	I	P	H	Y	S	E	A	L	A	N	L	U
K	T	I	B	I	A	B	M	L	O	M	A	X	E	L	S
S	O	S	T	E	O	C	L	A	S	T	N	D	I	A	O

Fill in the blanks

The humerus is the largest and longest bone of the upper arm. The head of the humerus is rounded and joined to the rest of the bone by the anatomic neck. The upper aspect of the bone has two prominences, the greater and lesser tubercles. The ulna is longer than the radius. The bones of the wrists are called the carpals; they are arranged in two rows of four each. The palms of the hands are made up of the five metatarsal bones. Metatarsals are small long bones; they each have a shaft and a head. The thumb has only a proximal and distal phalanx.

Match the bones to the shape

1. B, D, G
2. F
3. A, H, C, E

Chapter 6

Multiple choice questions

1. (a); **2.** (d); **3.** (c); **4.** (b); **5.** (a); **6.** (b); **7.** (d); **8.** (b); **9.** (d); **10.** (c).

True or false

1. False
2. False
3. False
4. True
5. True
6. True
7. False
8. True
9. False
10. True

Crossword

Across

1. Thick and thin filaments
3. Transverse tubules
4. Pyruvic acid
5. Generate heat
6. Insertion
8. Abduction
9. Myoglobin
10. Decrease

Down

2. Aerobic respiration
7. Rhomboid

Chapter 7

Multiple choice questions

1. (a); **2.** (a); **3.** (c); **4.** (d); **5.** (b); **6.** (a); **7.** (a); **8.** (b); **9.** (b); **10.** (c).

True or false

1. False
2. False
3. True
4. True
5. True
6. False

7. False
8. False
9. True
10. False

Blood groups

Blood type	Antigens	Agglutinins	Can donate to	Can receive from
Type A	Antigen A	Anti-B	A, AB	A, O
Type B	Antigen B	Anti-A	B, AB	B, O
Type AB	Antigen A	None	AB	A, B, AB, O
	Antigen B			
Type O	None	Anti-A	A, B, AB, O	O
		Anti-B		

Word search

P	X	D	M	H	S	Q	S	S	L	O	H	T	K	E
N	G	A	I	A	E	D	S	E	Y	S	A	P	M	Y
O	H	V	O	R	T	L	N	I	M	T	E	S	P	L
I	L	K	A	R	Y	I	I	R	P	E	M	L	L	M
S	M	S	V	R	C	H	E	A	H	L	O	F	A	N
U	N	O	S	E	O	P	V	L	O	E	G	L	S	J
F	S	G	I	T	N	O	V	L	I	T	L	E	M	U
F	E	N	S	Y	O	S	I	I	D	A	O	U	A	N
I	V	I	O	C	M	A	S	P	N	L	B	C	Y	W
D	L	T	M	O	Q	B	C	A	L	P	I	O	N	O
D	A	T	S	H	U	B	O	C	B	S	N	C	R	Y
O	V	O	O	P	S	T	S	O	C	R	B	Y	J	X
O	N	L	Y	M	E	F	I	D	R	A	M	T	C	U
L	H	C	H	Y	V	F	T	V	D	Q	C	E	A	O
B	R	M	L	L	V	O	Y	X	Z	S	F	S	R	F

Fill in the blanks

Blood

In adults, the most active bone marrow is found in the pelvic, shoulder bones, vertebrae, ribs, breastbone and skull. Immature blood cells found within the bone marrow are called stem cells. Stem cells can also be found in smaller amounts in the bloodstream. These are called peripheral blood stem cells.

The process of blood cell development is called haematopoiesis. In the earliest stage of blood cell development, stem cells begin to develop either along the lymphoid cell line or the myeloid cell line. In both cell lines the stem cells become blasts, which are still immature cells. During the last stage of cell development the blasts mature into three types of blood cells, called red blood cells, platelets and white blood cells.

Blood vessels

Arteries carry blood away from the heart to other organs. They can vary in size. The largest arteries have special elastic fibres in their walls. This helps to complement the work of the heart, by squeezing blood along when heart muscle relaxes. Arteries also respond to signals from our nervous system, either constricting or dilating.

Arterioles are the smallest arteries in the body. They deliver blood to capillaries. Arterioles are also capable of constricting or dilating and, by doing this, they control how much blood enters the capillaries.

Capillaries are tiny vessels that connect arterioles to venules. They have very thin walls that allow nutrients from the blood to pass into the body tissues. Waste products from body tissues can also pass into the capillaries. For this reason, capillaries are known as exchange vessels.

Lymphatic

The lymphatic system is like the blood circulation – the vessels branch through all parts of the body like the arteries and veins that carry blood. But the lymphatic system vessels are much thinner and carry a colourless liquid called lymph. Lymph contains a high number of lymphocytes. Plasma leaks out of the capillaries to surround and bathe the body tissues. This then drains into the lymph vessels.

Chapter 8

Multiple choice questions

1. (b); **2.** (c); **3.** (b); **4.** (c); **5.** (d); **6.** (a); **7.** (d); **8.** (d); **9.** (b); **10.** (b).

True or false

1. True
2. True
3. True
4. False
5. False
6. False

7. True
8. True
9. True
10. False

Word search

S	Z	Q	P	U	L	L	E	A	V	K	M	W	V	J	I	F	J	O	Q
I	H	R	E	F	R	A	C	T	O	R	Y	H	H	G	P	J	P	K	F
N	S	P	R	O	N	K	I	J	P	M	O	T	B	T	X	I	U	Y	L
O	R	T	I	O	M	R	H	I	L	U	F	J	D	R	F	G	L	K	A
A	W	R	C	N	O	V	D	C	A	O	I	U	H	I	K	Z	M	F	C
T	N	V	A	L	V	E	V	Y	A	D	B	I	M	C	N	D	O	M	L
R	G	F	R	G	E	N	D	O	C	A	R	D	I	U	M	G	N	M	D
I	Q	M	D	E	R	O	N	F	C	S	I	J	T	S	F	F	A	H	F
A	C	P	I	B	E	U	E	H	B	T	L	C	R	P	W	O	R	A	P
L	I	M	U	F	M	S	R	J	E	U	D	E	A	I	S	B	Y	I	S
X	S	P	M	G	O	D	P	R	N	K	M	J	L	D	M	F	T	R	A
A	Q	J	U	E	C	J	I	A	P	I	T	E	R	U	Y	U	X	U	R
C	L	T	C	F	R	S	S	N	A	Z	K	N	I	A	O	R	T	I	C
Y	T	D	E	Q	A	I	S	U	V	Y	T	R	W	G	C	N	H	K	O
A	S	I	N	U	S	Q	I	L	U	V	T	M	U	P	Y	X	O	K	L
B	C	B	K	O	S	R	C	I	R	A	C	U	S	P	T	B	R	T	E
Z	R	X	N	K	R	T	W	M	P	J	O	T	J	B	E	S	A	L	M
G	L	E	H	O	L	E	D	E	T	J	L	P	S	P	S	Q	C	B	M
B	T	P	O	R	D	I	A	S	T	O	L	E	Y	P	R	S	I	D	A
S	T	A	R	U	V	E	S	G	Z	Y	C	S	A	I	T	L	C	C	A

Fill in the blanks

Normal electrical excitation/distribution begins in the sinoatrial node, which is located in the right atrium, and is rapidly transmitted across the atria by fast pathways. The impulse is transmitted to the atrioventricular (AV) node where further transmission is delayed for approximately 0.1 seconds. This ensures that the atria have completely contracted before ventricular contraction is initiated. Once the impulse has been 'held' in the AV node it is then transmitted down the bundle of His (AV bundle) to the fast pathways of the two bundle branches. The bundles then divide into the smaller and smaller branches of the Purkinje system which transmits the impulses to the muscles of the ventricles.

Chapter 9

Multiple choice questions

1. (d); **2.** (b); **3.** (b); **4.** (c); **5.** (d); **6.** (a); **7.** (d); **8.** (a); **9.** (d); **10.** (a).

True or false

1. True
2. False
3. False
4. True
5. True
6. False
7. True
8. False
9. False
10. False

Crossword

Across	Down
1. Ascorbic acid	1. Amino acid
5. Incisor	2. Chyme
9. Elimination	3. Peristalsis
10. Amylase	4. Lysozyme
14. Lipid	6. Mastication
15. Mucosa	7. Parotid
17. Vitamin	8. Jejunum
18. Anus	11. Caecum
19. Pharynx	12. Pepsin
	13. Bile
	16. Gastrin

Fill in the blanks

The digestive system is also known as the alimentary canal. The action of enzymes on ingested food is known as chemical digestion. The churning of ingested food by the muscular activity of the digestive system is known as mechanical digestion. The digestive system is protected from invading pathogens by the presence of lysozyme in salivary amylase and hydrochloric acid produced by the parietal cells of the stomach.

Digestion of protein begins in the stomach. Amylase is the name of the enzyme involved in the breakdown of carbohydrates. Fat digestion relies on the presence of bile and lipase.

Chapter 10

Multiple choice questions

1. (c); **2.** (c); **3.** (a); **4.** (d); **5.** (a); **6.** (b); **7.** (d); **8.** (a); **9.** (c); **10.** (a).

True or false

1. True
2. True
3. False
4. True
5. False
6. True
7. False
8. False
9. False
10. False

Crossword

Across	Down
5. Aldosterone	**1.** Oliguria
6. Filtration	**2.** Renin
7. Urethra	**3.** Cystitis
11. Adrenal	**4.** Cystoscopy
12. ADH	**8.** Ureter
13. Urea	**9.** Capsule
14. Nephron	**10.** Bladder

Word search

592

R	K	N	F	U	L	A	M	I	X	O	R	P	O	E
E	E	M	U	R	E	T	E	R	N	K	O	M	U	J
N	O	N	O	I	T	A	R	T	L	I	F	N	R	X
I	R	R	O	Z	Y	U	I	Z	Q	J	N	N	C	G
N	F	E	O	R	D	Y	R	Z	A	B	L	I	R	C
S	P	I	N	V	E	D	R	E	L	E	W	L	E	Y
E	B	Y	Y	A	P	T	J	K	T	C	F	U	A	S
C	K	Z	V	K	L	G	S	I	C	H	W	N	T	T
R	I	I	L	U	R	E	M	O	L	G	R	I	I	I
E	D	I	O	G	B	L	A	D	D	E	R	A	N	T
T	N	E	P	H	R	O	N	J	T	L	G	T	I	I
I	E	I	N	F	E	C	T	I	O	N	A	R	N	S
O	Y	T	U	B	U	L	E	M	S	T	A	F	E	L
N	L	A	T	S	I	D	G	M	I	K	K	X	G	D
D	M	A	I	R	U	T	A	M	E	A	H	T	Q	N

Fill in the blanks

The kidneys, ureters, urinary bladder and the ureters form the normal urinary system. The kidneys filter the blood in order to remove the wastes and excess fluids from the body and form the urine. This travels to the urinary bladder via the ureters. The urinary bladder stores the urine until it is passed out of the body via the urethra.

Within the kidneys are nearly a million small filtering units called glomeruli. Blood flows through tiny tubes and intricate networks of blood vessels within the kidneys to the glomeruli in order to undergo the filtration process.

The function of the kidneys is, among other things, to get rid of the waste products that result from the body's metabolism. One of the major by-products of the metabolism of protein (muscle) is urea. The kidneys remove the waste products by extracting them from the blood and sending them along the ureter to the bladder, from where they are excreted in the urine. If the kidney function fails, the waste products accumulate in the blood and the body. The term for this build-up is azotaemia.

Chapter 11

Multiple choice questions

1. (c); **2.** (b); **3.** (a); **4.** (c); **5.** (a); **6.** (d); **7.** (d); **8.** (a); **9.** (d); **10.** (c).

True or false

1. True
2. False
3. True
4. True
5. True
6. False
7. False
8. True
9. False
10. False

Crossword

Across	Down
1. External respiration	**1.** Expiration
5. Alveoli	**2.** Trachea
7. Tidal volume	**3.** Surfactant
9. Hypoxia	**4.** Oxygen
10. Carbon dioxide	**6.** Vital capacity
13. Larynx	**8.** Lobes
14. Haemoglobin	**9.** Hypoxaemia
15. Fick's	**11.** Dyspnoea
16. Tachypnoea	**12.** Pleura

Word Search

```
G  N  S  T  I  M  H  A  A  N  I  R  A  C  S
A  O  D  P  V  J  U  X  R  C  W  K  L  A  M
Z  I  O  I  I  Y  L  T  I  U  K  L  O  R  M
Q  T  X  O  F  R  I  A  U  Y  E  C  V  B  G
W  A  Y  O  C  F  O  D  R  P  X  L  E  O  B
S  L  G  U  P  H  U  M  G  Y  S  B  P  N  A
G  I  E  T  R  Y  N  S  E  W  N  D  O  D  I
N  T  N  E  R  F  H  M  I  T  K  X  L  I  M
U  N  E  E  D  X  I  D  T  O  R  D  Q  O  E
L  E  N  R  Y  L  F  G  H  J  N  Y  H  X  A
A  V  B  R  O  N  C  H  I  O  L  E  S  I  X
Z  R  Y  E  I  T  R  A  C  H  E  A  H  D  O
X  V  V  O  R  O  P  H  A  R  Y  N  X  E  P
R  L  S  U  R  F  A  C  T  A  N  T  U  M  Y
A  D  N  O  I  T  A  R  I  P  S  E  R  B  H
```

Fill in the blanks

Lungs are divided into distinct regions called lobes. The heart sits in a space called the cardiac notch, which sits between both lungs. Each lung is protected by two membranes, called the visceral and parietal pleura. The lower respiratory tract starts at the trachea. At a point called the carina the airways subdivide into right and left primary bronchi, which divide again into secondary bronchi. The next branch of the bronchial tree is the tertiary bronchi, which all lead to a network of bronchioles. Eventually airways terminate at a terminal bronchiole. From this point forward this region of the airways is referred to as a lobule. Within this region the airways subdivide further into respiratory bronchioles, alveolar ducts and alveoli.

Chapter 12

Multiple choice questions

1. (b); **2.** (a); **3.** (a); **4.** (d); **5.** (b); **6.** (c); **7.** (d); **8.** (a); **9.** (d); **10.** (b).

True or false

1. False
2. False
3. False
4. False

5. True
6. False
7. True
8. False
9. False
10. False

Word search

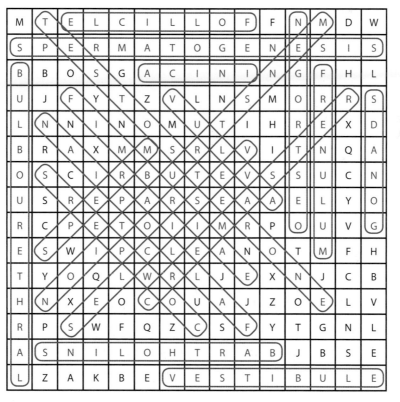

Fill in the blanks 1

Menstruation, or period, is normal vaginal bleeding that occurs as part of a woman's monthly cycle. Every month, the woman's body prepares for pregnancy. If no pregnancy occurs, the uterus (also known as the womb), sheds its lining. The menstrual blood is partly _____ and partly _____ _____ from inside the uterus. It passes outside of the body through the vagina.

Fill in the blanks 2

Menopause is a phase of life in women that signifies the end of their reproductive period. It signifies the end of menstruation. This means that the ovaries of the women stop producing an egg every four weeks and there is no monthly period. Beyond menopause a woman will no longer be able to have children.

Chapter 13

Multiple choice questions

1. (c); **2.** (a); **3.** (c); **4.** (a); **5.** (c); **6.** (c); **7.** (c); **8.** (a); **9.** (b); **10.** (b, c).

True or false

1. True
2. False
3. True
4. False
5. False
6. True
7. True
8. False
9. False
10. True

Crossword

Across

2. Neurone
4. Vagus
6. Optic
7. Arachnoid mater
9. Dura mater
10. Astrocyte
11. Pituitary gland
13. Olfactory
17. Involuntary
18. Medulla
19. Brain

Down

1. Somatic nervous system
3. Efferent
5. Acetylcholine
8. Hypothalamus
11. Potassium
12. Afferent
14. Pia mater
15. Microglia
16. Sodium

Chapter 14

Multiple choice questions

1. (a); **2.** (c); **3.** (a); **4.** (d); **5.** (b); **6.** (d); **7.** (c); **8.** (b); **9.** (b); **10.** (d).

True or false

1. False
2. True
3. True

4. False
5. False
6. True
7. True
8. False
9. True
10. True

Word search

L	K	N	Y	N	Z	A	P	H	O	T	O	R	E	C	E	P	T	O	R
Q	A	Z	Z	M	U	M	G	N	T	G	J	X	E	O	R	O	L	P	O
S	A	C	C	U	L	E	W	H	R	Q	L	K	W	C	N	V	D	T	S
C	Y	V	R	Z	O	R	X	L	I	U	A	P	G	H	B	H	L	I	A
A	V	B	A	I	N	O	C	O	T	A	T	S	R	L	Y	J	E	C	N
M	H	K	T	G	M	P	S	A	B	Y	C	Z	X	E	Z	U	O	X	O
M	S	Q	O	S	T	A	P	E	S	X	S	J	S	A	T	M	V	N	S
L	A	S	L	C	N	D	L	A	O	A	H	R	I	B	I	G	O	R	M
G	I	M	N	L	O	F	C	K	M	G	O	D	O	R	A	N	T	J	I
V	B	U	Q	E	S	H	I	S	N	T	K	G	I	A	V	T	Y	I	A
N	R	I	Y	R	M	K	Y	P	P	A	P	I	L	L	A	E	M	D	I
F	O	L	I	A	T	E	N	E	O	W	C	K	L	K	I	Q	P	A	L
O	B	E	P	U	O	N	C	H	O	R	O	I	D	I	A	D	A	B	P
V	M	H	U	D	T	E	A	Z	B	W	S	N	R	N	C	F	N	A	A
E	A	T	F	W	R	B	P	O	O	X	E	O	L	M	J	K	I	E	B
A	H	I	W	O	Y	I	D	L	G	G	B	C	F	F	A	D	C	S	F
O	G	P	M	A	O	J	K	I	N	O	C	I	L	I	U	M	B	N	V
S	T	E	S	T	P	Z	E	J	H	B	J	X	H	D	B	E	L	J	B
N	H	E	M	R	O	F	I	R	B	I	R	C	B	Q	G	M	Q	P	T
C	I	L	I	A	W	Z	A	H	U	S	O	R	C	X	I	T	X	S	T

Crossword

Across

1. Semicircular canals

5. Ossicles

6. Stapes

Down

1. Statoconia

2. Crista

3. Neural tunic

7. Lens

9. Conjunctiva

11. Ampulla

12. Cochlea

13. Iris

14. Perilymph

15. Vitreous humour

16. Central adaptation

4. Sclera

7. Ligaments

8. Vallate papillae

9. Cornea

10. Tympanic membrane

Fill in the blanks

Sound waves entering the external auditory canal travel along until they reach the tympanic membrane (ear drum), a thin translucent connective tissue membrane covered by skin on its external surface and internally by mucosa, and shaped like a flattened cone protruding into the middle ear. Sound waves that reach the tympanic membrane make it vibrate and this vibration is transmitted to the bones of the middle ear.

Look at the diagrams

1. (c); **2.** (b); **3.** (a); **4.** (d)

Chapter 15

Multiple choice questions

1. (a); **2.** (b); **3.** (d); **4.** (d); **5.** (b); **6.** (c); **7.** (b); **8.** (b); **9.** (b); **10.** (b).

True or false

1. False
2. True
3. True
4. False
5. True
6. True
7. True
8. False
9. True
10. False

Word search

B	Z	S	X	T	U	E	F	I	L	F	L	A	H	C	P	N	J	H	H
A	J	B	B	G	W	J	T	O	F	K	G	Y	P	H	H	E	O	G	C
G	L	Y	C	O	G	E	N	G	U	O	L	H	S	T	U	U	Q	R	R
L	O	J	I	E	S	Z	O	X	C	N	A	C	S	H	R	R	O	A	O
U	Q	R	V	W	E	X	O	C	R	I	N	E	A	Q	D	A	L	V	A
C	S	A	U	S	N	N	T	M	Y	M	D	N	T	D	G	L	I	E	A
A	R	F	V	H	I	H	O	W	L	A	G	B	S	U	M	H	T	S	I
G	A	V	N	C	X	G	U	R	E	K	K	L	G	A	K	P	B	U	N
O	F	I	V	H	O	H	I	S	E	B	I	O	E	T	E	R	C	E	S
N	H	V	O	Y	R	A	T	I	U	T	I	P	Q	K	O	P	G	M	U
W	H	I	I	J	Y	R	P	D	V	H	S	A	I	U	H	I	R	J	L
A	I	L	Q	K	H	K	B	C	H	Y	P	O	D	Q	E	N	O	S	I
N	P	C	O	R	T	I	S	O	L	P	C	W	D	F	B	F	T	R	N
T	M	O	J	I	D	S	C	R	E	E	E	B	O	L	P	M	P	R	A
O	N	R	H	U	R	L	D	T	C	R	K	U	B	J	A	L	E	J	S
M	R	T	Q	G	B	E	S	E	C	K	Q	R	B	A	C	M	C	L	K
L	P	E	H	T	B	T	P	X	B	J	N	I	M	M	U	N	E	S	L
H	R	X	C	I	E	N	T	M	U	Q	V	A	C	F	X	C	R	B	G
A	L	O	R	E	T	S	E	L	O	H	C	E	D	E	U	Z	P	T	B
N	O	R	S	M	A	S	T	R	E	S	S	W	W	Y	F	O	U	D	G

Fill in the blanks

The influence of a stimulus, from inside or outside the body, leads to the release of a hormone that has an effect on the stimulus; following this, some aspect of the target organ function then inhibits further reaction to the stimulus and thus further release of the hormone by the organ.

Chapter 16

Multiple choice questions

1. (a); **2.** (b); **3.** (d); **4.** (d); **5.** (a); **6.** (c); **7.** (d); **8.** (c); **9.** (c); **10.** (b).

True or false

1. False – phagocytes are white blood cells
2. True
3. True
4. False – they are descended from multipotent stem cells
5. False – it is monocytes and tissue macrophages that are included within the family of macrophages
6. False – it is some of the B-cells that develop into plasma cells
7. True
8. True
9. True
10. False – sneezing is a mechanical barrier

Fill in the blanks

Granulocytes are divided into three types; namely, neutrophils, eosinophils and basophils. These cells are called granulocytes because, under a high-powered microscope, they appear to be full of little granules. These, however, are actually vacuoles (or empty spaces) within the cells, and they are very importantly involved in the process of phagocytosis, which is the destruction of infectious organisms, such as bacteria and viruses. They work by first of all engulfing them and then they ingest them, so destroying the organisms and, at the same time, also providing the cell with nutrition.

Word search

P	H	A	G	O	C	Y	T	O	S	I	S	Z
L	X	V	N	W	Y	G	E	T	C	N	I	Y
A	J	K	E	X	T	D	N	Y	A	F	H	G
T	U	U	E	D	O	N	T	D	B	L	M	O
E	G	X	L	N	T	Y	H	L	M	A	R	N
L	Y	M	P	H	O	C	Y	T	E	M	R	T
E	W	A	S	T	X	Y	M	C	X	M	S	G
T	S	R	N	Z	I	T	U	D	N	A	R	N
S	C	E	P	T	C	Y	S	T	X	T	F	P
F	R	A	I	L	I	C	V	V	L	I	G	M
J	S	R	A	E	T	S	Q	U	A	O	L	W
K	R	Q	U	I	Y	V	E	Q	U	N	V	X
N	T	U	L	L	E	C	K	N	K	C	E	L

Chapter 17

Multiple choice questions
1. (d); **2.** (c); **3.** (d); **4.** (c); **5.** (b); **6.** (a); **7.** (d); **8.** (c); **9.** (d); **10.** (a).

True or false
1. True
2. False
3. True
4. False
5. False
6. True
7. True
8. False
9. False
10. True

Word search

S	N	G	S	E	V	R	E	N	C	L	H	T
U	I	L	I	P	R	O	T	C	E	R	R	A
B	N	A	S	S	K	I	N	S	L	U	W	E
C	A	N	R	I	A	H	Q	I	L	O	V	W
U	L	D	E	J	M	K	C	M	T	D	P	S
T	E	B	N	E	A	R	T	R	H	O	B	O
A	M	A	O	L	L	F	E	E	I	O	L	K
N	A	S	M	C	U	P	A	D	N	W	O	C
E	L	A	R	I	N	H	C	T	I	U	O	I
O	E	L	O	T	U	D	U	C	T	P	D	H
U	M	B	H	U	L	A	Y	E	R	S	E	T
S	U	O	E	C	A	B	E	S	O	L	I	P

Fill in the blanks
The skin has two layers. The outer layer is called the epidermis and the inner layer is the dermis. The dermal layer contains hair follicles, sebaceous glands, small blood vessels called capillaries and a pigment called melanin that helps to protect against ultraviolet light. The skin has a number of functions, and one of those functions is related to heat control; this is called thermoregulation. The skin can also protect from microorganisms invading the body. The skin is

the largest organ of the body. When a person becomes hot the blood vessels on the surface of the skin dilate. Sweat when released helps a person to cool down.

The epidermis is situated on the outside of the skin and is made from layers of cells with a basal layer. This layer drives through cell division. The newly divided cells gradually move towards the surface; this can take about 1–2 months. As the cells gradually die they become flattened, and keratin, the outermost layer of flat dead cells, is being continually eroded by friction. The keratin and oil from the sebaceous glands assist in making the skin waterproof.

Index

Page numbers in *italics* denote figures, those in **bold** denote tables.

Fundamentals of Anatomy and Physiology: For Nursing and Healthcare Students, Second Edition. Edited by Ian Peate and Muralitharan Nair.
© 2017 John Wiley & Sons, Ltd. Published 2017 by John Wiley & Sons, Ltd.
Student companion website: www.wileyfundamentalseries.com/anatomy
Instructor companion website: www.wiley.com/go/instructor/anatomy